THE
NURSING
EXPERIENCE

Trends, Challenges, and Transitions

THE
NURSING
EXPERIENCE

Trends, Challenges, and Transitions

Third Edition

Lucie Young Kelly, R.N., Ph.D., F.A.A.N.
Professor Emeritus
Public Health and Nursing
Columbia University
New York, New York

Lucille A. Joel, R.N., Ed.D., F.A.A.N.
Professor, College of Nursing
Rutgers, The State University of New Jersey
Newark, New Jersey

McGraw-Hill
Health Professions Division

New York   St. Louis   San Francisco   Auckland   Bogotá   Caracas   Lisbon
London   Madrid   Mexico City   Milan   Montreal   New Delhi   San Juan
Singapore   Sydney   Tokyo   Toronto

McGraw-Hill

A Division of The McGraw·Hill Companies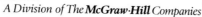

THE NURSING EXPERIENCE
Trends, Challenges, and Transitions

1234567890 DOC DOC 9876

ISBN 0-07-105483-9

This book was set in Times Roman by Keyword Publishing Services Ltd.
The editors were Gail Gavert and Mariapaz Ramos Englis.
The production supervisor was Rick Ruzycka.
The project was managed by Keyword Publishing Services Ltd.
R.R. Donnelley and Sons, Inc., was the printer and binder.
This book is printed on acid-free paper.

The cover photograph is courtesy of the Visiting Nurse Service of New York; the back cover photographs are by Anita Jones Horner.

Library of Congress Cataloging-in-Publication Data

Kelly, Lucie Young.
    The nursing experience: trends, challenges, and transitions /
Lucie Young Kelly, Lucille A. Joel.—3d ed.
      p.   cm.
    Includes bibliographical references and index.
    ISBN 0-07-105483-9
    1. Nursing—Vocational guidance. 2. Nursing. I. Joel, Lucille
A. II. Title.
    [DNLM: 1. Nursing. WY 16 K292n 1996]
RT82.K43 1996
610.73—dc20
DNLM/DLC
for Library of Congress   95-36827

Contents

PART 4: NURSING ETHICS AND LAW

Contents

Preface

It has always been a challenge to revise *The Nursing Experience*, first because of the many exciting, albeit sometimes disturbing, changes in the health care system in which nursing plays such a vital role, and second, because of my responsibility to meet the demands of the students and teachers who first urged me to write "something like *Dimensions of Professional Nursing*, but shorter." Given the times and the massive amount of potential content, a revision also means seeking new visual ways to highlight important aspects of the book. That in itself has always been a separate challenge. This year, for the first time, I have chosen a co-author for this book, and once more I have selected Dr. Lucille Joel, a distinguished nurse recognized nationally and internationally, who also co-authored the seventh edition of *Dimensions of Professional Nursing*. We worked well together, philosophically in harmony, but somewhat different in style and approach. I believe that our collaboration has enriched this third edition of *The Nursing Experience* and that the readers will find some interesting and provocative changes. We have both considered what was most important to the nurses of today, who are eager to be prepared to face what some consider a revolution in health care. (This is addressed particularly in Chapter 3, with extensive data on the major health occupations and professions in Appendix 2.)

Of course, each chapter and appendix has been updated, including information that readers might have difficulty in accessing themselves. Even nursing history has been given a different dimension. Chapter 2 has a new exhibit that puts the first hundred years of nursing in the context of what was happening in society, law, science, and medicine. This will enable the student to get a better idea of the times in which modern nursing originated and developed in the United States. In addition, the long requested biographies, "Distinguished Nurses of the Past" (Appendix 8), give today's students a human perspective on nursing's past. I fully expect some outcry: "Why didn't you include so and so?" Only limited space prevented me from adding another 50 or so who "made a difference." Meanwhile, I tried to present a cross-section. I only hope that this brief introduction to some remarkable nurses will stimulate readers to look for more information on this group, those omitted, and living nursing leaders. They are our past, our present, and our future.

Other innovations include a revised chart on nursing theories that offers new depth of understanding of nursing theorists, their work, and the application of such theories to practice (Chapter 4). The chapter on education and Appendix 3 acknowledge both the diversity of today's students and detail the educational programs available. This is followed by an expanded discussion of traditional, new, and emerging career opportunities, particularly useful in today's health care environment. Equally important are the new models of leadership and change presented in Chapter 7, including principles for analyzing the power nurses do hold.

Part 4 has been enlarged significantly, again by demand of the nurses we meet and talk to. Ethical dilemmas have increased with the growth of technology, paired with the move to limit resources. Moreover, ethics and the legal rights of people are more intertwined than ever, so the chapters on these topics are juxtaposed, with the latest issues reported and discussed. Equally in demand is information on the legal aspects of clinical nursing practice, and this topic too is enlarged upon, with the inclusion of the very latest court cases. Nurses are also concerned about their credentialing, particularly in relation to licensure and certification. Comparisons of key components of proposed licensure laws as seen by both the professional organization (ANA) and the nursing licensure boards (NCSBN) and details of specialty nursing certification opportunities and procedures (new Appendix 6) will be invaluable to all nurses. At a time in which the input of nurses to health policy and legislation is increasingly important, Chapter 10 provides both the "how-to-do-it" and an overview of legislation affecting nursing.

The all-important "Transition into Practice" section again gives practical guidelines for both job selection and termination (Chapter 14). Appendix 5 gives the most comprehensive information available in chart form about nursing and related organizations, with additional details in Chapter 13. The last chapter will be particularly meaningful to new graduates with new sections on the rights of nurses as employees, workplace hazards, and the problems and challenges these nurses may face.

Both the references and bibliography are almost entirely new, with citations dated 1990 and later. Generally only classic references are from earlier dates. The photos are also entirely new (with the exception of three in Chapter 1). They have been carefully selected from a variety of institutions and organizations and vividly illustrate specific topics.

Finally, let me repeat what I said in the last edition of *The Nursing Experience*, because it is the key to what Dr. Joel and I believe in. This book is unique. It is intended to give a large amount of important information in a compact, visual form that will have continuing value as the nurse becomes educated and practices. Most of all, it should stimulate thinking and discussion, to pique curiosity, and to encourage involvement in nursing. Knowledgeable nurses will create the future of nursing, and we hope that this book will help them.

Lucie Young Kelly

Acknowledgments

It is difficult to acknowledge everyone who has contributed in some way to this book. We have had feedback from both faculty and former students about what they like and what they needed more or less of. We have followed through and we certainly thank them. Many of those acknowledged in the seventh edition of *Dimensions of Professional Nursing* deserve a second thanks because much of what they provided one way or another was the basis for this edition of *The Nursing Experience*. Specific organizations that have allowed us to use their materials are credited throughout the book. In addition, we thank Winifred Carson, attorney, American Nurses Association, and Carolyn Yocum, National Council of State Boards of Nursing, for input into the chapter on credentialing; Anne Wojner, St. Luke's Hospital, Houston, for the model "critical path," and Yelena Vasilyeva, librarian, Sophia Palmer Library, American Journal of Nursing Company, for her support in our library research.

For assisting us in obtaining a fine selection of photos, we express our appreciation to the following: Constance Holleran and Nancy Vatre, International Council of Nurses; Lisa Wyatt and Mandy Mikulenchak, American Nurses Association; Al Foti, American Journal of Nursing Company; John Garde, American Association of Nurse Anesthetists; Robert Piemonte and Caroline Jaffe, National Student Nurses Association; Dorothy Fleming, New Jersey State Nurses Association; Brigadier General Irene Trowell-Harris and Colonel Nina Rhoton, US Air Force Nurse Corps; Major Constance Moore, US Army Nurse Corps; Gary Goldenberg, Columbia University School of Nursing; Eleanor Incalcaterra and Kathi Sengin, Robert Wood Johnson University Hospital; Ruben Fernandez, Newark Beth Israel Medical Center (New Jersey); Joyce Clifford and Jane Wandel, Beth Israel Hospital, Boston; Irma Goertzen, Magee-Women's Hospital (Pittsburgh); Jane Hirsch, Medical Center of the University of California, San Francisco; Joan Large, Museum of Nursing History (Philadelphia); Lyle Churchill, Visiting Nurse Service of New York; Eileen Freitag and Casey Cuthbert-Allman, Visiting Nurse Service of Boston; Catherine Wengerter and Caren Speizer, Daughters of Miriam Center (New Jersey); Margaret Harrington, Linda Diaz, and Jennifer Grey, Terence Cardinal Cooke Health Center (New York); Dale Evanson, Palisades General Hospital (New Jersey); Marge Taggart, Somerset Medical Center (New Jersey); Maris Lown, Brookdale Community College (New Jersey); Anne Miller and Susie Forehand, Valencia Community College (Florida); and Carla Thomas, Parke, Davis.

Finally, we thank Irene Tirella and Rosemary Britt for professional and timely typing.

THE
NURSING
EXPERIENCE

Trends, Challenges, and Transitions

The Evolution
of Nursing

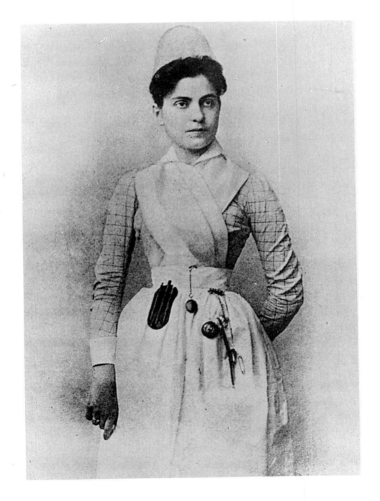

Lillian Wald, nursing leader and pioneer in public health nursing.
Courtesy of Visiting Nurse Service of New York)

1

Care of the Sick: How Nursing Began

OBJECTIVES

After studying this chapter, you will be able to:

1. Recognize the contributions of early civilizations to care of the sick.
2. Discuss how various nursing orders influenced the evolution of nursing.
3. Describe at least three ways in which Florence Nightingale influenced the development of nursing.

What does it matter whether or not we know anything about nursing history? A lot. Nursing today was formed by its history. Its development since ancient times, within the social contexts of those times, explains many things: its power or lack of power, its educational confusion, and the makeup of its practitioners. The changing relationships between nursing and other health care professions, nursing and other disciplines, and nursing and the public can be traced and better understood with the knowledge of past history. The impact of social and scientific changes on nursing and nursing's impact on society are ongoing processes that need to be studied; nursing does not exist in a vacuum.

Sometimes there is a repetition of history. For instance, 100 years ago, there were many arguments within and without the nursing profession about nursing education; this scenario is being repeated today. Seventy-five years ago, the question of nursing licensure was hotly debated; today, it is again a major concern. For 50 years, studies have documented reasons for nurses' discontentment with their jobs; only recently were some changes made.

These issues affect the practice of every nurse; in some cases, they are a factor in determining whether the nurse even chooses to stay in the profession. Understanding the past can be very useful in making decisions that shape the future.

CARE OF THE SICK IN EARLY CIVILIZATIONS

Undoubtedly, some form of nursing activity has existed since earliest civilization. Although for thousands of years concepts of health and illness were closely related to belief in the supernatural, there is evidence that plants were used as medicine, as well as heat, cold, and even some types of primitive surgery. In primitive times there were medicine men and women, but nursing care probably fell to the women of the family unit.

Records of the early known civilizations were sometimes written by the physicians of the time and provide interesting information on the care of the sick. There were also occasional references to nurses. In *Babylonia* for instance, one of the great civilizations that lay between the eastern Mediterranean and the Persian Gulf, a legalized medical system existed. There were even laws that punished physicians for malpractice. Some of the treatments included diet, rest, enemas, bandaging, and massaging (with or without incantations), and care was given by some type of lay nurse.

Although the ancient *Hebrews* attributed their illnesses to God's wrath, under the leadership of Moses they developed principles and practices of hygiene and sanitation. They performed various kinds of surgery and dressed wounds, using sutures and bandages. Nurses are mentioned in the *Old Testament*, but other than visiting and possibly caring for the sick in the home, their role is not clear.

Ancient *Egypt*, located along the Nile, also was noted for its laws on health and sanitation, which included regulations about diet and personal hygiene. There were medical schools and at least one school of midwifery for women, whose graduates taught physicians about "women's conditions." Excavated medical papyri have descriptions of nursing procedures, such as dressing wounds, but again, the nurses' duties are not clear.

The first hospitals were probably established in pre-Christian *India*. Records identify the first special nursing group: men who staffed the hospitals and performed some nursing functions. Actually, they may have been more like physicians' assistants. The Indian physicians were exceptionally skilled in surgery and used many drugs in their treatments, although, as in other civilizations, magic and evil spirits were part of medical belief.

In ancient *China*, both acupuncture and drug therapy were used. These were incorporated into the theory of yang and yin. Yang, the male principle, is light, positive, and full of life; yin, the female principle, is dark, cold, and

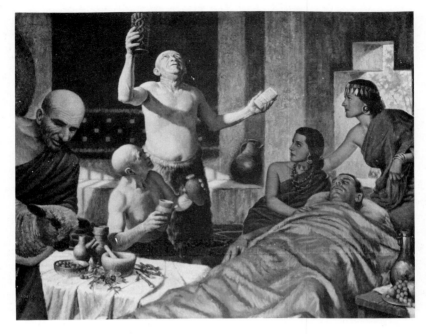

Physicians in ancient Babylonia treated the sick with a mixture of medicine and charms; nurses were probably the women in the family. (*Courtesy of Parke, Davis and Company.*)

lifeless. When the two are in harmony, the patient is in good health. The Chinese also refined ancient measures of hydrotherapy, massage, and other physical techniques, and promoted systematic exercise to maintain physical and mental well-being. Many of these treatments are still used effectively today.

Greece, too, had its demons, spirits, and gods related to illness, with Asclepios (Roman version: Aesculapius), the classic god of medicine, honored by the founding of temples for the sick, which were actually more like health spas. The staff of Asclepios, intertwined with the snakes or serpents of wisdom and immortality, are thought to be the basis of today's medical caduceus. The greatest name in Greek medicine is *Hippocrates* (about 400 B.C.), who developed patient assessment and recording and rejected the supernatural origins of disease. His establishment of high ethical standards is reflected in the Hippocratic oath still taken in some medical schools. For centuries after his death, the medical books he had written were the basis of medical knowledge. There is no account of nurses.

Rome's most lasting contribution to medicine may have been the founding of hospitals, at first primarily for the military as they conquered new territories. Both male and female attendants (nurses?) were used. Medical

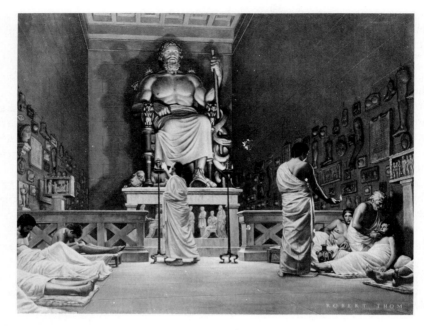

In the Greek temple of Asclepios (Aesculapius), the god of medicine, priests combined prayers and rituals with various treatments. (*Courtesy of Parke, Davis and Company.*)

care was in the hands of the Greeks, like the great *Galen* (about 200 to 130 B.C.), who lived in Rome.

CHRISTIANITY'S IMPACT ON NURSING

In the early Christian era, bishops were given responsibility for the sick, the poor, widows, and children, but the deacons and deaconesses carried out the services. It appears that there was a group of specially designated women (deaconesses, widows, virgins, and matrons) who cared for the sick. *Phoebe*, mentioned in the Bible by Paul, was the first deaconess actually identified as giving nursing care. There were other noted women in the first centuries of Christianity, frequently designated as saints later. *Olympias*, a rich aristocratic widow of Constantinople, erected a convent and with 40 deaconesses cared for the sick. *Marcella*, a wealthy Roman, converted her palace into a monastery and, among other things, taught the care of the sick to her followers. *Fabiola* was one of Marcella's group and became a Christian convert. Also wealthy, she founded the first free hospital for the poor and personally nursed the sickest and filthiest people who came to her. St. Jerome wrote letters of praise about both women.

The Middle Ages (about 500 to 1500 A.D.) has a mixed record in sick care. During the first half, called the *Dark Ages*, medical and nursing care, though needed, was barely available as wars, ignorance, famine, and disease flourished. The Christian church was obsessed with its belief that the main purpose of human beings on earth was to prepare for a future life and thus saw little need for science and philosophy. The teachings of hygiene and sanitation from earlier civilizations were discarded. Except for the eastern Roman and Moslem empires, medical knowledge stagnated.

During the Middle Ages, the deaconesses, suppressed by the Western churches in particular, gradually declined and became almost extinct. As the deaconesses declined, the religious orders grew stronger. Known as *monastic orders* and composed of monks and nuns (though not in the same orders), they controlled the hospitals, running them as institutions concerned more with the patients' religious problems than with their physical ailments. However, monks and some nuns were better educated than most people in those times, and their liberal education may well have included some of the medical writings of Galen.

Lay citizens banded together to form *secular orders*. Their work was similar to that of the monastic orders in that it was concerned with the sick and needy, but they lived in their own homes, were allowed to marry, and took no vows of the church. They usually adopted a uniform, or habit. Nursing was often their main work.

The *military nursing orders*, known as the *Knights Hospitallers*, were the outcome of the Crusades, the miliary expeditions undertaken by Christians in the eleventh, twelfth, and thirteenth centuries to recover the Holy Land from the Moslems. The most prominent of these three types of orders— religious, military, and secular—were the Order of St. Benedict, Knights Hospitallers, Hospital Brothers of St. Anthony, Third Order of St. Francis, Beguines of Flanders, Order of the Holy Ghost (Santo Spirito), Grey Sisters, and Alexian Brotherhood.

NURSING CARE IN EARLY HOSPITALS

Gradually, more hospitals in which the sick received care were established as the need increased. At the close of the Middle Ages, there were hospitals all over Europe, particularly in larger cities such as Paris and

Rome. In England, too, several hundred were established, some of which still remain. Hospitals in England during the Middle Ages differed from those on the Continent in that they were never completely church controlled, although they were founded on Christian principles and accepted responsibility for the sick and injured. The oldest and best-known English hospitals from a historical point of view are St. Bartholomew's, founded in 1123; St. Thomas's, founded in 1213; and Bethlehem Hospital, founded in 1247, originally as a general hospital, which later became famous as a mental institution, referred to frequently as *Bedlam*.

The Hotel Dieu of Paris, founded about 650, had an unfavorable record as far as nursing is concerned. Staffed by Augustinian nuns who did the cooking and laundry as well as the nursing, and who had neither intellectual nor professional stimulation, the hospital was not distinguished for its care of patients. The records of nursing kept by this hospital were well done, however, and have been a source of enlightenment for historians.

The nursing care in most early hospitals was essentially basic: bathing, feeding, giving medicines, making beds, and so on. It was rarely of high quality, however, largely because of the retarded progress of nearly all civilization and the shortsighted attitude toward women that was typical of the Dark Ages. Even after the Renaissance (1400 to 1550), during which Paracelsus, Vesalius, and Paré made major contributions in pharmaceutical

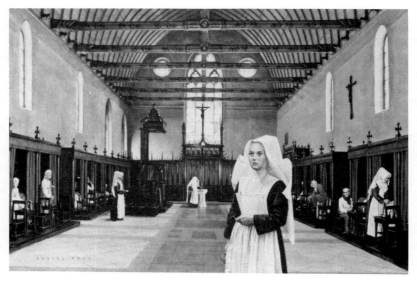

The Hotel Dieu of Paris was one of the earliest hospitals founded in the Middle Ages. (*Courtesy of Parke, Davis and Company.*)

chemistry, anatomy, and surgery, hospital nursing remained at the same basic level.

During the Reformation (beginning about 1500), which resulted in the formation of various Protestant churches, the Protestant leaders saw the vacuum in the care of the sick and urged the hiring of nurse deaconesses and elderly women to do nursing. By the end of the eighteenth century, nurses of some kind functioned in hospitals. Conditions were not attractive, and much has been written about the drunken, thieving women who tended patients. However, some hospitals made real efforts to set standards. Already a hierarchy of nursing personnel had begun, with helpers and watchers assigned to help the *sisters*, as the early English nurses were called.

In other parts of Europe, nursing was becoming recognized as an important service. Diderot, whose *Encyclopedia* attempted to sum up all human knowledge, said that nursing "is as important for humanity as its functions are low and repugnant." Urging care in selection, since "all persons are not adapted to it," he described the nurse as "patient, mild, and compassionate. She should console the sick, foresee their needs, and relieve their tedium."[1]

The dreary picture of secular nursing is not totally unexpected, given the times. Because proper young women did not work outside the home, nursing had no acceptance, much less prestige. Even those nurses not in the Dickens's Sairy Gamp mold or those desiring to nurse found themselves in competition with workhouse inmates, who were cheaper workers for hospital administrations. (Actually, most care was still given at home by wives and mothers). It was acceptable to nurse as a member of a religious order, when the motivation was, of course, religious and the cost to the hospital was little or nothing.

A startling development during the Reformation was the disappearance of male nurses. The Protestant nursing orders were female, and except for a few male orders like the Brothers Hospitallers of St. John of God, the Catholic nursing orders after 1500 were primarily made up of women. Among the most noted were the Sisters of Charity (France) the Irish Sisters of Charity and the Sisters of Mercy.

During the nineteenth century, several nursing orders were revived or originated that had substantial influence on modern nursing. In most instances, these orders cared for patients in hospitals that were already established, in contrast to the orders of earlier times, which had founded the hospitals in which they worked. Among the most influential orders was the Church Order of Deaconesses, an ancient order revived by Theodor Fliedner, pastor of a small parish in Kaiserswerth, Germany. (Florence Nightingale later obtained her only formal training there.) The Protestant Sisters of Charity, under Sister Elizabeth Fry, worked among prisoners and the physically and mentally ill.

Of the nursing orders established by the Church of England, the most noted were the Sisters of Mercy in the Church of England and St. Margarets of East Grinstead, both of whom were involved with "district" or home nursing. The Anglican order that did the most for hospital nursing in this period was St. John's House, founded in 1848 in London, whose purpose was to train members of the church "to act as nurses and visitors to the sick and poor."[2] The original plan required the order to be associated with a hospital in which women under training or those already educated could gain experience and exercise their calling. The program was very successful.

EXHIBIT 1.1

Three Centuries of Scientific Landmarks

William Harvey (1578–1657), England	First to describe completely (except for the capillary system) and accurately the circulatory system.
Thomas Sydenham (1624–1689), England	Revived the Hippocratic methods of observation and reasoning and in other ways restored clinical medicine to a sound basis.
Antonj van Leeuwenhoek (1632–1723), Holland	Improved on Galileo's microscope and produced one that permitted the examination of body cells and bacteria.
William Hunter (1718–1783) and his brother John (1728–1793), Scotland	Founded the science of pathology.
William Tuke (1732–1822), England	Reformed the care of the mentally ill.
Edward Jenner (1749–1823), England	Originated vaccination against smallpox.
René Laennec (1781–1826), France	Invented the stethoscope.
Oliver Wendell Holmes (1809–1894), United States	Furthered safe obstetric practice, pointing out the dangers of infection.

Many of the Catholic and Protestant orders went to the New World, founding hospitals in Canada, the United States, and Mexico. Cortez is credited with founding the first hospital in the New World, located in Mexico City, and within 20 years, most major Spanish towns had one. Hospitals in the New World were no better than those in Europe, and given the hard living conditions, there were numerous health problems.

Progress in medicine and science during these centuries (Exhibit 1.1) was accompanied by accelerated interest in better service and nurses'

EXHIBIT 1.1 (*continued*)

Crawford W. Long (1815–1878), United States	Excised a tumor of the neck under ether anesthesia in 1832 but did not make his discovery public until after Dr. William T. Morton announced his in 1846.
Ignaz P. Semmelweis (1818–1865), Austria– Hungary	Recognized that infection was carried from patient to patient by physicians and instituted preventive measures for puerperal fever in new mothers.
Louis Pasteur (1822–1895), France	Founder of microbiology and developer of pasteurization; developed preventive inoculations against anthrax, chicken cholera, and rabies.
Lord Joseph Lister (1827–1912), England	Developed and proved the theory of bacterial infection of wounds.
Robert Koch (1843–1910), Germany	Founded modern bacteriology; identified the tubercle bacillus.
Wilhelm Röntgen (1845–1923), Germany	Discovered x-rays in 1895 and laid the foundation for the science of roentgenology and radiology.
Pierre Curie (1859–1906), France, and his Polish wife, Marie (1867–1934)	Discovered radium in 1898.

training. Neither was achieved to a significant degree, however, despite the fine work of dedicated men and women who belonged to the nursing orders of the time. Limited in number and inadequately prepared for their nursing functions, the members of these orders could not begin to meet the need for their services. Such care as patients received in the majority of institutions was grossly inadequate.

In the mid-nineteenth century, therefore, the time was right—perhaps overdue—for the revolution in nursing education that originated under the leadership of Florence Nightingale and that influenced so greatly and so quickly (from a historical point of view) the nursing care of patients and, indeed, the health of the world.

THE INFLUENCE OF FLORENCE NIGHTINGALE

It has been said that Florence Nightingale, an extraordinary woman in any century, is the most written-about woman in history. Through her own numerous publications, her letters, the writings of her contemporaries, including newspaper reports, and the numerous biographies and studies of her life, there emerges the picture of a sometimes contradictory, frequently controversial, but undeniably powerful woman who probably had a greater influence on the care of the sick than any other single individual.

Called the founder of modern nursing, Nightingale was a strong-willed, intelligent woman who used her considerable knowledge of statistics, sanitation, logistics, administration, nutrition, and public health not only to develop a new system of nursing education and health care but also to improve the social welfare systems of the time. The gentle, caring lady of the lamp, full of compassion for the soldiers of the Crimea, is an accurate image, but no more so than that of the hard-headed administrator and planner who forced changes in the intolerable social conditions of the time, including the care of the sick poor. Nightingale knew that tender touch alone would not bring health to the sick or prevent illness, so she set her intelligence, her administrative skills, her political acumen, and her incredible drive to achieve her self-defined missions. In the Victorian age when women were almost totally dominated by men—fathers, husbands, brothers—and it was undesirable for them to show intelligence or profess interest in anything but household arts, this indomitable woman accomplished the following:

1. Improved and reformed laws affecting health, morals, and the poor.
2. Reformed hospitals and improved workhouses and infirmaries.

3. Improved medicine by instituting an army medical school and reorganizing the army medical department.
4. Improved the health of natives and British citizens in India and other colonies.
5. Established nursing as a profession with two missions: sick nursing and health nursing.[3]

The new nurse and the new image of the nurse that she created, in part through the nursing schools she founded, in part through her writings, and in part through her international influence, became the model that persisted for almost 100 years. Today, some of her tenets about the "good" nurse seem terribly restrictive, but it should be remembered that in those times not only the image but also the reality of much of secular nursing was based on the untutored, uncouth workhouse inmates for whom drunkenness and thievery were a way of life. It was small wonder that each Nightingale student had to exemplify a new image above reproach.

Early Life

Florence Nightingale was born on May 12, 1820, in Florence, Italy, during her English parents' travels there. The family was wealthy and well educated, with a high social standing and influential friends, all of which later would be useful to Nightingale. Primarily under her father's tutelage, she learned Greek, Latin, French, German, and Italian, and studied history, philosophy, science, music, art, and classical literature. She traveled widely with her family and friends. The breadth of her education, almost unheard of for women of the times, was also considerably more extensive than that of most men, including physicians. Her intelligence and education were recognized by scholars, as indicated in her correspondence with them.

Nightingale was not only bright but, according to early portraits and descriptions, slender, attractive, and fun-loving, enjoying the social life of her class. She differed from other young women in her determination to do something "toward lifting the load of suffering from the helpless and miserable."[4] Apparently, the encouragement of Dr. Samuel Gridley Howe and his wife, Julia Ward Howe (who wrote "The Battle Hymn of the Republic"), during a visit to the Nightingale family home in 1844 helped to crystallize Florence's interest in hospitals and nursing. Nevertheless, her intent to train in a hospital was strongly opposed by her family, and she limited herself to nursing family members.

Although remaining the obedient daughter, Nightingale found her own way to expand her knowledge of sick care. She studied hospital and sanitary

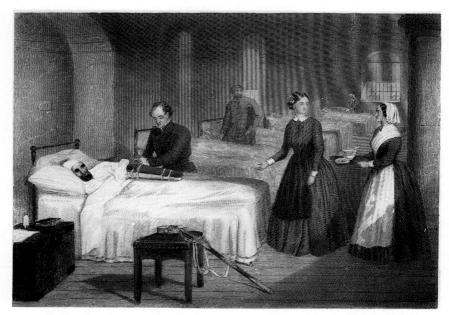

Florence Nightingale, the founder of modern nursing, in the hospital in Scutari. (*Courtesy of Lucie Kelly, private collection.*)

reports and books on public health. Having received information on Kaiserswerth in Germany, she determined to receive training there—which was more acceptable because of its religious auspices. On one of her trips to the Continent, she made a brief visit and was impressed enough to spend three months in training and observation there in 1851. Her later efforts to study with various Catholic orders were frustrated. However, she got permission to inspect the hospitals in various cities during her tours. She examined the general layout of the hospital, as well as ward construction, sanitation, general administration, and the work of the surgeons and physicians. Apparently, these observational techniques and her analytical abilities then and later were the basis of her unrivaled knowledge of hospitals in the next decades. Few of her contemporaries ever had such knowledge.

In 1853, Nightingale assumed the position of superintendent of a charity hospital (probably more of a nursing home) for ill governesses run by titled ladies. Although she had difficulties with her intolerant governing board, she did make changes considered revolutionary for the day and, even with the lack of trained nurses, improved the patients' care. And she continued to visit hospitals. Just as Nightingale was negotiating for a superintendency in the newly reorganized and rebuilt King's College Hospital in London, England and France, in support of Turkey, declared war on Russia in March 1854.

Crimea: The Turning Point

The Crimean War was a low point for England. Ill-prepared and disorganized in general, the army and the bureaucracy were even less prepared to care for the thousands of soldiers both wounded in battle and prostrated by the cholera epidemics brought on by worse than primitive conditions. Not even the most basic equipment or drugs were available, and, as casualties mounted, Turkey turned over the enormous but bare and filthy barracks at Scutari, across from Constantinople, to be used as a hospital. The conditions remained abominable. The soldiers lay on the floor in filth, untended, frequently without food or water because there was no equipment to prepare or distribute either. Rats and other vermin came from the sewers underneath the building. There were no beds, furniture, basins, soap, towels, or eating utensils, and few provisions. There were only orderlies, and none of these at night. The death rate was said to be 60 percent.

In previous wars, the situation had not been much different, and there was little interest on the battle sites, for ordinary soldiers were accorded no decencies. But now, for the first time, civilian war correspondents were present and sent back the news of these horrors to an England with a newly aroused social conscience. The reformers were in an uproar; newspapers demanded to know why England did not have nurses like the French Sisters of Charity to care for its soldiers, and Parliament trembled. In October 1854, Sidney Herbert, Secretary of War and an old friend of Florence Nightingale, wrote, begging her to lead a group of nurses to the Crimea under government authority and at government expense. Nightingale had already decided to offer her services, and the two letters crossed. In less than a week, she had assembled 38 nurses, the most she could find who met her standards—Roman Catholic and Anglican sisters and lay nurses from various hospitals—and embarked for Scutari. (One nurse who was not accepted was Mary Grant Seacole, who had nursed British soldiers in Jamaica. At her own expense she traveled to the Crimea, built and opened a lodging house for the comfort of the troops, and nursed sick officers with medicines, some of which were her own concoctions.)[5] Even under the miserable circumstances found there, Nightingale and her contingent were not welcomed by the army doctors and surgeons, who refused the nurses' services.

Nightingale chose to wait to be asked to help. To the anger of her nurses, she allowed none of them to give care until one week later, when scurvy, starvation, dysentery, exposure, and more fighting almost brought about the collapse of the British army. Then the doctors, desperate for any kind of assistance, turned to the eager nurses.

Modern criticisms of Florence Nightingale frequently refer to her insistence on the physician's overall authority and her own authoritarian approach to nursing. The first criticism may have originated with her situation in the Crimean War. In mid-century England her appointment created a furor; she was the first woman ever to be given such authority. Yet, despite the high-sounding title that Herbert insisted she have—General Superintendent of the Female Nursing Establishment of the Miliary Hospitals of the Army—her orders required that she have the approval of the Principal Medical Officer "in her exercise of the responsibilities thus vested in her."[6] Although no "lady, sister, or nurse" could be transferred from one hospital to another without her approval, she had no authority over anyone else, even orderlies and cooks. What she accomplished had to be done through sheer force of will or persuasion. Her overt deference to physicians was probably the beginning of the doctor-nurse game.

Whatever the limitations of her power, Florence Nightingale literally accomplished miracles at Scutari. Even in the week of waiting, she moved into the kitchen area and began to cook extras from her own supplies to create a diet kitchen, which for five months was the only source of food for the sick.

Nightingale had powerful friends and control over a large amount of contributed funds—a situation that gained her some cooperation from most physicians after a while. Through persuasion and the use of good managerial techniques, she cleaned up the hospital: the orderlies scrubbed and emptied slops regularly; soldiers' wives and camp followers washed clothes; and the vermin were brought under some control. Before the end of the war, the mortality rate at Scutari declined to 1 percent.

When the hospital care improved, Nightingale began a program of social welfare among the soldiers—among other things, seeing to it that they got sick pay. The patients adored her. She cared about them, and the doctors and officers reproached her for "spoiling the brutes." News correspondents wrote reports about the "ministering angel" and "lady with the lamp" making late rounds after the medical officers had retired— which inspired Longfellow later to write his famous poem "Santa Filomena." England and America were enthralled, and she was awarded decorations by Queen Victoria and the Sultan of Turkey.

But all did not go well. The military doctors continued in their resentment and tried to undermine her. There were problems in her own ranks, dissension among the religious and secular nurses, and problems of incompetence and immorality. No doubt Nightingale was high-handed at times. Despite praise of her leadership, she was also called "quick, violent-tempered, positive, obstinate, and stubborn."[7] Certainly she drove herself in all she did.

When the situation at Scutari was improved, she crossed the Black Sea to the battle sites and worked on the reorganization of the few hospitals there—with no better support from physicians and superior officers. There she contracted Crimean fever (probably typhoid or typhus) and nearly died. However, she refused a leave of absence to recuperate and stayed in Scutari to work until the end of the war. She supervised 125 nurses and forced the military to recognize the place of nurses.

On her return from the Crimea, Nightingale took to her bed, or at least to her rooms, and emerged only on rare occasions. There is much speculation on this illness—whether it was a result of the Crimea fever, neurasthenia, a bit of both, or whether she simply found it useful to avoid wasting time with people she did not want to see. For she was famous now and had been given discretion over the so-called Nightingale Fund, to which almost everyone in England had subscribed, including many of the troops.

From her experiences, and to support her recommendations for reform, Nightingale wrote a massive report entitled *Notes on Matters Affecting the Health, Efficiency, and Hospital Administration of the British Army*, crammed with facts, figures, and statistical comparisons. On the basis of this and her later well-researched and well-documented papers, she is often credited with being the first nurse researcher. Reforms were slow in coming but extended even to the United States when the Union consulted her about organizing hospitals. In 1859 she wrote a small book, *Notes on Nursing: What It Is and What It Is Not*, intended for the average housewife and printed cheaply so that it would be affordable. These and other Nightingale works are still amazingly readable today—brisk, down-to-earth, and laced with many a pithy comment. For instance, in *Notes on Hospitals*, written in the same year, she compared the administration of the various types of hospitals and characterized the management of secular hospitals under the sole command of the male hospital authorities as "all but crazy."[8]

Her knowledge was certainly respected, and she was consulted by many, including the Royal Sanitary Commission on the Health of the Army in India.

The Nightingale Nurse

In 1860, Nightingale utilized some of the 45,000 English pounds of the Nightingale Fund to establish a training school for nurses. She selected St. Thomas's Hospital because of her respect for its matron, Mrs. S. E. Wardroper. The two converted the resident medical officers to their plan, although apparently most other physicians objected to the school. The students were chosen; the first class in the desired age range of 25 to 35 years and with impeccable character references numbered only 15. It was to be a one-year training program, and the students were presented with what could be called terminal behavioral objectives that they had to reach satisfactorily. Students could be dismissed by the matron for misconduct, inefficiency, or negligence. However, if they passed the courses of instruction and training satisfactorily, they were entered in the "Register" as certified nurses. The Committee of the Nightingale Fund then recommended them for employment; in the early years, they were obligated to work as hospital nurses for at least five years (for which they were paid).

The students' time was carefully structured, beginning at 6 A.M. and ending with a 9 P.M. bedtime, which included a semimandatory two-hour exercise period (walking abroad had to be done in twos and threes, not alone). Within that time there was actually about a nine-hour work and training day (a vast difference from future American schools). This included bedside teaching by a teaching sister or the Resident Medical Officer and elementary instruction in "Chemistry, with reference to air, water, food, etc.; Physiology, with reference to a knowledge of the leading functions of the body, and general instruction on medical and surgical topics"[9] by professors of the medical school attached to St. Thomas's, given voluntarily and without payment.

The Nightingale school was not under the control of the hospital and had education as its purpose. The Nightingale Fund paid the medical officers, head nurses, and matron for teaching students, beyond whatever they earned from the hospital in carrying out their other duties. Both the head nurses and the matron kept records on each student, evaluating how she met the stated objectives of the program. The students were expected to keep notes from the lectures and records of patient observation and care, all of which were checked by the nurse-teachers. At King's College Hospital, run by the Society of St. John's House, an Anglican religious community, midwifery was taught in similar style and with similar regulations, again under the auspices of the Nightingale Fund Committee. And, at the Royal Liverpool Infirmary, nurses were trained for home nursing of the sick poor under a Nightingale protocol but were personally funded by a Liverpool merchant–philanthropist. As Nightingale said in 1863, "We have had to introduce an entirely new system to which the older systems of nursing bear but slight resemblance.... It exists neither in Scotland nor in Ireland at the present time."[10]

The demand for the Nightingale nurses was overwhelming. In the next few years, requests also came for them to improve the workhouse (poorhouse) infirmaries and to reform both civilian and military nursing in India. In response to these demands, Nightingale wrote many reports, detailing to the last item the system for educating these nurses and for improving patient care, including such points as general hygiene and sanitation, nutrition, equipment, supplies, and the nurses' housing conditions, holidays, salaries, and retirement benefits. (For India, she suggested that they had better pay good salaries and provide satisfactory working and living conditions, or the nurses might opt for marriage, because the opportunities there were even greater than in England.) She constantly reiterated that she could not supply enough nurses but, when possible, she would send a matron and some other nurses, who would train new Nightingale nurses.

Maintaining standards was a constant struggle. Even St. Thomas's Hospital slipped, and Nightingale, who had been immersed in the Indian reforms, had to take time to reorganize the program. What evolved over the years, from the first program, was one of preparation for two kinds of nursing practitioners: the educated middle- and upper-class ladies who paid their own tuition and the still carefully selected poor women who were subsidized by the Nightingale Fund. The first were given an extra year or two of education to prepare them to become teachers or superintendents; a third choice was district nursing. "This nurse must be of a yet higher class and of a yet fuller training than a hospital nurse, because she has not the doctor always at hand and because she has no hospital appliances at hand."[11] The special probationers were expected to enter the profession permanently. The second group were prepared to be hospital ward nurses.

In Nightingale's later years, she came into conflict with the very nurses who had been trained for leadership. In 1886, some of these nurses, now superintendents of other training schools, wanted to establish an organization that would provide a central examination and registration center, the forerunner of licensure. Nightingale opposed this movement for several reasons: nursing was still too young and disorganized; national criteria would not be as high as those of individual schools; and the all-important aspect of character could not be tested. She fought the concept with every weapon at her disposal, including her powerful contacts, and succeeded in limiting the fledgling Royal British Nurses' Association to maintaining a "list" instead of a "register."

Nightingale's prolific writings on nursing have survived, and some of them are still surprisingly apt. Often they reflected her concern about the character of nurses and her own determination that their main focus be on nursing. One principle from which Nightingale did not swerve was that nurses were to nurse, not to do heavy cleaning ("if you want a charwoman, hire one"); not to do laundry ("it makes their hands coarse and hard and less able to attend to the delicate manipulation which they may be called on to execute"); and not to fetch ("to save the time of nurses; all diets and ward requisites should be brought into the wards"). Then, as in many places now, status and promotion came through assumption of administrative roles, but Nightingale recognized that "many are valuable as nurses, who are yet unfit for promotion to head nurses." Her alternative, however, would not be greeted favorably today—a raise after 10 years of good service!

Nightingale also commented on other issues considered pertinent today. Continuing education was a must, for she saw nursing as a progressive art, in which to stand still was to go back. "A woman who thinks of herself, 'Now I am a full nurse, a skilled nurse. I have learnt all there is to be learned,' take my word for it, she does not know what a nurse is, and she will never know: she has gone back already."[12] Although there is no evidence that she took any action to help end discrimination against women, Nightingale believed that women should be accepted into all professions, but she warned them, "qualify yourselves for it as a man does for his work." She believed that women should be paid as highly as men, but that equal pay meant equal responsibility. In a profession with as much responsibility as nursing, she said, it was particularly important to have adequate compensation, or intelligent, independent women would not be attracted to it.

Until the end of her life, she was firm on the need for nurses to obey physicians in medical matters. However, she stressed the importance of nurse observation and reporting because the physician was not constantly at the patient's bedside, as the nurse was. She was adamant that a nurse (and woman) be in charge of nursing, with no other administrative figure having authority over nurses, including physicians. She knew the importance of a work setting that gave job satisfaction. In words that are a far-off echo of nurses' complaints today, she wrote:

> Besides, a thing very little understood, a good nurse has her professional pride in results of her Nursing quite as much as a Medical Officer in the results of his treatment. There are defective buildings, defective administrations, defective appliances, which make all good Nursing impossible. A good Nurse does not like to waste herself, and the better the Nurse, the stronger this feeling in her.[13]

Planner, administrator, educator, researcher, reformer, Florence Nightingale never lost her interest in nursing. At age 74, in her last major publication on nursing, she differentiated between sick nursing and health nursing, and emphasized the primary need for prevention of illness, for which a lay "Health Missioner" (today's health educator?) would be trained.

When Nightingale died on August 13, 1910, she was to be honored by burial in Westminster Abbey. However, she had chosen instead to be buried in the family plot in Hampshire, with a simple inscription: "F.N. Born 1820, Died 1910."

KEY POINTS

1. A certain amount of the ritualistic mystique and belief in spirits or gods pervaded care of the sick in early civilizations.
2. Records of early civilizations emphasize treatment given by those designated as physicians, but there appear to have been men and women fulfilling nursing roles of some sort.
3. In early Egypt, India, China, Greece, and Rome, as well as in the

lands of the Hebrews, setting rules of hygiene and sanitation, using herbs, and performing surgery were part of the care of the sick.

4. The Romans are generally credited with building the first hospitals, but in the Christian period, "houses for the sick" were available for the sick poor, often tended by men or women in religious and secular orders.

5. In 1860, Florence Nightingale founded modern nursing at St. Thomas's Hospital in London with organized training programs that included both theory and practice, careful selection of students, and freedom from hospital control.

6. In her careful observations and recording and her use of statistics in matters affecting health care and administration in the British army, in hospitals throughout Europe, and in the community, Nightingale is often credited with being the first nurse researcher.

7. Nightingale made many pertinent observations and recommendations on nurses and nursing practice, such as the need for nurses to be free from other duties so that they could concentrate on nursing, as well as the need for holistic care, for home care, for continuing education, for adequate compensation, and for a satisfactory working environment.

REFERENCES

1. Bullough B, Bullough V. *The Care of the Sick: The Emergence of Modern Nursing.* New York: Prodist, 1978, p 69.
3. Moore J. *A Zeal for Responsibility: The Struggle for Professional Nursing in Victorian England, 1869–1883.* Athens, GA: University of Georgia Press, 1983, p 3.
3. Barritt ER. Florence Nightingale's values and modern nursing education. *Nurs Forum* 12(4):7–47, 1973.
4. Bullough and Bullough, op cit, p 86.
5. Carnegie E. *The Path We Tread: Blacks in Nursing 1854–1984.* Philadelphia: J.B. Lippincott, 1986, pp 2–3.
6. Seymer LR. *Selected Writings of Florence Nightingale.* New York: Macmillan Publishing, 1954, p 28.
7. Barritt, op cit, p 8.
8. Seymer, op cit, pp 222–223.
9. Ibid, p 244
10. Ibid, p 234.
11. Ibid, p 316.
12. Pavey, AE. *The Story of the Growth of Nursing.* London: Faber and Faber, 1938, p 296.
13. Seymer, op cit, p 276.

2

Nursing in the United States: American Revolution to Nursing Revolution

OBJECTIVES

After studying this chapter, you will be able to:

1. Explain how early nursing schools in the United States were established and functioned.
2. Name at least five early nursing leaders and their contributions to nursing.
3. Identify factors that influenced major changes in the education of nurses in the period between 1900 and 1965.
4. Describe how major changes in the practice of nursing in the period between 1900 and 1965 were influenced.
5. Identify the key findings of major studies and reports about nursing before 1965.

The first 100 years of American nursing show an interesting pattern. At the close of the nineteenth century and the dawn of the twentieth, there was rapid establishment and expansion of the new training schools for nurses. Many exciting developments that included breakthroughs unheard of for a woman's occupation occurred just as rapidly, thanks to the intelligence, initiative, and risk taking of an extraordinary group of women. Then for most of the next 50 years, progress seemed slow, with a patient chipping away at the many obstacles to quality education and practice. However, after World War II, another rapid series of changes moved nursing into a new era, a revolution that created both opportunities and risks for the emerging profession.

THE VOLUNTEERS

Just as the Crimean War spotlighted the activities of Florence Nightingale and the importance of nursing, the Civil War was an impetus for the development of training programs for nursing in the United States. There had never been an organized system for the care of the sick and wounded in wartime. During the American Revolution, some basic care was given by camp followers, wives, women in the neighborhood and "surgeon's mates" who may have been employed by the army.[1]

When the Civil War began in 1861, untrained women quickly volunteered to become nurses. Dorothea Dix, well known by then, was appointed by the Secretary of War to supervise these new "nurses." Meanwhile, members of religious orders also volunteered, and nursing in some of the larger government hospitals was eventually assigned to them because of the inexperience of the lay volunteers.

Except for that group, almost none of the thousands of Northern women who served as nurses during the war had any kind of training or hospital experience. They can be categorized as follows:

1. The nurses appointed by Miss Dix or other officials as legal employees of the army for 40 cents and one ration a day.
2. The sisters or nuns of the various orders.
3. Those employed for short periods of time for menial chores.
4. Black women employed under general orders of the War Department for $10 a month.
5. Uncompensated volunteers.
6. Women camp followers.
7. Women employed by the various relief organizations.[2]

Because of the prejudice against the idea of Southern women as nurses in the terrible conditions in Confederate hospitals, only about 1000 served, mostly as volunteers, and they performed valiantly. As in the North, many nuns gave nursing care.

Some of the information on what the Civil War nurses did comes from the diaries of Northern and Southern women and the writings of Louisa May Alcott and Walt Whitman, both Northern volunteers. In her journal, Alcott described her working day, which began at six. After opening the windows, because of the bad air in the makeshift hospital, she spent her time "giving out rations, cutting up food for helpless boys, washing faces, teaching my attendants how beds are made or floors are swept, dressing wounds, dusting tables, sewing bandages, keeping my tray tidy, rushing up and down after pillows, bed linens, sponges, and directions...."[3] Volunteers also read to the patients, wrote letters, and comforted them. Apparently, even the hired nurses did little more except, perhaps, give medicines.

But so did the volunteers, sometimes giving the medicine and food of their choice to the patient, instead of what the doctor ordered. However, many of these women were very strong, and were outspoken about incompetence and corruption; sometimes one carried her complaints to the Secretary of War and got action.

By 1862, enormous military hospitals, some with as many as 3000 beds, were being built, although there were still some makeshift hospitals— former hotels, churches, factories, and almost anything else available. Floating hospitals were also inaugurated and served as transport units, with nurses attending the wounded. According to one army hospital edict, the nurses, under the supervision of the "Stewards and Chief Wardmaster," were responsible for the administration of the wards, but many of their duties appeared to be related more to keeping the nonmedical records of patients and reporting their misbehavior than to nursing care. If the patient needed medical or surgical attendance, the doctor was to be called.

Georgeanna Woolsey wrote that the often incompetent contract surgeons treated the nurses without even common courtesy because they did not want them and tried to make their lives so unbearable that they would leave. The formidable nurse Mary Ann (Mother) Bickerdyke attacked the surgeons and officers who were drunk, refused to attend the wounded, or injured them further because of their incompetence. She managed to have a number of them dismissed (in part because of her friendship with General Grant and General Sherman).[4] Another fighter was Clara Barton. One story told about her is that while supervising the delivery of a wagonload of supplies for soldiers, she neatly removed an ox from a herd intended for the Union Army, so that some starving Confederate wounded would have food.[5]

Only in recent years has attention been given to the black nurses of the Civil War or before. Harriet Tubman, the "Moses of her people," not only led many black slaves to freedom in her underground railroad activities before the war but also nursed the wounded when she joined the Union army. Similarly, Sojourner Truth, abolitionist speaker and activist in the women's movement, also cared for the sick and wounded. Susie King Taylor, born to slavery and secretly taught to read and write, met and married a Union soldier and served as a battlefront nurse for more than four years, although she received no salary or pension from the Union Army.[6]

There were other heroines, untrained women from the North and South, caring for the sick and wounded with few skills but much kindness, and, as in the Crimea, the soldiers were sentimentally appreciative, if not discriminating. On the other hand, given the circumstances, what they accomplished was amazing.[7] Altogether, some 10,000 women served.

Even when paid, Civil War nurses had little status and no rank. An investigative report by the United States Sanitary Commission noted that nurses had not been well treated or wisely used. Nevertheless, the

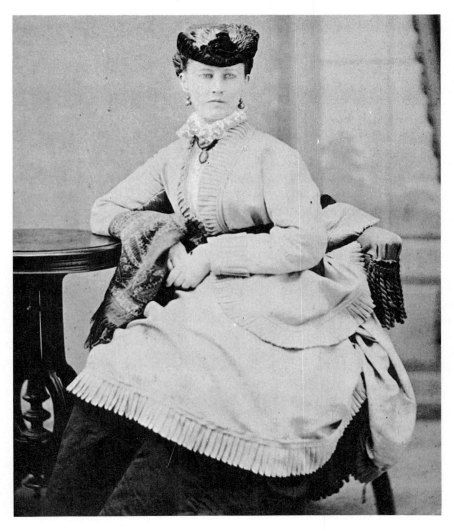

Jane Woolsey, Civil War volunteer nurse; she and her sisters were influential in the founding of early nurse training schools. (*Courtesy of Columbia University School of Nursing.*)

Civil War opened hospitals to massive numbers of women, well-bred "ladies," who would otherwise probably not even have thought of nursing. Some of these, such as Abby, Jane, and Georgeanna Woolsey, later helped lead the movement to establish training schools for nurses.

NURSING EDUCATION: THE FIRST 60 YEARS

The nursing role of women in the Civil War, however unsophisticated, and the fame of Florence Nightingale brought to the attention of the American public the need for nurses and the desirability of some organized programs of training.

More physicians became interested in the training of nurses and, at a meeting of the American Medical Association (AMA) in 1869, a committee to study the matter stated that it was "just as necessary to have well-trained, well-instructed nurses as to have intelligent and skillful physicians." The committee recommended that nursing schools be placed under the guardianship of county medical societies, although under the immediate supervision of lady superintendents; that every lay hospital should have a school; and that nurses should be trained not only for the hospital but for private duty in the home.[8]

Although a number of training programs for nurses and midwives existed before the Civil War, what is considered the first American school to offer a graded course in scientific nursing, based on guidelines set by Florence Nightingale, began in 1872 at the New England Hospital for Women and Children. Women physicians gave the twelve lectures that comprised the formal education of the 12-month course. The students, who received a small allowance after three months, worked from 5:30 A.M. to 9:00 P.M. and slept in rooms near the ward so that they were available when needed. One of the first graduates was Melinda Ann (Linda) Richards, thereafter called America's first trained nurse (probably because, of all the nurses who graduated from this primitive early program, she moved on to be a key figure in the development of nursing education). Richards, like some of the other students in the schools that evolved, had already been a nurse in a hospital. Some schools would not accept these students because they wanted to set a new image. Another outstanding graduate of the New England Hospital for Women and Children (1879) was Mary Mahoney, the first trained black nurse.

In 1873, three schools were established that were supposedly based on the Nightingale model. The Bellevue Training School in New York City was founded through the influence of several society ladies who had been involved in Civil War nursing, including Abby Woolsey. Although the school attempted to follow Nightingale principles and reported that it was attracting educated women, its overall purpose was to improve conditions in a great charity hospital, and much of the learning occurred on a trial-and-error basis. Nevertheless, Bellevue had a lot of interesting firsts: interdisciplinary rounds where nurses reported on the nursing plan of care; patient record keeping and writing of orders, initiated by Linda Richards, who became night superintendent; and the first uniform, by stylish and aristocratic Euphemia Van Rensselaer, which started a trend.

The Connecticut Training School was started through the influence of another Woolsey, Georgeanna, and her husband, Dr. Francis Bacon. Through negotiation with the hospital, the superintendent of nurses was designated as separate from, and not responsible to, the steward (administrator) of the hospital, and teaching outside the wards was permitted. Good intentions notwithstanding, the students soon were sent to give care in the homes of sick families, with the money going to the School Fund—and the school could boast that for 33 years it was not financed or directed by the hospital.

The Boston Training School was the last of that first famous trio. Again, a group of women associated with other educational and philanthropic endeavors spearheaded its organization, but this time their goal was to offer a desirable occupation for self-supporting women and to provide good private nurses for the community. After prolonged negotiations that allowed the director of the school rather than the hospital to maintain control, the Massachusetts General Hospital assigned "The Brick" building to the school because it (The Brick) "stands by itself; represents both medical and surgical departments; and offers the hard labor desirable for the training of nurses."[9] Apparently, there was rather poor leadership, and nurses continued to do menial tasks, with little attention given to training. When Linda Richards became the third director, she reorganized the work, started classes, and set out to prove that trained nurses were better than untrained ones.

Other major training schools that were to endure into the next century were founded in the next few years, somewhat patterned after Nightingale's precepts. Their success and the popularity of their graduates resulted in a massive proliferation of training schools. In 1880, there were 15; by 1900, 432; by 1909, 1105 hospital-based diploma schools. Hospitals with as few as 20 beds opened schools, and the students provided almost totally free labor. Usually the only graduate nurses were the superintendent and perhaps the operating room supervisor and night supervisor. Students earned money for the hospital, for after a short period they were frequently sent to do private nursing in the home, with the money reverting to the hospital, not the school. Except for the few outstanding schools, all Nightingale principles were forgotten: the students were under the control of the hospital and worked from 12 to 15 hours a day—24 if they were on a private case in a home. Lessons, if any, were scheduled for an hour late in the evening when someone was available to teach. (It wasn't necessary for all students to be available.) Moreover, if the "pupils" lost time because of sickness, which was almost always contracted from patients or caused by sheer overwork, the time had to be totally made up before they could graduate.

Why then did training schools draw so many applicants? Because the

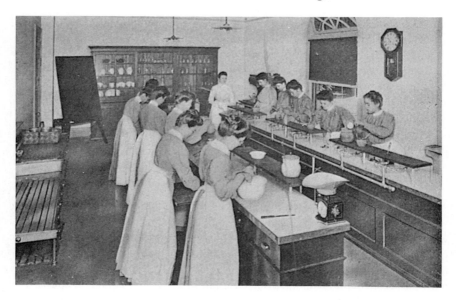

Nursing students in the better schools spent their time in formal classroom studies and laboratories like this class in domestic science. (*Courtesy of Columbia University School of Nursing.*)

occupational opportunities for untrained women were limited to domestic service, factory work, retail clerking, or prostitution. Higher education for women was limited to typewriting or teaching, but these were seldom taught in universities. Those colleges and universities that did admit women rarely prepared them for professions. Even with the strict discipline, hard work, long hours, and almost no time off, after a year or two of training (the second year consisting of unabashedly free labor to the hospitals), the trained nurse could do private duty at a salary ranging from $10 a week to the vague possibility of $20 (if she could collect it), a far cry from the $4 to $6 average of other women workers. Of course, on these cases, she was a 24-hour servant to the family and patient, lucky to have time off for a walk. And because there were necessarily months with no employment, even an excellent nurse was lucky to gross $600 a year.[10]

The more famous hospital schools, in particular, had hundreds and even thousands of applicants a year. On the other hand, there were a multitude of hospitals and sanitoriums of all kinds that were looking for students to meet their staffing needs, and for these, high-quality applicants were frequently lacking. Consequently, application standards were lowered rapidly. Apparently, most schools admitted a class of 30 to 35[11] (in some cases determined by their staffing and financial needs).

Attrition, caused in part by the extremely high rate of student illness and the unpleasant working and living conditions, was often 75 percent.

Student admission requirements varied, but all nurse applicants were female. Some hospitals accepted men in programs but gave them only a short course and frequently called them *attendants*. In 1888, at Bellevue Hospital, the Mills School for men was established with a two-year course, but for a long time its graduates were also called *attendants*. Other schools admitting men followed. Blacks were also generally silently excluded. Over the years, training schools for black nurses were founded, the first organized in 1891 at the Provident Hospital in Chicago.

The minimum age for all students was generally 21 years. Eight or fewer years of schooling were common, but usually good health and good character were absolute prerequisites. Obedience in training was essential, and a student could be dismissed as a troublemaker if the overworked girl grumbled, talked too much, was too familiar with men, criticized head nurses or doctors, or could not get along wherever placed. Married women and those over 30 were frequently excluded because they could not "fall in with the life successfully." And, of course, if they were divorced, they were totally unacceptable.

In the 1890s, only 12 percent of nurse training was theory, consisting of some anatomy and physiology, materia medica, perhaps some chemistry, bacteriology, hygiene, and lectures on certain diseases. The leading schools developed their own institutional manuals, but a few pioneering texts were also written by nurses before 1900.[12]

Even into the twentieth century, students continued to live a slavelike existence, without outward complaint, and were poorly housed, overworked, underfed ("rations of a kind and quality only a remove better than what we might place before a beggar," said a popular magazine), and unprotected from life-threatening illness (80 percent of the students in the average hospital graduated with positive tuberculin tests). If they survived all this, it was no wonder that they were expected to graduate as "respectful, obedient, cheerful, submissive, hard-working, loyal, pacific, and religious."[13] It was not professional education; it was not even a respectably run apprenticeship, because learning was not derived from skilled masters, but rather from their own peers, who were but a step ahead of them.

These principles of sacrifice, service, obedience to the physician, and ethical orientation are embodied in the Nightingale Pledge, written in 1893 by Lystra E. Gretter, superintendent of the school at Harper Hospital in Detroit, a pledge still sometimes recited by students today.

I solemnly pledge myself before God and in the presence of this assembly;
    To pass my life in purity and to practice my profession faithfully;
    I will abstain from whatever is deleterious and mischievous and

will not take or knowingly administer any harmful drug; I will do all in my power to maintain and elevate the standard of my profession, and will hold in confidence all personal matters committed to my keeping and all family affairs coming to my knowledge in the practice of my calling;

　　With loyalty will I endeavor to aid the physician in his work, and devote myself to the welfare of those committed to my care.[14]

Although the passage of the first licensure laws in 1903 (discussed later) set standards for nursing education, there was little improvement. The laws were not mandatory. Most training schools remained under the control of hospitals, and the needs of the hospital took priority over those of the school. For instance, it was not until 1912 that an occasional nurse received time from hospital responsibilities in order to organize and teach basic nursing, and superintendents were warned not to "neglect" patient care in favor of the school or they would face punishment. The hours were still long, and the students continued to give free service, with "book learning" as an afterthought. Only in California, where an Eight-Hour Law for Women was passed in 1911, was there any movement to include student nurses (not even graduate nurses). Yet, when the bill was introduced in 1913, it was fought bitterly not only by hospitals, as might be expected, but also by physicians and nurses.[15]

While the Flexner Report of 1910 was bringing about reform in medical schools, eliminating the correspondence courses and the weaker and poorer schools, Adelaide Nutting and other leaders were agitating for reform in nursing education. In 1911, the American Society of Superintendents of Training Schools for Nurses presented a proposal for a similar survey of nursing schools to the Carnegie Foundation. Ignoring nursing, the foundation directed a considerable amount of its funds to such studies in dental, legal, and teacher education.

Although women were having a little more success in being accepted in colleges and universities, there was only limited movement to make basic nursing programs an option in academic settings. The University of Minnesota program, founded in 1909 by Dr. Richard Olding Beard, a physician who was dedicated to the concept of higher education for nurses, became the first enduring baccalaureate program in nursing. Even this was more similar to good diploma programs than to other university programs. Although eventually the students had to meet university admission standards and took some specialized courses, they also worked a 56-hour week in the hospital and were awarded a diploma instead of a degree after three years. Similar programs were started by other universities that took over hospitals, in part to obtain student services for their hospitals. Just before World War I, several hospitals and universities, such as Presbyterian Hospital of New York and Teachers College, Columbia University, offered degree options. These developed into five-year programs with two years of college work and three years in a diploma school. This became a common pattern that lasted throughout the 1940s.

One of the more daring experiments of the times was the Vassar Training Camp. In the summer of 1918 a preparatory course in nursing was established at Vassar from which the students would move to selected schools of nursing to complete the program in little more than two additional years. A large percentage of the women completed the program and entered the nursing schools they had selected. Many of nursing's leaders arose from this group. Because this and similar programs were generally of considerably higher quality than those of the training schools, the movement of nursing education toward an academic setting received another nudge.

By the end of World War I, nursing had serious problems. There was a shortage of nurses, because many who had switched careers "for the duration" returned to their own field, and others appeared not to be attracted. In part, it was an image problem, one that was to continue to haunt nursing, but another important factor was that nursing education was in trouble. As Isabel Stewart said, "The plain facts are that nursing schools are being starved and always have been starved for lack of funds to build up any kind of substantial educational structure."[16] Later, this problem was clearly pinpointed by prestigious study committees (see Appendix 1).

In 1918, Adelaide Nutting had approached the Rockefeller Foundation to seek endowment for the Johns Hopkins School of Nursing, stressing the need for improvement in the education of public health nurses. The meeting resulted in a committee to investigate the "proper training" of public health nurses, an investigation that quickly concluded that the problem was nursing education in general. The finding of the 1923 Goldmark Report concluded that schools of nursing needed to be recognized and supported as separate educational components with not just training in nursing, but also a liberal education. Moreover, "Superintendents, supervisors, instructors, and public health nurses should in all cases receive special additional training beyond the basic nursing course."[17]

Although the report had little immediate impact, it did result in Rockefeller Foundation support for the founding of the Yale School of Nursing (1924), the first in the world to be established as a separate university department with its own dean, Annie Goodrich. Although a few other such programs followed, progress lagged, for many powerful physicians reached the public media with their notions that nurses needed only technical skills, manual dexterity, and quick obedience to the physician. Charles Mayo, for instance, deciding that city-trained nurses were too difficult to handle, too expensive, and spent too much time getting educated, wanted to recruit 100,000 country girls.[18]

This attitude was not new. Almost from the beginning, there were physicians who objected to so much education for nurses and devoted considerable medical journal space to raging about the "overtrained nurse."

One physician even suggested a correspondence course for training nurses to care for the "poor folks," and a New York newspaper editorial proclaimed, "What we want in nurses is less theory and more practice."[19] But then, this was at a time when a leading Harvard physician insisted that serious mental exercise would damage a woman's brain or cause other severe trauma, such as the narrowing of the pelvic area, which would make her unable to deliver children.[20]

However, there were also farsighted physicians who supported not "teaching a trade, but preparing for a profession," as Dr. Richard Cabot noted in 1901. But even popular magazines recognized that student nurses were being exploited by hospitals and that the kind of student being encouraged into nursing by school principals was one seen as not too bright, not attractive enough to marry, and too poor to be supported at home.

A study following close on the heels of the Goldmark Report soon reaffirmed the inadequacy of nursing schools and practicing nurses. *Nurses, Patients, and Pocketbooks*[21] pointed out that the hasty postwar nurse-recruiting efforts had not improved the lot of the patient or the nurse. In 1928, problems included an oversupply of nurses, geographic maldistribution, low educational standards, poor working conditions, and some critically unsatisfactory levels of care.

NURSING'S EARLY LEADERS*

In many ways, early nursing education and nursing leaders were intertwined. After graduating from one of the better training programs, these nurses often assumed dual positions as both superintendent of nursing in hospitals and superintendent of the training school. Since students provided almost all of the nursing service, with the exception of a few supervisors, the training school received much of the leaders' attention. They took the responsibility seriously. They were concerned with the quality of the students and the program, and much of what they did was directed at improving nursing education. In a male-dominated society, working in what was barely becoming an accepted, respectable occupation, these unusual women were not only talented but were also determined risk takers.

Before the new century was far along, they were responsible for setting nursing standards, improving curricula, writing textbooks, starting two enduring professional organizations and a nursing journal, inaugurating a teacher training program in a university, and initiating nursing licensure. They were a mixed group, but with certain commonalities: usually unmarried but, except for Lavinia Dock, not feminist. Almost all were involved in the

*See also Appendix 8.

early nursing organizations. Fortunately, most were also great letter writers and letter savers as well as authors, so that there are many fascinating insights into their lives. (See, in particular, the Christy series in *Nursing Outlook*, mentioned in the Bibliography.) Some highlights follow.

America's first trained nurse, Linda Richards, had a continuing impact on the training schools because she spent much of her career moving from hospital to hospital in what seems to have been an improvement campaign. In those earliest days, almost any graduate was considered a prime candidate for starting another program. Some undoubtedly lacked the intellectual and leadership qualities needed, so that the new schools, if not actual disasters, were frequently of poor quality. Linda Richards apparently had the skill and authority to upgrade both the school and the nursing service, which were, after all, almost inseparable. However, she seemed willing to accept school management that tied the economics of the hospital to student education, usually to the detriment of the latter.

One of the most noted nursing figures was Isabelle Hampton, who left teaching to enter Bellevue Training School in 1881. Not only was she attractive and charming, but she was "in every sense of the word a leader, by nature, by capacity, by personal attributes and qualities, by choice, and probably to some extent by inheritance and training; a follower she never was."[22] In her two major superintendencies, she made a number of then radical changes—cutting down the students' workday to 10 hours and eliminating their free private duty services. For the Johns Hopkins program, which she founded, she recruited feisty Lavinia Dock, who was still at Bellevue, to be her assistant. They must have made an interesting pair, for Lavinia, also a "lady," was outspoken and frequently tactless, particularly with physicians.

Adelaide Nutting graduated in that first Hopkins class, and the three became friends.[23] Nutting followed Hampton as principal of the school when in 1894 Isabel married one of her admirers, Dr. Hunter Robb, and, as was the custom, retired from active nursing. (Letters of the time reveal the anger, dismay, and even sadness of her colleagues at her marriage. They were sure Dr. Robb was not nearly good enough for her; besides, she was betraying nursing by robbing the profession of her talents.) Nevertheless, Isabel Hampton Robb maintained her interest in nursing and continued to be active in the development of the profession. In 1893, she had been appointed chairman of a committee to arrange a congress of nurses under the auspices of the International Congress of Charities, Correction, and Philanthropy at the World's Fair (Columbian Exposition) in Chicago. There, before an international audience of nurses, she voiced her concern about poor nursing education and stated that the term *trained nurse* meant "anything, everything, or next to nothing" in the absence of educational standards. At the same time, Lavinia Dock pointed out that the teaching, training, and discipline of nurses should not be provided at the discretion of doctors. Similar themes were repeated in other papers, as well as the notion that there ought to be an organization of nurses. Shortly after the Congress, 18 superintendents organized the American Society of Superintendents of Training School for Nursing, which was to become the National League of Nursing Education (NLNE) in 1912. Its purpose was to promote the fellowship of members, establish and maintain a universal standard of training, and further the best interests of the nursing profession. The first convention of the society elected Linda Richards president.[24]

Another attendee at those early meetings was Sophia Palmer, descendant of John and Priscilla Alden and a graduate of the Boston Training School, who, after a variety of experiences, organized a training school in Washington, D.C., over the concerted opposition of local physicians who wanted to control nursing education. She approved the actions that were taken by her colleagues but was impatient with what seemed to be the blind acceptance of hospital control of schools. "She had a very intense nature and, like all those who are born crusaders, had little patience with the slower methods of persuasion.... She was like a spirited racehorse held by the reins of tradition."[25]

Within a short time, Palmer and some of the others in the Society, including Dock and Isabel Hampton Robb, recognized the need for another organization for all nurses. Although some of the training schools had alumnae associations, they were restrictive; in some cases, their own graduates could not be members, and any "outsider" could not participate. Therefore, if a nurse left the immediate vicinity of her own school, there was no way in which she had any organized contact with other nurses. In a paper given in 1895, Palmer stressed that the power of the nursing profession depended on its ability to organize individuals who could influence public opinion. Dock also made recommendations for a national organization. In 1896, delegates representing the oldest training school alumnae associations and members of an organizing committee of the Society selected a name for the proposed organization: Nurses' Associated Alumnae of the United States and Canada (which became the American Nurses Association in 1911). They also set a time and place for the first meeting (February 1897 in Baltimore) and drafted a constitution. At the end of that February meeting, held in conjunction with the fourth annual Society convention, the constitution and by-laws were adopted, and Isabel Hampton Robb was elected president. Among the problems discussed at those early meetings were nursing licensure and the creation of an official nursing publication.

There were a number of nursing journals: the *British Journal of Nursing*, established by one of England's nursing leaders, Ethel Gordon Fenwick; and, in the United States, the short-lived *The Nightingale*, started by a Bellevue graduate; *The Nursing Record* and *The Nursing World*, also short-lived; and *The Trained Nurse and Hospital Review*, which Palmer edited for a time and which continued for 70 years. But the leaders of the new organizations wanted a magazine that would promote nursing, owned and controlled by nursing.

For several years there was discussion, but no action, until another committee on the ways and means of producing a magazine was formed. In January 1900, they organized a stock company and sold $100 shares only to nurses and nurses' alumnae associations. By May, they had a promise of $2400 in shares, and almost 500 nurses had promised to subscribe. Admittedly, they had overstepped their mandate, they reported to the third annual convention of the Nurses' Associated Alumnae, but they were given approval to establish the magazine along the lines formulated. The J. B. Lippincott Company was selected as publisher, and Sophia Palmer became editor, which she did on an unpaid basis for the first nine months. (She had become director of the Rochester City Hospital in New York.) As the first issues went for mailing in October, it was discovered that the post office rules prevented its being mailed because the journal's stockholders were not incorporated. M. E. P. Davis and Sophia Palmer assumed personal responsibility for all liabilities of the new *American Journal of Nursing*, and it went out. The *Journal* was considered the official organ of the nursing profession, but the stock was still held by alumnae associations and individual nurses. It was Lavinia Dock who donated the first share of stock to the association, and by 1912 the renamed American Nurses Association

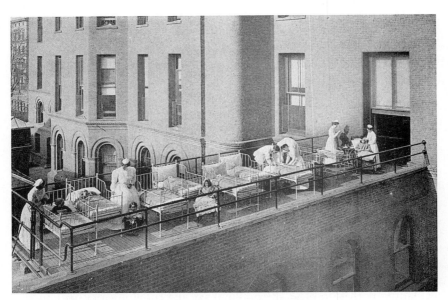

Much of hospital care in the early years of training schools was given by students, here tending to children in an open-air ward. (*Courtesy of Columbia University School of Nursing.*)

(ANA) had gained ownership of all the stock of the American Journal of Nursing Company, which it still retains.[26]

One other major organization, the American Red Cross, was established by a nurse, Clara Barton, the schoolteacher who had volunteered as a nurse and directed relief operations during the Civil War and served with the German Red Cross during the Franco-Prussian War in 1870. (The establishment of the International Red Cross as a permanent international relief agency that could take immediate action in time of war had occurred in Geneva in 1864 with the signing of the Geneva Convention guidelines.) After her return to the United States, Barton organized the American Red Cross and persuaded Congress in 1882 to ratify the Treaty of Geneva so that the Red Cross could carry on its humanitarian efforts in peacetime. Clara Barton, however, was not an active part of the nursing leadership that was molding the profession.[27]

That group had another immediate aim. The Society recognized that the nurses were at a disadvantage because they had no postgraduate training in administration or teaching, so a committee consisting of Robb, Nutting, Richards, Mary Agnes Snively, and Lucy Drown was formed to investigate the possibilities. At the sixth Society convention, they reported their success. James Russell, the farsighted dean of Teachers College, Columbia University, in New York, had agreed to start a course for nurses if they could guarantee the enrollment of 12 nurses, or $1000 a year. The Society agreed. Members of the Society screened the candidates, contributed $1000 a year, and taught the course—hospital economics. Later, the students were also allowed to enroll in psychology, science, household economics, and biology. Anna Alline, one of the two graduates of the first class, then took over the total administration of the course.

There was one more major goal to be reached: licensure of nurses. Not only did the hundreds of hospital-based schools vary greatly in quality, but the market was also flooded with "nurses" who had been dismissed from schools without graduating, "nurses" from six-week private and correspondence courses, and a vast number of those who simply called themselves nurses. It was inevitable that people became confused, for when they hired nurses for private duty in their homes, the "nurse" could present one of the elaborate diplomas from a $13 correspondence course that guaranteed that anyone could become a nurse, a real or forged reference, or a genuine diploma from a top-quality school. How could they judge? Therefore, because of the dreadful care given by individuals representing themselves as nurses, the public was once more disenchanted with nurses. Nursing's leaders were determined that there must be legal regulation, both to protect the public from unscrupulous and incompetent nurses and to protect the young profession by establishing a minimum level of competence, limiting all or some of the professional functions to those who qualified. Medicine already had licensing in some states, and many aspiring professions were also moving in that direction.

In September 1901, at the first meeting of the newly formed International Council of Nurses, which was held in Buffalo, a resolution was passed, stating that "it is the duty of the nursing profession of every country to work for suitable legislative enactment regulating the education of nurses and protecting the interests of the public, by securing State examinations and public registration, with the proper penalties for enforcing the same."[28]

Despite considerable opposition to nurse licensure from untrained nurses, managers, and proprietors of poor training programs, and some physicians, licensure was achieved and basic educational standards were set. In 1903, North Carolina, New Jersey, Virginia, and New York passed laws. However, New York's law was the strongest. For instance, New Jersey's law omitted a board of any kind; North Carolina had a mixed board of nurses and doctors and allowed a nurse to be licensed without attending a training school if vouched for by a doctor. It should be remembered, though, that all nurse licensure laws in those times were permissive, not mandatory. That is, only the registered nurse (RN) title was protected. Untrained nurses could continue to work as nurses as long as they did not call themselves RNs.

One of the key figures in community health nursing was Lillian Wald. After graduating from the New York Hospital School of Nursing and working a short time, she decided to enter the Women's Medical College. When she and another nurse, Mary Brewster, were sent to the Lower East Side to lecture to immigrant mothers on the care of the sick, they were shocked at what they saw; neither had known that such abject poverty could exist. Wald left medical school, moved with Mary Brewster to a top-floor tenement on Jefferson Street, and began to offer nursing care to the poor. After a short while, the calls came by the hundreds from families, hospitals, and physicians. People were cared for, whether or not they could afford to pay. The concern of these nurses was not just giving nursing care but seeing what other services could be made available to meet the many social needs of the poor.

After two years of such success, larger facilities, more nurses, and social workers were needed. In 1895, Wald, Brewster, Lavinia Dock, and other nurses moved to what was eventually called the Henry Street Settlement, a house bought by philanthropist Jacob H. Schiff. By 1909, the Henry Street staff had 37 nurses, all but 5 providing direct nursing service. Each nurse was carefully oriented to the customs of the immigrants she served and was able to demonstrate the value of understanding the family and the environment in giving good nursing care. Each nurse kept two sets of records, one for the physician and another recording the major points of the nurse's work. School nursing was also started by Lillian Wald, who suggested that placing nurses in schools might help solve the problem of the schools having to send home so many ill children.[29]

Another outstanding public health nurse was Margaret Higgins Sanger. She became interested in the plight of the poorly paid industrial workers,

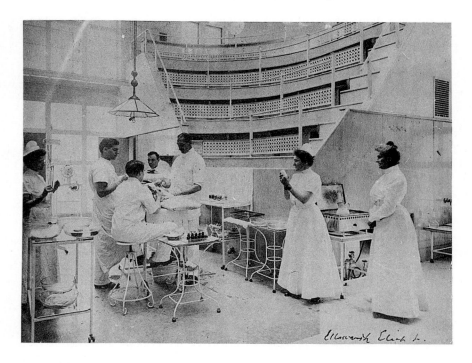

Nurses assisted physicians in the operating room early on (1903), here supervised
by Anna Maxwell, Superintendent of Presbyterian Hospital, New York City.
(*Courtesy of Columbia University School of Nursing.*)

particularly the women. She herself was married and had three children when
she decided to return to work in public health. She was assigned to maternity
cases on the Lower East Side of New York, where she found that pregnancy,
often unwanted, was a chronic condition. In 1912, one of her patients died
from a repeated self-abortion after begging doctors and nurses for information on how to avoid pregnancy. That was apparently a turning point for
Sanger. After learning everything she could about contraception, she and
her sister, also a nurse, opened the first birth control clinic in America in
Brooklyn. She was arrested and spent 30 days in the workhouse but
continued her crusade. She fought the battle for free dissemination of birth
control information for decades, against all types of opposition, until today,
birth control education is generally accepted as the right of women and as
one nursing role.[30]

   In the 23 years between World Wars I and II, nursing was affected
by the Great Depression and by adoption of the Nineteenth Amendment
to the Constitution in August 1920, granting women the right to vote.

Of the two, the latter had less immediate impact. Nurses showed relatively little interest in fighting for women's rights, and only one, Lavinia Dock, can be called an active feminist. "Dockie" was a maverick of the times. A tiny woman who loved music and was an accomplished pianist and organist, she also seemed to take on the whole worln in her battle for the underdog. Early on, she decided that nurses could have no power unless they had the vote. Her speeches and writings were brilliant, but she did not move her colleagues. Nevertheless, she devoted a good part of her life to working for women's rights. In England, she joined the Pankhursts and landed in jail. Back in the United States, she picketed the White House. Her colleague, Isabel Stewart, wrote, "They all went into the cooler for the night. I think it just pleased her no end."[31]

For all her devotion to women's rights, Dock remained committed to nursing. She was editor of the *Journal*'s Foreign Department from 1900 to 1923, during which she quarreled regularly with editor Sophia Palmer and managed to ignore World War I because she was a pacifist. She was also involved with the International Council of Nurses and was the author of a number of books, including *Health and Morality*, published in 1910, in which she discussed venereal disease. She was equally outspoken on this forbidden subject in open meetings. A number of nurses had become infected because physicians frequently refused to tell nurses when patients had the disease. Dock also regularly criticized her profession for withholding its interest, sympathy, and moral support from "the great, urgent, throbbing, pressing social claims of our day and generation."[32]

There were other nurses who put their mark on nursing in its first 60 years. Anne Goodrich reported on the poor nursing conditions in military camps during World War I, which resulted in the establishment of the Army School of Nursing. She became its first dean, and the high quality of the educational program, with only six to eight duty hours (unlike civilian hospitals), made it an overwhelming success. Isabel Stewart, who succeeded Adelaide Nutting (the first nurse ever to receive a professorship at Columbia University), in her 39 years at Teachers College set up a respected graduate program. In 1922, six nursing students at Indiana University founded Sigma Theta Tau, nursing's honor society, now an international organization. Then another pioneer, Mary Breckenridge, founded the Frontier Nursing Service in 1925; its staff was a mixture of British and British-trained American midwives.[33]

Little is known about either black or male nurses. However, after the Civil War, recognized black nurse leaders included Mary Mahoney, the first black nurse to graduate from a training program; Jessie Scales, the first district nurse; and Martha Franklin, founder of the National Association of Colored Graduate Nurses (NACGN). Adah Thomas led the fight to gain acceptance of black nurses by the army. She had corresponded extensively with Jane Delano, chairman of the national committee of the American Red

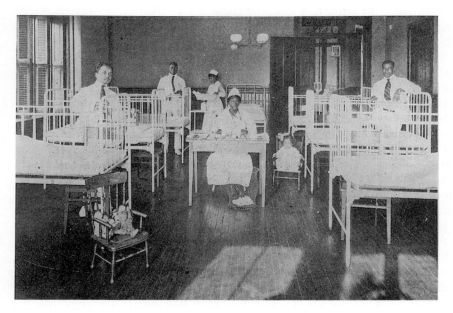

Generally "Negro" nurses and doctors cared for "Negro" patients, sometimes in hospitals such as here at Mercy Hospital-West, Philadelphia, *circa* 1910–1912. (*Courtesy of the Museum of Nursing History, Inc., Philadelphia.*)

Cross through which army nurses were enrolled at the time, and urged black nurses to enroll in the American Red Cross. Finally, a month after the armistice was signed in 1918 and in the midst of the flu epidemic, the first black nurses were assigned to army camps in Ohio and Illinois, with other assignments following. (However, it was not until World War II that black nurses were accepted into the military service.)[34]

THE NURSE IN PRACTICE

In the late nineteenth and early twentieth centuries, the graduate trained nurse had two major career options; she could do private duty in homes or, if she was exceptional (or particularly favored), gain one of the rare positions as head nurse, operating room supervisor, night supervisor, or even superintendent. The latter positions were, of course, much more available before the flood of nurses reached the market. Even so, in private duty, trained nurses often competed with untrained nurses who were not restrained from practicing in many states until the middle of the twentieth century. And, given the long hours and taxing physical work in home nursing, most private nurses found themselves unwanted at 40, with younger, stronger nurses being hired instead. Some of the more ambitious and perhaps braver nurses chose to go west to pioneer in new and sometimes primitive hospitals. There were a few in industrial nursing, and a limited but gradually increasing number in public health nursing.

The practice of nursing was scarcely limited to clinical care of the patient. Job descriptions of the time appear to have given major priority to scrubbing floors, dusting, keeping the stove stoked and the kerosene lamps trimmed and filled, controlling insects, washing clothes, making and rolling bandages, and other unskilled housekeeping tasks, as well as edicts for personal behavior (see Exhibit 2.1). Nursing care responsibilities included, in addition to carrying out the orders of the physician,

> making beds, giving baths, preventing and dressing bedsores, applying friction to the body and extremities, giving enemas, inserting catheters, bandaging, dressing blisters, burns, sores, and wounds, and observing secretions, expectorations, pulse, skin, appetite, body temperature, consciousness, respiration, sleep, condition of wounds, skin eruptions, elimination, and the effect of diet, stimulants, and medications.[35]

At the end of the nineteenth century, there was a marked growth of large cities in the United States. Although the cities had their beautiful public buildings, parks, and mansions, they also had their seamy sides—the festering slums where the tremendous flow of immigrants huddled. Between 1820 and 1910, nearly 30 million immigrants entered the United States, with a shift in numbers from Northern European to Southern European by the early 1900s. Health and social problems multiplied in the slum areas. Somehow, Americans did not seem to feel a great need to serve the sick poor in their homes; after all, there were public dispensaries and charity hospitals. Some visiting nurse groups were formed, but by 1900 it was estimated that only 200 nurses were engaged in public health nursing.

In 1912, the Red Cross established the Rural Nursing Service. Lillian Wald, at a major meeting on infant mortality, had cited the horrible health conditions of rural America, the high infant and maternal mortality rates, the prevalence of tuberculosis, and other serious health problems and suggested that the Red Cross operate a national service, similar to that of Great Britain. (Red Cross involvement gradually decreased until, with increased government involvement in public health, it discontinued the program altogether in 1947.)

However, in 1915, it is estimated that no more than 10 percent of the sick received care in the hospitals, and the majority of people could not afford private duty nurses. From this need, a public health movement emerged that increased the demand for nurses. At first most of these nurses concentrated on bedside care, but others, like those coming from the settlement houses, took broader responsibilities. Nevertheless, there were

---

EXHIBIT 2.1

Wanted: A Very Special Nurse to Care for 50 Patients at a Local Hospital

Duties and requirements:

- Daily sweep and mop the floors of your ward. Dust the patients' furniture and windowsills.
- Maintain an even temperature in your ward by bringing in a scuttle of coal for the day's business.
- Light is important to observe the patient's condition. Therefore, each day fill kerosene lamps, clean chimneys and trim wicks. Wash the windows once a week.
- The Nurses' notes are important in aiding the physician's work. Make your pens carefully. You may whittle nibs to your individual taste.
- Each nurse on duty will report every day at 7:00 A.M. and leave at 8:00 P.M. except on the Sabbath on which you will be off from 12:00 noon to 2:00 P.M.
- Graduates in good standing with the Superintendent of Nurses will be given an evening off each week for courting purposes, or two evenings a week if you go to church regularly.
- Each nurse should lay aside from each pay day a goodly sum of her earnings for her benefit in her declining years, so that she will not become a burden. For example, if you earn $30 a month, you should set aside $15.
- Any nurse who smokes, uses liquor in any form, gets her hair done at a beauty shop, or frequents dance halls will give the Superintendent of Nurses a good reason to suspect her worth, intentions and integrity.
- The nurse who performs her labors, serves her patients and doctors faithfully without fault for a period of five years will be given an increase by the Hospital Administration of five cents a day, providing there are no hospital debts that are outstanding.

Source: Reportedly an ad in a western newspaper in 1887.

no recognized standards or requirements for visiting nurses. Therefore in June 1912, a small group of visiting nurses, representing unofficially some 900 agencies and almost four times that many colleagues, founded the National Organization for Public Health Nursing (NOPHN), with Lillian Wald as the first president. It was an organization of nurses and lay people engaged in public health nursing and in the organization, management, and support of such work. The leaders of the group selected the term *public health nursing* as more inclusive than *visiting nursing*; it was also reminiscent of Nightingale's health nursing, which had focused on prevention. One of its first goals was to extend the services to working- and middle-class people, as well as to the poor.

By 1916, public health nurses were being called on to be welfare workers, sanitarians, housing inspectors, and health teachers as well. A number of universities began offering courses to help prepare nurses to fulfill this multifaceted role, and Mary Gardner, one of the founders of NOPHN and an interim director of the Rural Nursing Service, authored the first book in the field, *Public Health Nursing.* One of the observations she made was that although broad-minded physicians recognized that public health nurses helped them produce results that would not have been possible alone, the more conservative feared interference by nurses and

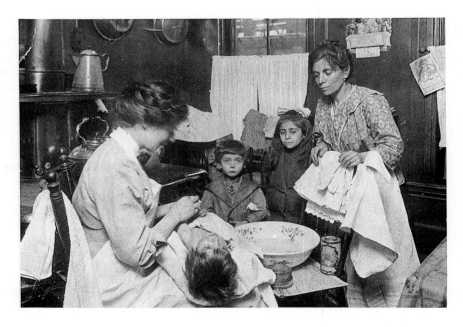

Turn of the century home care visits often included instructing parents in the care of their children. (*Courtesy of Visiting Nurse Service of Boston.*)

were resentful of them. She noted that a service had a better chance of success if it was started with the cooperation of the medical profession, and pointed out ways nurses could avoid friction with physicians and still be protected from the incompetents.

Gradually various other nursing specialties developed, such as anesthesia, industrial nursing, and nurse midwifery. However, it was the Great Depression, which followed the stock market crash in 1929, that helped alter nursing practice drastically. This was a period of high unemployment for nurses. As financial crises hit their clientele, private duty nurses found that there was little demand for their services. The situation worsened as nurses who were laid off in offices and industry, as well as married nurses, also looked for private duty cases. Both the Goldmark Report and *Nurses, Patients, and Pocketbooks* (Appendix 1) had warned that the overproduction and maldistribution of nurses would soon cause a problem, but no action had been taken. Now a reevaluation of nursing and nursing education was imperative. The result was the closing of many small schools and an increased concern for high standards, the setting of an eight-hour day for private duty nurses, and the employment of graduate nurses in hospitals. Unfortunately, the last also had long-lasting bad effects. By 1933, some nurses worked in hospitals for little more than room and board. It took many years for nurses to earn reasonable wages and to gain some autonomy in their practice.

Some help finally came with the Roosevelt Administration, when relief funds were allocated for bedside care of the indigent and nurses were employed as visiting nurses under the Federal Emergency Relief Administration (FERA). Ten thousand unemployed nurses were put to work in numerous settings under the Civil Works Administration (CWA) in public hospitals, clinics, public health agencies, and other health services. The follow-up Works Progress Administration (WPA) then continued to provide funds for nurses in community health activities.[36]

Of all the entrants into nursing, two groups got particularly short shrift—men and blacks. The prejudice against men was specially related to nursing and has persisted to some extent (see Chapter 4). As the distorted image of the female nurse evolved, men did not seem to fit the concepts held by powerful figures in and out of nursing. Therefore, although men graduated from acceptable, usually totally male nursing schools and attempted to become active members of the ANA, even forming a men's section, their numbers and influence remained small until the post-World War II era.

Black nurses were caught in the overall common prejudice against their race. Individual black nurses, as noted earlier, broke down barriers in various nursing fields. As early as 1908, they organized the National Association of Colored Graduate Nurses (NACGN), both to fight against discriminatory practices and to foster leadership among black nurses.

Although the ANA had a nondiscriminatory policy, some state organizations did not, and a rule that the nurse must have graduated from a state-approved school to be an ANA member eliminated even more black nurses. Finally, in 1951, the NACGN was absorbed into the ANA, which required nondiscrimination for all state associations as a prerequisite for ANA affiliation.

In 1924, it was reported that only 58 state-accredited schools admitted blacks, and most of these were located in black hospitals or in departments caring for black patients in municipal hospitals. Of these schools, 77 percent were located in the South. Twenty-eight states offered no opportunities in nursing education for black women. Most of the southern "schools" that trained black nurses were totally unacceptable, and many of those approved barely met standards. Moreover, there were some 23,000 untrained black midwives in the South, but no one made the effort to combine training in nursing and midwifery, which would have been a distinct service. In 1930, there were fewer than 6000 graduate black nurses, most of whom worked in black hospitals or public health agencies that served black patients. Opportunities in other fields either were not open to them or could not admit them because they did not, understandably, have the advanced preparation necessary. Middle-class black women were usually not attracted to nursing, because teaching and other available fields offered more prestige and better opportunities.

It was not until a 1941 executive order and the corresponding follow-through that any part of the federal government made any effort to investigate the grievances and deal with the complaints of blacks. Later, the Bolton Act opened the doors of participating nursing schools to blacks. Yet, overt and covert methods were used in both the North and the South to prevent the more able black nurses from assuming leadership positions— some as simple as advancing the least aggressive. And for all the desperate need for nurses, the armed forces balked at accepting and integrating black nurses. Not until the end of World War II and after some aggressive action by the NACGN and the National Nursing Council for War Service did this situation change.

WARTIME NURSING

Another influence on nursing was nurses' participation in American wars. Ironically, although the military was not prepared to care for its sick and wounded in the short but deadly Spanish-American War, once more the military physicians objected to the presence of women nurses. Finally, when men lay dying of malaria, dysentery, and typhoid, women from the training schools took over. Their letters and journals relate the horrible conditions under which they worked. Some literally worked themselves to death in the

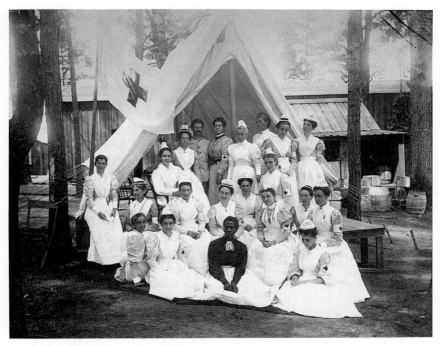

During the Spanish-American War, nurses, often led by the superintendents of the best training schools and hospitals, were responsible for saving the lives of many soldiers. (*Courtesy of Columbia University School of Nursing.*)

army hospitals in the South. One of the most serious diseases that nurses contended with was yellow fever, about which little was known. In testing the theory that the disease was caused by a certain type of mosquito, nursing gained its first martyr. Twenty-five-year-old Clara Maas of East Orange, New Jersey, volunteered to be bitten by a carrier mosquito. After being bitten several times, she died of yellow fever and is still considered a heroine in helping to prove the source of the disease.

The value of nurses in wartime was clear after the Spanish-American War, and recommendations were made that a regular corps of nurses ready for wartime duty be formed. Yet some military authorities were still hostile. So, although the number of women army nurses had reached 1158 by September 1898, by the next July there were only 202. Despite this setback, a group of influential women, including some prominent nurses, eventually lobbied through a bill, and the Army Nurse Corps was established on February 2, 1901.[37] It took longer for the Congress to act on a Navy Nurse Corps, although it had the support of the Navy's

Surgeon General, but finally it, too, became a reality in 1908.

World War I was different from other wars the United States had fought, both because of its international dimensions and the kinds of weapons that were used. The service of the nurse in the nightmarish battle conditions of World War I, coping with the mass casualties, dealing with injuries caused by the previously unknown shrapnel and gas, and then battling influenza at home and abroad, is a fascinating and proud piece of history.[38]

Both the Army and Navy Nurse Corps were expanded during this time, but not enough nurses were available and recruitment standards dropped. (Even though there were male nurses who volunteeered, they, like black nurses, were not accepted in the nurse corps.) Nursing leaders then formed a committee to devise methods of dealing with the problems related to care of the sick in the military, in hospitals, and in homes. Later the committee was given governmental status and very limited funding. The members found once more what had been true before and would be again: in wartime there are not enough nurses to meet the need. While efforts were made to recruit and produce nurses more rapidly, and they succeeded to some extent for the duration, there was inevitably a shortage afterward. When patriotic fervor faded away, the unpleasant conditions while "in training" and afterward, at

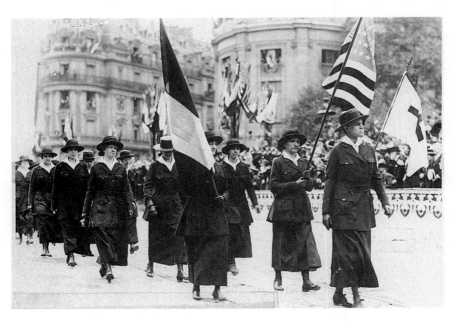

Colonel Julia Stimson, who became director of nursing services for the American Expeditionary Forces in World War I, leads a group of Red Cross Nurses down a street in Paris in 1918. (*Courtesy of the US Army Center of Military History.*)

a time when other working conditions were improving, made nursing a less desirable occupational choice. The high quality of students in the Rainbow Division of the Vassar Training Camp mentioned earlier was more the exception than the rule. The Army School of Nursing that emerged from World War I was also highly unusual.

In World War II, the role of nurses was even more extensive and perhaps even more dangerous. Once more nurses proved themselves able and brave in military situations.[39] Many were in battle zones, and some became Japanese prisoners of war.[40] Their stories have been told in films, books, plays, and historical nursing research and are well worth reading (see Bibliography). The war created opportunities, freedom, and also problems for nurses that proved to be long-lasting in both nursing education and practice. Some related to the nursing shortage that was again critical. There were not enough nurses for both the home front and the battle-field, even with stepped-up efforts to encourage women to enter nursing programs.

Finally, legislation was passed in 1943 establishing the Cadet Nurse Corps. The Bolton Act, the first federal program to subsidize nursing education for schools and students, was a forerunner of future federal

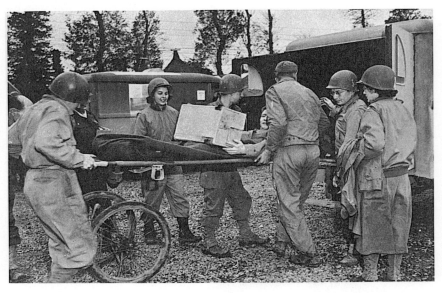

Nurses, here evacuating patients in Lison, France, *circa* 1944, were considered invaluable assets to care of the wounded. (*Courtesy of Columbia University School of Nursing.*)

aid to nursing. For payment of their tuition and a stipend, students committed themselves to engage in essential military or civilian nursing for the duration of the war. The students had to be between 17 and 35 years old, in good health, and with a good academic record in an accredited high school. This new law brought about several changes in nursing. For instance, it forbade discrimination on the basis of race and marital status and set minimum educational standards. The first standard, theoretically accepted, was not always implemented in good faith. The second, combined with the requirement that nursing programs be reduced from the traditional 36 months to 30, forced nursing schools to reassess and revise their curricula.[41]

Two other major efforts to relieve the nursing shortage had long-range effects in the practice setting. One was the recruitment of inactive nurses back into the field. For the first time, married women and others who could work only on a part-time basis became acceptable to employers and later became part of the labor pool. The other change was the training of volunteer nurse's aides. Although such training was initiated by the Red Cross in 1919, it was discouraged later by nurses, particularly during the Depression. During World War II, both the Red Cross and the Office of Civilian Defense trained more than 20,000 aides. At first, they were used only for nonnursing tasks, but the increasing nurse shortage forced them to take on basic nursing functions. After the war, with a continued shortage, trained aides were hired as a necessary part of the nursing service department. Their perceived cost effectiveness stimulated the growth of both aide and practical nurse training programs and eventually increased federal funding for both.

Finally, major changes occurred within the armed forces. Nurses had held only relative rank, meaning that they carried officers' titles but had less power and pay than their male counterparts. In 1947, full commissioned status was granted, giving them the right to manage nursing care. At the same time, as noted previously, discrimination against black nurses ended but, oddly enough, in the male-controlled armed services, it was not until 1954 that male nurses were admitted to full rank as officers.

When the Korean War broke out in 1950, the army again drew nurses from civilian hospitals, this time from their reserve corps. War nursing on the battlefront was centered to an extent on the Mobile Army Surgical Hospitals (MASH), located as close to the front lines as possible. Flight nurses, who helped to evacuate the wounded from the battlefront to military hospitals, also achieved recognition. When that war was over and nurse reservists returned to their civilian jobs, it is possible that their experiences increased their discontent with working situations at home. (For further readings on nursing during the Vietnam War, which is beyond this time period, see the Bibliography sources for Chapter 6.)

TOWARD A NEW ERA: STUDIES AND ACTION

The usual postwar nurse shortage occurred after World War II, but this time for different reasons. Only one of six army nurses planned to return to her civilian job, finding more satisfaction in the service. Poor pay and unpleasant working conditions discouraged civilian nurses as well. In 1946, the salary for a staff nurse was about $36 for a 48-hour week, less than that for typists or seamstresses (much less men). Salaries were supposed to be kept secret, and hospitals, in particular, held wages at a minimum, with such peculiarities as a staff nurse earning more than a head nurse. Split shifts were common, with nurses scheduled to work from seven to eleven and from three to seven, with time off between the two shifts. The work was especially difficult, because staffing was short and nurses worked under rigid discipline. Small wonder then that in one survey only about 12 percent of the nurses queried planned to make nursing a career; more than 75 percent saw it as a pin-money job after marriage or planned to retire altogether as soon as possible. Unions were beginning to organize nurses, so in 1949 the ANA approved state associations as collective bargaining agents for nurses. However, because the Taft–Hartley Act excluded nonprofit institutions from collective bargaining, hospitals and agencies did not need to deal with nurses. In addition, the ANA no-strike pledge took away another powerful weapon. As noted previously, one answer that administrators saw was the hiring of nurse's aides. The use of volunteers and auxiliary help—that is, anyone other than licensed nurses (practical nurses, aides, and orderlies)—increased tremendously.

One group of workers that proliferated in the postwar era was practical nurses, defined by ANA, NLNE, and NOPHN as those trained to care for subacute, convalescent, and chronic patients under the direction of a physician or nurse. Thousands who designated themselves as practical nurses had no such skills, and their training was simply in caring for their own families or, at most, aide work. Although the first school for training practical nurses appeared in 1897, by 1930 there were only 11, and in 1947 there were still only 36. With the new demand for nurse substitutes, 260 more practical nurse schools opened by 1954, mostly in hospitals or long-term care institutions and a few in vocational schools. Aiding the movement was funding under federal vocational education acts. There were, unfortunately, also a number of correspondence courses and other commercial programs that did little more than expose the student to some books and manuals and present her with a diploma. By 1950, there were 144,000 practical nurses, 95 percent of them women, and, although their educational programs varied, their on-the-job activities expanded greatly— to doing whatever nurses had no time to do. By 1952, some 56 percent of the nursing personnel were nonprofessionals, and some nurses began to fear that they were being replaced by less expensive, minimally trained workers.

Nevertheless, with working and financial conditions not improving, the nursing shortage persisted. Soon, a team plan was developed with a nurse as a team leader, primarily responsible for planning patient care, perhaps caring for patients with more complex problems, and less prepared workers carrying out the care plan for other patients. Although the team plan has persisted for years, it has done little to improve patient care, since generally it has not been carried out as originally conceived. Rather, it has kept the nurse mired in paperwork, away from the patient or required to make constant medication rounds. Often practical nurses have carried the primary responsibilities for patient units on the evening and night shift, with the few nurses available stretched thin, "supervising" these workers.

There were more nurses than ever at mid-century, but there were also tremendously expanded health services, a greater population to be served, growth of various insurance plans that paid for hospital care, a postwar baby boom with in-hospital deliveries, new medical discoveries that kept patients alive longer, and a proliferation of nurses into other areas of health care. Hospitals still weren't the most desirable places to work, and economic benefits were slow in coming. Moreover there were now more married nurses who chose to stay home to raise families. Studies done in 1941, 1948, and 1958 (Appendix 1), all of which pointed out some of the economic and status problems of nurses, particularly in hospitals, went largely ignored by administrators.

Nursing for the Future was a study conducted by Esther Lucile Brown, a social anthropologist, and related to both nursing education and nursing service. The report received mixed reviews. Many nurses felt threatened, and some physicians and hospital administrators considered it a subversive document, fearing that it had economic security implications for nurses. (Nor did they appreciate the fact that the authoritarianism of hospitals was pinpointed, as was the dilemma of the nurse caught between the demands of physicians and administrators.)

In the 1950s, Frances Reiter began to write about the *nurse clinician,* a nurse who gave skilled nursing care on an advanced level. This concept developed into that of the clinical specialist, a nurse with a graduate degree and specialized knowledge of nursing care, who worked as a colleague of physicians. At the same time, the development of coronary and other intensive care units called for nurses with equally specialized technical knowledge, formerly the sole province of medical practice. In Colorado in 1965, a physician, in collaboration with a school of nursing, was pioneering another new role for nurses in ambulatory care. As the nurses easily assumed responsibility for well-child care and minor illnesses, they called upon their nursing knowledge and skills, as well as a medical component. What emerged was the *nurse practitioner*. (These roles are described in Chapter 6.)

Nursing education was also going through a transition period in those decades. In the years immediately after World War II, the quality of nursing education was under severe criticism. There was no question that in the diploma schools, where most nurses were educated, there was frequently poor teaching, inadequately prepared teachers, and major dependence on students for services; often two-thirds of the hours of care were given by students. These were also the findings of Esther Lucile Brown, who had gathered her data by visiting nursing schools and health care facilities and consulting with many key people in the health care field, including nurses. Her findings were not much different from those in earlier reports, and 22 years later, in another national study, *An Abstract for Action*, the author noted that many of the recommendations in *Nursing for the Future* were still valid but unfulfilled. Brown particularly cited the poor quality of many schools and the fact that many diploma schools were operated for the staffing benefit of the hospital. (Even in the years of the Great Depression, when hospital administrators complained bitterly about the cost of nursing programs, their economic benefit was clear and most were kept.) One strong recommendation of the Brown report was "that effort be directed to building basic schools of nursing in universities and colleges, comparable in number to existing medical schools, that are sound in organizational and financial structure, adequate in facilities and faculty, and well-distributed to serve the needs of the entire country."[42]

The slow rate of growth of collegiate programs, even into the next decade, resulted in part from the uncertainty of nurses about what these programs should be and how they should differ from diploma education. Another factor was the anticollegiate faction in nursing that saw no point in higher education—a faction that was cheered and nurtured by a large number of physicians and administrators. While the Brown report did result in a reexamination of beliefs and attitudes about educational practices, it was also viewed as a threat to the comfortable status quo by hospital administrators, some doctors, and diploma nurses. However, both this report and the 1950 report *Nursing Schools at the Mid-Century*, a follow-up report sponsored by six nursing organizations, are credited with being the impetus for an established process of accreditation in nursing. Those schools that chose to go through the voluntary process and that met the standards were placed on a published list, which for the first time gave the public, guidance counselors, and potential students some notion of the quality of one school compared with another (Appendix 1).

Eventually, accreditation proved a significant force in improving good schools and closing poor ones (although it has also been accused of rigidity throughout the years). Actually the NLNE, which, as the National League for Nursing (NLN), later assumed responsibility for accreditation, had been involved in curriculum study and development since the publication of its 1917 *Standard Curriculum for Schools of Nursing* and its 1929 *A Curriculum for Schools of Nursing*. By 1937, these works were considered extremely helpful to those responsible for nursing programs, but their curricula were perhaps too inflexible. Out of this came *A Curriculum Guide for Schools of Nursing*, which was greatly influenced by a study directed by Isabel Stewart that had looked at "the most progressive ideas and practices" in basic nursing education. The new guide, intended, according to Stewart, for students of professional caliber preparing themselves for a profession, placed much greater emphasis on application of the sciences. The role of the clinical instructor was stressed, and all faculty members were encouraged to use newer and more creative methods of teaching. The guide was never revised again, but it was used in many schools for another quarter-century.

The study that probably changed nursing education more dramatically than any other was the doctoral research of Mildred Montag at Teachers College in New York. *Community College Education for Nursing*, published in 1959, was the report of a five-year project based on her dissertation. In this "action research" project, seven junior community colleges cooperated by establishing two-year associate degree (AD) programs for nursing. It was the right time for such programs with the rapid growth of community colleges and the availability of new types of students—mature men and women and the less affluent, who seized this opportunity for a college degree and a career. The project evaluation, including follow-up of the 811 graduates, presented persuasive arguments for the development of more such programs. (Chapter 5 discusses in more detail the original Montag dissertation and its effect on nursing education.) Twenty-five years later, associate degree programs made up the largest segment preparing nurses for RN licensure. AD education also had an effect on other nursing programs. It was probably partially the influence of the AD programs, which were nondiscriminatory and generally nonpaternalistic in their relations with students, that helped loosen the tight restrictions on nursing students' personal lives in both diploma and some baccalaureate programs. Still, even into the late 1960s, some diploma schools excluded married students and men. The growth of AD programs ultimately outran all others in nursing except practical nurse programs.

Federal funding of nursing education also had a major impact on nursing education. As noted earlier, nursing education was first subsidized during World War II with enactment of the Bolton Act in 1943. However, it was in effect only for the duration of the war, since its intent was to overcome the serious nursing shortage. There was no further funding of nursing education until the Health Amendments Act of 1956 provided traineeships, which did not have to be paid back, to prepare nurses for administration, teaching, supervision, and public health through both short-term and full-time study.

EXHIBIT 2.2

Nursing in the Context of the Times

1865 to 1885
Society at Large

- US population (1870): 38.5 million
- 1865: End of Civil War; Union restored; President Lincoln assassinated
- Ku Klux Klan founded
- Much Western railroad building
- National trade union movement; labor unrest
- Purchase of Alaska
- Wars against Indians in West
- Land booms in West
- Continuation of "old immigration" (Scandinavian, Irish, German)
- Chinese immigrant labor; other contract labor
- Beginning of petroleum industry
- Numerous political and financial scandals
- Panic of 1873 affects national income and leads to substantial unemployment
- Public schools free for all
- Booker T. Washington founds Tuskegee Institute for Blacks
- Spelman College opens to educate black women
- Illiteracy rate (1870) at 20 percent

Legislation, Supreme Court Decisions, Presidents

- 1863–65: Reconstruction Proclamation and Acts (ends 1877)
- 1865: 13th amendment, abolishing slavery, ratified
- Freedman's Bureau established
- 1875: Civil Rights Act bestows citizenship upon the "Negro"
- 1875: Civil Rights Act guarantees equal rights in public places; declared invalid by Supreme Court in 1883
- Supreme Court upholds Congress' power to punish as crime, private interference with right of citizen to vote (against Klu Klux Klan)
- Chinese Exclusion Act, prohibiting immigration of Chinese laborers for 10 years
- Contract Labor Act forbids importation of all but skilled, professional, and domestic labor
- Vice President Johnson becomes 17th president (remaining term)
- Grant becomes 18th president (2 terms)
- Hayes becomes 19th president (1 term)
- Garfield becomes 20th president (assassinated)
- Vice President Arthur becomes 21st president (remaining term)
- Cleveland becomes 22d president

*Medicine, Public Health,
Science, Technology*

- First practical intercity telephone lines
- Pioneer stages of motion pictures
- Practical application of electric arc lamps and incandescent bulb (Edison)
- Phonograph patented by Edison
- Advances in cameras and films made
- Development of automobiles
- Various electric home appliances and industrial equipment invented
- Advances in surgery, including methods for antiseptic surgery; advances in anesthesia
- Specialized medical journals published
- First state board of health established in Massachusetts
- Increased number of medical schools founded
- American Public Health Association founded (1872)
- Osteopathy founded
- *Index Medicus* and *Index-Catalogue* founded
- Sanitarium for tubercular patients founded in Saranac Lake, NY

Nursing

- Volunteer nurses in Civil War include Dix (superintendent of nurses) Bickerdyke, Barton, Tubman, Truth, Taylor and three Woolsey sisters (later influential in development of nurse training programs)
- 1872: First training school—New England Hospital for Women and Children; first graduate, Linda Richards
- 1873: Three schools founded on Nightingale principles: Bellevue Training School (New York); Connecticut Training School for Nurses (New Haven, CT); Boston Training School for Nurses at Massachusetts General (Boston); Richards, first superintendent
- First uniform designed
- Sister Mary Bernard (nurse) gives anesthesia at St. Vincent's Hospital (Erie, PA)
- First black trained nurse: Mary Mahoney
- 1880: 15 nurse training programs
- 1881: I. Robb heads training school at Johns Hopkins
- 1881: American National Red Cross founded under leadership of Clara Barton
- 1885: First district nurse (Buffalo, NY)
- Weeks writes textbook on nursing care for nurses and families.

(continued)

EXHIBIT 2.2 (*continued*)

Nursing in the Context of the Times

1886 to 1906

Society at Large

- US population (1900): 76 million; life expectancy 48–51
- North Dakota, South Dakota, Montana, Washington, and Utah admitted to Union
- "Coxey's Army" of jobless men march on Washington for work; disbanded when leaders arrested
- Panic of 1893: lasts 4 years; stock market crash; decline of US gold reserve
- Jane Addams founds Hull House in Chicago-settlement house for immigrants
- Klondike gold rush
- 1890: women in the labor force, 3.7 million; 14 percent married
- 1900: Illiteracy rate at 10.7 percent
- Growth of self improvement adult education
- 128 women's colleges founded by 1901
- Women make up about 25 percent of all undergraduate students
- 1898: Spanish American War; won by US. Spain cedes Philippines to US for 20 million dollars; also Puerto Rico and Guam (become territories)
- "New immigration" from eastern and southern Europe develops. Over one million immigrants in 1905
- Bureau of Immigration established
- Scott discovers Antarctic Plateau
- Carrie Nation leads crusade against liquor and saloons
- 1906: San Francisco earthquake

Legislation, Supreme Court Decisions, Presidents

- Sherman Antitrust Act; declares restraint of trade illegal
- Various legislation creates early conservation measures
- Plessy V. Ferguson (1896) rules that separate but equal facilities do not deprive Negroes of equal protection under 14th Amendment; legalizes segregation
- 1906: Pure Food and Drug Act enacted
- Meat Inspection Act enacted
- 23d president: Harrison (one term)
- 24th president: Cleveland (2d term)
- 25th president: McKinley (assassinated)
- Vice president Roosevelt becomes 26th president and is reelected; appoints Blacks and Jews to office, against Congressional pressure

Medicine, Public Health, Science, Technology

- Early stages of motion pictures
- Wright brothers make first heavier-than-air flight
- Mercury vapor lamp patented
- Rayon and Bakelite (plastic) patented
- Radio, flat disc phonograph, vacuum tube, telegraphy and battery invented
- Roentgen discovers X-rays
- Curies discover radium
- English physician Ross determines Anopheles mosquito transmits malaria; Dr. Reed determines Aedes mosquito transmits yellow fever
- Three biologists, working separately, rediscover Mendel's law of heredity
- X-rays used to treat breast cancer
- First Nobel prize awarded
- Introduction of rubber gloves in surgery
- Mayo Clinic founded
- Rockefeller Institute for Medical Research founded
- Chiropractic founded (1895)
- American Hospital Association founded.
- 112 Medical Schools founded (1873–95)
- States tighten medical licensure exams
- "Typhoid Mary" seen as evidence that typhoid can be carried by healthy people

Nursing

- Nursing journal, *The Nightingale*, edited by Bellevue graduate (dies of lack of support 1891)
- *The Trained Nurse and Hospital Review* considered first real nursing journal; lasts 70 years
- Dock writes materia medica textbook for nurses; Kimber writes anatomy book; Robb writes first substantial clinical nursing book; also ethics book
- First nursing school for men established (Mills School of Nursing at Bellevue), followed by others
- First nursing program for Blacks founded (Spelman Seminary) in 1886, followed by others, including diploma program at Howard University (1893)
- Jessie Sleet (Scales) first Black public health nurse
- 1893: American Society of Superintendents of Training Schools of Nursing founded; Richards, first president
- 1897: Nurses' Associated Alumnae of the United States and Canada founded; Robb, first president
- Wald and Brewster establish Henry Street Visiting Nurse (NY)
- First Industrial nurse, A. Stewart, employed by Vermont Marble Co.
- First school for training practical nurses
- Nurses, including Black nurses, serve in Spanish-American War
- Nurse Clara Maas dies: martyr to yellow fever research
- International Council of Nursing founded; Fenwick, first president (1899)
- Teachers College, Columbia University, first to offer college course to nurses (hospital economics)
- School nursing begins
- Permanent Army Nurse Corps established; headed by Kinney
- 1900: *American Journal of Nursing*, first nursing journal owned by nurses published; Palmer is editor
- 432 training schools in 1900; most graduates do private duty with few hired by hospitals
- 1903: First nurse licensure laws (NC, NJ, NY, VA)

(continued)

EXHIBIT 2.2 (*continued*)

Nursing in the Context of the Times

1907 to 1927
Society at Large

- US population (1910): 92.2 million
- US population (1920): 106 million
- Panic of 1907: stock market drop and business failures
- White House Conference on Conservation to educate public on importance of forest and water resources
- Arizona, Oklahoma and New Mexico admitted to Union
- Fist woman elected to Congress (Montana, 1916)
- First woman elected governor (Wyoming, 1925)
- W.E.B. Du Bois founds NAACP
- 1909: Peary flies American flag over North Pole
- 1914: Panama Canal opens to traffic
- Outbreak of World War I
- 1917: US declares war on Germany
- 1918: War ends; signing of armistice
- National League of Nations; no US government representation
- Number of Klu Klux Klan exposés: membership down
- Women in labor force 1920: 8.4 million; 23 percent married
- International Ladies Garment Workers Union founded
- Beginning of labor setbacks with recession 1920–
- Exposure of dishonesty in banking, railroads, finance, environment
- First nonstop flight, NY to Paris
- First transcontinental flight
- 1916: Fundamentalist religions gain converts

Legislation, Supreme Court Decisions, Presidents

- Mann Act (White Slavery Traffic Act) prohibits interstate transportation of women for immoral purposes
- Social legislation in states re: wages and hours, employment of women and children. Public assistance for women with children (1911); first state Workmen's Compensation law (MD)
- 16th amendment establishes income tax (1913)
- 17th amendment ratified: direct election of senators
- Workmen's Compensation Act for federal employees
- Selective Service Act (1917)
- 1920: Prohibition Act (18th amendment) goes into effect, prohibits manufacture and sale of liquor
- 1920: 19th amendment ratified (women's suffrage)
- 1921: Sheppard–Towner Act promotes welfare and health of mothers and children (lapsed in 1929)
- Clayton Act: Bill of rights for labor
- First seriously restrictive immigration law passed; sets quotas
- Veterans Bureau established
- Soldiers Bonus Act passed
- Army Air Corps established
- Japanese Exclusion Acts limit immigration of Japanese laborers
- 27th president: Taft (1 term)
- 28th president: Wilson (2 terms)
- 29th president: Harding (dies in office)
- 30th president: Coolidge (filled term plus 1)

Medicine, Public Health, Science, Technology

- Flexner Report exposes abuses in medical education and proposes reforms
- Number of medical schools and graduates decline
- Mental health movement founded
- Schick skin test for diphtheria developed
- Basic research in preventive medicine expands
- Vitamins discovered; increased research in deficiencies and related diseases
- Studies on hereditary conditions and traits; term "genes" first used
- Influenza epidemic (1918–19); 500,000 deaths in US
- Iron lung invented (used for polio)
- First commercial radio transmission (Pittsburgh)
- Einstein discloses formula for relativity
- Color photography, sound films invented
- First telephoto pictures sent over telegraph wires
- First Model T auto introduced
- First television images transmitted (London)
- World's first helicopter flight (France)
- Scopes Trial: teacher convicted of teaching evolution

Nursing

- 1105 diploma schools in 1909
- 1908: National Association for Colored Graduate Nurses founded
- 1909: First collegiate nursing program established at University of Minnesota by Dr. Beard
- Nutting becomes first nurse appointed to professorship in a university (Teachers College)
- First public health nursing course given at Teachers College
- National Organization for Public Health Nursing founded; Wald, first president
- Public health nursing journal published
- National League of Nursing Education publishes first *Standard Curriculum for Schools of Nursing*
- Nurses serve in World War I
- Army School of Nursing established; Goodrich, superintendent
- Vassar Training Camp (1918) provides preliminary course for college graduates for later shortened diploma programs
- Thom, Black nurse, succeeds in opening Army to Black nurses
- Studies: *Educational Status of Nursing*, 1912; *Nursing and Nursing Education* (Goldmark Report), 1923
- Breckinridge establishes Frontier Nursing Service in 1925, including midwifery school
- Sanger arrested for distributing birth control information; founds predecessor of Planned Parenthood
- Dock writes first nursing history book and book on venereal diseases; also active in women's suffrage movement
- Red Cross establishes rural nursing service
- Gardner writes first book on public health nursing
- Public health nursing section established in APHA
- Alpha Tau Delta, nursing sorority established (1921)
- Sigma Theta Tau, first national nursing honor society founded (1922) (later international)
- Harmon Plan: first annuity plan for nurses
- Yale School of Nursing, first autonomous collegiate school opens; Goodrich, dean (1924)

(continued)

EXHIBIT 2.2 (*continued*)

Nursing in the Context of the Times

1928 to 1948
Society at Large

- United States population (1930): 123.2 million
- United States population (1940): 132.2 million
- "Bonus Army" of veterans march on Washington to demand bonuses promised after World War I
- 1929: Stock market crash; beginning of the Great Depression with serious unemployment
- Manufacturing declines during Depression
- President Roosevelt initiates "Good Neighbor" policy for improved relations with Latin America
- Jehovah's Witnesses founded
- Educational testing developed
- Junior Colleges beginning to spread
- Illiteracy rate (1930) at 4.2 percent
- Illiteracy rate (1947) at 2.7 percent of population; rural farm 5.3 percent
- Earhart is first woman to fly Atlantic
- First woman elected to US Senate (Tennessee, 1932)
- Perkins becomes first woman Cabinet member (Labor, 1933)
- Hitler invades Poland: beginning of World War II (1939)
- Japanese bomb Pearl Harbor (1941); Germany declares war on US
- US declares war on Axis (Japan, Germany, Italy)
- Race riots erupt in Los Angeles and Detroit
- D-Day invasion of Normandy (1944); greatest amphibious assault ever
- US drops atomic bombs; destroy two Japanese cities
- Concentration camps in Europe liberated
- World War II ends (1945)
- United Nations Charter adopted; First General Assembly (1945); WHO established
- Cold War begins (1947)

Legislation, Supreme Court Decisions, Presidents

- Prohibition (Volstead Act) repealed (1933)
- National Housing Act insures home mortgages
- Number of "New Deal" laws passed to provide jobs; e.g. Works Project Administration (WPA), Federal Employment Relations Agency (FERA); Federal Relief Administration (FRA); Civil Works Administration (CWA)
- National Labor Relations Act passed; recognizes workers' right to organize and bargain collectively (1935)
- Fair Labor Standards Act passed
- Social Security Act becomes law (1935)
- Food, Drug and Cosmetic Act passed
- Selective Service Act makes men 21–35 eligible for military service
- 1943: Bolton Act creates Cadet Nurse Corps with full funding for basic nursing education; requires changes in educational programs
- Executive order to intern 120,000 Japanese on West Coast
- GI bill provides variety of benefits for veterans, including higher education subsidies and tuition
- First Clean Air Act passed
- Truman proclaims independence of Philippines
- 31st president: Hoover (1 term)
- 32d president: Roosevelt (4 terms, died in office)
- 33d president: vice president Truman (completed term plus 1 full term)

*Medicine, Public Health,
Science, Technology*

- Effectivensss of sulfanilamide and related drugs for variety of infections proved
- Use of insulin and electric shock for dementia praecox
- Advances in psychotherapy
- Fleming discovers penicillin; other antibiotics developed
- Massive attacks on crippling and killing diseases through research
- Antihistamines discovered
- Cortisone synthesized
- Patent issued for Nylon and other synthetics
- First binary calculating machine and other precursors to computers developed
- Instant camera, long-playing records and microwave oven developed
- Frozen food industry develops
- Polaroid glass invented
- Transistor and solar battery invented
- First jet engine produced

Nursing

- 1929: 2200 diploma programs
- Nursing schools close; Depression affects nurse employment in private duty; hospitals begin to employ more at a minimum wage
- New Deal agencies provide work for nurses in communities and governmental settings
- Studies and reports in the 1930s: *Nurses, Patients and Pocketbooks: An Activity Analysis of Nursing; Nursing Schools Today and Tomorrow; A Study on the Use of the Graduate Nurse for Bedside Nursing in the Hospital; A Curriculum Guide for Schools of Nursing; Studies of Income, Salaries and Employment Conditions affecting Nurses*
- American Association of Nurse-Midwives and American Association of Nurse Anesthetists founded
- First Nurse-midwifery school founded at Maternity Center in New York City
- Association of Collegiate Schools of Nursing founded
- USPHS employs first public health nurse
- First *Facts About Nursing* published
- 1936: 1500 diploma schools; 70 "collegiate"
- *RN*: commercial journal for nurses published
- Studies and Reports in the 1940s: *Administrative Cost Analysis for Nursing Service and Nursing Education; The General Staff Nurse; Hospital Care in the United States; Nursing for the Future; A Program for the Nursing Profession*
- Many changes in educational programs
- Nurses serve in all fronts in World War II
- Army and Navy nurse officers awarded permanent commission
- Chi Eta Phi sorority, American Association of Industrial Nurses; Association of State and Territorial Directors of Nursing, and Nurses' Christian Fellowship founded
- Major postwar nursing shortage

(continued)

EXHIBIT 2.2 (*continued*)

Nursing in the Context of the Times

1949 to 1965
Society at Large

- US population (1950): 151.3 million
- US population (1960): 179.3 million
- Baby boom peaks (1955)
- Korean conflict begins (1950); ends 1953
- Rosa Parks refuses to give up seat to white person in Montgomery AL; bus boycott begins
- "Freedom Riders" test segregation laws in deep South
- Voter registration drive begins in South
- King leads civil rights march to DC, later to Selma, AL
- Truman orders development of hydrogen bomb
- Alaska and Hawaii join the Union (49th and 50th States)
- Early gay rights organization founded in California
- Carson's *Silent Spring* launches environmental movement
- Major Black riots in Los Angeles
- Overcrowding in schools
- Expansion of higher education; major growth of community colleges
- President's Commission on the status of women recommends new educational opportunities for women
- Number of American troops in Vietnam escalated; opposition grows
- Postwar European refugees are the new immigrants
- Increase in Ku Klux Klan membership; about 40,000 in 1960s
- Gains in churches rolls seen
- Authorine Lucy, first Black to be enrolled in University of Alabama

*Legislation, Supreme Court
Decisions, Presidents*

- Immigration and Naturalization Act passed (1952), lifts last racial and ethnic barriers to naturalization
- Refugee Relief Act (1953) provides for entry into US on emergency basis outside regular immigration quota
- Brown *v.* Bd. of Education (1955); outlaws "separate but equal" educational systems; school segregation ends slowly
- 22d amendment ratified (presidential terms limited to two)
- Federal Nurse Traineeship Act; authorizes funds for baccalaureate and graduate education; also short-term continuing education
- Peace Corps established (1961)
- Johnson signs Civil Rights Act of 1964 and antipoverty bill prohibiting discrimination in voting, public housing, employment
- Beginning of "Great Society" and "war on poverty"
- Medicare bill passed
- Supreme Court holds that "right of privacy" covers use of contraceptives
- Supreme Court bans prayer in school
- 34th president: Eisenhower (2 terms)
- 35th president: Kennedy (1 term, assassinated 1963)
- 36th president: vice president Johnson (completed term plus one complete)

*Medicine, Public Health,
Science, Technology*

- Advances in medical technology creates changes in diagnosis and treatment of diseases
- Mechanical heart first used in human (1952)
- Increase in incidence of lung cancer due to cigarette smoking reported
- New discoveries in genetics
- Various hormones synthesized
- Oral Orinase for diabetes developed
- Tranquilizers synthesized; widespread use by 1955
- Salk develops vaccine for polio
- Sabin develops oral vaccine for polio
- First birth control pills sold
- Pandemic of Asian flu
- Dawn of space age: Russia launches Sputnik I, first artificial satellite (1957) and puts first man in space (1961)
- US launches first satellite into orbit (1958)
- Shepard travels on first US manned space flight (1961)
- Glen is first American to orbit earth (1962)
- "Mariner" completes first successful interplanetary mission
- Shortage of physicians
- Albert Schweitzer wins Nobel Peace Prize
- First human pregnancy induced with frozen sperm (1953)
- First color TV sold

Nursing

- Two practical nurse organizations founded
- Air Force gives nurse officers permanent commissions
- Male nurses granted full rank in armed services
- Code of ethics adopted by ANA
- Nurses serve in Korean War, including MASH units
- Structure study of nursing organizations results in two large nursing organizations (ANA, NLN), founding of National Student Nurses' Association, and dissolving of NACGN after ANA forbids membership discrimination against Black nurses
- American Nurses Foundation created, devoted to research
- *Nursing Research* published
- Studies and reports: *Nursing Schools at the Mid-century* (lists nursing programs meeting specific criteria); *Collegiate Education for Nurses* (suggests nursing education should be upper division college program); *Patterns of Patient Care* (describes team nursing); *Twenty Thousand Nurses Tell Their Story* (resulted in development of nursing functions, standards and qualifications); *Community College Education* (resulted in development and growth of associate degree nursing programs); *Toward Quality in Nursing: Needs and Goals* (noted need for more nurses with higher education and recommended federal financial assistance for nurses toward this end)
- *Nursing Outlook* published
- Reiter writes about clinical specialist
- Some increase in nursing doctoral programs
- Nurse practitioner role developed in Colorado, under direction of doctor and nurse
- 1965: ANA publishes *Educational Preparation for Nurse Practitioners and Assistants to Nurses: A Position Paper*, recommending baccalaureate education for professional nurses, AD education for technical nurses, and short preservice education for aides

However, useful as this was, even more far-reaching was the 1963 report *Toward Quality in Nursing, Needs and Goals.* It was prepared by a group of nurses, other health professionals, and members of the public appointed by the Surgeon General of the U.S. Public Health Service to advise him on nursing needs and the role the government should take in providing adequate nursing service for the public. The report, which cited major deficits in the number of nurses adequately prepared to meet the health needs for the future, had great influence. An obvious problem was the lack of qualified teachers; even in so-called university programs, nurses did not meet the usual requirements for teaching. Another was the almost total lack of educational background in management by nurses who held administrative and managerial positions. The enactment of the *Nurse Training Act of 1964* not only provided funding for students and schools for the next five years, but in its later forms, continued to provide a varied amount of support to nursing education and research until today.[43]

Such federal assistance was particularly important in the development of graduate programs in nursing education. Few such programs existed, and often nurses who sought graduate degrees turned to other disciplines such as education. However, even with the growth of graduate nursing programs, it was not until the 1960s that graduate education in clinical nursing was more readily available. This may have been due to the forms of federal funding. In fact, one outcome of such funding was the tendency for schools to develop educational programs according to the funding available—a great problem for the continuity of programs for minorities, continuing education, and clinical specialties when this "soft money" later diminished or evaporated altogether.

Nursing research also tended to make slow progress. Although there were studies of nursing service, nursing education, and nursing personality, most were done with or by social scientists. When nurses assisted physicians and others in medical research, it was just that—assisting. Nursing leaders realized that nursing could not develop as a profession unless clinical research focusing on nursing evolved. One of the first major steps in that direction was the 1952 publication of *Nursing Research*, a scholarly journal that reported and encouraged nursing research. The other was the ANA's establishment of the American Nurses Foundation in 1955 for charitable, educational, and scientific purposes. Of course, federal funding also had considerable impact.

With all of these changes, the professional organizations of nursing took varied and sometimes uncoordinated action. A study to consider restructuring, reorganizing, and unifying the various organizations was initiated shortly after World War II. In 1952, the six major nursing organizations—ANA, NLNE, NOPHN, NACGN, the Association of Collegiate Schools of Nursing (ACSN), and the American Association of

Industrial Nurses (AAIN)—finally came to a decision about organizational structure. Two major organizations emerged: the ANA, with only nurse members, and the renamed National League for Nursing (NLN), with nurse, nonnurse, and agency membership. The AAIN decided to continue, and the National Student Nurses' Association was formed. Practical nurses had their own organization. (See Chapter 13 for details of the organizations.) Although there was an apparent realignment of responsibilities, the relationships between the ANA and NLN ebbed and flowed: sometimes they were in agreement, and sometimes they were not; sometimes they worked together, and at other times each appeared to make isolated unilateral pronouncements. Some nurses wanted one organization, but there seemed to be mutual organizational reluctance to go in that direction. Yet, each had some remarkable achievements: NLN in educational accreditation and ANA in its lobbying activities, its development of a model licensure law in the mid-1950s, and its increased action regarding nurses' economic security.

In 1965, ANA precipitated (or inflamed) an ongoing controversy. After years of increasingly firm statements on the place of nursing education in the mainstream of American education, ANA issued its first Position Paper on Education for Nursing. It stated, basically, that education for those who work in nursing should be in institutions of higher learning; that minimum education for professional nursing should be at least at the baccalaureate level; for technical nursing, at the associate degree level; and for assistants, in vocational education settings.

Although there had been increasing complaints by third-party payers about diploma education, and although diploma schools had declined as associate and baccalaureate degree programs increased, there was an outpouring of anger by diploma and practical nurses and those involved in their education. It was a battle that persisted and became another divisive force in nursing. But then, so was the beginning of the nurse practitioner movement. There were nurses who feared it or saw it as pseudomedicine, detracting from pure nursing professionalism. The issues remain unresolved to some extent.

Therefore, whether or not 1965 can be considered the gateway to a new era of nursing, it was the beginning of dramatic and inevitable changes in the education and practice of nursing and in the struggle for nursing autonomy—a revolution in nursing.

KEY POINTS

1. The work and ongoing interest of the "lady" volunteers who acted as nurses in the Civil War were influential in the establishment of

the first training schools for nurses modeled (to some extent) on Nightingale principles.

2. Students in the early training schools worked long hours, did many menial nonnursing tasks, and gave almost all the nursing care in hospitals.

3. Twenty-five years after trained nursing had begun, nursing leaders in the United States were responsible for setting nursing standards, improving curricula, writing textbooks, starting two enduring nursing organizations and a nursing journal, inaugurating a teacher training program in a university, and initiating nursing licensure.

4. Studies about nursing that pointed out deficiencies in nursing education and practice were often ignored because of the students' economic benefit to the hospital, but they seem to have had a cumulative effect that eventually brought about change.

5. Because of the shortage of nurses that occurred during and after wars, reforms in both nursing education and practice were instituted.

6. The first baccalaureate program in nursing was founded in 1909, but for decades a common pattern was a combination of two years of college and three years in a diploma school.

7. AD nursing, initiated in 1952 as an action research project, produced a new kind of nurse and changed nursing education.

8. Before the Great Depression, most graduate nurses worked at private duty, but public health nursing, school nursing, industrial nursing, midwifery, and other specialties gradually emerged under the leadership of nursing pioneers.

9. Black nurses and men were often discriminated against in nursing but slowly gained status in the last half of the twentieth century.

REFERENCES

1. Selavan IC. Nurses in American history: The revolution. *Am J Nurs* 75:592–594, April 1975.
2. Kalisch P, Kalisch B. *The Advance of American Nursing*, 3d ed. Boston: Little, Brown, 1995, p 53.
3. Kalisch P, Kalisch B. Untrained but undaunted: The women nurses of the blue and gray. *Nurs Forum* 15(1):4–33, 1976; see p 17.
4. Kalisch and Kalisch (1995), op cit, p 47.
5. Dolan JA, et al. *Nursing in Society: A Historical Perspective*, 15th ed. Philadelphia: W. B. Saunders, 1983, pp 173–174.
6. Carnegie ME. Black nurses at the front. *Am J Nurs* 84:1250–1252, October 1984.
7. Culpepper MM, Adams PG. Nursing in the Civil War. *Am J Nurs* 88:981–984, July 1988.

8. Bullough V, Bullough B. *The Care of the Sick: The Emergence of Modern Nursing.* New York: Prodist, 1978, p 114.

9. Dolan et al, op cit, p 202.

10. Kalisch and Kalisch, 1995, op cit, pp 144–148.

11. Ibid, pp 109–110.

12. Flaumenhaft E, Flaumenhaft C. American nursing's first text books. *Nurs Outlook* 37:185–188, July–August 1989.

13. Kalisch B, Kalisch P. Slaves, servants, or saints: An analysis of the system of nurse training in the United States, 1873–1948. *Nurse Forum* 14(3):230–231, 1975; see p 228.

14. Kalisch and Kalisch (1995), op cit, p 114.

15. Ibid, p 206.

16. Ibid, p 243.

17. Kelly L. *Dimensions of Professional Nursing*, 5th ed. New York: Macmillan Publishing, 1985, p 71.

18. Bullough and Bullough, op cit, p 156.

19. Ingles T. The physician's view of the evolving nursing profession—1873–1913. *Nurs Forum* 15(2):123–164, 1976; see p 148.

20. Bullough B, Bullough V. Sex discrimination in health care. *Nurs Outlook* 23:40–45, January 1975; see p 43.

21. Kelly L, Joel L. *Dimensions of Professional Nursing*, 7th ed. New York, NY: McGraw-Hill, 1995, p 69.

22. Nutting MA. Isabel Hampton Robb: Her work in organization and education. *Am J Nurs* 10:19, January 1910.

23. Poslusny S. Feminine friendship: Isabel Hampton Robb, Lavinia Lloyd Dock and Mary Adelaide Nutting. *Image* 21:64–67, Summer 1989.

24. Benson E. Nursing and the World's Columbian Exposition. *Nurs Outlook* 34:88–90, March–April 1986.

25. Christy TE. Portrait of a leader: Sophia F. Palmer. *Nurs Outlook* 23:746–751, December 1975; see pp 746–747.

26. Flanagan L. *One Strong Voice: The Story of the American Nurses' Association.* Kansas City, MO: American Nurses' Association, 1976, pp 35–38.

27. Pryor EB. *Clara Barton, Professional Angel.* Philadelphia: University of Pennsylvania Press, 1987.

28. Kalisch and Kalisch (1995), op cit, p 193.

29. Christy TE. Portrait of a leader: Lillian D. Wald. *Nurs Outlook* 18:50–54 March 1970.

30. Ruffing-Rahal MA. Margaret Sanger: Nurse and feminist. *Nurs Outlook* 34:246–249, September–October 1986.

31. Christy TE. Portrait of a leader. Lavinia Lloyd Dock. *Nurs Outlook* 17:72–75, June 1969; see p 74.

32. Ibid.

33. Pletsch PK. Mary Breckenridge: A pioneer who made her mark. *Am J Nurs* 81:188–190, February 1981.

34. Carnegie ME. *The Path We Tread: Blacks in Nursing 1854–1984*. Philadelphia: J.B. Lippincott, 1986.

35. Kalisch and Kalisch (1995), op cit, p 137.

36. Fitzpatrick ML. Nursing and the great depression. *Am J. Nurs* 75:2188–2190, December 1975.

37. Gourney C. Military nursing: 211 years of commitment to the American soldier. *Imprint* 34:36–45, February–March 1987.

38. Kalisch and Kalisch (1995), op cit, pp 228–235.

39. Curtis D. Nurses and war: The way it was. *Am J Nurs* 84:1253–1254, October 1984.

40. Kalisch P, Kalisch B. Nurses under fire: The World War II experience of nurses on Bataan and Corregidor. *Nurs Res* 25:409–429, November–December 1976.

41. Kalisch B, Kalisch P. Nurses in American history: The Cadet Nurse Corps. *Am J Nurs* 76:240–242, February 1976.

42. Brown EL. *Nursing for the Future*. New York: Russell Sage Foundation, 1948, p 178.

43. Kelly and Joel (1995), op cit, pp 443–444.

Nursing in the Health Care Scene

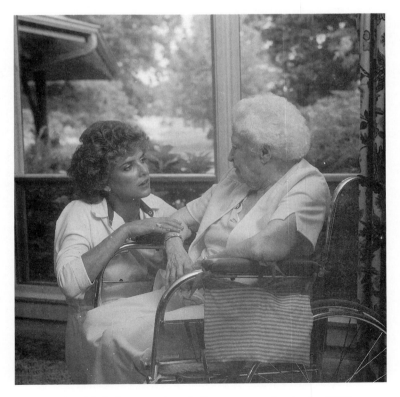

Care of the elderly is a growing challenge to nursing in the 1990s.
(*Courtesy of the American Nurses Association*)

3

The Health Care Delivery System

OBJECTIVES

After studying this chapter, you will be able to:

1. Explain how social and economic factors have affected health care delivery.
2. Describe the impact of cost containment on health care.
3. Define self-care, primary care, secondary care, and tertiary care.
4. Identify the major settings in which health care is given.
5. Distinguish the roles of major personnel who are part of the health care team.
6. Recognize changes that are common to many health occupations.
7. Understand how predictions for future health care are related to current trends.

Most people have no idea how complex health care is today, with its multiple settings and array of workers. Even those in the field often don't know much about what their colleagues do or how care is given in any place but their own. When a health "crisis" hits the headlines periodically, health workers are, naturally, more interested in how this affects them personally than in the larger picture. Yet, no part of health care is untouched when problems become big enough to be called a crisis. To remain ignorant or indifferent about what is going on is a luxury no one in health care can afford.

This chapter provides an overview of American health care, the settings, the people, the issues, and how outside factors influence the system.

WHAT INFLUENCES HEALTH CARE?

As a part of society and as one of the health professions, nursing is affected by the changes, problems, and issues of society in general, as well as those that specifically influence health care. Some of the changes, such as an emphasis on the civil rights of minority groups and women, have been occurring for almost 100 years. Others, such as the changes in social attitudes and the growth of economic pressures, have been building up but were ignored until they created a crisis. Still others, such as new lifestyles and technological and scientific advances, appeared to emerge with a suddenness that caused the shattering stress and disorientation common in individuals when they are subjected to too much change in too short a time. Yet, even though it might be tempting simply to do your job and never mind the outside world, people (or professions) that do not pay attention to economic and social trends find themselves scrambling to catch up, rather than planning to move ahead—reacting, rather than acting. When the public accuses the professions of unresponsiveness to their needs, it is, in part, because those professions have not been astute enough to observe patterns of future development or have been too self-centered to see the necessity to become a part of them. Among the major factors to consider are changes in population, people's health, technology and scientific advances, education and employment, and social movements.

THE AMERICAN PEOPLE: A TIME OF CHANGE

A census has been conducted in the United States every ten years since 1790, as mandated by the Constitution. There are additional interim projections, the latest of which estimates the US resident population at 262.2 million in October 1995. Although every attempt is made to be precise, there is undercounting which is verified by the Department of the Census, and ranges from 4.5 percent for native Americans to 0.7 percent for Caucasians.[1] There are also socio-economic lines which seem to be associated with undercounting, including people living in public housing projects and the homeless. The resident population grows even larger when we add undocumented aliens and migrant workers.

During the 1960s, population growth averaged 1.3 percent a year, but this reduced to 1.0 percent in the 1970s and 1980s. Even if growth declines to 0.5 percent by 2040 as predicted, a conservative population projection for that year is about 364 billion, an increase of 43 percent over 1992.[2] Numbers are an important ingredient in planning for health care needs, but only one aspect of the changing face of America.

The population will not be as white as before, and much less homogeneous. By the year 2000, one of every three Americans will be a member of an ethnic minority,[3] and by the middle of the twenty-first century, current minority peoples will become the numerical majority.[4] The influx of immigrants has added to this diversity.

Unlike the great European migration of earlier times, the new immigrants are primarily Hispanic, from the Americas, and Asian (particularly Korean and Filipino). This has affected the population mix in a number of states. The Asian population grew by 70 percent in the 1980s, and the Hispanic population is growing five times as fast as the rest of the population. It is predicted that, if current trends persist, non-Hispanic whites will be a minority in California by 2000. Hispanic-Americans are the youngest population group. One-third are under 18 years old, and half under 26.[5] Most Hispanics now live in Texas and California and other areas of the Southwest, although some cities such as New York and Miami are also favored. The largest number of Asians are in California and Hawaii.

Acceptance of the new immigrants has varied. One concern is their assimilation into the community. It has been noted that for the first time in our history, the majority of immigrants speak just one language—Spanish— and tend to live in ethnic enclaves served by media communicating in Spanish. Some Asians have also tended to cluster in ethnic neighborhoods and work in ethnic groups. The fact that foreign-born black and Hispanic people are more likely to have jobs than those native-born has caused resentment (although there is also resentment if the newcomers are receiving public assistance). The same is true of Asians, many of whom have the entire family working long hours to support a small shop or business and often pressure their children to perform well in school. There is no doubt that the diversity of our population enriches the nation. However, the American tradition of "one from many" will look more like a mosaic then a melting pot (an analogy commonly made and not originating with the authors). Each ethnic group is encouraged to retain its culture as a source of strength and identity. The implications for every aspect of life are staggering. Traditionalists who accept the reality of a multiracial society deplore a multicultural society, arguing that strong nations need a universally accepted set of values.

The graying of America is considered the single most significant factor affecting the future of the United States, with special emphasis on health care. In the year 2000, there are likely to be about 35 million Americans 65 years or older, with about 4.3 million 85 and older[6] (see Exhibit 3.1). Persons 85 or older are the fastest growing category of the US population. Over one-fifth of the elderly are poor or near-poor; women, Blacks, and Hispanics have a higher poverty rate, with social security the major source of support. Still, the economic level of the elderly varies widely, with income and assets from a variety of sources. Only about 5 percent live in institutions; but of those who do, disproportionate number are women, generally unmarried or

EXHIBIT 3.1

Aging of the Population

	1990	2000	Increase
Total US population (millions)	249.9	274.8	10.0%
Under 65	218.4	239.9	9.9%
% total	87.3%	87.0%	
65 and over	31.5	34.9	10.6%
% total	12.6%	12.7%	
85 and over	3.1	4.3	39.3%
% total	1.2%	1.6%	

Source: US Bureau of the Census.

widowed. One major impact that the elderly, better educated than ever, have had is in influencing legislation. With organizations such as the American Association of Retired Persons (AARP) as their lobbyists, and with politicians' appreciation of their voting power, the elderly have clearly influenced legislation affecting them.

Each generation is a product of its times. The aged of the mid-1990s faced the Great Depression as young adults, were patriots of World War II, knew economic deprivation in a period without social welfare programs, and were children of the liberalism and good times of the 1920s. Recent attention has been quick to focus on today's twenty-something young adults. They are alternately called the X generation, still defying classification, or the 13ers, being the thirteenth generation in American history.[7] Their relationship with their parents, the baby-boomers, sets the stage for the next generational crisis. They are a generation who inherit the repercussions of the excesses of their elders: a toxic environment, national debt, unemployment, economic recession, AIDS, recurrent TB. The fact that the cold war is over hardly seems an even exchange. Many were raised by grandparents of the silent generation of wartime America; while their parents, the boomers, were caught up in divorce or the super-mom phenomenon. These parents are still caught up in the work of mid-career, advancement in employment, buying a home, educating children, securing their financial future. They are the first generation where at least half are college-educated. By the turn of the century, their attention will be focused on public policy and the needs of the elderly. In contrast, the 13ers seem to suffer a loss in living standards when compared with their parents, a hard blow to Americans who were always expected to better their lot with each ensuing generation. Determined to regain what they have lost, the 13ers will strengthen the family, ask for very little governmental assistance throughout their lifetime, pursue conservative politics and investments, and favor the needs of the very young over the very old (mostly the boomers). Where the boomers were caught up in quick change and episodic relationships, the X generation will look to reestablish our traditional institutions and invest in our traditional social systems. This portends a whole new brand of volunteerism, a movement from "adhocracy" to a more long-term commitment, but with a no-nonsense attitude about what should be accomplished.

Americans have become more urbanized over time. The last census continues to show rural losses. Over 79 percent of the population lived in urbanized areas, compared with 63 percent in 1960 and 78 percent in 1980. The slowdown in the trend towards urbanization in the last generation should not be hastily interpreted. The decline of manufacturing and industry, the heavy concentration of rural elderly, more generous public assistance and agricultural subsidies and the negative image of many major cities may all have contributed. Whether this will change again with a Republican Congress set on cutting cost remains to be seen.

American households have shrunk to their smallest ever, 2.62 people in 1992, with projections for the year 2000 showing a continued drop, not as rapid. The decline slowed as the younger members of the "baby boom" generation began to start families, with women in their thirties and forties eager to plan for parenthood. The numbers of people living alone has declined as many young singles prefer to live with parents, given the cost of maintaining separate households. The increase of one-parent families continues to contribute to the low family size (defined as two or more people). Only 26 percent of all households with children under 18 include a married couple. The number of families maintained by a woman without a man increased to 11.7 percent of all households. Many in this group are also likely to be part of the 89 percent of US households receiving at least one noncash benefit such as food stamps and Medicaid. About one out of every four households with children under nineteen received such assistance.[8]

In general, there has been an increase in the number of women working; 47 percent of households with children had two parents who were employed. The number of women with children who work outside the home has increased tremendously, with single mothers even more likely to do so.[9] About half of the mothers with infants hold jobs, sometimes because of necessity, sometimes because of career demands. The need for child care arrangements and flexibility is becoming quite evident to employers.

About one in seven Americans live below the poverty level. Child poverty is particularly sad, with one in five children under 18 and one in four under 3 being poor. One of every two black children and two of every five Hispanic children are poor.[10] The fact that those who are already poor, undernourished, undereducated, and underemployed tend to have the most children increases the social consequences. Many of these families migrate to cities, where they become victims of drugs, AIDS, crime, prostitution, and other ills of the environment. Children of young, uneducated, unmarried mothers, little more than children themselves, may be born with crack addiction, AIDS or, all too often, low birthweight, leading to mental and physical problems. Their future is bleak, for while ideas for helping the poor abound, a consensus is wanting, as is funding. Today's solutions to poverty are often mean-spirited and dismiss constructive solutions.

But at least the majority of the poor have homes of a sort. An estimated 600,000 to 1.2 million Americans are homeless. Advocates of the homeless say that the figure is closer to 2 million.[11] Among these are youths who have come from chaotic or violent families, single males with alcohol or drug problems, and both men and women who are often mentally ill. Yet the fastest-growing segment are families, often single mothers and children, living in unsafe shelters and welfare hotels. Needless to say, the health problems of all the homeless are horrific, with tuberculosis (TB), accidents, drug-related conditions, violence, sexually transmitted diseases (STDs) including AIDS, and infections being common. Pregnancy occurs at twice the national average rate, and the babies are born with serious health problems. In many cities, and increasingly in suburban areas, soup kitchens are becoming common, and even those with homes come for food. Homelessness is not a simple phenomenon but is created and complicated by a variety of other social problems: unemployment, parental neglect, poverty, substance abuse, and so on. Where middle America once had a large quotient of sympathy for these people, that goodwill has turned into a backlash. The economic recession, unemployment, problems with health care, and crime on the streets have all tested our patience. Citizens want the streets and public buildings clean and uncluttered. The homeless are a reminder of our shortcomings as a society, and in times of personal stress our tolerance wears thin as our dollars for social welfare programs.

There is little doubt that the poor not only lack adequate housing, nutrition, and jobs, but they also have a multitude of health problems for which they may not seek help until the situation reaches crisis proportions. The need is for readily available health services, such as neighborhood family health centers, health workers who understand the problems of the people and are able to communicate with them, understandable health teaching, and coordination of the multiple social services. Even as a life of poverty is associated with complex health and social problems, poverty can be described in several ways. The poor who qualify for welfare may fare better than those who are medically indigent. The medically indigent earn too much to qualify for health care subsidies, but often have jobs which do not provide health benefits. Given even the least costly health care incident, their resources are exhausted.

The Nation's Health

Though Americans can boast about their scientific advancements in medicine and the specialists and sub-specialists who constitute the workers in the delivery system, fewer positive things can be said about this nation's health. The biggest killers of Americans are still heart disease, cancer, stroke, personal injury and chronic obstructive pulmonary disease.[12] The major contributing factors to death in this country are tobacco use, diet and activity patterns, substance abuse, firearms, risky sexual behavior, motor vehicles and toxic agents.[13] The status of the nation's health is the by-product of personal lifestyles, bad government, and a troubled social environment.

Convinced that health promotion and disease prevention are a much sounder investment than cure, the US Public Health Service authored *Healthy People 2000* which identified the major health challenges for the nation, and the opportunities which exist for gain in measurable terms. The basic goals of *Healthy People 2000* are to increase the years of healthy life for all Americans, decrease the disparities in health which exist among different populations in this country, and increase access to disease prevention and health promotion services.[14] An interim report on the progress made since 1990 shows some gains and other losses. Some of the outcome measures, their comparison to earlier years (for the most part 1987), and progress towards goals is presented in Exhibit 3.2.[15]

The gains that we see can be misleading. Aggregate data conceals the growing disparity in health indicators for minority populations. For Blacks there has been progress on prenatal care, infant mortality, deaths from coronary artery disease, cirrhosis and unintentional injury. Although the death rate has declined for black infants, progress has been greater for white infants, with the result that the gap has widened and the death rate among black babies is almost twice the rate for white babies. In 1990, 30 percent of the deaths from AIDS occurred among Blacks and 17 percent among Hispanics, although they only represented 12 percent and 9 percent of the population respectively.[16] In general, minority populations show an increase in homicides, overweight, tuberculosis and the incidence of AIDS. It becomes difficult to determine where these health indicators are more associated with poverty than with the ethnicity of any population.

Death from heart disease and cancer, except for smoking-related lung cancer and melanoma deaths, is down, but there is a slight increase in death from chronic obstructive pulmonary disease. Here again there is the minority distinction, showing death from heart disease 35 percent more prevalent in Blacks, and an 86 percent greater incidence of stroke deaths. The distinctions cannot be simplified or even fully presented, but the reader should be alerted to look for these disparities. The life expectancy of Blacks is 71.8 years, and 67.8 for black males as contrasted with 76.5 for Whites.[17]

EXHIBIT 3.2

Interim Report on the Goals of *Healthy People 2000*

Health habit	Baseline	Target	Update	Progress
Regular exercise	22%	30%	24%	Yes
Overweight	26%	20%	34%	No
Lower fat diets	36%	30%	34%	Yes
Cigarette smokers	29%	15%	25%	Yes
Youths who smoke	29%	15%	25%	Yes
Alcohol-related auto accidents (per 100,000 people)	9.8	8.5	6.8	Yes
Alcohol use among youths 12–17	25.2%	12.6%	18%	Yes
Teenage pregnancies (per 100,000 people)	71.1	50.0	74.3	No
Suicides (per 100,000 people)	11.7	10.5	11.2	Yes
Homicides (per 100,000 people)	8.5	7.2	10.3	No
Assault injuries (per 100,000 people)	9.7	8.7	9.9	No
Work-related injuries (per 100,000 people)	7.7	6.0	7.9	No
Low-birthweight babies	6.9%	5.0%	7.1%	No
Deaths (per 100,000 people) from:				
coronary artery disease	135	100	114	Yes
stroke	30.4	20.0	26.4	Yes
cancer	134	130	133	Yes
pneumonia/influenza	19.9	7.3	23.1	No

Adapted from the *Journal of the American Medical Association*.

Other quality-of-life behaviors have been monitored periodically by *Prevention* magazine through an independent telephone survey and are displayed in Exhibit 3.3. Though less rigorous than *Healthy People 2000*, this presents an image of Americans being concerned with healthy and safe living. It is also apparent that compliance is better as government imposes controls. Some examples are the strictly imposed drinking while intoxicated

EXHIBIT 3.3

Quality-of-Life Behaviors

	Percent practicing	
	1984	*1995*
Limit sodium in diet	53	47
Limit sugar in diet	51	40
Adequate vitamins, minerals	63	59
Wear seat belt (over 30 years old)	19	73
(under 30)	19	62
Avoid driving after drinking	72	85
Smoke detector in home	67	93
Obey speed limits	61	48
Control stress	59	70
Consume fiber	59	54
Get 7–8 hours sleep nightly	64	59

Adapted from *Prevention* magazine.

(DWI) penalties in many states; prohibitions against smoking in restaurants, public buildings and public transportation; smoke detector requirements; lower speed limits on the nation's highways (which are now rising again); and mandatory seat belt use. The cynic might say that we have to be protected from ourselves.

The shifting demographics in the US, the *Healthy People 2000* agenda, and environmental concerns are all reflected in 1995 data from the American Cancer Society:

1. Lung cancer remains the leading cause of cancer deaths in the United States for both sexes.
2. Breast cancer is still on the rise in all age groups.
3. Prostate cancer is increasing, principally because of the aging population.
4. Colon and rectal cancers are no longer among the four most frequent sites.
5. Skin cancer, especially the highly curable basal cell or squamous cell cancers, has an incidence of over 800,000 cases in 1995, by far the largest number of any cancer. The potentially fatal melanoma is increasing.

6. The cancer rate for Blacks is higher than for Whites; the death rate is also higher.
7. Hispanic-Americans are not adequately aware of most of the warning signals of cancer or ways to reduce risk. They tend not to seek early detection or treatment.
8. Eight million Americans are alive in 1995 who have had cancer; those diagnosed over five years ago can be considered "cured," that is, having the same life expectancy as someone without cancer.
9. Early detection and treatment is a major factor in survival.
10. Among hazards listed that might lead to cancer are smoking, excess sunlight, excess alcohol, smokeless tobacco, estrogen, radiation, occupational hazards such as industrial agents, and nutritional factors.
11. The greatest number of new cancer cases was found in California and Florida, the fewest in Wyoming and Vermont. (Environmental factors should be considered here.)

The major causes of death for Americans are for the most part incurable, but with lifestyle adjustments, a long and productive life is possible for most. For others, disability due to chronic disease is inevitable. In 1987, chronic disease disabled 9.4 percent of the population, but that incidence increased to 10.6 percent by 1993.[18] Chronic disease and disability is not only the result of the way we live but the sophisticated medicine we practice. In addition, there is concern about the increase in mental disorders: almost one in two Americans have experienced a mental disorder at some time in their lives, with 30 percent suffering from one in any given year.

Of all the diseases that affect Americans today, probably the most frightening is AIDS. Since AIDS was first identified in 1981, it has spread quickly and irrevocably. By June 1992, 230,000 cases of AIDS had been reported to the Centers for Disease Control and Prevention (CDCP); and there had been 150,000 deaths. By 1994, under an enlarged definition of AIDS that took effect in 1993, the estimated number of persons with AIDS ranged from 600,000 to 800,000 in the United States. Worldwide, the number that are HIV-infected is estimated to be 14 million. Though these statistics are staggering, it has been estimated that only 10 to 15 percent of the total number of people infected with HIV are reported.

Many stereotypes about AIDS have been shattered in recent years. AIDS and HIV are no longer diseases restricted to the largest metropolitan areas. AIDS cases have increased dramatically for heterosexuals, from about 1.9 percent in 1985 to 9 percent in 1995, particularly among Blacks and Hispanics. The number of women and children infected is growing significantly. AIDS is currently one of the leading causes of death for women between the ages of 25 and 45.[19] In August of 1994, the CDCP reported 51,235 women with AIDS in the United States. It is sobering to think that worldwide, each woman dying of AIDS will leave behind an average of two children. By the year 2000, nearly 10 million children will have been orphaned by the disease. Grandparents, many needing care themselves, bury their children and take on renewed responsibility for child rearing. There are also a rising number of infant and childhood deaths from AIDS. Many others will join the ranks of homeless children who are "throwaways," possibly infected themselves, and desperately trying to survive on their own.[20]

AIDS is not curable, but it is highly preventable. Because of the known relation between AIDS and substance abuse, as well as risky sexual practices, prevention programs have focused on the use of good-quality condoms as protection during sexual intercourse, discouraging needle-sharing among substance abusers, and establishing a rigorous standard in processing blood and blood products for transfusion. However, the human element remains. Many individuals are reluctant to demand the use of condoms in their sexual relationships, some religious groups object to publicizing safe sex, and drug users are often ignorant or indifferent. Teenagers continue to feel omnipotent and above harm and pursue risky behaviors. Given the length of time between infection and diagnosis, individuals with AIDS in their mid to late twenties were infected as teens. (It has also been noted that other viral sexual diseases are found in 1 of 5 in the United States.)

Even in the midst of this tragedy there has been progress. Though there is no cure, great strides have been made in palliative drug therapy. Individuals with AIDS are living longer and experiencing better quality of life. Persons with AIDS are a protected class under the Americans with Disabilities Act, therefore allowing them to continue in the American mainstream. Compliance with CDCP-approved universal precaution techniques is mandatory for every health care setting and provider. The health care community has held the line to diffuse the public tendency to panic by opposing mandatory testing and disclosure for any group, including health care workers or patients.

A nation's health is often evaluated in terms of its infants and children. According to a 1990 report by the House Select Committee on Children, Youth and Families, children in the United States are more likely than children in 11 other industrialized countries to live in poverty, live with one parent or be killed before the age of 2. At about the same time, the American Academy of Pediatrics emphasized such problems as crack babies (375,000 babies a year are born to mothers who use drugs); the effect of environmental hazards on children; the fact that injuries kill six times as many children as cancer, the second leading cause of childhood death; the increase of pediatric AIDS, now the ninth leading cause of death, and poor children's lack of access to care. Equal concern is expressed about the rising toll of child abuse and the resurgence of childhood diseases that could be prevented by routine immunization.

In 1994, adolescent sexuality and pregnancy continued to be major health and social problems. Since 1990, teenage pregnancy and birthrates in the

United States have exceeded those in most developed countries. There were one million pregnancies in women aged 15 to 19, over 50 percent resulted in births, and 95 percent of those pregnancies were unintended. Though the number of reported legal induced abortions has remained relatively stable since 1980 (varying within 5 percent), the national rate in 1990 was at its lowest point since 1977. The birthrate among teenagers continued to increase in 1991, as it had in previous years, with 65 percent of those births being out of wedlock (56 percent for Whites, 60 percent for Hispanics, 94 percent for Blacks). The typical woman selecting abortion is young, white, and unmarried with no previous live births, and having the procedure for the first time.[21] The Children's Defense Fund reported that Black teenagers were 2.3 times more likely, and Hispanic teenagers 1.9 times more likely, to give birth than White teenagers, although the level of sexual activity was about the same. Black, White, or Hispanic, one out of every five 16- to 19-year-old women with below-average academic skills, and coming from poor families, was a teenage mother. Frequent teenage pregnancy and the decline of abortions have significant implications for the future health of children and adults, and family structure. As of June 1992, 24 percent of single women aged 18 to 44 had borne children compared with 15 percent in 1982.

Physical and mental health are dependent on a supportive and nurturing environment. Despite public and governmental concern over our declining environment, progress is uneven and somewhat depressing. The emissions from the burning of fossil fuels are seen as a major cause of global warming. Despite this relationship, burning has increased almost 40 percent in the last 25 years. In the same period, there has been the same percentage increase in the number of trees harvested, and an increase in the numbers of US plant and animal species endangered from 109 in 1973 to 919 in 1995. On a more positive note, in 1972 only 36 percent of the rivers and lakes in the US were swimmable or fishable as compared with 62 percent in 1992.[22]

It is interesting to note that many of our gains in health and the environment have been associated with strong governmental positions (and perhaps many of our shortcomings associated with weak government). Landmark laws like the Clean Water Act, the Endangered Species Act and the Toxic Substance Control Act put muscle behind the environmental movement. Many advocates fear that the 104th Congress' Contract with America will gut many of these programs as it aims to reduce governmental control as a strategy to both cut cost and increase personal freedom.

Technological and Scientific Advances

The technological advances of the last quarter-century have been extraordinary. Some of the most significant advances affecting patient care can be categorized as follows:

1. Developments in diagnosis and patient care, such as automated clinical laboratory equipment; organ transplants; artificial human organs and parts; improved surgical techniques and equipment, such as microsurgery and laser beams; genetic engineering; and the use of the computer and new imaging techniques in diagnosis.

2. Hospital information management—mainly due to application of the computer for patient billing, accounting, and patient records. Methods are being developed to control the flow of information so that health care practitioners can have ready access to necessary data, and can have information transmitted quickly and accurately to all departments.

3. Developments affecting hospital supply and services, such as widespread adoption of plastic and other inexpensive disposable materials, and such equipment as specialized carts, conveyers, and pneumatic tubes.

4. Improvements in the management and structural design of health facilities aimed at more efficient utilization of personnel, equipment, and space. This involves improved concepts of management and construction of health facilities based on advances in the organization of health care services.

5. Mass communication, making possible speedy transmission of health information and new knowledge, and exerting a powerful influence in molding public opinion. It can bring about positive results, such as providing information on communicable diseases and ways in which to get help; it can provide knowledge about other social and health problems, and even provide formal educational programs.

Although there is undeniable progress in health care directly attributable to technology, there is also great fear that the more machines do, the less human interaction there will be. The high technology of the current day threatens to depersonalize health care, creating the need for a more humane delivery system (commonly called "high-touch"). Examples of "high-touch" are hospice care, birthing rooms, neighborhood clinics, and primary nursing. Even "high-tech" systems can be positioned to enhance "high-touch" services. Computers can allow for a more humanistic touch because of the ability to reach out and stay in touch with people and to share information. The information society has replaced the industrial society with new jobs being created in the information and service sectors, not the manufacturing fields.

Computers have had a definite impact on organizational structures such as hospitals. Hospital information systems (HISs) are expected to promote efficiency, but have proved in some cases that they can be both disturbing and disruptive to those already employed. If they are not appropriately selected, introduced, and used, communication can be less effective than expected. The greatest impetus to the development of nursing information systems (NISs) came about when Medicare–Medicaid coverage required nurses to provide data needed for reimbursement and to document the care given both in hospitals and in community health agencies. Effective use of computer systems in health care organizations requires that nurses be critical of the systems they evaluate and use, which means that they must learn about computers and what they can do. They must also help clarify and standardize the nursing database.

Over the last several years, a great deal has been written in the nursing literature about the use of computers in education and practice. The variety of uses continually increases, and more nurses are becoming computer experts. Nurses, like others, must find fast, effective ways to turn raw data into useful organized information. NISs can improve both the cost effectiveness and the quality of care as nurses can be helped to use their time in the most effective possible ways. Health care information systems (HCISs) can assist in patient assessment and classification, care planning and documentation, quality assurance, discharge planning, staffing and scheduling and tracking acuity, cost, and quality data. Computer terminals at the patient's bedside, in the examining room, and even in the patient's home can ease data entry, improve accuracy, and eliminate duplication of information. If used properly, computers can also improve exchange of information between nurses and other health care professionals and staff.

In addition, computer technology is increasingly being used in nursing education and research. Computer-assisted instruction (CAI) is used in such areas as drill and practice, simulations, and tutorials. Nursing informatics courses are being offered (or required) in many schools of nursing. Much nursing research also depends on competent use of computer technology, whether related to clinical data collection, retrieval of information from libraries, or the analysis of data. The increase in the use of electronic media is demonstrated in the new Sigma Theta Tau Center for Nursing Scholarship International Library in Indianapolis, where just about all information is in computerized form.

There is no question that the use of computers in health care institutions and agencies will escalate. Experts repeatedly identify computer technology as essential to improvement in health care. Particularly named are fully integrated information systems that link patient care with everything from accounting to materials management, computer-assisted clinical prescribing and monitoring of drug interactions, and computerized patient records, including bedside information systems.[23] The most useful systems link all the computers within a health care facility, thereby allowing multiple record correction from a single point of data entry. In simpler language, the nurse enters an order for a specific x-ray procedure which requires routine medication and dietary preparation. As the order is placed, the procedure is scheduled for the time of day that is most comfortable for the patient as

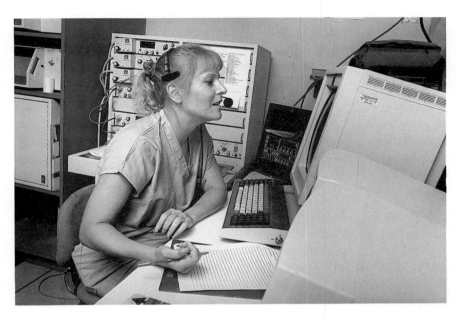

Computers are playing an important role in health care communication. (*Courtesy of Robert Wood Johnson Hospital, New Brunswick, New Jersey.*)

designated in the nursing history, the pharmacy receives the order for medication, transport is notified when to pick up the patient, diet is changed, inventories are updated where supplies were used, the episode enters the quality assurance loop, and the nurse is alerted to any possible adverse reactions.

Given the amount of nursing effort that is invested in coordination of services, the value of information technology is limitless. For nurses, this means learning to use the new technology for the benefit of the patient but continually maintaining the emphasis on individuality and human contact, which no machine can provide, as well as protecting the patient's privacy—that is, the question of security of information. In the last decade, computer experts have made headlines with their ability to invade the computers of banks, hospitals, industry, and even the government, in some cases changing or erasing data. While others had already used the computer to commit crimes (and were not always caught and punished), this new danger has reinforced earlier concerns about the confidentiality of computer-stored information. Would an employer, or simply a curious individual, be able to review another individual's credit record or hospital record? For that matter, would the record be accurate? Anyone who has had to deal with the unresponsive computers of businesses and the government knows the difficulty of catching and correcting errors; computer input still has a human component. All this has implications for nurses and their ethical responsibilities.

Education

Trends in education affect nursing in a number of ways: (1) the kind, number, and quality of students entering the nursing programs and the background they bring with them; (2) the development of educational technology, which frequently becomes a part of nursing education; and (3) the impact of social demands on education, which are eventually extended to education in the professions, including nursing. Usually it is not just one social or economic condition that brings about change in education, nor is there only one kind of change. For instance, overexpansion by most institutions of higher education when the baby boom was at its height created a large pool of unemployed college graduates in the early 1970s. Some of these, as well as college students with a worried eye to the future, looked for educational programs that seemed to promise immediate jobs with a future, among them nursing. Thus, what had once been a trickle of mature, second-degree students into nursing became a steady stream. As the baby boom group diminished, the overextended institutions of higher education and individual programs found it necessary to use marketing strategies of all kinds to attract enough students. They discovered the working adults in the community, who were a relatively untapped pool.

There were several definitive results. The diversity of age, background, education, and life experience in those seeking (or being sought for) advanced education has been an important factor in both social and political pressures for more flexibility in higher education. At the same time, providing such flexibility is one of the marketing strategies educational institutions are, after considerable resistance, relying on to attract the older prospective student. One focus is on liberalizing the ways in which individuals can receive academic credit for what they know, regardless of when, where, or how they acquired that knowledge. Credentials are viable currency in the struggle for upward mobility, and those in the health field are as eager as others in society to be a part of this movement. In general education, the concepts of independent study and credit by examination have been explored by an increasing number of colleges, and a variety of testing mechanisms are being used to grant credit, including teacher-made tests and standardized tests, which have wide acceptance. One example of the latter is the College Level Examination Program (CLEP), which includes tests of general education and numerous examinations in individual courses for which a number of colleges and universities award credit.

Other examples are the so-called external degree programs. While some of these are marginally legitimate operations that have given the whole concept a bad name with meaningless mail-order degrees, more and more respected, accredited educational institutions have established external degree programs using various modes: weekend, evening, summer, or other time periods for concentrated classes; outreach programs for isolated areas or even the workplace; self-study courses with examinations; and a process of combining educational credentials and examination results. A particularly successful example of the last is the Regents College Degrees, previously the New York Regents External Degree Program, which includes both associate and baccalaureate degrees in nursing. (See Chapter 5 for more detailed information on this and other open curriculum practices in nursing.)

It was predicted that an aid to these new educational or flexible patterns was the use of all types of audiovisual media, computers, programmed learning, and other new techniques that can enhance the teaching-learning process. Although these methods appear to be generally successful, they are expensive, and there is some argument as to whether the learning acquired is comparable to that gained by more traditional methods. One great asset appears to be that learning can be individualized more easily through the use of these techniques and also that satisfactory learning can occur in places other than the classroom and in the teacher's presence.

Equally significant are other happenings in higher education. Cost, to students and institutions, is an ongoing controversial issue. As governmental aid declines, costs go up for education, and there are not as many tax benefits in charitable giving. Colleges and universities have a major problem in balancing costs, quality, and service to students. Two-year colleges are under particular pressure because of their very low tuitions. There are also criticisms that relatively few students continue their education in a four-year college and that the dropout rate is high. On the other hand, despite the cry for higher quality, there is less state interest (and sometimes simply a lack of funds) for improving the public community colleges. Thus, many junior colleges have found it necessary to raise tuition and to market themselves vigorously to attract more students. There is renewed interest in the community college by the more traditional-age student, in part because of the relatively low costs and transferability of credits. The financial problems of some four-year colleges are also serious; many smaller colleges have been forced to close their doors, as have some nursing programs.

The cost of a college education is outpacing inflation. The nontraditional students, although welcomed by institutions of higher learning, have found costs particularly serious since they are often not eligible for funding, which is primarily reserved for full-time students. In testimony to Congress, the point was made that part-time students who must work often do not have the funds to pay high tuition. This had an impact on nursing when, in 1989, nurse traineeship funds were made available for the first time for part-time students. However, all students who need funding may have problems in the next few years, since federal funding has shifted from grants that do not have to be repaid to loans. Experts say that this will have a particular impact on the low-income group, since students from poor families are reluctant to go into debt for education. Consequently, many students take more than six years to complete a baccalaureate; over half of the Black and Hispanic students drop out for good.

Another point of interest is information about the attitudes and characteristics of today's undergraduates. The *Chronicle of Higher Education* publishes a survey of attitudes and characteristics of freshman every year. Today's undergraduate students consist of an equal number of men and women; Asians make up more than half of the foreign students. Most students entered college at age 18 or 19, are white and either Protestant or Catholic; their fathers and mothers had at least a high-school education and generally post-high-school education; fathers are in a business or profession; only 22 percent of mothers are homemakers or unemployed; over half have a family income of more than $40,000; about 62 percent of the men and 68 percent of the women plan graduate study; most drink beer, wine, or liquor, but do not smoke; most are middle-of-the-road politically. They think abortion should be legal; that there should be mandatory testing for AIDS and drugs; that a national health care plan is needed. They also support school busing; agree that the courts are too concerned about the rights of criminals; believe the government should do more to protect the consumer, control pollution, promote disarmament, and control the sale of handguns. They consider as very important objectives becoming an authority in one's own field, obtaining recognition from colleagues, raising a family, getting married, and being well-off financially.[24] Whether or not students' attitudes change during their college years has never been measured accurately, but it can be assumed that at least some changes will occur. Meanwhile, the data are, at the least, interesting to consider. Further, their attitudinal similarity to the X generation described earlier in this chapter cannot be dismissed, and holds implications for relationships with faculty, educational administrators and nursing students who are characteristically older. Many individuals select nursing for a midlife or later-life career change. Consequently, the average age of associate-degree students is almost 40 years old with baccalaureate enrollees in their mid and late twenties.

In recent years there has been much criticism of our basic educational system, including accusations of mediocrity and social promotion, and documentation of violence and disruption in the school. There have been repeated demands for better preparation in the basics and for school officials to restore order and discipline to the classroom. Teachers' unions have been criticized, and teachers point to the lack of public funds to improve education. Fewer than 5 percent of 17-year-olds possess the advanced reading skills to achieve excellence in academic or business environments; writing performance is deficient; math and science knowledge has improved but is far lower than that of students in Japan, as one point of comparison; knowledge of civics, geography, and history is abysmal, and rather disturbing since most of these students were approaching the voting age. Many critics point at the shallowness of the curriculum, minimum homework, and the short academic year. Serious concerns continue to be the drug problem and disruptive behavior in schools and the alarming dropout rate, particularly among Blacks and Hispanics. Eighty-six percent of Americans between the ages of 25 and 29 have completed high school, some through equivalency certificates.[25]

While this information might seem to be of only general interest, the reality is that such educational issues not only relate to the society in which we find ourselves, but for nurses, it has meaning for the kind of students who may or may not enter nursing as well as the kind of patients they deal with.

The Consumer Revolution

The consumer revolution, said to have begun when Theodore Roosevelt signed the first Pure Food and Drug Act in 1906, has been an accelerating phenomenon since the 1950s. Although various interpretations are given to the term, it might be broadly defined as the concerted action of the public in response to a lack of satisfaction with the products and/or services of various groups. The groups comprising the "public" are, of course, different, but they often overlap: a woman unhappy about the cost and quality of auto repairs might be just as displeased by the services of her gynecologist, the cost of hospital care, or the use of dangerous food additives.

There have always been dissatisfied consumers, but the major difference now is that many are organized and have the power, through money, numbers, and influence, to force providers to be responsive to at least some of their demands. The methods vary but include lobbying for legislation, legal suits, boycotts, and media campaigns. There is an increasingly strong force moving in that direction, especially with the better-educated and more aggressive baby boomers and elderly consumers. Consumers, who first concentrated their efforts against the shoddy workmanship and indifferent services offered in material goods, have now turned to the quality, quantity, and cost of other services, particularly in health care. Fewer patient/clients are accepting without protest the "I know best" attitudes of health care providers. The self-help movement, in which people learn about health care and help each other ("stroke clubs" and Alcoholics Anonymous, for instance), has extended to self-examination—sometimes through classes sponsored by doctors, nurses, and health agencies. Interest in health promotion and illness prevention has also been demonstrated by the involvement of consumers in environmental concerns.

The dehumanization of patient care, which is contrary to all the stated beliefs of the professions involved, is repeatedly cited in studies of health care. Although complaints often are directed at the care of the poor, it is a universal health care deficiency. The concerted action of organized minority groups led to the development of the American Hospital Association's Patient Bill of Rights. It received widespread attention in 1973, followed by a rash of similar rights statements specifically directed to children, the mentally ill, the elderly, pregnant women, the dying, the handicapped, patients of various religions, and others. In some cases, presidential conferences and legislation followed. The whole area of the rights of people in health care settings, which focuses to a great extent on patients' rights, has major implications for nurses (see Chapter 9).

An excellent example of the rise of a health consumer group is the women's health movement, which emerged from women's disenchantment with their personal and institutional health relationships. It came into existence around 1970 and is now worldwide. Among the best known of its activities are the various feminist health centers and their know-your-body and self-help courses and books.

Other consumers are also concerned with the power issue and are insisting on such rights as participation in governing boards of hospitals and other community health institutions, accrediting boards, health planning groups, and licensing boards. Their successes are increasing, and it is predicted that this trend will continue.

The nursing community has a history of supporting public policy that builds the strength of consumerism. These sentiments are prominent in *Nursing's Agenda for Health Care Reform*, organized nursing's directive for public policy reform.[26] Additionally in 1991, the American Nurses Association and the National Consumers League created a partnership called the "Community-Based Health Care Project." The project is funded by the Kellogg Foundation and supports the establishment of nurse–consumer coalitions in local communities. These coalitions bring pressure to bear for public policy changes and service projects that are responsive to local need.

The Women's Movement

Nursing, from its American beginning, was primarily made up of women, and some nurses have always been involved in the women's movement to some degree. However, feminist women and nurses have historically had an uneasy alliance. A group of nurse activists describe this relationship as follows:

Much of the energy in the women's movement has been directed toward opening up nontraditional fields of study and work for women. Nursing has been seen as one of the ultimate female ghettos from which women should be encouraged to escape. . . . Feminists have sometimes failed to look beyond the inaccurate sexist stereotypes of nurses and to acknowledge the multiple dimensions of professional nursing.[27]

Even today, there is a sense that many in the women's movement have been coopted into accepting men's values to define success and do not value traditional feminine values, such as caring.[28] Therefore, they look down on professions that consider caring an innate part of their practice. Obviously, nursing is one of these professions.

Women in all walks of life still face many formidable economic, social, and political barriers. But despite disagreements, the success of the women's movement attests to the fervor and commitment with which they have fought to improve women's status. It is no surprise that the women's movement has been considered one of the major phenomena of the mid-twentieth century. Over the years, there has been a proliferation of women's organizations concerned with women's rights. Among the most active groups is the National Organization for Women (NOW), founded in 1966 and made up of women and men who support "full equality for women in truly equal partnership with men" and ask for an end to discrimination and prejudice against women in every field of importance in American society.

The founding of NOW offered one of the most politically radical agendas of the twentieth century: men and women would share equally in public and private responsibilities—in paid work and in the rearing of children. NOW's activities are directed toward legislative action to end discrimination, and it attempts to promote its views through demonstrations, research, litigation, and political pressure. Among actions taken are the development of a model rape law and endorsement of health education for women in self-help clinics. It is interesting that the first president of NOW, Wilma Scott Heide, was a nurse and feminist, demonstrating that nursing and feminism can find common ground.

Another prominent women's organization is the National Women's Political Caucus (NWPC). It was founded in 1971 as the first national political organization to promote women's entry into politics at leadership levels. The main thrust of the NWPC is to ensure that women's issues are given more attention by facilitating the election of women to political office.

In addition to the League of Women Voters and the American Association of University Women, there are other important women's organizations such as the Women's Research and Education Institute, the National Women's Educational Fund, over 600 women's business organizations, and hundreds of women's sections and networks of major organizations.

Although many of the issues that women have confronted over the past 25 years remain unresolved, the women's movement has been the major catalyst in raising awareness of women's issues and opening discussions on sex discrimination and women's rights. The impact of the movement can be observed in newspaper reports, which show that both legal and social changes are occurring, slowly but surely, in relation to women's roles. A sudden, overwhelming about-face by men (and women) in terms of what women are, and can be, is not expected; attitudes are too deeply embedded. There is also insurmountable evidence that children are socialized into stereotyped male and female roles by books, use of toys, and influence of parents, teachers, and others—a problem that feminists and others continue to address. According to NOW, "A feminist is a person who believes women (even as men) are primarily people; that human rights are indivisible by any category of sex, race, class or other designation irrelevant to our common humanity; a feminist is committed to creating the equality (not sameness) of the sexes legally, socially, educationally, psychologically, politically, religiously, economically in all the rights and responsibilities of life."

Certainly these negative attitudes are not merely American. Reports from the United Nations' conference on women in 1995 show that discrimination and inequality are still widespread. In 1979, the United Nations General Assembly adopted "what is essentially an international bill of rights for women." However, the treaty, known as the United Nations Convention on Elimination of All Forms of Discrimination Against Women, has yet to gain worldwide recognition or acceptance. As of 1995, 128 countries had ratified the treaty, and few had made any significant efforts to eliminate discrimination against women. Notably, although the United States was part of the General Assembly consensus in adopting the convention, the US Senate has yet to ratify it.

In the years from 1975 to 1995, two UN-sponsored international conferences on women resulted in the following statement preceding the 1995 conference in Beijing:

> The picture is mixed: a greater proportion of women are literate and more of them are visible at high political levels. At the same time, many women are poorer than ever before, and women's human rights are being violated on an unprecedented scale. Despite the progress that has been made during the past 20 years, disparities between men and women, north and south, rural and urban, rich and poor, continue to concern women everywhere.[29]

In the United States, resistance to the women's movement is epitomized by the death of the proposed Equal Rights Amendment (ERA) to the Constitution, three states short of the 38 needed for ratification. Ten years after it was passed by Congress, and despite an extension of the deadline for ratification from 1979 to 1982, Indiana in 1977 was the last state to ratify it. More than 450 national organizations endorsed the amendment, and polls showed that more than two-thirds of US citizens supported it, but to no avail. The conservative opposition, including fundamentalist Christian churches, the so-called Moral Majority, the John Birch Society, the Mormon Church, and the American Farm Bureau, led a well-financed, smoothly organized, and politically astute campaign. Antiamendment forces assured state legislators that the Fourteenth Amendment offered sufficient protection to women and claimed that the ERA would cause the death of the family by removing a man's obligation to support his wife and children, would legalize homosexual marriages, would lead to unisex toilets, and most damaging, would lead to the drafting of women for combat duty. Advocates of the ERA were later criticized as lacking political finesse and alienating women who were potential supporters—Blacks, pink-collar (office) workers, and housewives. Amendment supporters lay heavy blame on men, particularly in legislatures and business. After the defeat, the 50,000-member Eagle Forum, and its founder, Phyllis Schlafly, the woman considered the leader of the anti-ERA forces, laid plans to campaign against sex education, the nuclear freeze, and "undesirable" textbooks. These activities are indeed being carried out.

In the 1980s and early 1990s, feminists determined to concentrate women's new consciousness and resources in building legislative strength to eventually pass the ERA and to mount a campaign for reproductive freedom, democratization of families, more respect for work done in the home, and comparable pay for the work done outside it.

Some 25 years after Betty Friedan published *The Feminine Mystique* (called by the futurist Alvin Toffler "the book that pulled the trigger of history") changes can be clearly identified, even though some of the results have varied. In terms of the ERA, Congress voted down another ERA bill in 1983. The bill was defeated by six votes. Yet, both friends and foes of equal rights note that the campaign for the amendment, along with other social forces, made a definite impact on American life. For example, labor force participation has become the norm for most women. More women than ever before are combining responsibilities of raising children, keeping up a household, and working outside of the home. Seventy-five percent of working women work full-time. These female labor force participation rates seem to be increasing, and projections to the year 2000 call for continued increases and further convergences of male and female labor force patterns over the life cycle.

Although women's wages are still not commensurate with men's, they are improving in that regard. The ratio between what the average woman earns and what the average man earns has risen in recent years to 75 cents on the dollar, up from 62 cents in the late 1960s. In terms of education, young women aged 25 to 29 have just about closed the gap in educational attainment between men and women.

On the downside, many women and men report dissatisfaction with the toll that women's work outside the home takes on family and personal lives. In a 1989 survey, 48 percent of all women respondents said that they had to sacrifice too much for their gains, especially with regard to time spent with children and family. More recent surveys reiterate this concern. The labor force participation of women can be viewed as a further disadvantage when one considers the many single mothers who have no choice but to work outside of the home because they are facing severe financial hardships. These problems seem to be intensifying as the proportion of families maintained by women alone increases.

Finally, despite the narrowing of the wage gap between women and men, 59 percent of women work in low-paying "pink-collar" jobs because they are trained for nothing else, some because such jobs tend to be more compatible with childrearing. It is harder to explain why the higher women advance, the larger the wage gap between men and women. Corporate women at the vice-presidential level and above earn considerably less than their male peers.

A growing number of lawsuits and union negotiations have challenged the male–female pay ratio based on the *comparable worth* theory. This theory, going beyond equal pay for equal work, calls for equal pay for different jobs of comparable worth. The intent is to revalue *all* jobs on the basis of the skills and responsibility they require. Neither the Equal Pay Act nor the Civil Rights Act brought about reform at any level of the workforce. A landmark case resulted in the state of Washington being ordered in 1984 to pay female workers up to $1 billion in back wages and increases because of such pay inequity. However, shortly thereafter, the decision was reversed on appeal.

Generally, federal and state governments, as well as the courts, have not been supportive of the comparable worth concept. For example, in 1985, the US Civil Rights Commission rejected it. That same year, a US Court of Appeals ruling written by Judge Anthony M. Kennedy, who was later appointed to the Supreme Court, approved a state's relying on market rates in setting salaries even if it knowingly paid less to women as a result.

More recently, a federal judge in California ruled that California had not deliberately underpaid thousands of women in state jobs held predominantly by women, a serious blow to the country's largest lawsuit on this issue. Nonetheless, industry and business are becoming more interested in job evaluation studies, with presumably equal pay following. Also important are a series of Supreme Court rulings that ban employers from offering retirement plans that provide men and women with unequal benefits. As one justice wrote, "An individual woman may not be paid lower monthly benefits simply because women as a class live longer than men."

Despite the advances women have made over the past 30 years, the burdens of childrearing still fall disproportionately on the shoulders of women. For example, slightly less than 9 out of every 10 one-parent families are maintained by women, and the number of single mothers increased to 7.7 million in 1990 from 5.8 million a decade earlier.

Furthermore, the feminization of poverty is a very serious problem facing American society. In 1991, 54 percent of all poor families were maintained by a woman with no spouse present. Among poor Black families, 78 percent were headed by a woman; among poor Hispanics, 46 percent; among poor White, 44 percent.[30]

Therefore, political and economic gains women have achieved cannot obscure (in fact they even intensify) the need for a national consensus on family policy. A major step forward was made when President Bill Clinton signed the family leave bill into law, which gives employed parents the right to a leave after the birth or adoption of a child and be ensured of job security. In addition, childcare initiatives from the private and public sector are also important in easing the dual responsibilities of family and career that so many women face. For several years, Congress has wrestled with legislation for both parental leave and childcare. Now that parental leave has been enacted, the time seems ripe for daycare legislation as pressure from women's organizations and other groups intensifies. ANA has lobbied for these bills, because of its predominantly female constituency and because of the importance of these bills for the health and welfare of the American people. In the meantime, some state legislatures and private companies have launched programs that assist families, and most often women, with regard to childcare and parental leave. None of these initiatives would have evolved without the force and appeal of the women's movement.[31]

In fact, the success of the movement is evidenced by John Naisbett, the author of *Megatrends 2000*, who referred to the 1990s as the "Decade of Women in Leadership."[32] He based his prediction on his belief that women were ready to break through the "glass ceiling," the invisible barrier that has kept them from the top, because their talents and abilities are being recognized and because they have already taken two-thirds of jobs in industries of the future. He also pointed out that the tendency to want to balance the top priorities of family and career along with other interests, once attributed to women, is becoming increasingly important in these times. He sees the emergence of a new leadership style, which focuses on quick responses to change and the ability to bring out the best in people, as symbolic of women's influence in the workplace. (These are certainly attributes that most nurses have mastered!) He describes a new type of work environment due to the growing numbers of women who work out of the home and the values they bring to their places of employment. In addition to citing the importance of the critical mass that women have reached in the professions, he predicts that benefits such as day care will increasingly be used as recruitment and retention strategies because of their importance to men and women alike.

The issue of women's rights is closely related to the problems, activities, and goals of women working in the health service industry. From 75 to 85 percent of all health service workers are women, and the largest health occupation, nursing, is almost totally female. These women-dominated occupations are also expanding most rapidly, but men continue to dominate the positions of authority within the health care system.

The reasons for so many women in health care is that, first, they are an inexpensive source of labor; second, they are available; and third, they are safe, that is, no threat to physicians. The rise of nurses as autonomous practitioners certainly is a threat to that traditional power base.

Labor, Industry, and Economics

It is expected that the political pendulum that swung from liberal to conservative with the beginning of the Reagan administration will continue in that direction for some years, even with a more liberal president, since the 1994 Congress was highly conservative. There are a number of other responses that are also expected to continue. One is more support for business and less for labor. As early as 1978, labor was losing members, primarily due to its inability to adjust to changing work patterns—a growth switch from industry to the white-collar, wholesale, and retail trades and service industries. Their loss of numbers meant a loss of political power, especially since they seemed to have less ability to influence their own members to vote a certain way. Legislators, therefore, have felt more free to vote for business interests and have done so, particularly since so many were heavily supported by business and religious conservatives. While union lobbying is still influential, the economic and political climate has emboldened employers in dealing with unions.

What has also made it easier for management is the growing tendency of people to prefer to work part time, a trend that is predicted to increase. Although this is particularly true of women, including nurses, who have young families or simply need to contribute to the family's income, there are also a surprising number of men who make this choice. Both women and men may be attending school, beginning their own businesses, testing a different field, working at a second job, or simply looking for more flexibility and independence. Some like the variety and the fact that they need not get involved in the politics and problems of the workplace. On the other hand, wages may be lower (not necessarily true for nurses), there is little opportunity for career advancement, and some temporary workers complain of being "dumped on" by regular employees. Industry has found these "contingency workers" economically advantageous. Employers do not usually pay for any benefits, which can be a considerable saving, and they can bring in these workers at busy times while maintaining a minimum workforce. Employing part-timers provides a way around union work rules and, at times, a way to confront striking unions. The negative side is that part-time or short-term workers may not have the same commitment to the company, and unless they return to the same place frequently, they need orientation and perhaps even training. Yet, it is quite possible that the availability of these workers as replacements has made strikes less effective. However, an executive order signed by President Clinton in 1995 makes it illegal for industries with government contracts to hire permanent replacements for striking workers. This action strengthens the value of the strike as a tool against management.

Despite these problems, by the beginning of 1990 there was some optimism in the ranks of labor. For the first time in over a decade, younger, more sophisticated labor leaders had replaced nearly all the old guard. Also, both labor and industry were stressing the need for harmony. The year 1989 had seen union membership grow, although with a greater growth in the workforce, the percentage continued to diminish (16.4 percent as opposed to the previous low of 23 percent in 1977). There was considerable growth in governmental unions, but the service industries, accounting for most of the growth in the labor force, had only 6 percent union participation. All seemed to be good candidates for organization. Because women are a large part of the latter group (they are also considered easier to organize), the unions are beginning to tackle women's issues such as abortion, and the safety of women on the job. However, their interest has not extended to placing women in the top echelon of the labor federation's hierarchy.

Management, criticized for its authoritarian approach, is trying new techniques to increase worker satisfaction. While far from widespread, there does seem to be growing interest in involving workers in decision making. Most American companies have reform programs in which workers and supervisors discuss operations.[33] In industry these may be called quality circles; in health care they may be shared governance. Some labor experts say that these "reforms" (also known by such names as *job redesign, work humanization, employee participation, workplace democracy,* and *quality of work life*) are more cosmetic than real, since few workers participate in the companies' most important decisions, and that in a difficult situation most managers revert to an authoritarian stance. Others say that this new management style is necessary now that the nation is engaged in vigorous international competition. Similar techniques have been used in Europe and Japan for some time, and production success, particularly in Japan, has concerned American industry. Whether there will be backsliding when economic times are better is the question.

In summary, American unions have been in decline since 1980, with the presence of a federal administration that favored big business and created incentives for the country's financial recovery to occur through the development of small business and industry. This antilabor sentiment was acted out through management-friendly appointments to the Supreme Court and the National Labor Relations Board, the governmental unit critical to facilitating efforts at organizing and unionization. At the same time, more basic employee guarantees were being provided through legislation and regulations, decreasing the need for union protection. A final observation is that the American union tradition had been built on an adversarial relationship between labor and management. This has proved to be inconsistent with the employee–employer relationships that have produced quality outcomes in other countries. American labor is in a state of transition. This transition will be further discussed in Chapter 15.

Anticipating the Future

Nursing and health care must exist within the context of the socio-economic and technological changes described here. The professions must identify patterns that allow us a glimpse of the future. There is a story to tell beyond today's reality. Some accurate predictions are possible.

1. The complexity of our human problems demands that we accept the fact that health care, housing, education, workplace safety, and a host of other concerns interrelate in the search for quality of life and vie for the same resources.
2. Health care is provided within a cultural context with its unique value system.
3. In the United States, demographics are our destiny; we are faced with an aging and chronically ill population.
4. The declining presence of the traditional family in this culture demands the creation of new services, programs, and public policy.
5. A fragile environment requires we take every caution to prevent its further deterioration.
6. "High-tech" advances will not stop but must be counterbalanced by a conscious and generous dose of caring and humanism.
7. Nurses stand at the center of an information-rich environment, the most strategic position for the 1990s.
8. Americans are demanding personal expression in their work, hours that complement a private life, and participation in decisions that impact the quality of their workplace. Yet the "downsizing" in business, industry, and health care that has created layoffs at all levels has also made the employee nervous about job security and perhaps a little less anxious to press these demands.
9. We are in an era of active consumerism.
10. Americans will live with less, they will sacrifice, but never give up their right to choose.

The reader is urged to test these predictions in the light of what is said in following chapters.

ISSUES IN HEALTH CARE

Before describing where and by whom health care is delivered, it is essential to understand some of the changes that have occurred in the last several decades—changes that relate directly to the public's concern about the cost and quality of health care. As often happens, the public's dissatisfaction with something becomes translated into legislation by those they elected. In this case, because the cost of health care was (and is) rising so rapidly, executive branch regulations, both on the national and state levels, also began to clamp down on the people (providers) and places delivering health care. (See Chapter 10 on how laws are made and how legislation affects health care.) The reason governmental impact is so great is that most health care facilities and many providers are funded, one way or another, by the government. Moreover, others who pay for health care (payers) such as health insurance companies, including the well-known Blue Cross and Blue Shield, tend to follow the patterns of payment set by the government.

Health care in the United States (frequently criticized as more likely to be "sick care") devours almost 15 percent of the gross national product (GNP), with a steady, sometimes massive increase in the last decades that exceeds that of any other advanced country. A variety of factors have been blamed. Both Medicare and Medicaid and most health insurance plans traditionally have paid for the "full and reasonable" cost of care on a retrospective basis, that is, whatever the provider said it cost, within certain limits. (Medicare/Medicaid law and its changes are described more fully in Chapter 10.) With the high cost of new technology used for both diagnosis and treatment, consumer demand for the biggest and the best, and the tendency of providers to over-order to protect themselves from being sued, costs soared. In 1983, because of fear that Medicare funds would run out, a new form of payment for hospital service was devised. Under this system, disorders of the human body were divided into major diagnostic categories (MDCs) with hundreds of subgroups called diagnosis-related groups (DRGs). The hospital receives a predetermined amount for each case based on the patient's principal diagnosis, and the presence or absence of complications/comorbidity and surgery. The dollar amount represents the usual length of stay for a patient with these characteristics and the diagnostic and therapeutic services which would usually be ordered. Some hospitals are exempt from the system, and special provisions are made for patients who have needs that are costly and extraordinary (outliers).[34] One problem for health care institutions, public health agencies, physicians, and the public is that reimbursement can be denied retroactively, after the service has been given, and the amount of documentation needed is both specific and voluminous. Another concern has been whether the relative severity of the patient's illness is considered, especially in relation to the nursing care needed.[35] On the other hand, if the patient is discharged more rapidly, hospitals may keep the full amount of the designated reimbursement. This has resulted in accusations that patients are being discharged "sicker and quicker," with more complex and highly technological care required in the home or nursing home. (Both of these settings are also under tight fiscal constraints.) Hospital utilization has been greatly reduced, and patients are considerably sicker since there are no grace periods of early admission for tests, now to be done on an outpatient basis, and no leisurely postacuity or postsurgical recovery before discharge.

Since the Reagan administration encouraged competition and the introduction of cost-saving approaches, several changes resulted as some hospitals found themselves in a financial bind. One was aggressive marketing, aimed particularly at self-paying patients and those with insurance. From nothing in 1980, $1 *billion* a year was spent on marketing by 1990. Although it is sometimes denied, administrators encouraged physicians to admit patients who were likely to be dischargeable early. Some hospitals, particularly the for-profit chains, closed units that were costly and unlikely to be fully reimbursed, such as burn units and trauma units. "Patient dumping," transferring certain patients to public hospitals, was another cost-saving technique, although in 1989 a law was enacted penalizing hospitals that dump. Hospitals looked for other ways to fill beds with paying patients, such as those requiring long-term care. As described later, hospitals formed satellite clinics, emergicenters, surgicenters and home care services. These services were not subject to the DRG model. They used helicopters to bring in emergency patients from distant areas and advertised their services and their physicians in media campaigns. Some created profit-making components that included equipment rental, health promotion and teaching classes, and even hotels and contracts with noted fast-food companies. They merged with other hospitals or agencies to share services, sometimes even developing into national chains. Even some academic health science centers began to look to other, like institutions to create merger or other sharing arrangements. In these activities, all hospitals mimicked the more businesslike for-profit hospitals or hospital chains. These had long used those tactics to increase profitability, even creating health-care malls, which include doctors' offices, a hospital, ambulatory care, laboratory, pharmacy, optometry, physical therapy and physical fitness services, as well as home care services, restaurants, gift shops, banking, and parking. While such "copy-cat economics" was criticized, nonprofit hospitals maintained that these approaches were needed for survival. In fact, since the 1980s, many small hospitals, especially in rural areas, have gone out of business, despite the needs of the population, and closures and downsizing (reducing the total number of beds) continue.

Even with these limitations on reimbursements, health care costs continue to soar faster than the inflation rate. There are still too many empty beds and too much expensive technology used. To add to the costs, AIDS patients continue to fill hospital beds and draw on complex home care services. The CDCP estimates that in January 1995 there were 120,000 living people in the United States diagnosed with AIDS. The estimated lifetime cost of health care for a person with HIV infection is $119,000: $50,000 from infection until the development of AIDS, and $69,000 from AIDS until death. One factor influencing cost is the length of periods of hospitalization. The average number of hospital days for a person with HIV/AIDS and a related opportunistic disease is 19 days per year, compared with 6.5 days per year for people with all other diseases.[36] Even though palliative care is improving, this will only continue to increase cost by extending the time the person will be in the health care system. In 1991, the cost of care for all people with HIV was estimated at $5.8 billion.[37] Given the impoverishment that accompanies AIDS and the difficulty in securing private sector insurance, many of these dollars will come from government. Only care for automobile accident victims and cardiac patients will be more costly, and it has been said that AIDS will be with us forever.

Another major problem for private hospitals is the care of the uninsured, estimated by some at more than 41 million nationwide in 1995. These people are not unemployed but are the working poor, not covered by health insurance or federal programs and unable to afford private health insurance, or those with very limited insurance. Then there are the homeless who come to emergency rooms, also without Medicaid, even though they may be eligible.

Hospitals have always given free care, and usually the cost was absorbed by increasing the bills of paying patients. Now this practice, too, is backfiring, since most of these patients are insured. The health insurer (third party payer) is refusing to subsidize the medically indigent—those neither poor enough for Medicaid, nor old enough for Medicare, with inadequate or absent private insurance, and limited personal dollars. Health insurers have put a variety of strategies into place to control cost escalation which eventually means higher premiums. Preapproval of payment for an elective procedure is common. Many employers have become self-insured to better control the health care spending of their employees. Self-insured programs are not as tightly regulated by state laws. Smaller companies may simply drop this employee benefit, or increase the copayment and deductibles to keep premiums affordable. Other employers encourage employees to choose managed care plans. There are a number of versions, but the principle is to enter into an agreement with a limited number of providers, hospitals, home care agencies and so on who will offer service to a number of potential patients at a discounted price or for a periodic all-inclusive fee (called a capitation fee, a nonvarying amount no matter how much service you need).

In cases where health benefits are offered through the workplace, the law requires that employees have a choice between managed care options and more traditional fee-for-service plans (choose whatever provider you want and pay separately for each service). Premiums are generally higher for those choosing the fee-for-service option.

A combination of all these factors has brought back interest in national health insurance, a concept that has not been popular since the Great Society years of the Johnson administration. Except for South Africa, the United States is the only industrialized nation that does not guarantee its citizens universal access to health care. Nevertheless, the government expected to spend $156 billion on Medicare and Medicaid in 1991. While there seems to be a trend in those other countries to privatize a portion of their health care, and certainly there are problems, including high costs, several national polls of Americans showed that they were interested in a national health plan such as Canada's, although it also has growing deficiencies. Actually, both the ANA and the NLN, as well as the American Public Health Association (APHA), have supported this concept for years, but the American Medical Association (AMA) and other powerful groups that influence health policy have opposed it. It is predicted that there will be no national health plan in the foreseeable future. However, given the burden of caring for the uninsured, there is a movement to guarantee basic health care services for everyone. Massachusetts and Hawaii were the first states to provide near-universal access for their citizens, requiring employers to provide insurance while providing some state support. Yet, financial problems plague many of these plans.[38] Meanwhile, just about everyone agrees that unnecessary use of health care should be curbed, and some of the power figures insist that the way to do that is to shift more of the financial burden to the workplace. Regrettably, there is some evidence that those who are insured make little effort to limit utilization or search for the best services for the least cost. Of course, such information is not always easy to come by, although consumer advocates are making some progress in having providers or the government present cost and quality information. Meanwhile, the issue of access to care—that is, who gets what when resources are limited—is becoming a serious ethical problem. (This is explored in more depth in Chapter 8.)

Perhaps because of this limited access for many groups, including the uninsured and Medicaid patients, there has been a surge of interest in plans to expand health care coverage. Some have been suggested by physicians, some by consumer groups, some by congressional committees, and some by nursing groups. They range from recommendations to expand Medicaid and Medicare, to employer-based financing approaches, to shared public-private financing. *Nursing's Agenda For Health Care Reform* developed by the Tri Council for Nursing made up of the NLN, the ANA, the American Association of Colleges of Nursing (AACN), and the American Organization of Nurse Executives (AONE), was presented to the public in February 1991.

Its major components were (1) a federally defined "standard package" of essential health care benefits, including primary care and prevention, available to all citizens and residents of the United States, and provided and financed by a mix of public and private sources; (2) improved consumer access by delivering primary care services in convenient settings such as schools, the workplace, the home, and others; (3) control of health care costs through managed care and incentives for consumers and providers, consumer freedom of choice concerning providers, settings, and delivery arrangements, reduced administrative costs via simplified bureaucratic controls and administrative procedures, and payment policies tied to the results of effectiveness and outcomes research; and (4) implementation of the plan through incremental steps, with priority status in allocation of resources given to pregnant women, infants, and children. Initial focus on these groups was seen as a cost-effective investment in the future health and prosperity of the nation.[39]

The strategy was to involve consumers, who are often left out of such planning, and to position nurses as "cost-saving providers," who, as gatekeepers in a managed care system, would encourage more appropriate care. Needless to say, there were criticisms of this plan, as well as of the others, based to a large extent on the questions of funding and cost. Even when there is no agreement about *which* plan is most feasible, almost no one believes that things can go on as they are. The federal government predicts that national health care expenditures will reach $1.5 *trillion* by the year 2000, 15 to 17 percent of the GNP. The task is formidable, especially for a country that prides itself on its autonomy, diversity, and pluralism in relation to health care delivery.

Another serious issue is quality of care. Accusations that quality is not commensurate with cost are heard from many sources. Beyond state licensing of hospitals and other health care facilities and agencies, which presumably represents some screening for quality, the Joint Commission on Accreditation of Healthcare Organizations (JCAHO), described later, puts its stamp of approval on institutions and agencies that meet specific criteria of quality. There is some cynicism as to whether this is simply a paper tiger, but the value of accreditation is certainly evident in some circumstances: federal funding of certain kinds may require accreditation. A number of consumer groups, some formal, some loosely organized, some interested in specific kinds of care, such as nursing homes, and some servicing a large group such as the AARP, which see high-quality health care as one of their concerns, are also active in evaluating health care and/or lobbying for improvements. In addition, the federal government has released the names of hospitals with high mortality rates, which some have said is unfair because certain hospitals have more at-risk patients. There are predictions that quality of care will be a major issue in the next decade and that the public expects health practitioners to take responsibility for ensuring high-quality care. Although both physicians and nurses have peer review systems in place, to one extent or another, the warning is that unless improvements are made, government oversight, such as the federally funded peer review organizations (PROs) that assess medical necessity, appropriateness, and quality of care provided to Medicare patients to determine if Medicare should pay the hospital, will increase.

Meanwhile, health care experts continue to present varying proposals to change what many call the disarray of the American health care system (although others maintain that it has never been otherwise). These include development of or increased use of alternative systems of delivering care, most of which are discussed in the following sections. Nevertheless, the quick demise of President Clinton's health care plan in 1994, and much talk but little agreement by a newly-elected Congress, demonstrates that a successful plan is not easy to come by.

HEALTH CARE DELIVERY: AN EXPANDING MAZE

Health care is big business, sometimes said to be the second or third largest industry in the United States, with over $2 billion spent on health care per day. There are now about 5916 hospitals, 19,100 long-term care facilities, and almost 13,951 home care agencies.[40] Uncounted but growing are a wide variety of ambulatory care services, besides the physician's single and group practice that has been traditional. Among these are surgicenters and other "centers" for urgent care, mental health, alcohol/drug addiction, renal dialysis, women's health, childbearing, adult/geriatric day care, and wholistic health. HMOs and hospices, more concepts than places, are also on the rise, while free clinics and community health centers may come and go, depending on the economy and support. Add to this an estimated 11 million health-related employees, one of every 10 American workers,[41] and it is easy to see why people are confused and sometimes frightened about who and what to select for their health care needs. Even nurses, who can be found in every setting, are not always clear about the system and the choices available. Following is an overview of current health care delivery, its organization, and its workers. Specific details on how the nurse may function in these various settings are presented in Chapter 6.

SELF-CARE

Obviously, most people spend most of their lives in a relative state of health or in a state of self-care. The World Health Organization (WHO) defines health as a "state of complete physical, mental, and social well-being, and not merely the absence of disease or infirmity." Although it serves as a broad philosophical declaration, this definition is more an optimum goal than a reality. Also frequently quoted is Parson's definition: "a state of optimal capacity of an individual for effective performance of the roles and tasks for which he has been socialized."[42] On a practical level, the Public Health Services' National Center for Health Statistics defines health implicitly in its use of "disability days," when usual activities cannot be performed.

Self-care can be defined as "a process whereby a lay person can function effectively on his own behalf in health promotion and (disease) prevention and in disease detection and treatment at the level of the primary health resource in the health care system."[43] The self-care concept is not new, and ranges from simply resting when tired to a more careful judgment of selecting or omitting certain foods or activities, or a semiprimary-care activity of

---

EXHIBIT 3.4

Definitions

Primary care: "(a) a person's first contact in any given episode of illness with the health care system that leads to a decision of what must be done to help resolve his problems; and (b) the responsibility for the continuum of care, i.e., maintenance of health, evaluation and management of symptoms, and appropriate referrals."[a]

Secondary care: the point at which consulting specialty and subspeciality services are provided in either an ambulatory, residential, or community hospital inpatient setting.

Tertiary care: the point at which highly sophisticated diagnostic, treatment or rehabilitation services are provided, frequently in university medical centers or equivalent situations.

Acute care: "those services that treat the acute phase of illness or disability and has as its purpose the restoration of normal life processes and function."[a]

Long-term care: "those services designed to provide symptomatic treatment, maintenance, and rehabilitative services for patients of all age groups in a variety of health care settings."[a]

---

[a] US Department of Health, Education, and Welfare: *Extending the Scope of Nursing Practice.* Washington, DC: The Department, 1971, pp 3–11.

taking one or more medications self-prescribed or prescribed by a physician at some other point of care. Health care advice comes from family, friends, neighbors, and the media (often with a product to sell). People also seek information from a health professional acquaintance, but self-care often becomes a matter of trial and error. Increasingly, with the consumer mentality, people turn to others with similar conditions. The individual gets support and reinforcement as needed but can also detect at what point he or she needs professional help. There are even programs and courses teaching specific knowledge and skills that a lay person can learn and use. Included are such aspects as taking vital signs, use and abuse of medications, when to call a doctor, and methods of health risk appraisal. The sale of do-it-yourself medical tests, stethoscopes, blood pressure devices, and other medical devices for home use has become a rapidly growing big business.

Health promotion and health education also play a large part in maintenance of health. Lifestyle has a major influence on most serious illnesses, and those who know what risk factors are at least have the choice of making decisions leading to better health. Experts note that the role of parents as early models for children's health beliefs is undisputed and that early experiences structure people's personal beliefs and shape their attitudes. Because this learned behavior may be deep-seated, it is often resistant to reeducation. Thus, changing undesirable eating patterns, smoking and drinking, and other aspects of a lifestyle takes more than simple information. Other determinants influencing health attitudes and behavior are both cultural and socio-economic. Evaluative research on health education, health promotion, and self-care is being done and is expected to provide helpful information on overcoming some of these obstacles.

Various polls seem to indicate that business, industry, and the public in general believe that the health care system should give more emphasis to preventive rather than curative medicine. However, reimbursement for health education is still not common, in either the public or the private sector, despite the rhetoric. And there is evidence that interest in healthy living is primarily a middle-class and upper-class concern.

Besides consumerism, another factor that encourages self-care is the cost of health care. It has been estimated that perhaps 85 percent of all health care could be self-provided and might be necessary to avoid flooding parts of the health care system. For instance, emergency rooms are frequently filled with patients who have minor conditions that could have been prevented or self-treated at home at an earlier stage.

One interesting movement closely associated with self-care is *holistic* or *wholistic* health care, which incorporates a number of precepts of the consumerist ethic. These include providing physical, psychological, and spiritual care, therapeutic approaches that involve the patient and encourage the patient's independence and capacity for self-healing, emphasis on self-care and education, consideration as an individual, and an environment that encompasses other activities besides health care. *Wholistic health care centers* were so named as a protest against the fragmentation of care. These centers are often primary care doctors' offices or parish nurse practices located in a church, which offer pastoral counseling and health education as well as physical care.

AMBULATORY CARE

It is not practical to discuss the institutions involved in the various types of health care delivery under the headings of primary care and so on, because there is considerable overlap of functions. For instance, hospitals and HMOs may deliver all levels and types of care, even encouraging or sponsoring self-care activities on the part of individuals and community groups. Therefore, institutions and agencies are presented as units.

Ambulatory care is generally defined as that care rendered to patients who come to physicians' offices, outpatient departments, and health centers of various kinds.

Physician Office Practice

The vast majority of care given by physicians is on an ambulatory basis; only about 10 percent of the people seen are admitted to a hospital. Most patient visits for health (or sick) care have been made to health care practitioners in solo, partnership, or private group practice. This is the major mode of organization for physicians and other health care providers generally acknowledged to be licensed to practice independently, such as dentists, chiropractors, podiatrists, and optometrists. Although there is a growing acceptance of nurses practicing independently, most people must be educated to that concept.

Nurse Private Practice

Nurses have been in private practice since formal nursing programs were started (see Chapter 2). In a manner of speaking, private-duty nursing was and is a professional practice for which the individual has professional and financial responsibility.

In an emerging concept of nurse private practice, the nurse has an office where patients are seen, although he or she may also make house calls. In this form of independent practice, nurses have the same economic and managerial requirements as physicians, with the added concern that reimbursement by third-party payers is somewhat limited. Most nurses in private practice are advanced practice nurses. They are discussed more fully in Chapter 6.

Community Health Centers (CHCs)

Out of the social unrest of the 1960s and early 1970s emerged the *neighborhood health center* (NHC), an ambulatory facility based on the concepts of full-time, salaried physician staffing, multidisciplinary team health practice, and community involvement in both policy making and facility operations. The NHC movement was stimulated by funding from the Office of Economic Opportunity (OEO) during the Johnson administration. Now more commonly called *community health centers* (CHCs), they serve some 6 million people at about 2000 primary care sites. They may be freestanding, with a backup hospital for special services and hospital admissions, or legally part of a hospital or health department, functioning under that institution's governing board and license, but with a community advisory board.

CHCs are primarily found in medically underserved urban areas. Often they are at least partially staffed by the ethnic group served, so that communication is improved. A real effort is made to provide services when and where patients/clients need them in an atmosphere of care and understanding. Use of nontraditional workers such as family health workers and an emphasis on using a health care team have been characteristics of CHCs. Starting and maintaining CHCs is extremely expensive, and most patients can pay only through Medicare or Medicaid, if at all. Few are self-supporting. When external funds are not available, severe program and personnel cuts are often necessary. The future of CHCs remains uncertain, in part because of a sociological question: are they perpetuating a separate kind of care for the poor? Nevertheless, variations of CHCs are present in different parts of the country. *Rural health centers*, developed under federal financing or funded by communities or foundations, serve people, usually the poor, in medically underserved areas (MUAs). Recent federal regulations have created a class of CHCs which are designated as federally qualified health centers (FQHCs). The government requires that advanced practice nurses (APNs) be regular participants in the delivery of care in these sites. FQHCs are qualified to serve Medicare and Medicaid recipients and will become central in Medicare and Medicaid managed care plans which are beginning to dominate, especially for the poor. Whether this new federal designation creates more bureaucracy or improves quality is yet to be determined. Care in CHCs is often given by APNs and physicians' assistants (PAs).

Nurse Managed Centers

Nurse managed centers (NMCs) offer "the ultimate autonomous practice opportunities (to nurses) as managers and primary caregivers."[44] NMCs may also be called community nursing organizations (CNOs), community nursing centers (CNCs), or nurse run clinics. They guarantee direct client access to nursing services, offer services that are reimbursable, place the accountability for both the services and the management of the center with nurses, and allow nurses to practice to the fullest extent of their legal scope of practice.

NMCs are not new creations, but can trace their roots to the turn of the century and the tradition of the visiting nurse and public health nursing. Neither must all NMCs be community based. A modern-day example of a NMC can be observed in the Loeb Center established at Montefiore Hospital in New York by Lydia Hall in the early 1960s. Hall characterized Loeb as a nursing center with the qualities of public health being offered in an institutional setting.[45] (Unfortunately, Loeb Center, as described, was discontinued by a new hospital administration.) It should be noted that some of the most successful NMCs have been birthing centers established by certified nurse midwives (CNMs). Models for NMCs have also been developed by clinical nurse specialists within such areas as cardiovascular, oncology, low-birthweight babies, patients with chronic obstructive pulmonary disease, diabetics, and so on. Despite these highly focused exceptions, the majority of NMCs pursue primary care as their major agenda.[46]

NMCs have a tradition of serving our most vulnerable populations. Further, RNs employed with NMCs are significantly more educated than the nursing staff complement in other health care settings, with 31 percent holding a baccalaureate degree and 37 percent with a masters.[47] The future of NMCs will depend on their success as participants in managed care, and in making strategic decisions to diversify or focus their services. Further, nursing's commitment to the underserved is consistent with our history, but to grow and flourish the vast middle class must become our consumers.

A 1992 survey estimates 250 NMCs in the United States. A few exemplary programs are summarized here:

- Genesis/Tampa General Health Center for Women and Children is affiliated with Tampa General Hospital and has an annual budget of $40 million.
- University of Rochester School of Nursing Community Nursing Center is a vehicle for faculty practice with both education and research goals accomplished through a diversified range of direct and subcontracted services.
- Alcorn State University Division of Nursing, Nursing Center in Natchez, provides care of adolescents and their families living in rural southwest Mississippi.

- The Block Nurse Program in Cleveland is a neighborhood-based home care service for older persons which integrates formal health care and informal support services.
- Community Health Clinic of Lafayette, Indiana, provides comprehensive family focused care to women, children, and male adults to age 65 and concentrates on the uninsured.
- Mercy Mobile Health Program of Atlanta brings primary care, HIV testing, substance abuse counseling, and other services to underserved populations in a fully equipped van.
- UCLA School of Nursing Health Center, Union Rescue Mission, is a large facility bringing primary care to the homeless.
- Community Health Services of Scottsdale provides family health care for individuals of all ages, and at least half are privately insured.

Ambulatory Sites for Surgical and Emergency Care

The 1980s brought increased complaints about the expense of health care, particularly in hospitals, and ushered in the *competitive model*. The idea is that consumer choice and market forces rather than regulation should be used to control health care costs.

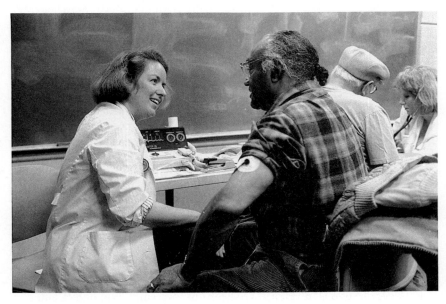

A stroke prevention program is an example of primary care. (*Courtesy of the University of California San Francisco Medical Center.*)

As a result, alternative health care delivery modes, particularly in ambulatory care, developed and expanded. Among these are the *surgicenters*, originally independent proprietary facilities. Some are specialized, such as plastic surgery centers, but in general, the centers can perform any surgery that does not require prolonged anesthesia. Because of their low overhead, surgicenters can charge as little as one-third of hospital costs for the same procedure. Patients like being able to return to home, or even work, the same day. Surgicenters were seen to be the most cost-saving innovation in health care. However, because the unregulated fees soon soared, the government is now stepping in, with DRG-type payment pending. Tentatively, 2509 ambulatory patient groups (APGs) are being suggested, with payment accordingly for all types of ambulatory care.

Private, for-profit, freestanding emergency centers (FECs), also called *emergicenters* or *urgicenters*, first appeared in 1976. Designed to treat episodic, nonurgent health problems, they are among the fastest-growing forms of US health care. The term *freestanding* may refer either to an independent, physician-owned emergicenter or to one that is hospital sponsored or affiliated. Typically, the emergicenters are located in shopping centers or commerical and industrial areas, have a high patient turnover, a short (15- to 20-minute) waiting period, and a cost that may be 30 to 40 percent lower than that of hospital emergency rooms.

Birth Centers

Although some women are again turning to home births attended by midwives, a more popular and growing alternative to hospital births is the *childbearing center*, also called *birth center* or *childbirthing center*. These centers appeared in 1973, when the alienated and questioning middle class became disenchanted with hospital maternity care. The demonstration nurse-midwifery model was the Maternity Center of New York, which was established much earlier. Now out-of-hospital centers are operating in an increasing number of states. About one-third are operated by or utilize nurse-midwives; others are sponsored by physicians and/or lay midwives. There are freestanding centers or variations of them in hospitals. Both allow for more humane care in a high-quality, homelike setting with the father and other children present—all costing considerably less than regular hospital care.

Renal Dialysis Centers

Renal dialysis centers were spurred into massive growth by their inclusion in the 1972 Medicare amendment. Once, the treatment of those with chronic kidney disease by using expensive artificial kidneys was a sensitive matter of deciding who shall live. When Congress decided that all patients should have that opportunity and funded it, the cost rose to unexpected millions of dollars. Many centers are freestanding, mostly physician owned or developed by proprietary organizations, but they also exist in hospitals. A whole new group of specialists at all levels has developed. The desired alternative now is less expensive home dialysis.

Women's Clinics/Family Planning

Women's clinics are usually owned and operated by women concerned about women's health problems and dissatisfied with the quality of care for women and the attitudes of many male health care providers. Most emerged out of the women's movement, along with the consumer and self-care movements. Services may include routine gynecological and maternity care and family planning, as well as some general health care. Emphasis is on self-help, mutual support, and noninstitutional personal care. Both nurse-midwives and lay midwives are used, as are NPs and supportive physicians, although many staff are lay people. In a number of cities and towns, the clinics have been harassed by conservative groups and medical societies, and some have had to become involved in lengthy and expensive legal suits. These should not be confused with women's health care centers developed and operated by hospitals to target this specific clientele.

Family-planning clinics, of which the clinics of Planned Parenthood are most notable, provide a spectrum of birth control services and information. *Abortion clinics* are sponsored by community and other groups, as well as proprietary organizations, or may be a physician's private practice. However, harassment by antiabortion activists, including picketing and sometimes violent action, and a shortage of physicians willing to do abortions, as well as some cutbacks in funding by the government and external funding services, have resulted in limitation of services and even closings in the last few years. A recent US Supreme Court decision considered the harassment of patients and professionals and came down in favor of the public's right to access these facilities.

Mental Health Centers

Mental health centers or *community mental health centers* are intended to provide a wide range of mental health services to a particular geographic catchment area. They may be sponsored by state mental departments, psychiatric hospitals or departments of hospitals, or the federal government. They are staffed by teams of mental health personnel, such as psychiatrists, clinical psychologists, psychiatric nurses, social workers, marriage and family counselors, and community workers. They may consist of single physical entities or networks but are usually for short-term care, including crisis intervention. These centers were originally intended, in part, to prevent the warehousing of mental patients and assist their reintroduction into the community. Unfortunately, deinstitutionalization moved faster than the available community services, and even today there are mentally ill patients living on the streets (estimated at one-fourth to two-fifths of the homeless population), or in deplorable, but less available, single-room occupancy hotels (SROs). While there are good halfway houses, day-care centers, and semi-supervised living services, the services have not caught up with the demand.

There is general agreement that what is needed is a spectrum of services ranging from providing suitable housing to managing serious psychiatric and physical illness, and adequate coordination of these multiple community services. A particular concern is management of the chronically mentally ill, who need psychosocial services of mental health professionals as well as social workers. The noninstitutionalized mentally ill must be reached in many settings, including the streets, shelters, board-and-care facilities, and jails. A recent emphasis is the need for mental health services in rural areas.

Treatment for Substance Abuse

It would be irresponsible to omit some mention of treatment and rehabilitation for substance abuse. Both drug and alcohol abuse are ugly and destructive problems which are more comfortably dismissed in a discussion of the health care delivery system. The antisocial behaviors that often result cloud the health issues and move the platform into the courts as the primary arena for resolution.

Treatment can take the form of a range of possibilities, both residential and outpatient. Methadone maintenance programs (substituting methadone for heroin along with certain rehabilitative measures) have achieved some credibility in the health care community. Drug and alcohol-free programs which combine withdrawal with self-help and a therapeutic residential experience, halfway houses, counseling centers and "hot lines" are all options. Despite these efforts, the problems are frequent and the answers evasive. Some of the best outcomes have been achieved by Alcoholics Anonymous (AA), combining withdrawal and maintenance of abstinence with support from those who have experienced the same pain, self-help, and a good dose of reality therapy (public disclosure and personal confrontation of what you are). Detoxification units have also become common in local hospitals where substance abuse has penetrated every stratum of American society. For referral to one of these programs, local chapters of AA are listed in the phone book.

Adult Day Care

Adult day-care centers are agencies that provide health, social, psychiatric, and nutritional services to infirm individuals who are sufficiently ambulatory to be transported between home and center. Psychogeriatric daycare centers were first opened in 1947 under the direction of the Menninger Clinic. Studies ordered by Congress in 1976 showed daycare centers to be cost-effective, but no national policy on reimbursement followed. Funding now comes from uncoordinated disparate sources, and therefore some communities have set priorities as to who can use the services. Yet, daycare has been shown to be superior to nursing homes to eligible individuals because of lesser cost, improved health and functional outcomes, and an increased quality of life. Unresolved issues are related to their use for young adults with debilitating diseases, the feasibility of rural centers, and the need for regulation and licensing. Currently governmental distinctions exist between medical and social day care. The former requires some presence of health care personnel or some available health care services.

HOSPICES

Another humanistically oriented as well as cost-saving type of care is the *hospice*. The hospice movement was pioneered in Great Britain. The first widely recognized hospice in the United States was Hospice, Inc., established in 1971 in New Haven, Connecticut. Modeled after St. Christopher's in London, it concentrated on improving the quality of patients' last days or months of life so that they could "live until they die."

The Hospice Association of America estimates that there are between 1700 and 1900 hospices in the United States; about 1158 hospitals have hospice services. Medicare classifies hospices into four types: hospital based; home health agency based; skilled nursing facility based; and independent. The first three are part of a larger institution; the independents, of which there are very few, are corporate entities. Hospices may offer inpatient care, home care, or a mix of the two. But whatever the setting, in reality it is a concept, an attitude, a belief that involves support of the family as well as the dying patient. Patients must be aware of their diagnosis and prognosis to qualify for a hospice. Two-thirds of the patients die at home, surrounded by their families and free of technological, life-prolonging devices. Symptom control is a vital first step, and pain-relieving medications are not withheld.

The hospice functions on a 24-hour, 7-day-a-week basis; backup medical, nursing, and counseling services are always available. The typical hospice team consists of a physician and some combination of nurses; medical social workers; psychiatrists; nutritionists; pharmacists; speech, physical, and occupational therapists; and clergy or pastoral counselors. Most hospices serve cancer patients primarily, but many also care for patients with progressive neurological diseases and, now, AIDS. Except for the latter two groups, the majority of hospice patients are elderly. Any patient whose physician certifies that he or she has a life expectancy of less than six months is eligible for hospice care. Studies show that hospice care is less expensive than traditional care, and slowly reimbursement is being offered. Most major private insurance companies and some HMOs reimburse at least partially; however, since hospice care can be an "add-on" benefit, very few patients receive full reimbursement. In 1986, hospice care became a permanent Medicare benefit and an optional Medicaid benefit, but at least 80 percent of the care is supposed to be provided in the home.

GOVERNMENT FACILITIES

In the federal government, at least 25 agencies have some involvement in delivering health services. Those with the largest expenditures in direct federal hospital and medical services are the Department of Veterans Affairs (VA), which operates the largest centrally directed hospital and clinic system in the United States, the Department of Defense (members of the military and dependents), the Indian Health Service (IHS), and the Health Resources and Services Administration (HRSA) of DHHS, which operates one Public Health Service (PHS) hospital and provides care for federal prisoners and Coast Guard personnel. Other DHHS agencies provide indirect funding or contracts for a variety of clinics and the National Health Service Corps.

State and local governments also have multiple functions and multiple services in health care delivery, directly through grants and funding to finance their own programs, and indirectly as third-party payers. Although most states have some version of a state health agency (SHA) or department of public health, health services are often provided through other state agencies, a situation that has created territorial battles, duplication, and gaps.

In providing direct services, some states operate mental, tuberculosis, or other hospitals and alcohol and drug abuse programs, provide non-institutional mental health services, fund public health nursing programs and laboratories, and provide services for maternal and child health, family planning, crippled children, immunization, tuberculosis, chronic respiratory disease control, and venereal disease control. All are considered traditional public health services, in addition to environmental health activities.

On a local level, services offered by a health department depend a great deal on the size, needs, and demands of the constituency. Some large municipalities operate hospitals that provide for the indigent or working poor who are not covered by Medicaid or private insurance. Some health departments run school health services and screening programs. Some duplicate services offered by the state.

There are few data on how much state and local agencies coordinate their services to avoid publication or omission, but lack of coordination or cooperation is not uncommon. Although there is a great deal of criticism of most local health services in relation to high cost, waste, corruption, and poor quality, attempts to terminate any of them, particularly hospitals in medically underserved areas, become political conflicts, with representatives of the poor complaining that no other services are available and that the loss of local jobs will create other hardships. With all the politically sensitive issues involved, most health care experts are pessimistic about reorganization or major improvement of the health systems at any governmental level. Sale of city hospitals to the private sector is being initiated by some mayors, with the intent of saving money. Another emergent trend that may predict an exception to this statement is the recent tendency to privatize both Medicare and Medicaid. Several states have chosen to give their poor a "voucher" to buy into the managed health care plan of their choice. This in fact forces government health care facilities to rise to the cost-efficiency and attactiveness of the private sector. In the same spirit of seeking simplification, talk on Capitol Hill questions whether the existing federal systems should continue to exist as separate entities or should continue to exist at all, the option being to award vouchers for use in the private sector to all individuals having a right to government entitlement programs.

HOME HEALTH CARE

Home health care is probably more of a nurse-oriented health service than any other, originating with Florence Nightingale's "health nurses" and the pioneer efforts of such American nurses as Lillian Wald. (Today the term *public health nurse* or *community health nurse* may also be used here.) Moreover, what Wald worked for in the late nineteenth century—comprehensive services for the patient and family that extend beyond simple care of the sick—is even more pertinent today.

Home care includes a broad spectrum of services from home birthings to hospice care. Medical services are primarily provided by the individual's private or clinic physician, although in some instances agencies will employ or contract for a physician's services. In addition, there are homemaker–home health aide services, required in addition to (or sometimes following) nursing and therapy and consisting of providing personal grooming needs, helping with the practice of self-help skills, and general housekeeping services. Among the other home health services that may be available are medical supplies and equipment (expendable and durable), nutrition, occupational therapy, physical therapy, speech pathology services, and social work. Other services, which may be provided through coordinated efforts of the agency and the community, include audiological services, dental services,

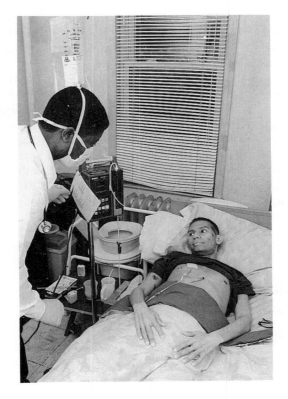

Home care is much more complex today as patients are sent home earlier. (*Courtesy of Visiting Nurse Service of New York.*)

home-delivered meals (Meals on Wheels), information and referral services, laboratory services, ophthalmological services, patient transportation and escort services, podiatry services, prescription drugs, prosthetic/orthotic services, respiratory therapy services, and x-ray services. Home health agencies may also operate adult daycare centers, wellness clinics, hospices, and Meals on Wheels programs.

Agencies that provide home care have various organizational bases. They may operate under public auspice (in many instances linked to health department services), be proprietary (profit making), private non-profit, hospital based or visiting nurse associations (VNAs).

Home care has been a dramatic growth market since the advent of DRGs, and the discharge of patients from hospitals who are sicker and in need of a variety of continuing services. Between 1988 and 1991, Medicare home care expenditures alone increased at an annual rate of 40 percent.[48] There are also some very observable patterns in the growth of Medicare-certified home health agencies. In 1967, before DRGs, over 36.6 percent of agencies were VNAs and 53.6 percent were publicly sponsored; by 1987 only 9.5 percent were VNAs and 18.5 percent public. The most rapid growth was in hospital-based and proprietary agencies, dominating 24.9 percent and 31.9 percent of the market respectively.[49] The National Association for Home Care (NAHC) identified a total of 17,561 "home care agencies" in the United States as of June 1995. These consisted of 8747 Medicare-certified home health agencies, 1795 Medicare-certified hospices, and 7019 home health agencies, home care aide organizations and hospices that do not participate in Medicare.[50]

There has also been a dramatic shift in the sources of payment for home health care. In 1987, 43 percent of these services were paid with out-of-pocket dollars and 46.2 percent through public entitlement; by 1991 personal pay had been reduced to 12.7 percent and governmental sources paid 71.8 percent. This comparison is presented in Exhibit 3.5.

Visiting nurse associations (VNAs) of various names, which are nonprofit voluntary agencies, have been the classic providers of home care. VNAs

EXHIBIT 3.5

Payer Sources for Home Care, 1987 and 1991

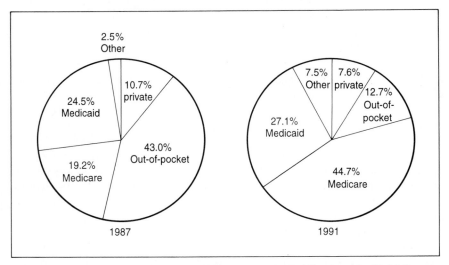

1987   1991

Sources: Agency for Health Care Policy Research, Publication No 93-0040, Rockville, MD, 1993.

Letsch SW, et al, National health expenditures, 1991; in Lee PR, Estes CL (eds): *The Nation's Health.* Boston: Jones and Bartlett, 1994, pp 252–262.

ensure quality care by being overseen by professional advisory committees composed of local physicians, nurses, and other health professionals. They are governed by voluntary boards of directors. Community volunteers assist the VNAs by serving on the board of directors, raising funds for indigent care, visiting patients in their homes, assisting at wellness clinics, delivering meals to patients, running errands for patients, doing VNA office work, and providing support by frequent telephone calls.

The mission of VNAs is to provide quality care to all people, regardless of their ability to pay. Because for-profit agencies dump patients who are no longer reimbursable, which the VNAs then pick up (such as terminal AIDS patients and long-term stroke patients), many VNAs find themselves functioning under tight financial constraints. Nevertheless, VNAs are noted for their high quality of care. They were among the first home health agencies to seek accreditation. Accreditation is offered by both the Community Health Accreditation Program (CHAP), described in Chapter 13, and the Joint Commission on the Accreditation of Health Care Organizations (JCAHO).

Other home care providers are hospital-based home health services, the "hospital without walls" concept. A prototype program was established at Montefiore Hospital in New York City in the late 1940s. Since then, a large number of hospitals have initiated such programs, but the number of services may be limited. In some cases, most services, including nursing, are contracted for, using established voluntary or proprietary agencies already in operation. At times, the program is little more than a coordination of services for continuity of care, which is nevertheless a vast improvement over what is still common—discharge with no follow-up except for a clinic or physician appointment. In part because of the prospective reimbursement system and the consequent pressure to discharge patients as soon as possible, more hospitals have become interested in setting up home care programs as a means of increasing income.

Most aggressive in providing services are the large number of proprietary agencies that are springing up throughout the country. Some offer comprehensive services; others concentrate their efforts on training and deploying home workers and home health aides. In these agencies, operated for profit, marketing is brisk and sophisticated. Although there have been complaints of poor-quality care, the readily available services on a 24-hour-a-day, 7-day-a-week basis have proved to be highly competitive (VNAs are now also providing this round-the-clock service in many places).

One reason for the increase in the interest is the financial support of Medicare/Medicaid. On the other hand, the complex restrictiveness of the regulations, particularly in relation to reimbursable services, leads to quality problems and severe financial burdens for the homebound patient and sometimes the agency. Determining the need for home care is not a simple matter, and varies in terms of both the patient and the environment; in addition, retroactive cost adjustment according to new Medicare rules has sometimes caused severe losses. Some of the VNAs and other agencies that have survived best now plan on a more businesslike basis, and new organizational patterns have emerged. One includes the development of a holding company or major corporation with both a nonprofit (traditional VNA) and a for-profit subsidiary, and others as necessary, somewhat similar to the new hospital models. The for-profit corporation may provide a variety of profitable services, such as home-health aides, chore services for the frail elderly, presurgery counseling before hospital admission, equipment rental, pharmacies, and vocational rehabilitation. The after-tax profits from this corporation are then donated to the nonprofit corporation to provide the free services that have sometimes kept VNAs on the point of bankruptcy.

Both voluntary and official (governmental) agencies have been affected by the financial squeeze, and although total restructuring is not always possible, approaches have been used that were never even considered previously. Some have successfully marketed health teaching–health promotion services to industry and the public. Another developed a new market and gained increased economy by establishing "neighborhood nurse" offices. Other variations are block nursing[51] and nurses working out of the home. Computers have become essential for keeping records and statistics and for case management. Seen as the key by many is marketing of services based on the needs of the consumer. More recently, a number of VNAs are competing to be part of managed care groups. This is a matter of survival, since many of their patients are forced into managed care by their employers.

Comprehensive home health care is being hailed as less expensive than institutional care and as a more effective, humane approach, especially for the elderly and chronically ill. Whether it is indeed cheaper may depend on what supportive services are needed, an issue that is now the focus of serious study.

EMERGENCY MEDICAL
SERVICES (EMS)

Ambulance services, originally a profit venture of funeral directors, are a vital link in transporting accident victims or those suffering acute overwhelming illnesses (such as myocardial infarctions) to a medical facility. In most cases, providing for such services, either directly or through contracts, has now become the responsibility of a community, a responsibility that is not consistently assumed. The unnecessary deaths due to delayed and/or inept care have received considerable attention, which was probably responsible for some important federal legislation.

With continued federal and state funding and regulation, the previous diverse ambulance and rescue services of volunteers, firemen, police, and commerical companies are being coordinated with regional systems. Several hundred are now in place. Criteria include training of appropriate personnel; education of the public; appropriate communication systems, transportation vehicles, and facilities; adequate record keeping; and some participation by the public in policymaking.

Under these laws, a variety of emergency medical technicians (EMTs) have been trained and staff many ambulance services, including mobile intensive-care units, which have very sophisticated equipment.

HOSPITALS

Hospitals are generally classified according to size (number of beds, exclusive of bassinets for newborns); type (general, mental, tuberculosis, or other specialty, such as maternity, orthopedic, eye and ear, rehabilitation, chronic disease, alcoholism, or narcotic addiction); ownership (public or private, including the for-profit, investor-owned proprietary hospital or not-for-profit voluntary hospital, which may be owned by religious, fraternity, or community groups); and length of stay (short-term, with an average stay less than 30 days, or long-term, 30 days or more). Hospitals vary from fewer than 25 to more than 2000 beds. The most common type of hospital has been the voluntary, general, short-term hospital. In September of 1994, these facilities represented 892,126 beds. This is compared with 918,786 beds in 1993. A restructured delivery system will require even fewer beds, and 1994 levels may be reduced an additional 54 percent over time,[51A] according to the American Hospital Association (AHA) many small hospitals have closed for reasons including financial cutbacks in federal funding, pressure by insurance companies and business to reduce health expenditures, and changing health care practices (such as those described earlier). If not closed, the small hospitals are likely to become part of a multi-institutional system, a major trend in health care delivery. These systems may comprise two or more hospitals owned, leased, sponsored, or contract-managed by a central organization. They can be for profit or nonprofit. Advantages can include improved access to capital markets, shared purchasing and technology, economics of scale, and use of technical and management staff. In 1994, there were about 5916 hospitals in the United States.

The primary purpose of hospitals is to provide patient services. However, many also assume a major responsibility for education and research. The term *teaching hospital* is applied to those hospitals with accredited medical residency programs in which medical students and/or residents and specialty fellows (house staff) are taught. It does not include those that provide educational programs or experiences for other health professionals or allied health workers.

Administrative organization of services varies greatly according to administrative philosophy and types of services. Exhibit 3.6 shows a common

EXHIBIT 3.6

One Pattern of Hospital Organization

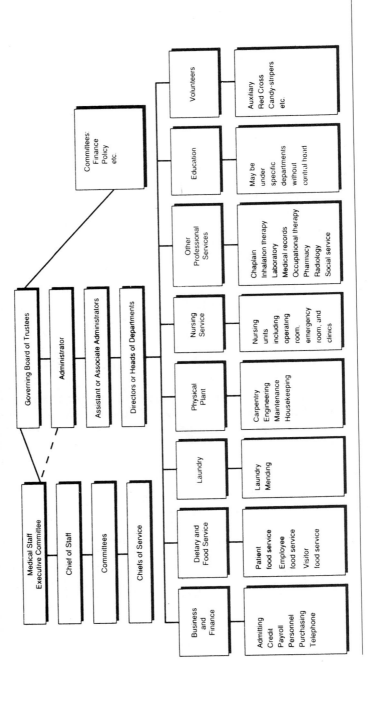

organizational pattern of a general hospital, which illustrates both the lines of authority and the kinds of services available. However, not all of these services or units exist in all hospitals. Size is a factor, but another is the fact that hospitals that are part of a chain sometimes purchase certain services, like food and laundry. The nursing service has the largest number of personnel in the hospital, in part because of round-the-clock, 7-days-a-week staffing. Other departments, such as radiology and clinical laboratories, may maintain some services on evenings and weekends and may be on call at night. There is a trend toward having other clinical services available at least on weekends.

The physical layout of a hospital varies from one-story to high-rise, and may include large or small general or specialized patient units, special intensive care units, operating rooms, recovery rooms, an emergency department, offices (sometimes including doctors' private offices), space for diagnostic and treatment facilities, storage rooms, kitchens and dining rooms, maintenance equipment workrooms, meeting rooms, classrooms, a chapel, waiting rooms, and gift and snack shops. To expand, build, or remodel extensively, hospitals need a certificate of need (CON) from the state. The approval of the pianning agency is based on specific criteria and community need.

Hospitals are licensed by the state and presumably are not permitted to function unless they maintain the minimum standards prescribed by the licensing authority. ("Presumably" because the process of closing a hospital

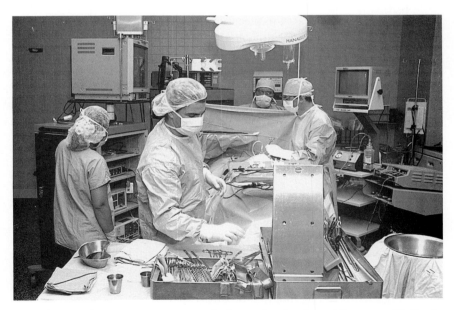

Today's operating rooms are centers of advanced technology. (*Courtesy of Palisades General Hospital, North Bergen, New Jersey.*)

due to inadequate facilities and/or staff is long, difficult, and not always successful.) However, to be eligible for many federal funding programs, such as Medicare, and to be affiliated with educational programs, including medical residency programs, accreditation is necessary. Accreditation by JCAHO is voluntary and is intended to indicate excellence in patient care. Specific standards, usually more rigorous than those of the state, are set to measure hospital efficiency, professional performance, and facilities, and must be met in all facets of health care services (including nursing). Visits are made by an inspection team (that may or may not have a multidisciplinary makeup) that reviews various records and minutes of meetings, interviews key people, and generally scrutinizes the hospital. Reports are made that include criticisms and recommendations for action. Accreditation may be postponed, withheld, revoked, granted, or renewed on the basis of the inspection and review of the hospital's report and self-evaluation. Nurses are now usually included on the inspection team, and there is nursing input into the standards for nursing service. Another external quality check is the federal PRO program. An internal *utilization review committee* is expected to monitor the quality of care (and cost) of federally insured patients (and in some states all patients), using chart reviews. Nurses are often employed in these positions.

Voluntary hospitals are usually organized under a constitution and by-laws that invest the board of trustees with the responsibility for patient care. This governing board is generally made up of individuals representing various professional and business groups interested in the community. Although unsalaried and volunteer (except for proprietary hospitals, in which members are often stockholders), board members are usually extremely influential citizens and are often self-perpetuating on the board. This type of membership originated because at one time administrators of hospitals did not have a business background, and because of the still-present need to raise money to support hospitals. (Most trustees still see recovery of operating costs as their most crucial hospital problem.) Some consumer groups have complained that most members are businessmen, bankers, brokers, lawyers, and accountants, with almost nonexistent representation of women, consumers in general, and labor. Physicians also complain of lack of medical representation, although they work closely with the board and are subordinate to it only in certain matters. Because of these pressures, boards are gradually acquiring broader representation.

It is also possible that there will be some lessening of trustee power as hospitals adopt the corporate model, integrating the board of trustees and the administration of the hospital, with the board having full-time and salaried presidents and vice-presidents. The growth of mergers, consortia, and holding companies that are creating new business-oriented hospital systems may also change the role of trustees.

Public hospitals usually do not have boards of trustees. Hospital administrators are directly responsible to their administrative supervisors in the governmental hierarchy, which may be a state board of health, a commissioner, a department such as the VA, or a public corporation with appointed officials. All are ultimately responsible to the public.

Although *administrator* is still the generic term for the managerial head of a hospital, in recent years this title has included a variety of designations such as *president* and *chief executive officer*, usually called CEO. The hospital administrator, the direct agent of a governing board, implements its policies, advises on new policies, and is responsible for the day-to-day operations of the hospital. Department heads or supervisors are next in the line of authority; these individuals are also gradually becoming specialists by education and experience in their area of responsibility. Nurses, in charge of the largest department, are either department heads or assistant/associate administrators or vice-presidents.

The medical staff organization is made up of selected physicians and dentists who are granted the privilege of using the hospital's facilities for their patients. They, in turn, evaluate the credentials of other physicians who wish to join the staff and recommend appointment to the hospital's governing board, which legally makes the appointments. In some institutions, nurse-midwives, NPs, and other health professionals, such as podiatrists, have been given these practice privileges, which can include the right to admit, treat, or consult about patients.

LONG-TERM CARE FACILITIES

Long-term care services for chronic diseases and conditions are one of the fastest-growing areas of health care. In part this is due to the success of medical science in saving those who once might have died, and in part to the fact that the nuclear family has no place for those who, years ago, were simply cared for at home with no public help. While the use of ambulatory care facilities and a return to home are being recommended, such care requires a considerable number of social and health-related backup services. These are not easy to organize or coordinate and are even less easy to be reimbursed for. Therefore, institutional care for long-term patients, while considerably more expensive and often lessening the individual's quality of life, still appears to be necessary for part of the population.

There are two major categories of long-term care institutions: long-stay hospitals (for example, psychiatric, rehabilitation, chronic disease, and tuberculosis hospitals) and nursing homes. There are about 300 long-term stay hospitals, mostly psychiatric and mostly government owned. According to the American Health Care Association (AHCA), in 1994 there were approximately 16,608 nursing homes that are certified for Medicare and Medicaid, about 67 percent of which were proprietary. There were about 1.5 million persons receiving care in nursing homes in 1993, 13 percent less than 1990.[52]

This does not include residential facilities that may provide some degree of nursing services over and above room, board, and personal care or "custodial" services. About 66 percent of nursing homes have fewer than 100 beds; only 5 percent have more than 200. Although over half are still independently owned and operated, this is decreasing, as chains buy more and more.

Nursing homes can be classified according to the level of care offered and whether they are certified for the Medicare and/or Medicaid programs. According to these regulations, a skilled nursing facility (SNF) which provides inpatient skilled nursing and restorative and rehabilitative services must provide 24-hour nursing services, have transfer agreements with a hospital, and fulfill other specific requirements. An intermediate care facility (ICF) provides inpatient health-related care and services to individuals not requiring SNF care. Nursing homes may be certified for either or both levels; about 25 percent are not certified at all. If certified, PROs monitor them; some are also JCAHO accredited.

The organizational structure of a nursing home is often much like that of a hospital, but there are fewer diagnostic and therapeutic departments, depending on the major purpose of the institution. Usually both short-term and long-term care are offered. The nursing home may or may not be associated with a particular hospital. Some extended-care facilities have expansive services providing a continuum of care from skilled nursing to home care. For those who can afford it, there are complexes in which older people can live in their own apartments for life; health care services, including skilled nursing, are made available when needed. Sometimes a nursing home and even a hospital are on site.

Most of the 1 million employees who care for nursing home residents are aides, sometimes trained and certified, sometimes not. Almost no direct hands-on care is given by licensed nurses, although at least one RN must be employed by every licensed nursing home. That one RN may also be the director of nursing and probably has no degree. Neither do most nursing home administrators. Medical care is also minimal, with few physicians employed by nursing homes. Although it represents a minority of the elderly, the nursing home population is very old, with 85 percent over 75 years and more than 10 percent over 90. Patients usually have three to four chronic illnesses; half have psychiatric diagnoses. However, a major predictor of nursing home admission is inability to manage activities of daily living (ADL). The majority of residents are poor, white, unmarried, or widowed women, whose sole significant source of income is a survivor (not retiree) Social Security check. The lack of Hispanics and Blacks is seen as due to inequity in access to services, not cultural preferences. In almost all cases, residents in a nursing home lack financial resources and/or family members to care for them outside. Over half of the patients stay less than six months, but after three years, discharge is usually to a terminal hospital stay or "discharged dead." Except in the best nursing homes, there is minimal social activity.

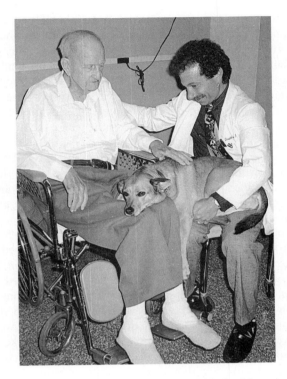

Pet therapy can be a meaningful experience for the elderly. (*Courtesy of Daughters of Miriam Center/Rutgers Teaching Nursing Home, Clifton, New Jersey.*)

The cost of nursing home care is quite high on a long-term basis, and often the patient and spouse must "spend down" their assets until the patient is eligible for Medicaid. About 69 percent of nursing home residents are financed by Medicaid. Not long ago, this practice could have reduced the spouse to poverty, but recent legislation allows the spouse to keep both assets and a monthly income at a more reasonable (but still not generous) level. Some elderly people are still often upset that their hard-earned savings, which they have hoped to leave to their children, are almost wiped out when nursing home care is necessary. Whether or not another law like the Catastrophic Coverage Act (enacted in 1988 and repealed in 1989, because some elderly people objected to the surcharge all would need to pay) will eventually cover long-term care is questionable. It is difficult to get agreement on what people need and what the government and taxpayers are willing to pay.

Nursing homes are considered good business opportunities for investors, many of whom believe that more elderly people will have good investments in years to come and can pay the ever-increasing rates. And these are the kinds of clients they seek—not the Medicaid patients, with relatively low reimbursement and more governmental oversight. There are now some insurance plans (rather expensive) that cover nursing home care, but Medicare covers very little. This situation may change, since a number of SNFs now care for patients who require complex care and technology that was once seen only in hospitals. Giving intravenous (IV) fluids is common, as are tube feedings. Some extended-care facilities have set up geriatric intensive-care units (GICUs) for ventilator-dependent patients. Caring for these patients usually requires coordination with the hospital, where the nursing home staff may receive appropriate training. For such GICUs, the staff mix is different, with more nurses and often a geriatric nurse practitioner (GNP). The variation in care needed by LTC patients will also probably affect the prospective payment and classification systems used by some states, such as the Resource Utilization Groups (RUGs) which includes multiple categories to reflect patient needs.

Aside from the cost, another issue is the quality of nursing homes. In 1989, the Health Care Financing Administration (HCFA) released a 75-volume report on the 15,000 nursing homes that then participated in Medicare and Medicaid programs. This, like earlier investigations, revealed many serious discrepancies in both the environment and care. Regulations for the 1987 OBRA nursing home reform law were then finally put into effect, but they drew fire from almost everyone: nursing homes said they were too tough and expensive, health groups that they were too weak. One key element was the requirement for 24-hour "licensed nurse" coverage, with an RN on duty on the day shift. Coupled with a generous waiver clause, it was possible that nursing home patients could be entirely without an RN. One happier note was that physicians could designate an NP (or PA) to make some of the required visits to nursing home residents, and that nurses' aides must be given a minimum of 75 hours of training. Nurses' aides give up to 85 percent of the care and are often given little or no training. Among other improvements were requirements for a full-time social worker in facilities with more than 120 beds; rehabilitation and dental services; no admissions of mentally ill patients except those with Alzheimer's or related dementia; and residents' guarantee of freedom from abuse, excessive medication, and punitive physical or chemical restraints. Other rights were also spelled out. These regulations do not apply to noncertified facilities.

There will probably still be complaints about the quality of life, if not always the quality of physical care, in nursing homes. In some areas, voluntary ombudsmen regularly make checks to prevent or detect abuses. There are also a few adopt-a-grandparent or similar programs that give the residents caring social contacts outside the home. The factors generally listed by residents as important to quality of care are an adequate, competent, caring staff, a homelike environment, properly prepared and varied food, activities, and medical care. No doubt, if these were present in most nursing homes, people would not be as reluctant, even frightened, to be admitted to them.[53]

Experts disagree on the future of nursing homes. Nursing homes chiefly serve socially isolated women, a group that is increasing, but no one seems to want to expand the nursing home system because of concerns about cost and quality of care. Yet if all home care and support services were reimbursed, the latent demand might cause a financial catastrophe, since almost all of that care is now given by family and friends without reimbursement. As the older population increases, so does the need for a reasonable plan for their long-term care needs.

Managed Care

It is impossible to speak of health care in the mid-1990s without giving significant attention to managed care: what it is, what it is not, what it hopes to accomplish.

Managed care is not a place, but an organizational structure. More correctly, it is a variety of organizational structures that use active risk sharing to provide the best value in health care to a defined group of enrollees or members of a plan. The goal of managed care is to require the decision makers, who are the consumers, payers, and providers, to carefully consider the merit of services, procedures, and treatments in view of the resources available to them. Because of the rapid growth of managed care plans and their intent to cut costs, the question of whether the care is of high quality is being raised with increasing frequency.

Managed care includes three basic types of arrangements: the health maintenance organization (HMO), preferred provider organization (PPO), and managed indemnity health insurance plans. In addition, there are growing variations on each of these themes, so that no one definition remains totally pure. Two common features being inserted into managed care systems are the "point-of-service" option and the "single point of entry."[54] The former guarantees the right to select a nonparticipating provider any time you wish without prior approval. This privilege usually includes higher premiums, copayments, or deductibles. The latter requires system entry through a point designated by the entity at risk (the plan) and is usually a primary health care provider. Extensive data collection proves that nurses in advanced practice are especially suitable for this role.[55]

The HMO combines the delivery and financing of services into one system. The HMO assumes an explicit contractual responsibility to provide a stated range of services. There is an enrolled, defined population who agree to a fixed periodic payment (capitation rate) that is established independent of the actual utilization of services by the enrollees. The HMO assumes financial risk but exerts control on the use of services. These services may be provided in facilities which they own, most usually for the ambulatory care component, or at sites where they have contractual arrangements. The name *health maintenance organization* evolved from the fact that priority is accorded to teaching, counseling, and self-care activities that promote health and independence, therefore reducing the cost to the plan for more complex medical services. It is to the HMO's advantage to avoid hospitalization as the most expensive component of the health care industry.

In comparison, the PPO is somewhat between the HMO and standard indemnity plans in the degree to which it shapes prescribing (the provider) and consumption (the consumer) behaviors. The PPO offers financial incentives for membership by creating a network of providers who agree to reduced fees for enrollees. Because of the lower cost, you are tempted to select from the panel of preferred providers. In most plans, the enrollee maintains the right to go "out of network" for services if desired (point of service option), and on those occasions the indemnity plan "kicks in." In essence, the PPO is an agreement among a limited group of providers to reduce fees for individuals intending exclusive (more or less) use of their services.

Indemnity plans (financial protection against the cost associated with covered service) have incorporated some techniques of managed care. Preauthorization, second opinion for surgery, continued stay certification, discharge planning, and even copayment and deductibles are strategies of managed care. The decision lies with the consumer, but the goal is to introduce an incentive to be prudent.

THE CAREGIVERS: A GROWING NUMBER

A hundred years ago, trained caregivers consisted of physicians, dentists, some pharmacists, and nurses. Now there are more than 250 acknowledged health occupations, with more being developed every day. In 1990, the number of health-related employees was over 8.7 million, one of every twelve workers in the United States. This figure includes certain supportive services. Health care facilities, like other places of business, employ secretaries, clerks, accountants, receptionists, messengers, and others to carry on business operations. In addition, institutions need laundry workers, dietary workers, cooks, plumbers, electricians, carpenters, maids, porters, and similar kinds of employees to function in the hotel-keeping aspect of their services. Not included in any category are faith healers, root doctors, or certain untrained healers who rely on herbs, meditation, or other semi–self-care techniques of healing. Nor does it include independent practitioners or others who are self-employed.

The overwhelming growth of personnel is in direct health services. Many of the health occupations and suboccupations have emerged because of increased specialization in health care, others on the peculiar assumption that several less-prepared workers can substitute for one scarcer professional. Some of these workers can be employed in almost any health setting—hospitals, nursing homes, clinics, doctors' offices, occupational health, and school health. Some work primarily in one setting. Most of these workers are not licensed; many are trained in on-the-job programs, and even more are trained in a variety of programs with no consistent standards. Others have standardized programs approved by the AMA and/or other health organizations. This entire group, categorized as *allied health manpower* (AHM) by the federal government, includes almost any health worker engaged in activities that support, complement, or supplement the professional functions of physicians, dentists, and registered nurses.

Services rendered by AHM range across the entire spectrum of service delivery and include every aspect of patient care, as well as services provided as part of community health promotion and protection. AHM range from personnel with complex functions and the highest educational degrees, who have always had a great deal of autonomy, to those who function in relatively simple assisting roles and must be supervised, sometimes by others categorized as AHM. Because of this diversity, as well as changes in health care, there are also many changes occurring within occupations/professions so identified. Since such a large percentage of health care personnel are AHM, it is ironic that there are so little fundamental data. This is blamed on the elasticity of supply and the constant evaluation of the roles and responsibilities of certain occupations.

At one time, most AHM were educated in almost apprentice-like programs in hospitals. Many AHM programs are now offered in a junior college setting, with the hospital remaining as a clinical practice site. Credentialing of health care providers and their educational programs is under a variety of auspices: the state, a single professional organization, or a coalition of professional organizations, such as the Commission on Accreditation of Allied Health Education Programs (CAAHEP), a collaborative effort of national health organizations and medical specialty organizations with the American Medical Association (AMA). CAAHEP accredits the educational programs of seventeen allied health occupations. Practitioners who are not licensed may become certified or registered on a voluntary basis by the occupation's national organization or a parent medical group. The inconsistency of these various processes is the focus of some of the complaints about health care credentialing. The following health personnel are licensed in every state: nursing home administrators, chiropractors, dentists, dental hygienists, practical nurses, professional nurses, optometrists, pharmacists, physical therapists, physicians (MD and DO), podiatrists, psychologists, and veterinarians, but many others are licensed in *some* state. This does not necessarily mean that licensure is required, only that it is available (see Chapter 11).

The largest categories of health workers, in order, are nursing (all types, including aides), physicians, dentists and their allied services, clinical laboratory workers, pharmacists, and radiological technicians. As feminists are the first to point out, *manpower* is a misnomer; from 75 to 85 percent are women. However, they are, or have been, in the lower-paid and less powerful positions. Except for the independent practitioners who are primarily self-employed, the mass of health workers are employed in institutions and agencies, with the greatest number concentrated in hospitals.

It would be unrealistic to attempt to describe all the professional and technical workers with whom nurses work or interact. However, an introduction to the most prevalent health occupations should provide a better understanding of the complex relationships in health care. Appendix 2 puts these in a format that allows comparison of numbers, education, credentials, and issues.

The organization of this section is primarily alphabetical, although two closely related groups may be described in logical succession. The education of RNs and practical nurses is described in Chapter 5 and the practice of nursing in Chapter 6.

Administration

Health services administrators manage organizations, agencies, institutions, programs, and services within the health care delivery system. They may work in any setting but are probably more visible in hospitals, academic medical centers, nursing homes, neighborhood health centers, and community health agencies.

Other positions in the operation of health facilities and plants are the usual business positions, finance, data processing, personnel, public relations, and admissions, with all types of jobs and educational levels.

Chiropractic

Chiropractic is described by the American Chiropractic Association (ACA) as "a branch of the healing arts which is concerned with human health and disease processes. Doctors of chiropractic are physicians who consider man as an integrated being, but give special attention to spinal mechanics and neurological, muscular, and vascular relationships." Chiropractors use standard diagnostic measures, but treatment methods, determined by law, do not include prescription drugs and surgery. Essentially, treatment includes "the chiropractic adjustment, necessary dietary advice and nutritional supplementation, necessary physiotherapeutic measures, and necessary professional counsel." Most chiropractors are in private practice. All 50 states, the District of Columbia, and Puerto Rico recognize chiropractic as a health profession and authorize these services for workmen's compensation. They are also reimbursable by Medicare and Medicaid.

Clinical Laboratory Sciences

There are a number of technicians or technologists working in the clinical laboratories in such specialties as immunohematology, hematology, clinical chemistry, serology, microbiology, and histology. The physician in charge is a pathologist, although technologists may have specific responsibilities for technicians. *Medical technologists* are prepared for all phases of clinical laboratory work. *Certified laboratory assistants*, who perform routine laboratory tests, and *histological technicians*, who prepare body tissues for microscopic examination by pathologists, are usually prepared in one-year hospital programs.

Dentistry

Dentists treat oral diseases and disorders. They may fill cavities, extract teeth, and provide dentures for patients. About 15 percent of dentists specialize, selecting orthodontics (straightening teeth), oral and maxillofacial surgery (operate on mouth and jaw), pediatric dentistry, periodontics (treating gums), endodontics (root canal therapy), oral pathology, public health dentistry, or prosthodontics (making artificial teeth). These specialties usually require two or more additional years of training and a specialty board examination. Nine out of ten dentists are in private practice; the others practice in institutions, the armed forces, and health agencies, teach, or do research. An increasing number of minorities and women are entering the field.

Dental hygienists, almost all women, provide dental services under a dentist's supervision. They examine and clean teeth, give fluoride treatments, take x-rays, and educate patients about proper care of teeth and gums. In many states, hygienists' responsibilities have been expanded to include duties traditionally performed by dentists, such as giving local anesthetics.

Dental assistants maintain supplies, keep dental records, schedule appointments, prepare patients for examinations, process x-rays, and assist the dentist at chairside, but their functions are also expanding.

Dental technicians or *denturists* make and repair dentures, crowns, bridges, and other appliances, usually according to dentists' prescriptions. They are lobbying to work directly with patients and have become licensed in some states.

Dietetics and Nutrition

Nutritionist is a general occupational title for health professionals concerned with food science and human nutrition. They include dietitians, home economists, and food technologists.

Dietitians may have a general dietary background or preparation in medical dietetics. Medical or therapeutic dietitians are responsible for selection of appropriate foods for special diets, patient counseling, and sometimes management of the dietary service. More and more are becoming licensed and are seeking third-party reimbursement.

Clinical dietitians work with patients not only in the hospital, but in clinics, neighborhood health centers, or in the patient's own home.

Dietetic technicians graduate from one of two kinds of ADA-approved technical programs with an associate degree. A program with food service management emphasis allows the individual to serve as a technical assistant to a food service director and, with experience, to become a director. The program with nutritional care emphasis enables the individual to become a technical assistant to the clinical dietitian.

Most *dietetic assistants* serve as *food service supervisors* in hospitals, schools, and nursing homes. However, a number of food service supervisors currently functioning in that position lack such preparation.

Health Educators

Community health educators help identify the health learning needs of the community, particularly in terms of prevention of disease and injury. They may then plan, organize, and implement appropriate programs, for example, screening, health fairs, classes, and self-help groups. Some health educators are employed by the state as consultants, others by insurance companies, voluntary health organizations such as the American Heart Association, the school system (school health educators), and, occasionally, industry.

A number of hospitals are employing *patient educators* or health educators to develop and direct programs of both patient education and community health education. Frequently, these people are nurses with or without training in health education and administration. In a few states, health educators are registered and/or certified.

Medical Records

Medical record administrators are responsible for preparation, collation, and organization of patient records, maintaining an efficient filing system, and making records available to those concerned with the patient's subsequent care. They may also classify and compile data for review committees and researchers.

Medical record technicians assist the physician and the administrator in preparing reports and transcribing histories and physicals. They also work closely with others using patient records.

Medical record transcriptionists have specialized courses in terminology, in addition to typing and filing.

Medicine

Doctors of medicine and osteopathy practice prevention, diagnosis, and treatment of disease and injury. *Doctor of medicine degrees* (MDs), awarded in more than 100 allopathic medical schools, are considered the first professional degree. Some physicians may later decide to acquire advanced degrees (master's or doctorates) in an advanced science or public health.

The formalized program of education after the MD degree is titled *graduate medical education* and consists primarily of the residency, which involves preparation for specialties, a period of two to five years. On completion of the specified years of residency, the physician may take certification exams in the specialty and is board-certified. If exams are not taken (or failed), he or she is board-eligible. In some cases, continuing medical education is required for recertification. Ninety percent of American physicians choose specialties as their field of practice; however, this is changing slowly, since there is an oversupply of specialists and many are not being accepted into managed care plans because the need is for primary care physicians. In medical centers, a *fellow* is a postresidency physician who enters even more advanced, highly specialized, or research-oriented programs, although presumably still involved in teaching and patient care. Graduate medical education is under the direction of medical school faculty recognized as specialists or subspecialists.

Physicians practice in every setting where medical care is provided, as well as in medical or public health education, public health practice, and research. About 50 percent are now employees (not in private practice), with the number increasing as HMOs enroll the physicians' patients, cutting down on their practice. Some positions, such as that of medical director, are primarily administrative and are beginning to be recognized as such.

The number of women in medical schools has increased and there has been a slight increase in under-represented minorities.

Doctors of osteopathy (DOs) are qualified to be licensed as physicians and to practice all branches of medicine and surgery. DOs graduate from colleges of osteopathic medicine, accredited by the Bureau of Professional Education of the American Osteopathic Association (AOA). After graduation, almost all DOs serve a 12-month rotating internship, with primary emphasis on medicine, obstetrics/gynecology, and surgery, conducted in an approved osteopathic hospital. Those wishing to specialize must serve an additional three to five years of residency. Continuing education is required by the AOA for all DOs in practice.

Osteopathic physicians are considered separate but equal in American medicine; they are licensed in all states and have the same rights and obligations as allopathic (MD) physicians. The "something extra" they claim is emphasis on biological mechanisms by which the musculoskeletal system interacts with all body organs and systems in both health and disease. They prescribe drugs, use routine diagnostic measures, perform surgery, and selectively utilize accepted scientific modalities of care. DOs comprise about 5 percent of all physicians; most are general practitioners who provide primary care, usually in small cities and towns and rural areas. Osteopathic physicians are chiefly located in states with osteopathic hospitals. In 1994, 4 out of 5 DOs were practicing in 16 states, most were in Michigan followed by Pennsylvania, Ohio, Florida, Texas and New Jersey.[56]

Medical assistants (MAs) are usually employed in physicians' offices, where they perform a variety of administrative and clinical tasks to help the doctor; however, some work in hospitals and clinics. They perform tasks required by the doctor and are supervised by the doctor. The medical assistant, among other things, answers the telephone; greets patients and other callers; makes appointments; handles correspondence and filing; arranges for diagnostic tests, hospital admissions, and surgery; handles patients' accounts and other billings; processes insurance claims, including Medicare claims; maintains patient records; prepares patients for examinations or treatment; takes patients' temperature, height, and weight; sterilizes instruments; assists the physician in examining or treating patients; and, if trained, performs laboratory procedures. Most are trained in one- or two-year programs.

Physician Assistants (PAs)

In 1965, Dr. Eugene A. Stead, Jr., of Duke University inaugurated a program for *physician's assistants* (PAs), later called *physician's associates*, designed to assist physicians in their practice, either to enable them to expand that practice, or to give them time to pursue continuing education, or to have more time for themselves and their families. The generally accepted name now is *physician assistant*.

PA programs are found primarily in schools of allied health, four-year colleges, and allopathic medical schools, with a few each in community colleges, teaching hospitals, and federal facilities. All these accredited programs have medical facilities and clinical medical teaching affiliations of some kind. The clinical rotations or preceptorships introduce the student to potential areas of expertise, including family medicine, internal medicine, surgery, pediatrics, psychiatry, obstetrics/gynecology, and emergency medicine. This is intended to prepare the PA to:

1. Elicit a comprehensive health history.
2. Perform a comprehensive physical examination.

3. Order and interpret simple diagnostic laboratory tests.
4. Develop diagnoses and management plans.
5. Provide basic treatment for individuals with common illnesses.
6. Provide clinical care for individuals with commonly encountered emergency needs.
7. Develop treatment plans and explain them to patients. They may recommend medications and drug therapies and, in more than one-half of the states, have the authority to write prescriptions.

In addition to specific technical procedures that PAs perform, which vary with the practice setting, they carry out a variety of minor surgical procedures. They also may provide pre- and postoperative care. Surgeon assistants (graduates of specialized training programs) and PAs with surgical training often act as first or second assistants in major surgery. By law, all activities must be done under the supervision of a physician.

In recent years, PA residency programs ranging from 9 to 12 months have been developed that provide further classroom and clinical education in various specialties. Some offer certificates and a few offer a master's degree. PA education is not seen as part of a career ladder leading to MD licensure, although some PAs may go to medical school later, just as they may turn to schools of public health or nursing in a career change. Lack of career choices without shifting to another discipline is a PA complaint.

Most PA graduates take the certification exam given by the National Commission on Certification of Physician Assistants (NCCPA), which requires that educational programs be accredited by CAAHEP. Although not all PAs are certified, most states (and employers) require certification in order to practice. About 92 percent were certified in 1992. The statutory provisions for utilization of PAs vary from state to state, but because PAs cannot practice without the supervision of a physician, licensure is almost unheard of. This may change; the Federation of State Medical Board's model Medical Practice Act includes PAs.

Most PAs are employed in one of three specialty areas: family medicine; surgery, including subspecialties; and internal medicine. Surgery is increasingly favored. Although about 35 percent work with physicians in private or group offices and another 30 percent in a variety of clinics, the trend is toward employment by hospitals. One reason is that medical residents' hours are being limited and PAs are being hired to fill in the gap for patient care, especially in the emergency room and in assisting the doctor in the operating room (OR). There are still a large percentage practicing in rural areas or small towns (mostly men), but hospital employment in larger cities and suburbs is becoming more common, especially for women. (About 40 percent are women, 9 percent of all practicing PAs are from minority ethnic groups.) Some say that demand is a major factor; others point out that PAs must go where there is a doctor to supervise them, and doctors prefer urban and suburban areas over rural ones. In reality, though, those in rural clinics are "supervised" from a distance. Salaries of PAs have increased in the last few years differing with the specialty, setting, and geographic location. Women consistently earn less than men, even when they have the same education and experience. (Sometimes PAs earn more than NPs in the same setting.) Medicare and Medicaid policies governing coverage for PA services in hospitals and other institutions encourage their employment. PAs often care for underserved populations in rural areas, inner-city neighborhoods, substance abuse clinics, prison systems, and long-term care facilities. They are also actively involved in the treatment of HIV-infected persons at all levels, from ordering tests to counseling patients. Thirty-eight states grant prescription authority to PAs.

There are still many unresolved issues related to PA practice, particularly in relation to role and functions. The AHA has published a statement on PAs in hospitals, which, overall, indicates that the medical staff and administration should formulate guidelines under which the PA can operate, with the request for the PA to be permitted to practice in the hospital being handled by the medical staff credentials committee. Emphasis is on medical supervision; however, current reality has shown that PAs go unsupervised in busy urban hospitals where they handle many emergency and other ambulatory patients. This has created a problem for nurses, for the authority of the PA *vis-à-vis* the nurse is frequently not clear. Although the nurses' associations, some state boards, some courts, and attorneys general have indicated that nurses do not take orders from PAs, in other states the rulings are the reverse. Because the PA usually functions according to a protocol specified by the employer-physician, an operational agreement may be reached similar to the basis on which a nurse carries out standing orders or some verbal orders from the physician. Nevertheless, there is frequently interdisciplinary conflict when roles are not clarified.

Emergency Medical Technicians

Emergency medical technicians (EMTs) recognize, assess and manage medical emergencies involving acutely ill or injured persons in prehospital settings. They may administer cardiac resuscitation, treat shock, provide initial care to poison or burn victims, and transport patients to a health facility.

In addition to the EMT-Ambulance (EMT-A), the entry level worker, there are two other levels of EMTs, known in most places as EMT-Intermediates (EMT-Int) and EMT-Paramedics. The former may assess trauma patients, administer intravenous therapy, use antishock garments and esophageal airways. They are widely used in rural areas. EMT-Paramedics are trained in advanced life support. Working in radio communication with a provider professional, they may in most states administer drugs, interpret EKGs, perform endotracheal intubation, and defibrillate.

EMTs are employed by community fire and police departments, by private ambulance services, and in hospital emergency departments.

Nursing Support Personnel

Nursing assistants, nurse's aides, orderlies, and *attendants* functioning under the direction of nurses are all part of the group of ancillary workers prepared to assist in nursing care, performing many simple nursing tasks, as well as other helping activities besides nursing. Usually training occurs on the job and is geared to the needs of the particular employing institution, but there has been some increase in public school programs within vocational high school tracks or as outside public education services. The program may vary in length from six to eight weeks or more and costs little or nothing. Commercial programs usually cost the student an unreasonable amount, make unrealistic promises of jobs, and frequently give no clinical experience; therefore these "graduates" are seldom employed. Sometimes students who drop out of certain practical nurse programs after six weeks receive a certificate as aides. In-service education during employment is relatively common. The difference in training, patient care assignment, and ability may be enormous on both an individual and an institutional basis. These workers are not licensed but must be certified to work in long-term care if the facility expects Medicare reimbursement.

Under a change in the Medicare law, assistants employed in LTC nursing facilities participating in Medicare and Medicaid programs must complete 75 hours of training and pass a competency exam. This awards a *certification* as a *long-term care aide.* One program, introduced by AHCA, uses interactive video, with practice exams (since nursing assistants often are not accustomed to test taking). There is also considerable concern that these "chronic care workers," usually middle-aged, the sole support of a family, and a dispro-portionate minority, are not only undertrained but underpaid, with few benefits available. The turnover is great because of these reasons as well as their low status, few opportunities for advancement, and with sicker patients, a stressful working environment. Consequently, there is an increased tendency to seek union representation.

The major concern about the use of unlicensed assistive personnel (UAP) seems to be focused on the hospital. Since the salaries of professional nurses have increased and, in the wake of the recent shortage, considerable restructuring of nursing care has occurred, UAPs seem to be used more extensively in acute care hospitals. Often, there are no consistent criteria for training or responsibilities nor were there any studies on cost-effectiveness.

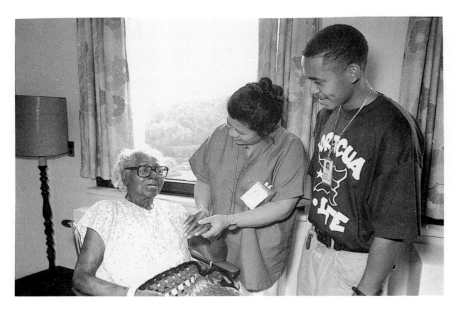

Nurses' aides and volunteers add a great deal to the well-being of patients in nursing homes. (*Photo by Joe Vericker. Courtesy of Terence Cardinal Cooke Health Care Center, New York.*)

Issues of competence, motivation, security, and supervision have been raised.[57] Staff nurses say that they need more "help," yet UAPs generate fear, distrust, and a perception of inadequate preparation. Nursing must move to clarify these issues.[58]

Community health aides of various kinds are found in ambulatory care settings, especially in disadvantaged areas. Community residents are sometimes recruited and trained as health aides. There is usually a limited period of education with ongoing supervision and on-the-job instruction. Certain technical skills are learned, such as auditory and visual screening, but the primary purpose is to identify health problems or deficiencies, such as lack of immunization, poor oral hygiene, dermatological problems, and child development problems, and to assist and encourage families to seek and continue necessary medical, nursing, and other services. Community health aides may also go into the community to do case finding rather than wait for the client to appear in the formal health facility.

As more attention is focused on keeping people at home rather than in institutions, the services of *homemaker/home health aides* have become reimbursable by Medicaid, Medicare, or other governmental funding sources under certain circumstances. The aide is assigned to the home of a family or individual when home life is disrupted by illness, disability, or other problems, or if the family unit is in danger of breakdown because of stress. Specific tasks include parenting, performing or helping with household tasks, providing personal care such as bed baths or helping with prescribed exercises, and providing emotional support. Educational programs are usually developed by the employing agency in a 60-hour (or less) course. Most aides already have housekeeping skills; even so, there is some question as to how effectively they can be prepared in the limited time suggested. In 1989, New Jersey was the first state to certify this group, requiring certain criteria. As others follow, educational requirements will probably be raised.

There is an increasing tendency for proprietary agencies to offer homemaker/home health care services and to contract these workers out to voluntary agencies. Although there is evidence that a well-trained, conscientious home/health aide can be extremely helpful to a sick person or disrupted family, there are also some serious problems in the selection of workers, the quality of training, and supervision. There are also some reimbursement problems when the homemaking part of the aide's function is reimbursable and the health part is not, or vice versa. Most often, a combination of the services is needed by the client. Ongoing assessment by health professionals is intended to evaluate the need of the family/client for specific services. The lack of reimbursement often prevents the use of homemaker/home health aides, for this can cost hundreds of dollars a month. Still, it is a less costly health service than institutional care.

Surgical technicians or *surgical technologists* function in the operating room and sometimes the delivery room. Under the direction of the operating room supervisor, an RN, they perform required tasks, such as setting up for surgery, preparing instruments and other equipment before surgery, "scrubbing in" for surgery (assisting the surgeons by handing instruments, sutures, and so on), and otherwise assisting in the operating room.

The psychiatric/mental health technician is found in psychiatric and general hospitals, community mental health centers, and the home, working with the mentally disturbed, disabled, or retarded under the direction of a physician and/or nurse. In hospitals, he or she is concerned with the patient's daily life as it affects his or her physical, mental, and emotional well-being, including eating, sleeping, recreation, development of work skills, adjustments, and individual and social relations. In the community, the focus is on social relationships and adjustments. In the hospitals, psychiatric technicians are expected to give some routine and emergency physical nursing care, but their close contact with patients makes observation and reporting of the patient's behavior particularly important. In some institutions they function almost independently in group therapy and counseling, seeking consultation as necessary. They may be skilled in nursing, communication techniques, counseling, training techniques, and group therapy.

Ward (unit) clerks or *ward (unit) secretaries* are usually trained on the job in an inservice program to assist in the clerical duties involved in the administration of a nursing unit. Ward clerks order supplies, keep certain records, answer telephones, take messages, attend to the massive amount of routine paperwork and, in some cases, copy doctors' orders.

Unit managers take even broader responsibilities in the management of a patient unit (usually in a larger institution) and may report directly to the hospital administration instead of the nursing service administration. Unit clerks often function under the direction of unit managers. In some institutions, unit management is an early step in an administrative career, and managers have full administrative responsibilities.

Pharmacy

Pharmacists are specialists in the science of drugs and require a thorough knowledge of chemistry and physiology. They may dispense prescription and nonprescription drugs, compound special preparations or dosage forms, serve as consultants, and advise physicians on the selection and effects of drugs.

With the increase of prepackaged drugs and the use of pharmacy assistants, pharmacists in hospitals and clinics are becoming interested in a more patient-oriented approach to their practice. They may be involved in patient rounds, patient teaching, and consultation with nurses and physicians. Pharmacists working in (or owning) drugstores have also been encouraged to increase their client education efforts in terms of explaining medications.

Besides the traditional responsibilities of pharmacists, the doctor of pharmacy (Pharm D) or clinical pharmacist provides consultation with the physician, maintains patient drug histories and reviews the total drug regimen of patients, monitors patient charts in ECFs and recommends drug therapy, makes patient rounds, and provides individualized dosage regimens. In some states, such as California, clinical pharmacists may also prescribe (as do NPs and PAs), with certain limitations.

Podiatry

Podiatrists, doctors of podiatric medicine (DPM) (once called *chiropodists*), are professionally trained foot care specialists who diagnose, treat, and try to prevent diseases, injuries, and deformities of the feet. Treatment may include surgery, medication, physical therapy, setting fractures, and preparing orthoses (supporting devices that mechanically rearrange the weightbearing structures of the foot). Podiatrists may note symptoms of diseases manifested in the feet and legs and refer the patient to a physician. Most podiatrists are in private practice; others practice in institutions, agencies, the military, education, and research.

Podiatric assistants aid podiatrists in office management and patient care.

Mental Health Practitioners

Besides the physician (the psychiatrist), clinical psychologists, psychotherapists, nurses, social workers, and a variety of semiprofessionals trained in mental health participate in individual and group therapy. Psychologists may also give and interpret various personality and behavioral tests, as might a *psychometrician*, who is skilled in the testing and measuring of mental and psychological ability, efficiency, potentials, and functions.

Public Health

Industrial hygienists deal with the effects of noise, dust, vapor, radiation, and other hazards common to industry on workers' health. They are usually employed by industry, laboratories, insurance companies, or government to detect and correct these hazards.

Sanitarians, sometimes called *environmentalists*, apply technical knowledge to solve problems of sanitation in a community. They develop and implement methods to control those factors in the environment that affect health and safety, such as rodent control, sanitary conditions in schools, hotels, restaurants, and areas of food production and sales. Most work in government under the direction of a health officer or administrator.

Biostatisticians apply mathematics and statistics to research problems related to health. *Epidemiologists* study the factors that influence the occurrence and course of human health problems, including not only acute and chronic diseases but also accidents, addictions, and suicides.

Radiology

Radiologists are physicians who deal with all forms of radiant energy, from x-rays to radioactive isotopes; they interpret radiographic studies and prescribe therapy for diseases, particularly malignancies. A number of technicians work under the direction of a radiologist in radiology departments. They operate equipment, prepare patients, and keep records. These include the *radiologic technologist*, sometimes called *x-ray technician* or *radiology technician*; *radiation therapy technician* or *technologist*; and *nuclear medicine technologist*.

Rehabilitation Services

Occupational therapy is concerned with the use of purposeful activity in the promotion and maintenance of health, prevention of disability, and evaluation of behavior. Persons with physical or psychosocial dysfunction are treated using procedures based on social, self-care, educational, and vocational principles. One important responsibility is helping patients with activities of daily living. Adaptive tools such as aids for eating or dressing may also be provided.

Occupational therapists (OTs), the professional workers, and *occupational therapy assistants and aides* are usually employed in rehabilitation settings. However, OTs may also work in private practice or for nursing homes, community agencies, or hospitals.

Physical therapy (PT) is concerned with the restoration of function and the prevention of disability following disease, injury, or loss of a body part.

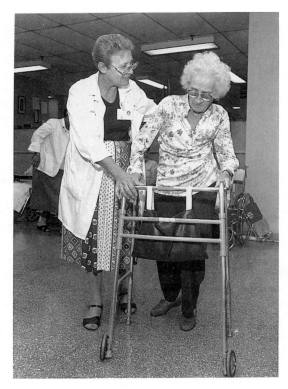

Rehabilitation services aim to restore independence. (*Courtesy of Daughters of Miriam Center/Rutgers Teaching Nursing Home, Clifton, New Jersey.*)

The goal is to improve circulation, strengthen muscles, encourage return of motion, and train or retrain the patient with the use of prosthetics, crutches, walkers, exercise, heat, cold, electricity, ultrasound, and massage. Most *physical therapists* (PTs) and *PT aides* work in hospitals, but PTs may also work in private practice or for other agencies. The physical therapist designs the patient's program of treatment, based on the physician's stated prescription of objectives. He or she may participate in giving the therapy and/or evaluate the patient's needs and capacities and provide psychological support. The aides work directly under the PT's supervision, with limited participation in the therapeutic program.

Prosthetists make artificial limb substitutes. *Orthotists* make and fit braces. Both work with physicians and other therapists, and have direct patient contact to promote total rehabilitation services. *Orthotic/prosthetic technicians* make and repair devices but usually have no patient contact.

Rehabilitation counselors help people with physical, mental, or social disabilities begin or return to a satisfying life, including an appropriate job. They may counsel about job opportunities and training, assist in job placement, and help the person adjust to a new work situation. Others assisting in patient rehabilitation include *art therapists*, *dance therapists*, and *music therapists* who work primarily with the emotionally disturbed, mentally retarded, or physically handicapped. *Recreational therapists* or *therapeutic recreationists* may plan and supervise recreation programs that include athletics, arts and crafts, parties, gardening, or camping.

Respiratory Therapy

Respiratory therapy personnel perform procedures essential in maintaining life in seriously ill patients with respiratory problems and assist in the treatment of heart and lung ailments. Under medical supervision, the *respiratory therapy technician* administers various types of gas, aerosol, and breathing treatments; assists with long-term continuous artificial ventilation; cleans, sterilizes, and maintains equipment; and keeps patients' records. The *respiratory therapist* may be engaged in similar tasks, but exercises more judgment and accepts greater responsibility in performing therapeutic procedures. Respiratory therapy personnel usually work in hospitals and clinics.

Social Work

The *social worker* attempts to help individuals and their families resolve their social problems, using community and governmental resources as necessary. Social workers are employed by community and governmental agencies as well as hospitals, clinics, and nursing homes. If the social worker's focus is on patients and families, he or she may be called a *medical* or *psychiatric social worker*. When patients are being discharged to go home or transfer to another health care facility, these social workers assist the patient and family in making suitable arrangements.

Social workers also have assistants and aides, who sometimes carry a client load in certain agencies. There may be only on-the-job training available for these workers, but in order to move up, they must acquire additional education.

Speech Pathology and Audiology

Speech therapists and *audiologists* are specialists in communication disorders. Speech pathologists or therapists diagnose and treat speech and language disorders that may stem from a variety of causes. Speech therapists are particularly valuable in assisting patients whose speech has been affected by a cerebrovascular accident or patients with laryngectomies. Audiologists often work with children, and may detect and assist with the hearing disorder of a child who has been mistakenly labeled as retarded.

Vision Care

Ophthalmologists are physicians who treat diseases of the eye and perform surgery, but they may also examine eyes and prescribe corrective glasses and exercises. *Opticians* grind lenses, make eyeglasses, and fit and adjust them. *Optometrists*, doctors of optometry (OD), are educated and clinically trained to examine, diagnose, and treat conditions of the vision system, but they refer clients with eye diseases and other health problems to physicians. They describe their focus as maximizing visual ability, and therefore often use therapeutic programs such as eye training. After a variety of diagnostic tests, they may prescribe corrective lenses, contact lenses, and special optical aids, as well as corrective eye exercises, to provide maximum vision. Some may specialize in such areas as prescribing and fitting contact lenses. The majority of optometrists are in private office practice; but they are increasingly found in institutional settings. All of these professionals are aided by technicians and assistants.

Other Health Workers

There are a number of other health workers not described in this chapter, such as those in science and engineering: anatomists, biologists, biomedical

engineers (who design patient care equipment such as dialysis machines, p...
makers, and heart-lung machines), biomedical technicians (who maintain and...
repair the equipment), and technicians dealing with instrumentation. There
are also diagnostic medical sonographers, electrocardiograph (EKG/ECG)
technicians, electroencephalographic (EEG) technologists and technicians;
clinical perfusionists, who operate equipment to support or replace
temporarily a patient's circulatory or respiratory functions; specialists in
dealing with the visually handicapped; biological photographers; medical
illustrators; patient advocates; acupuncturists; health science librarians; and
computer specialists, to name just a few. In addition, volunteers provide
many useful services.

All of these specialties are part of what the federal government calls *health
manpower* and for which federal funds are often distributed for educational
programs. The fact that this list is not complete and is expanding may help
to explain why the public often becomes angered by the fragmentation of
services. It is clear that if the public is to receive the services it requires,
expects, and deserves, direction must be given through the health care
delivery maze.

ISSUES IN HEALTH MANPOWER

Many of the most serious issues in health manpower—numbers, distribution, proliferation, and especially quality of care—have been focused on
credentialing. This complex process is discussed in Chapter 11. However, the
problem of health manpower planning has even greater priority. Why, over
and over, are there shortages and then oversupplies of health care workers?
Is it because administrators encourage the training of quickly prepared
assistants without thinking ahead to their future place in health care? Does
the government artificially expand the growth of certain categories by
providing funds for education and reimbursement of services? The answer
to both questions is probably yes, but for many reasons, predicting demand
and supply is not easy. The data used are often inexact and out of date.
When the need for a certain kind of worker is met, there are still many
students in the educational pipeline. Lobbying for continued funding,
perhaps unnecessary, is powerful because those who have started programs
don't want to lose them. The need may shift because of unexpected social
or economic changes. Because of costs, administrators now look for a multipurpose worker. For the least-educated, lowest-paid workers this may mean
increased union activity or even unemployment, because there is little job
mobility. For the highly educated, it is a shaky start to a career that
may need to go in a totally different direction. For all those employed,
oversupply also affects salaries and job security. The climate of competition
has added to the pressures, with practitioners in and across various health

with their colleagues for a piece of the health care

the 1960s improved salaries were a major budget
.o move from what were often below-poverty wages
largely responsible for the jump. Since that catch-up
of workers have gained a new aggressiveness that affects
y considerations but also power issues. Some are not
, best interests of the consumer. Nevertheless, one of the
trends .. been widely predicted is aggressive action by unions to organize every type of health worker—professional, technical, aide, clerical, maintenance, and housekeeping. The likelihood that this will be successful is now in doubt because of the tight economic constraints of health care institutions and their preference for multipurpose workers.

The issue of maldistribution is also not easily resolved. Maldistribution of professionals, toward more attractive urban and suburban areas and away from isolated, poor, or ghetto areas, is a major problem. In some cases, nurses, PAs, physician-nurse, or physician PA and/or nurse teams are giving care that is as good as or better than that provided by solo practitioners, but the service gap still exists. Even federal intervention, such as requiring service in medically underserved areas (about 30 percent of the United States) in return for supporting the practitioners' education, has had only short-term results—practitioners leave after their required service.

Health workforce education is a major issue. How many? What kind? Prepared where? Financed by whom? The education for all levels of health service practitioners is under scrutiny. Why is this education so costly? Could institutions develop more economical teaching–learning methods? Are minority groups being actively recruited? Are the types of workers in proper proportion? Should the government continue to subsidize the education of high-earning professionals? How much should any health profession be subsidized, and for whom—the programs or students? Are the practitioners appropriately prepared to give safe and effective care?

Another concern is the workability of the health care team. It is naive to expect that bringing together a highly diverse group of people and calling them a team will cause them to behave like a team. One obvious gap is their lack of communication and "practice" together, either as students or as full practitioners. Sports teams practice together intensively for long periods of time, both to develop a team spirit and to enhance and coordinate their individual skills to produce a functioning unit. Not only do health care teams not have (or take) time to practice together, but often there are serious territorial disputes as areas of responsibility overlap more and more. As for patients, who should be members of the team, unless they are assertive, their only participation is as recipients of care.

Theoretically, legally clear distinctions of each profession would be helpful; practically, it is impossible. Successful coordination depends on collegial behavior, trust, and full, frequent, open communication; otherwise, valuable participants in health care will continue to be underutilized. It has also been said that society can no longer afford, and does not need, to use the physician as gatekeeper to control the flow of patients in and out of the health system. Physician services should be saved to assist patients who need that level of services. In other words, there must be other fully acknowledged practitioners in primary health care. This is slow to happen.

A review of the issues that each occupation sees as vital makes it clear that the struggle between medicine and other health care groups to expand or limit the scope of practice will continue and perhaps escalate. And with the current economic pressures that are not expected to let up, various types and levels of workers may fight even harder to get and keep territory. The trend to increase educational criteria seems to permeate each occupational group, but almost all face the questions asked by the cost-conscious: "Will it cost the consumer more? Will it keep out the poor? Is it really necessary, or is it a status ploy?"

The nursing shortage (or more accurately, supply and demand) will be discussed in Chapter 6, but solutions proposed by AHA and AMA present a picture of their involvement (not to be seen as always bad). In 1989, the AHA co-sponsored a pilot project with the Illinois Hospital Association to test a new employee group, an all-purpose worker to make beds, empty trash, serve meals, and take over other nonclinical chores to help nurses. The idea was to cross-train staff to handle anything from transport to housekeeping. (How the unions reacted was not reported.) It was expected that other hospitals would replicate this plan, and some did. Meanwhile, some hospitals produced other kinds of assistants called general medical technicians or unit helpers to do all the non-nursing tasks nurses are forced to do. The idea has merit, but will it create one more set of low-paying jobs that go nowhere? And how clear is it to both the public and health care personnel, just what the responsibilities of these unlicensed workers are, how safe they are, and who supervises them?

On the other side of the shortage issue is oversupply, a reality for physicians, dentists, nurses, and some administrators; given the uncertainties of the health care future, others could be included. The reactions of those concerned follow a pattern: denial or prediction of a later shortage as in medicine; a tendency to warn off potential students; disillusionment with the field; an attempt to hold on to their own territory and resist others' encroachment, but also an attempt to encroach on still others; efforts to expand their services to meet previously unnoted or unattractive needs (serving the elderly); or making some aspect of their services attractive to consumers (cosmetic dentistry). Because real health care needs may begin to be met, there are good aspects to the situation; however, the dissension and the cost to the public are not desirable.

EXHIBIT 3.7

Predictions for Health Care in a New Century

- Technology will have a dramatic impact:
  More accurate diagnoses
  Treatment selection based on history of effectiveness
  Less invasive procedures
  Genetic screening and engineering

- Ethical dilemmas associated with cost, quality, access, and use of certain technology, will escalate

- There will be universal access to a minimum standard of health care through increased workplace involvement and governmental programs for the poor and unemployed

- A two-tiered system will be even more apparent

- There will be decreased federal control over health care with increased state involvement

- Personal responsibility for health care through the use of over-the-counter diagnostics and therapeutics, electronic information systems for problem definition and self-help groups will grow

- Better understanding of the difference between cost-efficiency and cost-control will emerge

- The medical domination of the delivery system will wane

- Dominance of the health care industry by managed care will escalate

- There will be more private/public sector partnerships in delivering services, administering plans, and every other conceivable means

- Hospitals will continue to shrink, essentially becoming giant intensive care units

- Consumers, even the poor, will have control over their health care choices; marketing will become critical and consumer satisfaction will become a major ingredient for industry success

- There will be increased concern over the effects of environment on health

- The decisive movement towards community services, including home care, will continue

- The age for Medicare eligibility will be raised, and a means test will be put into place (the well-to-do will get less)

- Mandatory AIDS testing will become more common regardless of logic, including marriage licenses, immigration, insurance policies

- Alternative treatment for illness will challenge traditional medicine: behavioral and wholistic medicine, biofeedback, meditation, acupuncture, homeopathy, therapeutic touch

- A business orientation to health care is seen as essential for industry survival

- There will be industry emphasis on primary care, health promotion, a basic standard of quality

- Disputes among health care providers about overlapping roles will create public intolerance of turf battles

- Education for practice will prepare future providers for this era of change and for the predictable direction of change, or their area of practice will self-destruct

Another major issue is quality of care. This inevitably involves health care personnel. Related to this issue is not only practice but education. Health care personnel, experts say, must develop some special skills to deal with the future and educators should take note.

If there are any good answers to these questions and issues, they have not been found or accepted. Consumers' restlessness with professional indecision and evasion of their concerns and complaints is reaching a critical stage. Armed with the information and discussion contained in this chapter, we should be a little wiser and more strategic. Major predictions that flow from these observations are presented in Exhibit 3.7.

KEY POINTS

1. Being aware of population patterns, as well as social and economic trends, helps in anticipating the kinds of patients who will enter the health care system and how to give the best care.

2. Social trends like the women's movement and changes in the economy affect not only health care delivery but also the economic security of the workers.

3. The prospective payment method of reimbursement has changed the way patients are admitted to and discharged from hospitals, resulting in shorter stays and a greater likelihood of their going home sicker.

4. Competition and cost containment in the health care system have resulted in marketing of services, a trend toward conglomerates, and the growth of investor-owned health care corporations and nonprofit chains.

5. Health care services are now being provided in many places besides traditional doctors' offices and institutional agency settings. There is increased emphasis on more cost-effective delivery modes such as community nursing centers, surgicenters, and emergicenters.

6. The large numbers of caregivers and the overlapping of their activities add to the public's confusion about the selection and cost of services.

7. Health manpower needs are seldom predicted accurately, with a resulting cycle of shortage and oversupply.

8. Many of the common issues that concern health care providers are related to competition—the desire of some to expand their scope of practice and others to hold on to their territory. Therefore many of those striving for a better place in the system are looking to further education and credentialing.

9. Predictions about health care focus on economic issues, public demand, and the conflicting pull of health promotion ideals, on the one hand, and the complex, expensive treatments made possible by technology on the other.

REFERENCES

1. Kovner A. *Health Care Delivery in the United States*, 5th ed. New York: Springer, 1995, p 39.
2. Ibid.
3. Furula B, Lipson J. Cultural diversity in the student body revisited. In McCloskey J, Grace H (eds): *Current Issues in Nursing*, 4th ed. St. Louis: Mosby, 1994, p 665.
4. Bullough B, Bullough V. *Nursing Issues*. New York: Springer, 1994, p 187.
5. Population growth strips earlier US census estimates. *New York Times*, A1, D18, December 4, 1992.
6. US Bureau of the Census (USBOC). *Statistical Abstract of the United States: 1993*, 113th ed. Washington, DC: USBOC, 1993.
7. Howe N, Strauss B. *13th Generation: Abort, Retry, Ignore, Fail?* New York: Vintage Books, 1993.
8. *The World Almanac and Book of Facts 1994*. Mahwah, NJ: Funk & Wagnalls, 1994.
9. Ibid.
10. *The World Almanac*, loc cit.
11. Foster C, et al. *Homelessness in America*. Wylie, TX: Information Plus, 1993.
12. *Health Care Delivery in the United States*, op cit, p 42.
13. McGinnis J, Foege W. Actual causes of death in the United States. *JAMA* 270:2207–2122, 1993.
14. Institute of Medicine, National Academy of Science. *Healthy People 2000: Citizens Chart the Course*. Washington, DC: National Academy Press, 1990.
15. McGinnis JM, Lee PR. *Healthy People 2000* at mid decade. *JAMA* 273:1123–1129, 1995.
16. Ibid.
17. Ibid.
18. Ibid.
19. The National Commission on AIDS. Americans living with AIDS: Transforming anger, fear and indifference into action. In Lee P, et al (eds): *The Nation's Health*. Boston: Jones and Bartlett, 1994, pp 391–397.
20. UNICEF progress report on programme activities in prevention of HIV and in reducing the impact of AIDS on families and communities. *Policy Review* 26, February, 1993.
21. *Abortion Surveillance*. Atlanta, GA: CDCP, December 17, 1993.
22. Earth Day. *The Sunday Record* NJ-1, April 16, 1995.
23. Hannah KJ, et al (eds). *Computers in Health Care: Introduction to Nursing Informatics*. New York: Springer-Verlag, 1994.

24. Almanac Issue. *Chronicle of Higher Education* 41, September 1, 1994.

25. Ibid.

26. American Nurses Association and National League for Nursing. *Nursing's Agenda for Health Care Reform.* Washington, DC: ANA, 1991.

27. Vance C, et al. An uneasy alliance: Nursing and the women's movement. *Nurs Outlook* 33:281–285, November–December, 1985.

28. Gordon S. *Prisoners of Men's Dreams.* Boston: Little, Brown, 1991.

29. United Nations Department of Public Information: *Conference to Set Women's Agenda into the Next Century.* New York: United Nations, 1993.

30. *The World Almanac,* loc cit.

31. Quinn J. The luck of the Xers. *Newsweek* 73:66–67, June 6, 1994.

32. Naisbett J, Aburdene P. *Megatrends 2000: Ten New Directions for the 1990s.* New York: Morrow, 1990, pp 216–240.

33. Hoerr J. What should unions do? *Harvard Business Review* 30–45, May–June, 1991.

34. *Dimensions of Professional Nursing,* op cit, p 130.

35. Joel L. Reshaping nursing practice. *Am J Nurs* 87:793–795, June, 1987.

36. American Nurses Association. *Nursing and HIV/AIDS.* Washington, DC: American Nurses Publishing, 1994.

37. Harrington C, Estes CL. *Health Policy and Nursing.* Boston: Jones and Bartlett, 1994.

38. Braunstein J. National health insurance: Necessary but not sufficient. *Nurs Outlook* 39:54–55, March–April, 1991.

39. *Nursing's Agenda for Health Care Reform,* loc cit.

40. *Health Care Delivery in the United States,* op cit, pp 165, 198, 202.

41. Ibid, p 55.

42. Parsons T. Definition of health and illness in the light of American values and social structure. In Jaco EG (ed): *Patients, Physicians, and Illness.* Glencoe, IL: Free Press, 1958, p 176.

43. Levin L. Self care: Towards fundamental changes in national strategies. *Int J Health Ed* 24:219–228, 1981.

44. Sharp N. Community nursing centers coming of age. *Nurs Manage* 23:18–20, August, 1992.

45. Hall L. A center for nursing. *Nurs Outlook* 11:805–806, 1993.

46. Phillips DL, Steel JE. Factors influencing scope of practice in nursing centers. *J Prof Nurs* 10:84–90, March–April 1994.

47. Barger S, Rosenfeld P. Models in community health care. *Nurs Health Care* 14:426–430, October, 1993.

48. Bishop C, Skwara KC. Recent growth of Medicare home health. *Health Affairs* 12:95–107, 1993.

49. National Association for Home Care. *Basic Statistics about Home Care.* Washington, DC: NAHC, 1995.

50. Ibid.

51. Jamieson MK. Block nursing: Practicing autonomous professional nursing in the community. *Nurs Health Care* 11:250–253, May, 1990.

51A. Immigration Nursing Relief Advisory Committee: *Report to the Secretary of Labor on the Immigration Nursing Relief Act of 1989.* Washington, DC, March, 1995.

52. Infeld D, Kress J. *Crisis of Quality: Management for Long-Term Care.* Arlington: Association of University Programs in Health Administration, 1990.

53. Kayser-Jones J. The environment of life in long-term care institutions. *Nurs Health Care* 10:125–130. March, 1989.

54. Hicks L, et al. *Role of the Nurse in Managed Care.* Kansas City, MO: National Center for Managed Health Care Administration, 1992.

55. American Nurses Association. *Nurse Practitioners and Certified Nurse-Midwives: A Meta-Analysis of Process of Care, Clinical Outcomes, and Cost-Effectiveness of Nurses in Primary Care Roles.* Washington, DC: ANA, 1993.

56. *Health Care Delivery in the United States*, op cit, p 102.

57. Manuel P, Alster K. Unlicensed personnel: No cure for an ailing health care system. *Nurs Health Care* 15:18–21, January, 1994.

58. Huber D, et al. Use of nursing assistants: Staff nurse opinions. *Nurs Mgt* 25:64–68, May, 1994.

4

The Discipline of Nursing

OBJECTIVES

After studying this chapter, you will be able to:

1. Give a definition of nursing that is based on your beliefs about nursing.
2. Give examples of how well nursing meets the criteria for being considered a profession.
3. List nursing functions common to all nurses.
4. Describe the nursing process and nursing diagnosis.
5. Name five major nursing theorists.
6. Describe how today's image of nursing differs from the reality and how it might be accurate.

THE NEW-OLD QUESTION: WHAT IS NURSING?

If asked what a nurse does, probably most people entering nursing would, like the general public, say "Take care of the sick." That is a common dictionary definition, a common media image, and a large part of reality. That nurses do health teaching and want to keep people well is also part of the reality. So is the fact that they hold nursing positions in education, administration, research, and publication in many settings that aren't too different in basic responsibilities from similar jobs in other fields. And more are becoming entrepreneurs. Yet the historical orientation of nursing has been one of mother surrogate, of tending and watching over a dependent ward, of a helping person. Perhaps because the caring, helping part of the role is basic to nursing, it is confusing to some that nurses can also be powerful, assertive professionals cutting out a piece of the health care pie for *nursing*, controlled by *nurses*.

Some nurses cherish a traditional image and are uncomfortable as they move into new roles. Others, as they enter this changing field, have more contemporary ideas about what nursing is, without discarding the caring concept, which is seen as the heart of nursing. Thus, there are many interpretations of nursing. Why not? There are many facets to nursing, and perhaps it isn't logical or accurate to settle on one point of view. All nurses must eventually determine their own philosophies of nursing, whether or not these are formalized. The public and others outside nursing will probably continue to adopt an image that is nurtured by contact, hearsay, or media representations of the profession. The first may be the most powerful influence. This chapter presents an overview of the components of nursing, the theory, the image, and the reality.

PROFESSIONS AND PROFESSIONALISM

An ongoing debate centers on whether or not nursing as a whole is an occupation, rather than a profession, in the same sense that medicine, theology, and law have been called professions since the Middle Ages. The classic work on the topic was done in a 1915 study of medicine by Flexner.[1] Flexner proposed six criteria, characterizing professions as: intellectual, possessing an expanding body of knowledge, unique and socially necessary, taught through a system of professional education as opposed to an apprenticeship, internally organized in a manner which allows peer accountability and independence, and motivated through altruism. These statements ring just as true today as they did some 80 years ago, but they must be reinterpreted for contemporary use. Later day scholars have added their own perspectives and enriched our understanding.[2,3,4] In total, there is little disagreement. Neither is there any profession, even the most historically recognized that can claim to be untouched by our changing terms. Synthesizing the best of thinking on the topic, professions are distinguished by the following qualities:

1. *Their work is intellectual.* A profession is distinguished by a substantial body of knowledge. The artfulness of professionals is cognitive; it is predominately in their heads, not in their hands.
2. *Each is unique, providing the answer to a very vital social problem.*

Professions exist at the pleasure of the society. This privilege requires that the organized profession guarantee adequate numbers in their ranks to address the purpose for which they were created. It is not enough that the professionals understand their uniqueness and are convinced of their importance and usefulness; the public must concur.

3. *An expanding body of knowledge* honors the responsibility to maintain practice that is state-of-the-art. The spirit of this quality is seen in individuals and in the profession as a collective. This requires an appreciation of the relationship of research to practice, and the commitment to establish research as a priority.

4. *Personal responsibility* for the services offered to the public overshadows any allegiance to an employer. This is an important element as more professionals become employees. The professional–client relationship fosters trust, should guarantee confidentiality, and requires an individual license (where governmental licensure is the standard).

5. *A long period of education* for practice is expected. That education should involve both theory and practice, and should be entrusted to the educators of the profession. This position of maintaining a closeness yet independence between professional practice and education is not new. Rather, it was strongly advised by both Nightingale in the 1800s and Flexner in 1915. This practice–education relationship should not be construed as any devaluation of experience. The art of the professional is enriched with exposure to multiple variations of the human condition. Experience counts here.

6. *Autonomy* has always been offered as a hallmark of the professions. Autonomy infers the ability to develop policy about your discipline and control the activity of your members. The growing presence of governmental regulation reduces our degrees of freedom. We can expect that the policies of the profession will be the basis of regulatory decisions and that members of the discipline will be well represented on governmental panels which speak to our practice (Boards of Nursing).

7. Members of the profession share *a common identity.* They are socialized into the values and attitudes of the discipline during the educational process. There is a conscious decision to "buy into" a way of thinking, and a way of life. This collective identity was once reinforced by what nurses wore. Now it is reinforced by what we do. It is seen in the desire to socialize with colleagues, to search out role models and mentors, to look to the more seasoned members of the profession for wisdom built on experience, to seek solidarity and comradery through membership in alumni and professional associations.

8. The career choice of a profession is *motivated by altruism*, and it

signifies a long-term, if not life-long, commitment. From another perspective, the profession as a whole also emphasizes public service above personal inconvenience, continuing education, responsibility to monitor the service delivered to the public, and so on.

9. The public are provided with reassurance of the profession's credibility through a *Code of Ethics*. Nursing has further documented its contract with the public in *The Social Policy Statement*, describing the nature of its work, its systems of specialization and advanced practice, and the manner in which the profession monitors its practice and its practitioners.

It has also been popular to use the term *semiprofession*, with the implication that there are steps that a group must go through to become professional. Caplow describes a first step as the formation of a membership organization with explicit criteria for belonging. The name of the area of work is changed to create a new identity and begin to stake-off both the title and the area of service. A code of ethics comes next and the lobbying to secure legal statutes which eventually make licensure and the broader presence of the profession mandatory. During this same period, education for the profession is being either directly or indirectly upgraded by the professional society.[5] This scenario is highly descriptive of nursing. Each of the state nurses associations (the state affiliate of the ANA) was established for the express purpose of seeking regulation of nursing practice through licensure and title protection. The battle to increase nursing's presence in health care (for the public good) is the continuing governmental agenda: more nurses in nursing homes, direct access to nurses by the public without the physician's approval, the right to have nurses do school physicals. These are but a few examples. The *Code of Ethics* was completed in 1950. The ANA has been vigorously lobbying the profession since 1965 to standardize our system of education. All of these things will be discussed in more detail in subsequent chapters.

Looking objectively at the criteria associated with the professions, nursing does not fulfill all of them. It has been pointed out that nursing's theory base is still developing, the public does not always see the nurse as a professional, not all nurses are educated in institutions of higher learning, not all nurses consider nursing a lifetime career, and in many practice settings, nursing does not control its own policies and activities. This lack of autonomy is considered the most serious weakness. Sociologists have long contended that an occupation has not become a profession unless the members of that occupation are the ones who make the final decisions about the services they provide.

The public has deferred to the profession to establish its standards and monitor the practice of its members. This is a courtesy given to experts in a complex area of work who exercise unquestioned integrity and respect the client–provider relationship above all others. This tradition has seriously eroded in recent years. Surveys tell us that Americans have developed a significant suspicion about professionals. Given this discomfort with individuals who provide very essential services, the public has looked to government for more oversight. There are many examples: consumer presence on professional boards, setting of fee schedules for reimbursement, the development of guidelines for the management of certain disease conditions, the governmental requirement to advise patients of their right to execute a living will.

Autonomy and immunity from governmental intrusion has always been the strongest in areas of specialty practice, where consumers feel least qualified to challenge the judgment of professionals. The recent movement to license nurses in advanced or specialty practice is both an example of eroding autonomy and a cue that we are arriving too late to apply traditional models.[6]

Declining autonomy may well be associated with the changing client–provider relationship. For nurses that relationship is further challenged by a US Supreme Court decision of May 1994.[7] In that opinion, the court creates the potential for any nurse who supervises assistive personnel to be considered management. This could rob nurses of their employee protections and of the autonomy that has enabled them to be patient advocates first and employees second. These critical incidents provide beginning evidence to cause us to rethink or at least reinterpret our criteria for professionalism.

A second point of debate is associated with the uniqueness of the services provided by professionals. The service of any group of providers must be timely, relevant, and offered with an appreciation of what each discipline can contribute. Resistance to change and refusal to move with the times is not only counterproductive but a violation of the public trust. Examples abound as professionals strain to protect their turf. The very public and negative response of the American Medical Association to the role of nurses as primary care providers is one instance.[8]

In recent years, there has been progress in both achieving autonomy and, perhaps more important, nurses' recognition that this is important to both the profession and to themselves in terms of how they practice. This mental turnaround has something to do with the fact that more nurses are seeking higher education and that more are planning nursing careers as opposed to taking nursing jobs. Nurses are also becoming more aggressive about getting recognition for what they *have* accomplished. Both nurses and others are convinced that the fact that nursing is predominantly female is also a factor in why nurses have had difficulty achieving high professional status. If nursing is not considered a profession in the strictest sense of the word, it is well on the way to becoming so. One author commented thoughtfully, "On the continuum of professionalization, qualitatively nursing and many individual nurses excel far beyond contemporary recognized professions in many areas. Quantitatively, the road ahead is very long."[9]

Never forget that the term *profession* is essentially a social concept and has no meaning apart from society. Society decides that for its needs to be met in a certain respect, a body undertaking to meet these particular needs will be given special consideration. The contract is that the individuals of that favored group continually use their best efforts to meet those obligations, constantly reexamining and scrutinizing their functions for appropriateness and always maintaining competence. When they fail to honor these obligations and/or slip into demanding status, authority, and privileges that have no connection with carrying our their professional work satisfactorily, society may reconsider.

Violation of this agreement eventually brings retribution from society, as seen today in the tightening of laws regulating professional practice and reimbursement. Certain behaviors, such as unprofessional conduct, may be specifically punished by removal of the practitioner's legal right to practice—licensure (see Chapter 11).

The stereotype of idealized professionals who are guaranteed economic security by the public in exchange for a lifetime of dedicated service to their work is a rarity. This does not make these individuals any less, but only a product of their times. First, economic security is a relative term and open to a range of definitions. No group will be guaranteed income, most especially those in the health care field, as we move into models of managed care with providers as employees more commonly than as entrepreneurs. Perhaps even more telling is the trend for members of the American workforce to demand more personal and private time. More Americans are also enjoying the opportunity to change careers or at least enjoy some variety in their work life. Midlife and later-life career changes are not rare, and the professionals are not immune to these trends. Further collective bargaining, unionism, and strikes, once seen as unprofessional, have been gradually accepted as legitimate activities by professionals who are employed. One of today's most challenging issues is for the professional employee to distinguish obligations as an employee from those as a professional.

And so the debate continues, and we are lost in a sea of confusion over whether we have achieved some degree of professionalism. The danger lies in taking too much time to decide who we are, while much work remains to be done. In these changing times, the qualities of professionalism are being redefined. Rather than taking our cues from tradition, we may be better served by looking internally. Establish our own standard, herald our uniqueness, look to the public need and our own sense of purpose. There was a time when nurses never doubted their professionalism. Do we have more time to flail at windmills today?

DEFINITIONS OF NURSING

Causing almost as much disagreement as the question of whether nursing is a profession is "How do you define nursing?" Definitions of nursing vary according to the philosophy of an individual or group. How people see the roles and functions of nursing is based on what they think nursing is. Exhibit 4.1 gives an overview of some of the best-known definitions. Most nurses would probably accept any of these in principle, although they might argue that some are more ideal than real. In the ANA position paper of 1965, the concepts *care, cure,* and *coordination* were part of a definition of *professional practice,* and have since become commonly associated with nursing.

As nurses expanded their functions into the new nurse practitioner role, *cure* acquired a different meaning for some nurses, including aspects of what has been medical diagnosis and treatment. Some nurses were adamant that medical (not nursing) diagnosis and treatment diminishes the role of the nurse as a nurse. (The same opponents also usually reject the term *nurse practitioner* or *NP.*) However, Ford, a pioneer of the NP movement, immediately responding, called this "semantic roulette" and added, "I'm not so concerned about the words. I'm convinced that nursing can take on that level of accountability of professional practice that involves the consumer in decision making in his care and also demands sophisticated clinical judgment to determine levels of illness and wellness and design a plan of management."[10]

Coordination and integration of the therapeutic regimen have historically been the province of nursing. We did it in the home and in the community within our early models of practice, and took these traditions into hospitals. Our 24-hour presence and holistic philosophy suited us well to this responsibility. Active coordination on behalf of our patients has always been a nursing hallmark and is more critical today as nurses are often the only human link between patients and an intimidating experience in the health care delivery system.

Although the definitions included in Exhibit 4.1 are interesting and some are provocative, day-to-day practice is directly shaped by legal, professional and institutional definitions. Each may be different. Consistency one to the other is a goal. The institutional definition will most likely be incorporated in the introductory paragraph of your job description. The professional and legal definitions are promulgated by the ANA and the National Council of State Boards of Nursing (NCSBN) respectively. They are compared in Chapter 11. For the purpose of this section it is interesting to note the evolution of our professional definitions over the years, especially if we expect the profession's definition, in the true spirit of autonomy, to directly or indirectly drive practice. The 1965 definition was bold in its

EXHIBIT 4.1

Definitions of Nursing by Nurses

- "(to have) charge of the personal health of somebody ... and what nursing has to do ... is to put the patient in the best condition for nature to act upon him." (Florence Nightingale, 1859)
- Nursing in its broadest sense may be defined as an art and science which involves the whole patient—body, mind, and spirit; promotes his spiritual, mental and physical health by teaching and by example; stresses health education and health preservation as well as ministration to the sick; involves the care of the patient's environment—social and spiritual as well as physical; and gives health services to the family and the community as well as to the individual. (Sister M. Olivia Gowan, 1944)
- The unique function of the nurse is to assist the individual, sick or well, in the performance of those activities contributing to health or its recovery (or to peaceful death) that he would perform unaided if he had the necessary strength, will, or knowledge. And to do this in such a way as to help him gain independence as rapidly as possible. This aspect of her work, this part of her function, she initiates and controls; of this she is master. In addition she helps the patient to carry out the therapeutic plan as initiated by the physician. She also, as a member of a medical team, helps other members, as they in turn help her, to plan and carry out the total program whether it be for the improvement of health or the recovery from illness or support in death. (Virginia Henderson, 1961)
- ... to facilitate the efforts of the individual to overcome the obstacles which currently interfere with his ability to respond capably to demands made of him by his condition, environment, situation and time. (Ernestine Wiedenbach, 1964)
- The essential components of professional nursing are care, cure, and coordination. (ANA Position Paper, 1965)
- Nursing's first line of defense is promotion of health and prevention of illness. Care of the sick is resorted to when our first line of defense fails. (Martha Rogers, 1966)
- Nursing is the diagnosis and treatment of human responses to actual or potential health problems. (New York State Nurse Practice Act, 1972)
- The first level nurse is responsible for planning, providing, and evaluating nursing care in all settings for the promotion of health, prevention of illness, care of the sick and rehabilitation; and functions as a member of the health team. (International Council of Nursing, 1973)

EXHIBIT 4.1 (*continued*)

- Nursing is an essential service to all of mankind. That service can be succinctly described in terms of its focus, goal, jurisdiction, and outcomes as that of assessing and enhancing the general health status, health assets, and health potentials of all human beings. (Rozella Schlotfeldt, 1978)
- A service of deliberately selected and performed actions to assist individuals to maintain self-care, including structural integrity, functioning and development. (Dorothea Orem, 1980)
- The "Practice of Nursing" means assisting individuals or groups to maintain or attain optimal health, implementing a strategy of care to accomplish defined goals, and evaluating responses to care and treatment. (Model Practice Act, National Council of State Boards of Nursing, 1994)

---

incorporation of the concepts "cure, care and coordination," but risked the ire of those opposed to any repositioning of the boundaries between professions. In the early 1970s, nursing was defined as "... the diagnosis and treatment of human responses to actual or potential health problems." The somewhat obscure definition made what we do less than totally clear to some nurses, and totally confusing to nonnurses.

The intervening years have rewarded us with more internal solidarity and the consequent ability to be flexible and live with uncertainty. The boundaries between profession will shift, with those things that were the exclusive domain of one group becoming the day-to-day work of another. To accommodate a rapidly changing world of practice the 1995 revision of *Nursing's Social Policy Statement* avoids a precise definition of nursing, but cautions that "... nursing (has) been influenced by a greater elaboration of the science of caring and its integration with the traditional knowledge base for diagnosis and treatment of human responses to health and illness."[11] Given this environment, ANA does not offer any specific definition, but observes that definitions of nursing increasingly acknowledge four essential features of current practice:

1. Attention to the full range of human experiences and responses to health and illness without restriction to a problem-focused orientation.
2. Integration of objective data with knowledge gained from an understanding of the patient or group's subjective experience.
3. Application of scientific knowledge to the processes of diagnosis and treatment.
4. Provision of a caring relationship that facilitates health and healing.[12]

These statements allow flexibility and confer many liberties. They:

- Remove any restriction to a problem-focused relationship (nursing may be intervening in a good situation to make it better).
- Recognize subjective experience as a valid source of information on which to design care (a critical admission as we enter a multicultural era, and additionally opens the door to give credibility to intuition as a quality in nursing practice).
- Use language which returns the profession to a recognition of our caring relationship, and link that caring to outcomes, building a case for a science of caring.
- Talk of diagnosis and treatment without the modifier "nursing," thereby recognizing that as we bridge the boundaries of other professions, new role functions are valid.

As a class, all of these definitions (personal, professional, legal) portray nursing as a comprehensive, holistic health service working to empower patients on their own behalf through teaching, counseling, surveillance of physical and mental status, intimate personal care, and participation in interdisciplinary practice. The most recent renditions infer diagnosis and treatment of illness.

NURSING FUNCTIONS

The question remains just what do nurses do? Building on their definitions of nursing, members of the profession have detailed the functions of the nurse in broad or specific terms. Noteworthy differences appear when comparing iterations over time. Schlotfeldt's proposal is accurate and complete for the 1970s, with the trepidation we felt then to speak out too honestly:

1. Interviewing to obtain accurate health histories.
2. Examining, with use of all senses and technological aids, to ascertain the health status of persons served.
3. Evaluating to draw valid inferences concerning individuals' health assets and potentials.
4. Referring to physicians and dentists those persons whose health status indicates the need for differential diagnoses and the institution of therapies.
5. Referring to other helping professionals those persons who need assistance with problems that fall within the province of clergymen, social workers, homemakers, lawyers, and others.

6. Caring for persons during periods of their dependence to include:
   - compensating for deficits of those unable to maintain normal functions and to execute their prescribed therapies;
   - sustaining and supporting persons while reinforcing the natural, developmental, and reparative processes available to human beings in their quest for wholeness, function, comfort, and self-fulfillment;
   - teaching and guiding persons in their pursuit of optimal wellness;
   - motivating persons toward active, knowledgeable involvement in seeking health and in executing their needed therapies.
7. Collaborating with other health professionals and with persons served in planning and executing programs of health care and diagnostic and treatment services.
8. Evaluating in concert with consumers, other providers, and policymakers the efficacy of the health care system and planning for its continuous improvement.[13]

More recent lists of functions have noteworthy changes which are consistent with the patterns found in definitions of the discipline:[14,15]

1. The medical and nursing regimens are seen as separate and distinct. Where it was once common to call for the provision of nursing care based on a medical regimen, such sentiments are absent from contemporary definitions.
2. Performing acts of medical diagnosis and treatment are commonly mentioned.
3. Collaborative practice is consistent.
4. Caution is taken to include the nurse's right to delegate.
5. Language mentions the right to manage, supervise and teach the practice of nursing.

The degree of expertise with which nurses carry out these functions depends on their level of knowledge and skills, but the profession has the responsibility of setting standards for its practitioners. In its 1991 *Standards of Clinical Nursing Practice*, the ANA incorporated standards of care and standards of professional performance.

THE NURSING PROCESS AND NURSING DIAGNOSIS

Yura and Walsh state that the term *nursing process* was not prevalent in the nursing literature until the mid-1960s, with limited mention in the 1950s.[16] Orlando was one of the earliest authors to use the term, but it was slow to be adopted. In the next few years, models of the activities in which nurses engaged were developed, and in 1967, a faculty group at the Catholic University of America specifically identified the phases of the nursing process as *assessing, planning, implementing,* and *evaluating.* The nursing process is described as "an orderly, systematic manner of determining the client's health status, specifying problems defined as alterations in human need fulfillment, making plans to solve them, initiating and implementing the plan, and evaluating the extent to which the plan was effective in promoting optimum wellness and resolving the problems identified."[16] In fact, the nursing process adheres to the steps in logical thinking or problem solving. The fact that it is used in nursing has gained it the label of the nursing process.

At this point, there is considerable information in the nursing literature about the use of the nursing process, and many schools of nursing use it as a framework for teaching. However, there are those who feel that other approaches are more suitable to today's complex care. More specifically, we are not proposing the abandonment of logical thought, but to incorporate in our educational systems and practice the most cutting edge of cognitive techniques. There is promise of great gain from incorporating some recent work on critical thinking, diagnostic reasoning, and skill acquisition.[17,18]

Nursing diagnosis is part of the nursing process. It is the title given to the act of identifying a problem and labeling it. A diagnostic system has been in development since 1973. It is developing currently under the direction of the North American Nursing Diagnosis Association (NANDA) and may serve as a major communication tool among nurses. It could also facilitate public understanding of what nurses do; just as physicians can pinpoint what they do in relation to treating diseases, nurses can point out nursing diagnosis as the patient problems they try to resolve.

In the late 1980s, the ANA initiated an era dedicated to recognition of the work nurses do as reflected in their classification systems. A formal appeal to the World Health Organization to incorporate the NANDA system into the next revision of the International Classification of Diseases (ICD) was rejected on the basis that the taxonomy was not internationally useful or relevant. Simultaneously the ANA became responsive to several other classification systems for nursing, and was successful in having all of them accepted for incorporation into the National Library of Medicine's database; these include the NANDA system,[19] Bulechek and McCloskey's classification of nursing intervention,[20] and the Omaha[21] and Saba[22] systems for home care. Work to increase the international usefulness of nursing diagnosis currently continues under the auspices of the International Council of Nurses (ICN) and the Kellogg Foundation.[23]

It will remain to be seen whether the nursing diagnosis movement has been a strategy to bring us to maturity as a profession, or a sign of our maturity. The trends in health care restructuring move us towards interdisciplinary practice. Should our language also reflect a unity of practice?

MAJOR NURSING THEORIES

As nursing has developed in professionalism, nursing scholars have developed theories of nursing based on research, and the science of nursing is coming of age. A scientific body of knowledge unique to nursing is important to provide a basis for clear differentiation between medicine and nursing, on the one hand, and nursing and nurturing on the other. Research and theory building unique to a discipline are elements required for that discipline to be recognized as a profession.

Although Florence Nightingale identified a body of knowledge specific to the nursing of her time and used this as the basis for instruction in the Nightingale schools, it was not until the 1950s and 1960s that there was a proliferation of nursing concepts and theories. Nursing scholars argued that without research and theory building, nursing would be unable to carve out a role for itself in the future health care system, and would thus allow itself to be defined, instructed, and controlled by other disciplines.

A theory is a system of concepts and relationships which allows nurses to describe, understand, predict and prescribe in their practice. Theory (for nursing or anything else) can take one of three forms, each with its distinct purpose. There are nursing philosophies or *philosophical theories* which give meaning to situations requiring nursing. This is accomplished through the cognitive skills of analysis, reasoning and often divergent thinking. Grand theories are the most comprehensive, applying to the entire domain of nursing, and more properly called models because they are so all-encompassing. *Mid-range theories* are built on the work of supportive sciences (natural, behavioral), earlier nursing theories or grand theories. Mid-range theories have a narrower focus, are more concrete and target specific practice questions. They are essential to the development of specialty knowledge, which in turn allows cutting-edge practice in general nursing and in education for entry into practice. Each theory for nursing has its own concepts, definitions, assumptions and derives from different more basic scientific models or theories. Exhibit 4.2 provides an overview of selected nursing theories which have significantly influenced practice. The common theme of wholism and patient–client empowerment through the nurse–patient relationship is noteworthy. Further, each theory is organized around its view of man (human beings), health, society (environment) and nursing.

Exhibit 4.2 is but a representative sample of grand, mid-range and philosophical theories. The information contained is only a very limited

EXHIBIT 4.2

Theorist, theory and date of early work[a]	Concepts/definitions/ assumptions	Influential models or sciences
Florence Nightingale: adaptation/ environmental, 1859	• Disease is a reparative process • Rejected germ theory • Inbalance between patient and their physical environment frustrates energy conservation and decreases the capacity for health	Environment/ sanitation
Dorothy Johnson: behavioral systems, 1959	• Seven behavioral subsystems which can be analyzed in terms of structure and function	Ethological systems
Dorothea Orem: self-care model, 1959	• Constituted from three related theories: self-care, self-care deficit and nursing systems • People have a need for the provision and management of self-care actions on a continuing basis to sustain life and health and to recover from disease • When an individual's self-care agency is not adequate to their requirement or that of their dependents, deficit is created	Henderson
Virginia Henderson: developmental model, 1961	• The patient is a person who requires help towards independence	Thorndike Rehabilitation principles Orlando Maslow
Ida Jean Orlando: interpersonal theory, 1961	• Distinguishes automatic from deliberate actions • Perception, thoughts and feelings are not explored in automatic actions • Deliberate actions yield solutions and prevention of problems	Eclectic

Nursing role	Theory type	Major contribution
• Manipulation of the external environment, such as ventilation, warmth, light, diet, cleanliness and noise would contribute to well-being and the reparative process • Patient is relatively passive • Nursing places patients in the best condition for nature to act upon them • Saw nursing role in health as well as illness • Stressed nurses' use of observation	Philosophical	• Pioneered nursing's domain as the patient/environment relationship • Statistical analysis for health and nursing
• Maintain or restore balance and equilibrium, or • Help person achieve a more optimum level of function if possible or desirable	Grand	• Strong philosophical statements related to model • Strong influence on Roy, Neuman, and others
• Self-care deficit is the target of nursing • The nursing system is designed as wholly or partially compensatory or supportive–educative as dictated by the agency of the patient	Grand	• Pragmatic and comfortable concepts
• Acts in the patient's behalf to do those things that they would do for themselves had they the strength, knowledge or willingness to do so • Identifies 14 components of basic nursing care corresponding to Maslow's hierarchy of needs	Philosophical	• Delineates autonomous functions • Stresses goals of interdependence with the patient • Self-care concepts that influenced later theorists
• A nursing situation consists of patient behavior, nurse reaction, and nursing actions • Nurse provides assistance to patients to deal with helplessness • Physician's orders directed to patient, and nurse helps patient comply or decide not to comply	Mid-range (psychiatric nursing)	• Advanced nursing to a disciplined practice

(continued)

EXHIBIT 4.2 (*continued*)

Theorist, theory and date of early work[a]	Concepts/definitions/ assumptions	Influential models or sciences
Imogene King: open systems model, 1964	• The dynamic nature of life assumes continuous adjustment to life's stressors • The self is a person's total subjective environment, and is a distinctive center of experience and significance for each • Adjustment entails three open systems interacting with the environment: personal, individual and social	Highly eclectic Piaget Erikson Etzioni Bennis (among others)
Myra Levine: conservation model, 1966	• Focuses on the person as a wholistic being • The life process is characterized by unceasing change that has direction, purpose and meaning • The organism retains integrity through adaptive capability	Borrowed from a range of natural and behavioral sciences
Joyce Travelbee: human-to-human relationship, 1966	• The self-actualization aspect of illness is a natural and commonplace life experience	Peplau Orlando
Lydia Hall: core, care, and cure model, 1969 (clinical work dates to 1950s)	• Illness and rehabilitation are learning experiences	Carl Rogers
Martha Rogers: science of unitary man, 1970	• The person is a unified energy field continually interacting and exchanging matter and energy with the environment • This exchange results in increased complexity and innovativeness of the person • Well-being is reflected in pattern and organization	Systems Electromagnetic theory

Nursing role	Theory type	Major contribution
• Nursing's goal is to help individuals maintain their health so that they can function in their roles • The nurse enters the situation when the client can no longer perform their usual daily activities, yet • The domain of nursing includes health promotion and maintenance	Grand	• The Theory of Goal Attainment is a product of this model, and describes the nature of the nurse–client encounter • Emphasis on the derivation of nursing knowledge from other disciplines
• The goal of nursing is promotion of wholeness • Nursing intervention provides help in adaptation based on the principles of conservation of energy, and structural, personal and social integrity	Grand	• Distinctive and extensive vocabulary that makes it complex • Logically consistent and wholistic • Great influence on later theorists
• A major goal of nursing is helping the patient find meaning in illness	Mid-range (psychiatric nursing)	• Early emphasis on caring
• Stressed the autonomous function of nurses • The nurse guides and teaches in the process of personal care-giving • The nursing role consists of therapeutic use of self (core), the treatment regimen within the health care team (cure), nurturing and intimate bodily care (care)	Philosophical	• The eventual base for primary nursing • Applied to practice in a large metropolitan setting
• Acts to promote symphonic interaction between man and environment • Achieve maximum health potential by repatterning the human and environmental fields	Grand	• Strong voice for the development of nursing as a basic science

(continued)

EXHIBIT 4.2 (*continued*)

Theorist, theory and date of early work[a]	Concepts/definitions/ assumptions	Influential models or sciences
Sister Callista Roy: adaptation model, 1970	• Individual adapts behavior to cope with stimuli from environment that are stressors • Stressors disrupt dynamic state of equilibrium and illness results • Adaptive modes focus on physiological needs, self-concept, role function, and interdependent relations • A positive response to stress is determined by whether the simulation exceeds the level that can be accommodated by the individual	Systems Stress Adaptation
Betty Neuman: systems model, 1972	• Stressors as well as reaction and reconstitution can be viewed as intra-, inter- and extra-personal • Each individual has a usual range of responses to stress which maintains equilibrium and is called the normal line of defense • A flexible line of defense also exists to protect against unusual stress • Should a stressor break through the normal line of defense, lines of resistance attempt to stabilize the situation	Gestalt theory
Jean Watson: theory of caring, 1979	• Caring is a universal social behavior • Care for the self is necessary before care for others • Care and love are the cornerstones of humanness	Leninger Existential phenomenology
Patricia Benner: caring, 1984	• Describes caring as a common human bond	Dreyfus model of skill acquisition

[a] As determined by published work.

Nursing role	Theory type	Major contribution
• Nurse assesses the adequacy of the patient's coping, and if needed changes the patient's response potential by bringing the stimuli to the point where positive response is possible	Grand	• Excellent example of how knowledge can become unique in nursing; an eclectic view including stress, systems, adaptation
• Nursing aims at the reduction of stress factors and adverse conditions which threaten optimal functioning in a given situation • This is accomplished by identifying stress factors and assisting individuals to respond by strengthening their normal and flexible lines of defense	Grand	• Potentially useful in a variety of health care disciplines
• Emphasizes the humanistic dimension of nursing which can only be practiced interpersonally	Philosophical	• Makes the humanism in nursing scientific and credible
• Primary focus of the model is nursing • Through a qualitative process describes five stages of competency development: novice, advanced beginner, competent, proficient and expert • Gives credibility to the role played by intuition in practice	Philosophical	• Recognizes the value of experience in a practice discipline

glimpse. A concept, definition or assumption has been chosen because it depicts the distinctiveness of each theorist's work. In some instances, they are very subtle variations on a theme. There are other observations that are even more telling. Chronologically the early theorists were more philosophical, searching to give form and meaning to nursing, and they were successful. In many contemporary situations, we go back to their work for a clarity which has been lost over the years. Later theorists became highly abstract, applying behavioral, systems and developmental models to nursing. For all the difficulty in sometimes translating their work to practice, they have given us credibility as scholars. Swept away as we have been in the allure of high technology and the search for precise scientific explanations for our practice, the humanness of nursing often became lost. Our most recent theorists bring us full circle to our roots, reminding us that health and illness are personal experiences and that nurses serve the public best by their commitment to caring.

NURSING'S IMAGE: TRUE OR FALSE

Considering how much responsibility nurses have in health care, their constant presence in every place that care is given, and their numbers, you might expect that people would have a reasonably accurate idea about what nurses do. Yet they don't. One reason may be the extreme diversity of nurses' responsibilities. There simply isn't just one kind of nurse. Therefore, people's image of the nurse is formed in many ways and from many sources: personal acquaintance, contact during their own or someone else's illness, or the media—books, magazines, newspapers, radio, and television.

In the last few years, the nursing profession has been disturbed about the inaccurate picture of nursing in the media to the point where various nursing groups have made image making a priority. The Kalisches have presented an excellent overview of how nurses have been portrayed over the years in all the media, especially television. (See the partial list in the Bibliography.) The nurse, almost always a woman, is everything from angel to devil, sexpot to sexless, stupid to brilliant, tender to terrible—much like characters representing any other field. Although sometimes these nurses do seem to function as autonomous practitioners, more frequently they are physicians' handmaidens, technology tenders, and pillow plumpers. The storylines about personal relationships, problems, and successes are what is important; the rest is background. What is surprising is why anyone should really expect any other priority. Other disciplines are probably treated just as well or badly in fiction and are just as unhappy about it. At times doctors, nurses, and others in the health field are pleased with their images in shows where real issues are tackled (not always realistically). That does not mean that the nurses are shown as what we'd like nurses to be.

Books about nursing, from simplistic preteenage novels to those such as *One Flew Over the Cuckoo's Nest*, are also seen to impress the public. The Kalisches have also done an interesting analysis of movies and novels about nursing.[24] Both media seemed to follow similar patterns. In six time periods from 1854 to the late 1980s, nurse stereotypes ranged through the stages of angel of mercy, girl Friday, heroine, mother, sex object, and, finally, careerist, which is seen as the ideal image for this decade. Needless to say, this was not necessarily consistent in each time period. In fact, Dorothy Canfield Fisher, who ranked with the most noted authors of the time and was published from 1907 to 1953, "wrote with clarity and compassion about nursing and its contribution to the well-being of individuals and society."[25] A former public health nurse administrator, Mary Sewall Gardner, wrote realistic novels about public health nurses in the 1940s (as well as textbooks).

Yet, perhaps because television is so pervasive in almost everyone's life today, attracting all age groups, there is some fear that, of all the media, this one is most likely to influence the public concerning the image of nurses. Nursing was concerned enough that in the late 1980s it took massive action against a TV show called *Nightingales*, which portrayed nurses as promiscuous birdbrains and tinsel handmaidens.[26] Nursing organizations and individuals offered to provide script consultation and other help, and were turned down. The surge of nursing protests led commercial sponsors to back out, and eventually the show was canceled. (Lone's lucid "op-ed" commentary in the *New York Times*, widely reported, was seen as particularly useful in affecting public opinion.) At the same time, another series, *China Beach*, was praised as a realistic and sensitive portrayal of nurses in the Vietnam War. Its star later did commercials to promote nursing as a career. Ironically, however, this program, too, was eventually canceled, and the protests of nurses could not revive it.

Does the public believe that such fiction is reality? Probably not. Even children are beginning to regard some aspects of television cynically. More serious might be the nonfiction or news programs and articles that show what is new in medicine and health care, and where nurses are shadowy background figures or have limited exposure, to show what they do to help patients recover. In addition, when nurses become involved in criminal cases related to patients, the news coverage can be unfair or slanted toward the sensational.

Magazines publishing feature stories have often taken a "pity the poor nurse" point of view, although more recently the emphasis has been on new nursing roles. In fact, in nonfiction of all kinds, the portrayals of nurses have become more positive and up-to-date (while not totally eliminating the "poor nurse" aspect). No breakthrough seems to have come from greeting card manufacturers, who often portray nurses as devastating cartoons in get-well cards. Some have complained that the protesters had no sense of humor.

The power of the media and the numerous shows that continue to portray nurses in a negative and unrealistic manner led to the organizing of a group called Nurses of America (NOA) and their publication, *Media Watch.* NOA was sponsored by the Tri-Council organizations (see Chapter 13). It was funded by a grant from the Pew Charitable Trusts and administered by the NLN. NOA described itself as "a national, multi-media effort designed to inform the public about the role contemporary nursing plays in the delivery of high quality, cost-effective health care services. ... NOA's media efforts are designed to demonstrate the real drama of nursing; the vital work that nurses do every day."

NOA worked with a variety of media, ranging from newspapers and magazines to TV and community forums. A large component of their activities included monitoring the media for health-related issues and the portrayal of nurses and nursing practice.[27] Although its funding ceased in 1991, the nurses involved hope for continued support from the Tri-Council.

Does all this have any effect on how the public sees the nurse? Hard data are not easy to come by. Questions have been raised as to how much a prestige rating is influenced by personal contact and how much by reputation or image. Overall, the public seems to have a positive view of nurses and see them as an untapped resource for the nation's health. A 1990 survey found positive public sentiment:[28]

1. Nurses were far and away the health care provider that the public most respects and supports.
2. The public was impressed with nurses, and saw them as competent and caring.
3. The public saw nurses as underutilized.
4. Americans were receptive to nurses performing more routine health care services such as physical examinations and prescribing medications.

A national sample of 1000 adults were polled by the Gallup Organization in July 1993 about their receptiveness to advanced practice nurses assuming some of the role activities currently associated with physicians. They were asked if they would allow nurses to perform physical examinations, deliver prenatal care, immunize, and treat illnesses such as colds and infections. They responded as follows:[29]

1. Eighty-six percent were willing to receive everyday primary care services from a nurse.
2. Over half of the respondents were very willing.

3. One-third, or 34 percent, were somewhat willing.
4. Only 12 percent said they would be unwilling to use the advanced practice nurse as their primary health care provider.

A survey conducted by the Kellogg Foundation and completed in April 1994 demonstrates that Americans believe it is important to have nurses involved in their care.[30] Half of the 1000 respondents had been treated by a nurse practitioner in the last year. In a Gallup poll of the same year, consumers saw reduced RN staffing in hospitals as the most detrimental among cost-cutting strategies commonly used in health care today.[31]

The enhanced public image of nursing may be at least partly attributed to the image campaign launched between 1989 and 1992 by the National Commission on Nursing Implementation Project (NCNIP) and the Advertising Council of New York. The Ad Council guaranteed a minimum of $20 million in creative development and media exposure over a three-year period. The idea was to portray nursing as a "discipline that offers excitement, clinical substance, and authority and responsibility, all tied up in the richness of interpersonal closeness with patients."[32]

In addition to the image of nursing in the media and the public's viewpoint, another concern of nurses is how physicians perceive them and their profession. It is clear that the perceptions of some physicians are as confused as they were 100 years ago. However, now, as then, there are physicians and leaders in organized medicine who see and applaud the changes in nursing toward full professionalism; others find this trend either threatening, incongruent with what they think a nurse's role should be, or not as desirable as the situation in the "good old days."[33] A descriptive study on nurse–physician collaboration reports less of what was interpreted as collaboration, with nurses claiming more practice areas and patient care goals as their sole responsibility and physicians willing to delegate more shared areas to the nursing domain. This may indicate more assertiveness on the part of nurses, and ultimately clearer lines of responsibility.[34]

What about the impact of the "real" nurse on the *perception* of the nurse? Emerging research indicates that direct contact with a group, like nurses, may be the most influential factor in image making. Such contact may actually not provide a more objective view. Personal acquaintance almost always introduces the factors of liking or disliking, with little relation to, or knowledge of, professional performance. For others, emotionalism involved in contacts during illness is inevitable, because neither patient nor family and friends can be objective at such times. People do have expectations about what they want from a nurse, most often competence and caring. If their expectations aren't met, a bad image may replace a good one. For instance, whether a nurse is pleasant or unpleasant, patient or hurried, gentle or rough are factors. If buzzers aren't answered promptly or a patient is left in pain or discomfort, an image of uncaring nurses is formed and often communicated to others. It does not help that some caregivers today are difficult to identify and that the "nurse" may not be an RN. Moreover, unimportant as it may seem, *how* a nurse looks makes an important first impression. It is critical to make an impression that communicates professionalism. Kalisch and Kalisch wrote about the changes in nursing uniforms over time, and they were quick to note that "clothing is a form of nonverbal communication that stimulates judgmental or behavioral responses in others. Our clothing makes it possible for a stranger to categorize us—at least tentatively—and set the stage for further interactions. ... For better or worse, clothing communicates. Now, as before, it is important that nurses dress for success. Other points that are made about how nurses can improve their image are these: they should be more visible and active in community activities and organizations; converse more easily on a broad range of subjects, rather than be focused on nursing alone; and learn how to handle the media and communicate with the public.[35]

THE REALITY: FACTS, FIGURES, GUESSES

The information we have about the *real* nurse can also cause confusion. Demographic data, such as numbers, age, marital status, and employment, are usually acquired by taking a sample and then projecting to the total number. By the time that these and other facts are published, they may be somewhat outdated. However, by comparing them with earlier data, a trend or a change can be detected. Exhibit 4.3 shows some of the latest information available on nurses. Some of the interesting trends in the employed population over the last 10 years are a slow increase in the number of men, no significant increase in nonwhite nurses, more married nurses, and nurses as a group are getting older. A dramatic drop in the number of nurses with a diploma as the highest degree reflects educational trends, as does the older average age. Hospitals have consistently employed the largest number of nurses, with the percentages not varying much in this time period; private duty has decreased the most dramatically. Even though the percentage of NPs and clinical specialists has remained quite small in the last several years, this category was not even listed before the 1977 surveys.

A Nursing Profile

The most current, general, comprehensive demographic data about nurses comes out of the Division of Nursing of the Department of Health

EXHIBIT 4.3

Who Are the Nurses?

	1992	1988	1980
Total RN population	2.2 million	2.0 million	1.7 million
Employed in nursing[a]	83.2%	80.0%	76.6%
	(about 31% part time)		(about 32% part time)
Sex			
Female	96.0%	96.6%	96.1%
Male	4.0%	3.3%	3.0%
Ethnic-racial background			
White/non-Hispanic	91.4%	91.7%	90.4%
Black	4.0%	3.6%	4.3%
Asian/Islander	3.4%	2.3%	2.4%
Hispanic	1.4%	1.3%	1.4%
American Indian/ Alaskan Native	0.4%	0.4%	0.28%
Age			
Under 25	2.1%	3.9%	9.6%
25–34	23.6%	29.8%	36.2%
35–44	34.7%	29.5%	23.3%
45–54	20.6%	19.1%	17.2%
55–64	12.7%	12.3%	15.7%
65 or over	5.6%	5.0%	4.5%
Marital status			
Married	71.5%	70.6%	70.6%
Divorced, separated, widowed	16.5%	15.4%	13.8%
Never married	11.1%	13.0%	14.8%
Places of employment			
Hospital	66.5%	67.9%	65.6%
Nursing home	7.0%	6.6%	8.0%
Community health	9.7%	6.8%	6.6%
Physician's office/ ambulatory care	7.8%	7.7%	5.7%[b]
Nursing education	2.0%	1.8%	3.7%
Student health service	2.7%	2.9%	3.5%
Occupational health	1.9%	1.3%	2.3%
Private duty nursing	0.6%	1.2%	1.6%
Other	3.0%	3.6%	1.7%

(continued)

EXHIBIT 4.3 (*continued*)

Who Are the Nurses?

	1992	1988	1980
Type of position			
Staff nurse	61.6%	66.9%	65.0%
Head nurse and supervisor	9.6%	10.9%	13.1%
Administration (service and education)	6.2%	6.6%	4.8%
Instructor	3.5%	3.8%	4.7%
Clinical specialist/ clinician	1.9%	2.9%	2.1%
Nurse practitioner/ midwife	1.4%	1.5%	1.3%
Nurse anesthetist	1.0%	1.0%	1.1%
Other	6.5%	6.6%	6.8%
Higher educational preparation			
Doctorate	0.5%	0.3%	0.2%
Master's	7.5%	6.2%	5.1%
Baccalaureate in nursing	27.3%	25.1%	20.7%
Other baccalaureate	2.6%	2.3%	2.6%
Diploma	33.7%	40.4%	50.7%
Associate degree	28.2%	25.2%	20.1%

Source: DHHS Division of Nursing, National Sample Survey of Registered Nurses, 1988, 1992.
[a] Data refer to *employed* nurses. Some figures do not total 100% because of no response and rounding of figures.
[b] Refers to physician's office only.

and Human Services. The most recent was published in February 1994, and reports 1992 data from the *National Sample Survey of Registered Nurses*. Exhibit 4.3 summarizes data from the 1992 survey and includes comparisons with the 1980 and 1988 surveys. There are easily discernible trends. In March 1992, an estimated 2,239,815 individuals held licenses to practice as registered nurses in the United States. This was a 10 percent increase from March 1988. There was a 4 percent increase in the proportion employed in nursing. This "activity rate" was accompanied by a decrease in the numbers of nurses working part-time. In 1988, 32 percent of employed nurses were part-timers, while in 1992 this had decreased to 31 percent. All areas of the country, with the exception of New England, showed an increase in the numbers of employed nurses.[36]

The predominant setting for the employment of nurses continued to be the hospital. The overall number of nurses employed in hospitals increased from 1988 to 1992, although they represent a declining proportion of the nursing profession. The number of nurses providing bedside care to inpatients increased only 6 percent, while there was a two-thirds increase of nurses in outpatient departments and a 17 percent increase in the operating room, labor and delivery, and postoperative recovery. Rapid development in less intrusive techniques that decrease the need for major surgery, and the prevalence of managed care programs that often discourage elective surgery, will have implications here. There was a 30 percent increased employment of nurses in community settings.[37]

The "aging" of the registered nurse population continues. In 1992, the average age of the registered nurse was 43, compared with 42 in 1988. Put a different way, in 1992, 60.4 percent of the nurse population was under 45 years of age, as compared with 63.3 percent in 1988 and 69.1 in 1980.[38] Not only is the current nursing workforce aging, it is being augmented by RNs who are older. In Knopf's 1962 study, over 86 percent of nurses prepared at the diploma and baccalaureate level started nursing school when they were 19 years old or younger.[39] The average age of a new RN in 1992 was 33.7 years. The average age for an associate degree graduate is 35.7 years, 31.3 years for the diploma graduate, and 29.2 for the baccalaureate.[40] It is obvious how the discipline's appeal to the more mature student or the person looking for a midlife or retirement career change will shape the average age and even the expectations of the incumbents of the role of nurse.

In 1992, the majority of nurses received their basic nursing preparation in an academic as opposed to a service setting. In the first sample survey of 1977, 75 percent of nurses were originally diploma school graduates. In 1992, only 42 percent came from this origin. The greatest growth was among associate degree graduates, who were 11 percent of all nurses in 1977. In 1992, one-third of the universe of registered nurses received their initial nursing preparation in associate degree programs. In total, 30 percent of registered nurses in 1992 had baccalaureate degrees, 8 percent had advanced degrees, 28 percent had associate degrees, and a little over a third had a diploma.[41]

Salary gains for registered nurses from 1988 to 1995 were significant, between 28 and 38 percent on a regional basis. The mean annual salary in 1995 was $40,900.[42]

Another comprehensive study on nursing is the National League for Nursing (NLN) newly licensed nurse survey.[43] It provides details on the employment, mobility, and demographic characteristics of all newly licensed nurses in the country on a regional basis. In 1992, each nurse who was newly licensed after taking the July 1991 licensure exam, received a questionnaire covering demographic, employment, educational, and geographic characteristics. Over 34,000 nurses responded, for a response rate of 63.5 percent.

New RNs were overwhelmingly eager to work in hospitals for their first job (90.5 percent), but fewer than in 1990 (92.3 percent). Their major reason for choosing their current job was that they were able to work in their desired specialty. Salary and benefits was the second reason for choosing employment. In 1992, the percentage separating these two responses was much less than in 1990. In a related item, only 37 percent of the sample found "many jobs" available in 1992 as compared to 70 percent in 1988, and 63 percent in 1990. These results are not surprising and reflect the patterns of surplus and shortage discussed in Chapter 6.

As in previous years, the overwhelming number of new graduates, although generally older than previously, are still white women. Although the second-degree students may account for some of the older group (19 percent of graduates), the AD programs also attract older students. Over 18 percent of AD graduates held a college degree before nursing school, and 32 percent held LPN/LVN licenses (down from 41 percent in 1990). The majority of AD graduates have children living at home (62.9 percent); the BSN graduates are mostly single. This may also account for the fact that most AD nurses tended to choose a nursing program close by, whereas baccalaureate students were more mobile. Most RNs stayed in the same locale after graduation.

Minority Groups in Nursing

Studies on the general population of nursing students and graduates are inevitably influenced by the fact that the majority of nurses are both women and white. There is increasing interest in both the ethnic minority groups in nursing, such as Blacks, native Americans, and Hispanics, and the male minority. One question is why minorities do or don't enter nursing and why they often do not complete nursing education programs. Reasons given to explain why many of the racial and ethnic minorities, who are often also considered socioeconomically deprived, do not enter nursing include lack of role models, lack of understanding of what nursing is, lack of proper counseling, and inability to qualify because of poor academic records. The Advertising Council compaign, in cooperation with the National Commission on Nursing Implementation Project (NCNIP), made a special effort to recruit men and minorities (see Appendix 1). A very positive factor in the increase of doctoral minority nurses has been the ANA Minority Fellowship Program that began in 1974. It provides stipends and other forms of support to ethnic-minority students seeking doctoral education.

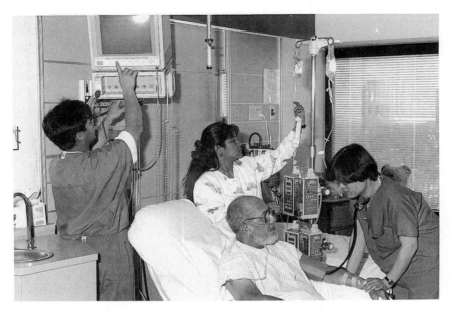

An increasing number of men and ethnic minorities are entering nursing. (*Courtesy of Beth Israel Medical Center, Newark, New Jersey.*)

In 1992, 13.3 percent of new graduates and 9.2 per cent of all nurses were members of a racial or ethnic minority group, as compared with 14.9 percent and 7.6 percent respectively in 1990.[44,45] These statistics represent more than a drop in minority recruitment to the profession, they represent a shift. The proportion of black graduates has dropped since 1990, and the proportion of Asians has grown substantially. This trend may be linked to a strong economic undercurrent. The federal dollars available for minority education have dwindled, and the current attitude of the Congress on domestic social welfare programs, including education, does not promise any more substantial funding in the near future. This absence of nurses from minority groups is of particular concern as we approach a future in which minority peoples will become the majority in the United States. There is a very noticeable absence of minority presence among the ranks of nursing leadership. Carnegie notes a number of blacks who hold doctorates, serve in high offices in nursing organizations, and hold very prestigious positions in the academia and health institutions,[46] but these are too few among many.

Men have been neglected as potential sources of nurse power, although male nurses have existed almost as long as female nurses in the United States. By 1910, about 7 percent of all student and graduate nurses were men, but in succeeding years the percentage declined, until by 1940 it had dropped to

2 percent. Most men were graduates of hospital schools connected with mental institutions; not many schools (for men) were affiliated with general hospitals, and few coeducational ones existed (see Chapter 2). By 1960, male nurses (not including students) comprised 0.91 percent of the nursing workforce. The current 4.0 percent level reflects a significant increase in the number of male nurses and a gradual increase in their proportion of the total employed RN population over the past 30 years. In 1992, the number of men in basic RN educational programs reached 11.1 percent.[47]

Men suffered the same discrimination in nursing that women encountered in male-dominated fields, although this was not always the fault of nursing. For instance, male nurses were kept in the enlisted ranks in the regular armed services until 1966, when, with the continuous pressure of the ANA, commissions were finally available to them in the Regular Nurse Corps.

Some surveys and studies show that overall, female nurses recognize that male nurses are accepted by both patients and physicians and believe that they can make a valuable contribution to nursing. Discrimination has been highlighted primarily in assignment of private duty nurses and in the care of women in obstetrics and gynecology.[48] Some men have gone to court, with varied results. (See Chapter 12.) One serious concern is that men comprised 18 percent of the disciplinary cases reported by state boards, most relating to substance abuse.[49]

Men in allied health roles or with other health care experience represent a major recruitment pool for nursing. They should not be expected to choose traditional male specialties, such as emergency, anesthesia, or intensive care, but should be urged to consider a whole range of career choices. They should be supported in career mapping to build a future in the profession.[50]

When looking at the issues regarding the role of minorities in nursing, it is important to remember that cultural differences stem from a myriad of components in all our backgrounds—gender, religion, ethnicity, and even geographic locale. The same biases and insensitivities that thwart our attempts to increase the ethnic, racial, gender, and religious diversity among the ranks of nurses hamper our ability to minister to those who are different from ourselves. Thus, it is important to be aware of and sensitive to minority issues in nursing but not to give them greater weight than the human issues that affect all people and are the mainstay of nursing care.

Attitude and Opinion

The tendency now is for nursing journals to publish surveys. These are often popular with readers because nurses like to know what other nurses think about an issue. Over a period of time, if the same issue is addressed, such as baccalaureate education, differences in attitude can also be detected.

However, interesting though they may be, results should be taken with the proverbial grain of salt. First, all survey questions are subject to varied interpretation, and some are slanted to get a certain type of answer. Most of all, unlike a scientific sample, only those who are interested and happen to find that particular survey interesting will answer, leaving hundreds of thousands of nurses whose opinion is not known.

One kind of research on nurses that has been done continually explores their attitudes about nursing in general, work situations, and reactions toward certain kinds of patients. The finding of the NLN study previously cited, indicating that individuals entered nursing because they wanted to help others, has been consistent over the years. Therefore, because it is evident that a number of students left nursing before completing the program, or did not work in nursing after graduation, and because nurses have also been accused of some indifference to quality care, the basic question arises: why? A number of writers have cited "disillusionment with nursing" as a major reason why nurses leave jobs or nursing itself. Yet, further investigation seems to show that the disillusionment, for graduates as for students, is related more to the practice setting than to the practice. This is discussed more fully in Chapter 6. Whether the study is almost 20 years old or one of the many new studies (see Appendix 1), nurses still appear to find their greatest satisfaction in caring for patients. As in any field, there are some who are primarily interested in nursing as a job or as a way to earn money—the so-called utilizer, migrant, or appliance nurse (one who works only long enough to buy a new home appliance). However, the majority of nurses still apparently have some of the same motivations with which they entered nursing. This is reinforced in a 1991 survey showing that a desire to help people was the primary reason most nurses entered the field; providing high-quality care ranked first in importance in their practice.[51]

A word should be said about nurses' attitudes toward certain types of patients. There has been some evidence that nurses do not view all types of patients equally favorably; for example, they tend to be more negative toward the elderly, alcoholic, criminal, mentally ill, or those with certain kinds of conditions. A number of studies, usually small, have been done on these topics. The purpose is primarily to determine what these attitudes are and why, how they affect patient care, and how to encourage or change particular attitudes. Several researchers have explored nurses' attitudes and concerns regarding AIDS. A number of nurses described a negative attitude in caring for AIDS patients, despite the perceived control of any occupational risk.[52] Another study found that avoidance of patients was linked to a negative attitude toward homosexuality.[53]

Finally, it is necessary for nurses to acknowledge the importance of our attitudes toward each other, especially when such attitudes affect clinical care, the advancement of the profession, and an individual nurse's practice. We need to question whether we govern our professional interrelationships

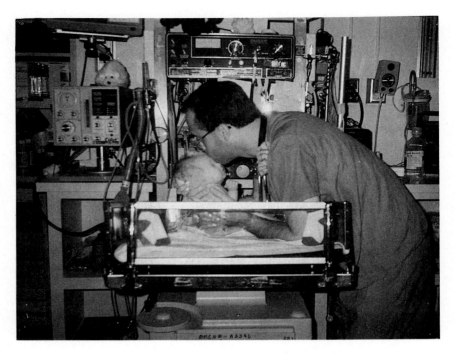

Nursing requires intellectual ability, technical competence, and the capacity to continue to care. (*Courtesy of US Army Center of Military History.*)

with the same guidelines that regulate our performance in patient care. Other areas to consider are attitudes toward nurses who are impaired, handicapped, or of different ethnic or national origin, and even nurses of different educational backgrounds.

SO, WHAT IS NURSING?

It can easily be seen that there may not be a single definition of nursing. Perhaps there never will be, since nursing is a multifaceted profession. Nevertheless, at some point, every nurse has to decide what nursing is to him or her and how to interpret it to others. The last point is by far the most important for the future of the profession. Too many people are uninformed or left with unflattering stereotypes about nursing. Each nurse owes it to their profession to assume the role of emissary of nursing. Take an active role in educating your patients and your public.

KEY POINTS

1. The basic criteria of professionalism include the concepts of autonomy, altruism, a defined body of knowledge, research, career commitment, social value, and ethics.
2. Nursing is defined in many ways, but the concept of caring for the individual as a whole is generally consistent.
3. Basic nursing functions include interviewing, examining, evaluating, treating, referring, collaborating, and caring for persons during their periods of dependence.
4. The nursing process and nursing diagnosis are a way of organizing data for nursing care.
5. The emphasis of nursing on the wholistic approach is evident in the work of nursing theorists, beginning with Florence Nightingale.
6. The image of nursing in the media is often distorted, but the public may also form a more lasting image, whether positive or negative, through direct contact.
7. Nurses must take some responsibility for creating a true, positive image of nursing.
8. Changes in the growing RN population include an older average age for working nurses and a higher level of education.
9. Since nursing is a large profession made up of a diverse population, information about the background and attitudes of subgroups, as well as of the majority, helps nurses understand one another better.

REFERENCES

1. Flexner A. Is social work a profession? *Proceedings of the National Conference of Charities and Correction.* New York: New York School of Philanthropy, 1915.
2. Pavalko R. *Sociology of Occupations and Professions.* Itasco, IL: Peacock, 1971.
3. Levenstein A. The Road to Professional Growth. *Nurs Mgmt* 15:7, 1985.
4. Truog R, et al. The problem with futility. *New Engl J Med* 12:326, 1992.
5. Caplow T. *The Sociology of Work.* Minneapolis: University of Minnesota Press, 1954.
6. King CS. Second licensure. *Ad Prac Nurs Quart* 1:7–9, Summer, 1995.
7. ANA Disturbed by Supreme Court Decision on Nurses as Supervisors. *News Release.* Washington, DC: ANA, May 24, 1994.
8. O'Neill SP, et al. APNs breaking down the barriers to provide primary care. *Nurs Spect* 4–5, February 7, 1994.

9. Beletz E. Professionalism—A license is not enough. In Chaska N (ed): *The Nursing Profession: Turning Points.* St. Louis: Mosby, 1990, pp 16–23.

10. The nurse practitioner question. *Am J Nurs* 74:2188, December, 1974.

11. American Nurses Association. *Nursing's Social Policy Statement.* Washington, DC: American Nurses Publishing, 1995, p 2.

12. Ibid.

13. Schlotfeldt R. The professional doctorate: Rationale and characteristics. *Nurs Outlook* 26:303, May, 1978.

14. NCSBN. *Model Nursing Practice Act.* Chicago: NCSBN, 1994.

15. ANA. *Model Practice Act.* Washington, DC: American Nurses Publishing, 1995.

16. Yura H, Walsh M. *The Nursing Process: Assessing, Planning, Implementing, Evaluating.* Norwalk, CT: Appleton–Century–Crofts, 1988.

17. Lunney M. Divergent productive thinking and accuracy of nursing diagnoses. *Res Nurs Health Care* 15:303–311, 1992.

18. Miller M, et al. Critical thinking in the nursing curriculum. *Nurs Health Care* 11:67–73, February, 1990.

19. Warren JJ. Nursing diagnosis taxonomy development. In McCloskey JC, Grace HK (eds): *Current Issues in Nursing*, 4th ed. St. Louis: Mosby, 1994, pp 122–128.

20. Bulechek GM, et al. Report of the NIC Project: Nursing interventions used in practice. *Am J Nurs* 94:59–66, October, 1994.

21. Martin KS, Sheet NJ. *The Omaha System: A Pocket Guide for Community Health Nursing.* Philadelphia: W.B. Saunders, 1992.

22. Saba VK, et al. A nursing intervention taxonomy for home health care. *Nurs Health Care* 12:296–299, June, 1991.

23. National Databases/Sets to Support Clinical Nursing Practice. *A Report to the Nursing Organizational Liaison Forum.* Kansas City, MO: American Nurses Association, November, 1991.

24. Kalisch PA, Kalisch BJ. *The Changing Image of the Nurse.* Palo Alto, CA: Addison-Wesley, 1987.

25. Benson ER. An early 20th century view of nursing. *Nurs Outlook* 38:275, December, 1990.

26. Lone P. TV's Nightingales—or birdbrains? *New York Times*, April 7, 1989, p A31.

27. What nurses of America is all about. *Media Watch* 1:1–2, Winter, 1990.

28. National League for Nursing. *A Nationwide Survey of Attitudes toward Health Care and Nurses.* New York: NLN, 1990.

29. American Nurses Association. Consumers willing to see a nurse for routine "doctoring," according to Gallup poll. *News Release*, September 7, 1993.

30. Kellogg Foundation. *How People View Their Providers.* Report of a survey, June 24, 1994.

31. American Nurses Association. Consumers believe RN cutbacks hurt quality of care in hospitals according to Gallup survey. *News Release*, June 14, 1994.

32. Joel L. NCNIP/Advertising Council campaign challenges resistant stereotypes. *Am J Nurs* 22:13, February, 1990.

33. Stein LI, et al. The doctor–nurse game revisited. *Nurs Outlook* 38:264–268, November–December, 1990.

34. Jones RAP. Nurse–physician collaboration: A descriptive study. *Holistic Nurs Pract* 38–53, April, 1994.

35. Gordon S, Buresh B. Nursing in the right words. *Am J Nurs* 95:20–22. March 1995.

36. Moses EB. *The Registered Nurse Population.* Rockville, MD: US Department of Health and Human Services, February, 1994, pp 10–22.

37. Ibid, p 8.

38. Ibid, p 14.

39. Knopf L. *From Student to RN.* Bethesda, MD: US Department of Health, Education and Welfare, 1972.

40. Rosenfeld P. *Profiles of the Newly Licensed Nurse*, 2nd ed. New York: NLN, 1994, p 14.

41. Moses, op cit, pp 17–18.

42. Begany T. 1995 earnings survey. *RN* 58:49–56, October, 1995.

43. Rosenfeld, loc cit.

44. Ibid, pp 16–17.

45. Moses, loc cit.

46. Carnegie ME. Blacks in America: An update. *Am Nurse* 22:6, February, 1990.

47. NLN. *Nursing Data Review 1994.* New York: NLN, 1994, p 20.

48. Halloran EJ, Welton JM. Why aren't there more men in nursing? In McCloskey JC, Grace HK (eds): *Current Issues in Nursing.* St. Louis: Mosby, 1994, pp 683–691.

49. Lewis JD, et al. Men in nursing: Some troubling data. *Am J Nurs* 90:30, August, 1990.

50. Perkins J, et al. Why men choose nursing. *Nurs Health Care* 14:34–38, January, 1993.

51. Yeast C. Nurses: Who are we and what motivates us? *Am Nurse*, Supplement 23:14, October, 1991.

52. Jemmott LS, et al. Predicting AIDS patient care intentions among nursing students. *Nurs Res* 5:172–177, May, 1992.

53. Jemmott JB, et al. Perceived risk of infection and attitudes towards risk groups: Determinants of nurses' behavioral intentions regarding AIDS patients. *Res Nurs Health Care* 15:295–301, 1992.

Nursing Practice

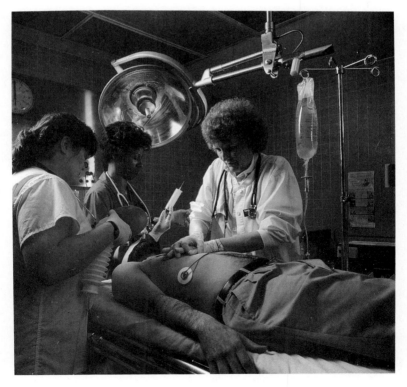

They saved a life today. (*Courtesy of the American Nurses Association*)

5

Education and Research for Practice

OBJECTIVES

After studying this chapter, you will be able to:

1. Identify four ways in which nursing education programs are alike.
2. Compare the major types of education programs leading to RN licensure.
3. Explain briefly the various alternatives for RNs seeking a baccalaureate.
4. Discuss the controversies surrounding continuing education.
5. Present the key points in landmark actions related to entry into practice.
6. Give the pros and cons of a two-tier educational system for nursing.
7. Define nursing research.
8. Identify the problems in putting nursing research into practice.
9. Describe briefly two trends or issues in nursing education and how they may affect future education.

Unlike most professions, nursing has a variety of programs for entry into the profession (also called *basic, preservice,* or *generic education*). This situation confuses the public, some nurses, and employers. The three major educational routes that lead to RN licensure are the diploma programs operated by hospitals, the baccalaureate degree programs offered by four-year colleges and universities, and the associate degree programs usually offered by junior (or community) colleges. The master's degree program for entry into practice was never widely available, and has now all but disappeared. The student with a nonnursing undergraduate degree is expected to complete nursing baccalaureate requirements. Many programs give the opportunity for these students to progress directly to the master's degree and specialization. There are a few professional doctorate programs that admit students with baccalaureate or higher degrees in fields other than nursing.

Although at one time diploma schools educated the largest number of nurses (more than 72 percent of the total number of schools in 1964 were diploma schools), the movement of nursing programs into institutions of higher learning has been consistent. Between 1964 and 1994, associate degree (AD) programs expanded from 130 to 868; BSN programs grew from 187 to 509. At the same time, diploma programs decreased from 833 to 124. Admission rates vary. Such unpredictable factors as a sudden shortage of nurses or a decreased amount of federal aid to schools often change the picture.

This chapter gives an overview of the various educational programs in nursing, continuing education, the open curriculum, research, and related issues and trends. Appendix 3 presents a comparison of programs, including what each type of graduate is prepared to do after completion.

PROGRAM COMMONALITIES

There are certain similarities that all basic nursing programs share, in part because all are affected by the same societal changes.

1. Nursing education is becoming more expensive, and financial support is less available for schools and students. Both state and federal governments have been tightening the financial reins on programs. Tuition seldom covers the cost of education, but, even so, it has been rising consistently. Students are finding it more and more difficult to receive scholarships, loans, and grants, particularly with the great cutback in federal funds. Also, because of both costs and social trends, fewer students live in dormitories, and those who do, pay for room and board.

2. The student population is more heterogeneous. Few, if any, schools refuse admission or matriculation to married students with or without families. It is not unusual to have a grandparent in a class as more mature individuals look for a new or better career. The tight job market in many fields brings to nursing individuals with degrees and sometimes careers in related or unrelated fields. All programs are including more men, by a small but definite percentage. Overall the

percentage of minority students has not increased, although the profession as a whole sees the recruitment of minority students and the development of minority leadership in nursing as a priority. In all cases, the diploma programs admit the lowest percentage of men and minority students.

3. Educational programs are generally more flexible. Trends in this direction, plus the admission of a very mixed student body, including aides, LPNs, and RNs seeking advanced education, have required a second look at proficiency and equivalency testing, self-paced learning, new techniques in teaching, and the external degree program.

4. State approval is required and national accreditation is available for all basic programs. Every school of professional nursing which prepares for entry into practice, as well as practical nurse programs, must meet the standards of the legally constituted body in each state authorized to regulate nursing education and practice within that state. These agencies are usually called *state boards of nursing* or some similar title. Without the approval of these boards, the graduates of the school would not be eligible to take the licensing examination. In addition, many schools of nursing seek accreditation by the National League for Nursing (NLN). Accreditation by the League is a voluntary matter, not required by law. Increasing numbers of schools seek it, however, because it represents nationally determined standards of excellence, and nonaccreditation may affect the school's eligibility for outside funding or impede the graduates' entrance into BSN or graduate programs or their ability to obtain grants and loans. Today, most schools are accredited. Nevertheless, accreditation is often criticized. (See Chapter 11.)

5. Faculty and clinical facilities are scarce resources. Faculty with the recommended doctoral degree for baccalaureate and graduate programs and the master's degree for other programs are increasing in number, but the total need has not been met. Clinical facilities are at a premium. Most schools, including diploma programs, use a variety of facilities. In large cities, several schools may be using one specialty hospital or clinical area (particularly obstetrics and pediatrics) for student experience. In rural areas, distance, small hospitals, and fewer patients are problems. Community health resources are very limited. Schools are also searching for new types of clinical experiences with various ethnic groups and in new settings such as hospices and community nursing centers.

6. There is a slow but perceptible trend toward involving students in curriculum development, policymaking, and program evaluation. Social trends and the maturity of students, with their demands to have a part in shaping the educational program, are making some inroads on faculty and administrative control of schools.

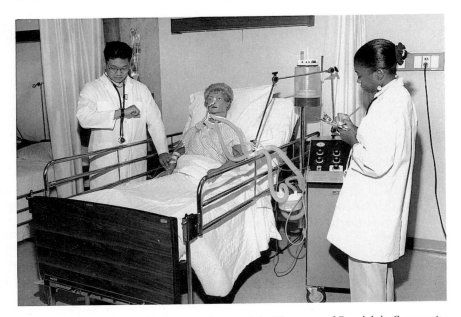

Students practice their skills in a nursing arts lab. (*Courtesy of Brookdale Community College, Lincroft, New Jersey.*)

7. All nursing students have learning experiences in clinical settings. Somewhere a myth arose that only practical nurse and diploma students gave "real" patient care in their educational programs, that AD students barely saw patients, and that baccalaureate students prepared only for teaching and administration. In fact, the time spent in the clinical area differs among programs within a particular credential as much as it does among various types of programs. In all good programs, students care for selected patients in order to gain certain skills and apply theoretical content.

8. It is generally agreed that the standards by which nursing education programs are judged should all include the same basic criteria related to the administration of the institution; facilities and resources; quality of faculty; student selection; retention and evaluation; and appropriateness and quality of the program.

THE NURSING ASSISTANT

It has been traditional that nurses are helped in their work by individuals called nursing assistants, aides or unlicensed assistive personnel (UAPs).

This category of workers has received added attention lately because of their increased presence in hospitals, often for the purpose of reducing the numbers of registered nurses needed to give care. The result has been an often adversarial relationship between RNs and management with UAPs caught in the middle.

This group of caregivers was traditionally prepared through on-the-job training. In 1987, the dissatisfaction with the quality of care in this nation's nursing homes resulted in a series of amendments to the Omnibus Budget Reconciliation Act. One of these amendments required that nursing aides in facilities qualifying for Medicare reimbursement be certified, and that certification be based on 75 hours of instruction including an examination to verify competency in both theory and practice. Though this process is handled by the state, there are specific federal guidelines. Many states have requirements that exceed those of Medicare. By 1990, all nursing assistants in long-term-care facilities were required to either have had a competency evaluation or completed an approved course.[1] Evaluation programs are offered by both the National Council of State Boards of Nursing (NCSBN) and the National League for Nursing (NLN). In each state the certification is awarded by a different administrative agency, but for the most part it is the Board of Nursing, Department of Health and Human Services or the Department of Health. Long-term-care aides were singled out for this degree of scrutiny because of the vulnerability of the population they serve, the frail elderly, and the token amount of supervision from the RN. In some ways, this was to compensate for unsuccessful legislative attempts to increase the numbers of RNs required in nursing homes.

There are similar certification requirements for home health aides, although the evaluation requirements seem to be less stringent. To some degree there is the assumption that the home-bound are more in control because they are candidates for community living. The skeptic would say they can be even more isolated and potentially open to abuse and victimization. Though the incidents of unloving care are few, they do exist.

Though the functions of nurses' aides are governed by state law and there is a great deal of inconsistency, some comments are possible. Nurses' aides are generally responsible (under the direction and supervision of the RN) to maintain a safe environment, perform basic nursing skills, grooming, helping with feeding, elimination, and mobilization. The most important thing for the RN to remember is that the aide functions under his or her license. It is the RN who supervises and determines the appropriate utilization of any unlicensed worker involved in direct patient care.[2] The basic education course for this assisting role may be given by a health care facility, high school, vocational/technical school, community college or a privately owned program which may run for profit and guarantee no employment. Many licensed practical nurse programs will award some credit for a formal nursing assistant course, thereby creating the first rung in a career ladder. Certification of assistive personnel has never been an issue for hospitals where patient contact is more limited and the RN presence is intense enough to honor the true meaning of supervision and delegation.

PROGRAMS FOR PRACTICAL NURSES

Professional nurses work closely with practical nurses (PNs) in many practice settings. Both PN education and licensure are different from those of RNs, but because of changes in health care, an increasing number of PNs have been entering RN programs at either a beginning or an advanced level.

PNs (called *vocational nurses* in Texas and California) fall into four general groups: (1) those whose only teacher has been experience and who are not licensed to practice (this type of PN is disappearing); (2) those with experience but no formal education who have taken state-approved courses to qualify them to take state board examinations and become licensed; (3) those who have been licensed through a grandfather clause; and (4) those who have graduated from approved schools of practical nursing and, by passing state board examinations, have become licensed in the state or states in which they practice. There are also a few who were enrolled in RN programs and were permitted by their state law to take the PN examination after a certain number of courses. The large majority of LPNs/LVNs are licensed by examination (NCLEX-PN). Although LPNs in the second and third categories can be legally employed, employers with a choice usually prefer graduates from an approved school who have been licensed by examination. (A grandfather clause is a legal device that allows persons who can show evidence that they have been practicing in a field to attain or maintain licensure even though the requirements have been changed and made more stringent.)

Formal PN education actually came later than that of the trained nurse. Although many women who nursed family and friends in the last 100 years were probably considered a type of PN, the first formal training programs were started by the Brooklyn, New York, YMCA in 1893. The three-month course taught home care of chronic invalids, the elderly, and children. Included were cooking, care of the house, dietetics, simple science, and simple nursing procedures. The program's success inspired similar courses in other states, but the first school was not organized until 1897. By 1947, there were only 36 schools, and only a few states had any kind of legislation regulating PN practice. After World War II, the nursing shortage and considerable amounts of federal vocational education funds set the stage for extraordinary expansion. Most of the early postwar programs, of about one year's duration, were in public schools, with practical experiences supervised by graduate nurses in cooperating hospitals. Generally no tuition was charged, although exploitive trade schools often charged much and gave little. By the 1950s there was more pressure for regulation, with states gradually requiring licensure.

Today the LPN programs are distributed throughout the nation, although most are in the South (45 percent) and fewest in the West (15 percent). LPN education takes place primarily in vocational/technical schools and community colleges, with fewer programs offered in secondary schools and hospitals, and is commonly one year in length. Most programs are publicly funded. Interestingly, tuition at community colleges is about the same per year for LPN and ADN programs. In 1984, "concern for job safety" due to the layoffs that followed DRGs prompted the National Federation of Licensed Practical Nurses (NFLPN) House of Delegates to endorse two levels of nursing (RN and LPN) and the expansion of the PN curriculum to at least 18 months. An implementation date of 10 years was set, but no real action followed. In 1986, North Dakota changed its educational requirement for LPN licensure to a two-year community college program.

Not all LPNs or LPN faculty agreed with this decision. However, some programs began planning to phase into an AD level. Already existing are PN programs that are the first year of a two-year AD program. A student may exit at the end of the year, become licensed and work, or become licensed and not work and continue into the second year and eventually become eligible for the RN licensure examination (NCLEX-RN). Some RN programs, particularly for the AD, give partial or total credit for the PN program (often only if the PN has also passed the licensing examination). Actually, over 25 percent of newly licensed RNs in 1992 already held LPN licenses.[3] A concerted effort has also been made to upgrade nurses' aides, home health aides, and other paraprofessional health care workers to LPN status through career ladders (discussed later).

Legitimate PN programs must be approved by the appropriate state nursing authority and may also be accredited, usually by the NLN. Upon graduation, the student is eligible to take the licensing examination (NCLEX-PN) to become an LPN or LVN. The licensing law is now mandatory in all states.

PN programs emphasize technical skills and direct patient care, but a (usually) simple background of the physical and social sciences is often integrated into the program. Clinical experience is provided in one or more hospitals and other agencies. The number of skills that are taught increases each year, probably because of employers' demands. The NLN has published statements on LPN entry-level competencies; the key points are found in Appendix 3.

LPNs work primarily in hospitals, extended care facilities, doctors' offices, private homes, and other health facilities, including to some extent community health agencies. They care for patients of all ages, but mostly adults.

Recent studies on the role activities of the LPN show a tendency for LPNs to expand their practice once they become experienced. This is accomplished through a sequence of events: an educational program appropriate to the activity, supervised practice, documented competency, continued supervision, and state board approvals. However, despite the fact that many activities have become a usual part of LPN practice, they are not included in the basic educational program. LPNs report administering IV medications, starting IVs, hemodialysis monitoring, pronouncing death, inserting GI tubes, ventilator care, central line management, management of total parenteral nutrition (TPN), as some examples.[4] These situations are of great concern to the RN, who is not only legally responsible but bound by a code of ethics.

The decline of LPN programs from a peak of 1319 in 1982 appears to have reached its limit for the time being. With the significant increase in RN salaries, employers seem to feel that the LPN carrying out technical tasks will free the more expensive RN to perform those vital tasks that only a professional nurse can do. On the other hand, LPNs, who are often forced to do more complex nursing tasks than they were trained for, and who are frequently in charge of a unit (when, legally, they shouldn't be), will probably also demand better salaries. They are more highly unionized than RNs and a target for more unionization. Furthermore, the federal government predicts an increased need for LPNs because of the growing elderly population; LPNs are a significant part of the nursing labor force in long-term care. Currently, it is estimated that there are over 500,000 LPNs. It is, and will be, a diverse population in terms of age and racial background. A larger percentage of black, Hispanic, and native American students enter LPN programs as opposed to RN programs (almost 27 percent compared with 16 percent). Where once more men were admitted to LPN than RN programs, this is no longer so (9.9 percent and 12.0 percent respectively).[5] There is some conjecture that LPN education is seen by many as a quick, inexpensive, and useful first step on a nursing career ladder, so this diversity will also affect the RN population in the future.

DIPLOMA PROGRAMS

The diploma or hospital school of nursing was the first type of nursing school in this country. Before the opening of the first hospital schools in the late 1800s, there was no formal preparation for nursing. But after Florence Nightingale established the first school of nursing at St. Thomas's

Hospital, England, in 1860, the idea spread quickly to the United States.

Hospitals, of course, welcomed the idea of training schools because, in the early years, such schools represented an almost free supply of nurse power. With some outstanding exceptions, the education offered was largely of the apprenticeship type; there was some theory and formal classroom work, but for the most part students learned by doing, providing the majority of the nursing care for the hospitals' patients in the process.

Gradually these conditions improved, faculty were better educated, and students had more classroom teaching. Yet, even as late as the 1950s, many classes were taught by doctors, and the focus was on giving care in the hospital, with the how sometimes more important than the why. When sciences were taught by a nearby college, courses were designed especially for nurses, often at a lower level than for other students. The student was typically a white, single, 18-year-old female who had to live in the dormitory. Breaking rules about curfew, smoking, drinking, and especially marrying meant dismissal, no matter how excellent the student.

This is no longer true. Today, in order to meet standards set in each state for operation of a nursing school and to prepare students to pass the licensing examinations, diploma schools must offer their students a truly educational program, not just an apprenticeship. Hospitals conducting such schools employ a full-time nurse faculty, offer students a balanced mixture of coursework (in nursing and related subjects in the physical and social sciences) and supervised practice, and look to their graduate nursing staff, not their students, to provide the nursing service needed by patients. The educational program has been generally three years in length, although most diploma schools have now adopted a shortened program. Upon satisfactory completion of the program, the student is awarded a diploma by the school.

This diploma, it should be understood, is not an academic degree. Because most hospitals operating schools of nursing are not chartered to grant degrees, *no* academic (college) credit is routinely given for courses taught by the school's faculty. (Exceptions are some external degree programs and some nonnursing baccalaureate programs that offer "blanket credit" to RNs. The latter type of degree may be a problem when seeking graduate education.) For this and economic and educational reasons, large numbers of diploma schools enter into cooperative relations with colleges or universities for educational courses and/or services. It is not uncommon for diploma students to take regular physical and social science courses and, occasionally, liberal arts courses at a college. If these courses are part of the general offerings of the college, college credit is granted. Credit is usually transferable if the nursing student decides to transfer to a college or continue in advanced education. If the course is tailored to nursing only, it is often not transferable to an advanced nursing program but is sometimes counted as an elective.

The primary clinical facility is the hospital, although the school may contract with other hospitals or agencies for additional educational experiences. Advocates of diploma education usually say that early and substantial experiences with patients seem to foster a strong identification with nursing, particularly hospital nursing, and thus graduates are expected to adjust to the employee role without difficulty.

Hospital schools usually provide other necessary educational resources, facilities, and services to students and faculty, such as libraries, classrooms, audiovisual materials, and practice laboratories. When it was taken for granted that students would be housed, good schools had dormitory and recreational space, as well as educational facilities in a separate building. Such housing must now be paid for and may also be used by others educated in or involved with the hospital.

The perceptible shift away from diploma school preparation for nursing can be explained (in an oversimplified way) by three factors: (1) some hospitals are terminating their schools, either because of the expense involved in maintaining a quality program and the objections of third-party payers, such as insurance companies and the government, to having the cost of nursing education absorbed in the patient's bill or because of difficulty in meeting professional standards, particularly in employing qualified faculty; (2) increasing numbers of high school graduates are seeking some kind of collegiate education; and (3) the nursing profession is becoming more and more committed to the belief that preparation for nursing, as for all other professions, should take place in institutions of higher education.

These social and educational trends will probably continue, but it is expected that diploma programs will be on the scene for some time and that quality programs will continue to prepare quality graduates. In fact, diploma schools have reported a dramatic increase in admissions in the last several years. Indeed, the vast majority of current diploma programs are NLN accredited, and many of the schools that dissolved or were "phased into" AD or baccalaureate programs were also accredited. The 1970 National Commission study recommended that strong, vital schools be encouraged to seek regional accreditation and degree-granting status, but only a few have done so. Another recommendation, that other hospital schools move to effect interinstitutional arrangements with collegiate institutions, has been acted upon more readily.

Although hospitals are less likely to operate schools, they continue as the clinical laboratories for nursing education programs. In the communities where new AD or baccalaureate programs are opening, there is often planning for the new programs to evolve as diploma programs close—a phasing-in process. This cooperation enables prospective candidates for the diploma program to be directed to the new program, qualified diploma faculty to be employed by the college, and arrangements made to use space in the hospital previously occupied by the diploma school. Cooperative planning provides for continuity in the output of nurses to meet the needs of the community.

ASSOCIATE DEGREE PROGRAMS

A relative newcomer to the scene of nursing education is the associate degree (AD) program that is usually offered by a junior or community college, is two years in length, and prepares graduates for the RN licensing examination. This type of program, offered in a college setting but not leading to a baccalaureate degree, was not even envisioned by nursing educators of the late nineteenth and early twentieth centuries.

The AD program is the first nursing education program to be developed under a systematic plan and with carefully controlled experimentation. In 1951 Mildred Montag published her doctoral dissertation describing a nursing technician able to perform nursing functions seen as considerably more prescribed and narrower in scope than those of the professional nurse and broader than those of the PN. This nurse was intended to be a bedside nurse who was not burdened with administrative responsibilities. Montag listed the functions as (1) assisting in the planning of nursing care for patients, (2) giving general nursing care with supervision, and (3) assisting in the evaluation of the nursing care given.[6] Previous experiences with the Cadet Nurse Corps supported the concept of providing a shortened nursing program. The emerging community college was seen as a suitable setting for this education since it would place nursing education in the mainstream of education, and the burden of cost would be on the public in general rather than on the patients, as was the case with diploma programs. An AD would be awarded at the end of the two years. As originally conceived, the program was considered to be terminal and not a first step toward the baccalaureate.

A five-year project to test this idea was started in 1952, with seven junior colleges and a diploma school participating. The results of the project showed that AD nursing graduates could carry on the intended nursing functions, that the program could be suitably set up in junior colleges with the use of clinical facilities in the community at no charge, and that the program attracted students. The success of the experiment plus the rapid growth of community colleges combined to give impetus to these new programs.

Over the years there have been changes in philosophy as to what the graduate of these programs is prepared to do. Many AD deans do not see the program as terminal or technical, perceiving a difference in amount rather than kind of education for practice. The entire concept of the AD nursing program as terminal has changed over the last 25 years. Obviously, no educational program should be terminal in the sense that graduates cannot continue their education toward another degree. Trends have developed toward enhancing articulation opportunities for AD–RNs into baccalaureate nursing programs. However, the AD nurse need not continue formal education to hold a valuable place in the health care system.

The practice of the AD graduate has often been called technical, as differentiated from professional. Montag viewed nursing functions on a continuum, placing technical training in the middle of the continuum[7] (see Exhibit 5.1). The boundaries of the continuum are not totally fixed, and some overlap. Many nurse educators at all levels agree that there is a common core of knowledge drawn upon by all RN education.

Whether the term *technical* will continue to be used is not clear. The concept of a technical worker, honored in other fields, has not been fully accepted in nursing, possibly because it is considered a step down from the *professional* label that has been attached to all nurses through licensing definitions and common usage over the years. Montag, noting the difficulty of choosing an appropriate term for the new type of proposed nurse, said, "It is also probable that the term 'nursing technician' will not satisfy forever, but it is proposed as one which indicates more accurately the person who has semi-professional preparation and whose functions are predominantly technical."[8]

The use of the term *technical* was rejected by the NLN Council of Associate Degree Programs in a 1976 action and the term *associate degree*

EXHIBIT 5.1

Montag's Continuum of Nursing Functions

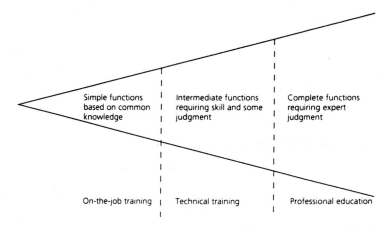

nurse (AD nurse) was suggested. This term is frequently used now.

More important than the name are the role and functions of the AD nurse. Because of nursing shortages, as well as lack of understanding of the abilities and preparation of technical nurses, a tendency to use the diploma nurse of previous years as a standard, and general traditionalized concepts of nursing roles, employers have often not assigned AD nurses in the manner that best suits their preparation. Like nurses throughout the centuries, AD nurses have been placed quickly as team leaders and charge nurses, positions in which they were not intended to function.

The NLN has published a role and competencies statement for AD nurses, which provides guidelines for identifying their expected level of practice at graduation and six months later. The document is very comprehensive. The introduction notes that AD education is still based on Montag's "middle range" of nursing functions and states: "the goal of associate degree nursing programs continues to be preparation of registered nurses to provide direct client care. Although associate degree nursing students receive preparation to provide care for clients across the life span, the majority of the graduates are employed in settings where the focus of care is on adult clients."[9]

Over the years, as Montag predicted, the AD course of studies has varied and changed. For instance, when college policies permit, there is a tendency to put a heavier emphasis and more time on the nursing subjects and clinical experiences, sometimes through the addition of summer sessions or clinical preceptorships. Some programs are also adding team leadership and managerial principles because their graduates are put in positions requiring these skills. Today, most AD programs are between 18 and 24 months in length, but some require that all science and general education courses be completed before the nursing program is begun, which may lengthen the AD program considerably. The Council of Associate Degree Programs of the NLN, the AD accreditor, has set 108 quarter hours or 72 semester credits as the maximum number of credits for any program.[10] This should allow completion in four semesters of full-time study.

Although there has been some complaint that AD nurses are not proficient in certain technical skills and require too much orientation to the responsibilities of a staff nurse, many AD educators believe that the need for additional clinical experiences is not suggested more frequently than for graduates of other programs. It is generally unrealistic for new graduates or their employers to expect newcomers to function as seasoned practitioners. Almost everyone agrees that AD graduates have a good grasp of basic nursing theory, have inquiring minds, and are self-directed in finding out what they don't know. It is also generally agreed that a good orientation program is the key to satisfactory adjustment to the work setting by new graduates from any type of RN program. One realistic concern is that the majority of AD programs do not appear to teach their students how to carry

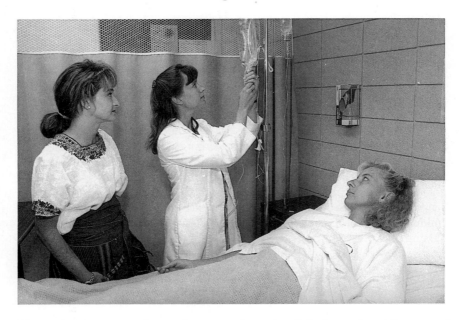

All nursing programs give students experience in clinical practice. (*Courtesy of Valencia Community College, Orlando, Florida.*)

out complex technological procedures that both staff nurses and nurse executives consider an essential part of nursing practice, even for a new graduate. Yet it is expected that a similar situation exists in other kinds of nursing programs.

AD programs are the fastest-growing segment of nursing education for a variety of reasons. Clearly, the availability of AD programs in a community; the low cost of $1500–$1800 a year (most programs are publicly funded); the fact that this is usually the shortest way to RN licensure; the increasing possibilities of educational career ladders; and the reality that most employers do not differentiate much, if at all, in salaries for RNs with different kinds of education, are all important factors. AD programs are distributed throughout the United States, with most in the Midwest and the South; however, they make up the majority of nursing programs in *all* regions. The makeup of AD students (and graduates) is distinctly different from that of the other programs. In relation to minority enrollment, there is little significant difference in AD and BSN programs. The African-American enrollment is 8.5 percent (AD) versus 9.0 percent (BSN); for Hispanic students 3.2 percent to 2.8 percent; Asians 2.8 percent to 3.9 percent.[11] There are a larger number of Hispanics in two-year institutions as opposed to Asian-Americans and Blacks, who gravitate to baccalaureate programs. AD students are also more likely to be older, married with children, and working part-time. There is some indication that they are more likely to continue to work in the community. An interesting point is that AD programs have been attracting second-career students and second-degree students, perhaps, in part, because of the brevity of the program. The long-term implications of all these factors for nursing in general are discussed later.

BACCALAUREATE NURSING PROGRAMS

The first baccalaureate program in nursing was established in 1909 under the control of the University of Minnesota, through the efforts of Dr. Richard Olding Beard. Since then, these programs have become an increasingly important part of nursing education and have grown steadily in numbers.

The baccalaureate graduate obtains both a college education with a bachelor's degree and preparation for licensure and practice as a registered professional nurse. The most notable differences between baccalaureate education and the other basic nursing programs are related to liberal education, development of intellectual skills, and the addition of community health practice and teaching and management concepts, although some of the other programs do include a limited amount of such content. Baccalaureate nurses have the opportunity to become liberally educated; almost all programs allow free electives in the humanities and the sciences, as well as nursing courses. Nursing students are able to participate in the college/university cultural and social activities throughout their whole program and develop relationships with professors and students in other disciplines. Nursing majors meet the same admission requirements and are held to the same academic standards as all other students. The nursing program is an integral part of the college or university as a whole and is usually four years in length.

The baccalaureate degree program includes courses in general education and the liberal arts, the sciences germane to and related to nursing, and nursing. In some programs, the student is not admitted to the nursing major (nursing courses) until the conclusion of the first two years of college study. In most programs, courses in the nursing major are concentrated in the upper division, the last two years of the program.

As in the other nursing programs, the baccalaureate program has both theoretical content and clinical experience. The baccalaureate student who takes courses in the physical and social sciences will have greater depth and breadth, because students majoring in nursing take the college courses in the sciences and humanities with students majoring in biology or English literature.

Although technical skills are essential to nursing, learning activities that assist students to develop skills in recognizing and solving problems, applying general principles to particular situations, and establishing a basis for making sound clinical judgments are also emphasized. This enables the nurse to function more easily when a familiar situation takes an unexpected turn or when it is necessary to deal with an unfamiliar situation.

Like other nurse educators, those in baccalaureate programs constantly review (and often revise) their nursing curriculum, but they have given relatively little attention to the liberal arts component, even though this part of the program is supposed to be important in making the baccalaureate nurse an educated person as well as a clinical practitioner. In 1986, an interdisciplinary "Panel for Essentials of College and University Education for Professional Nursing" reported the recommendations of its two-year study to the American Association of Colleges of Nursing (AACN), its sponsor. The report had two components, one related to nursing knowledge and the other to liberal education. The panel members noted that a liberally educated person can responsibly challenge the status quo and anticipate and adapt to change. Their recommendations were that the education of the professional include (among other things) the ability to write and speak effectively, think analytically, understand a second language and multi-cultural traditions, interpret qualitative data, use computers, and appreciate the social role of the fine and performing arts.[12] Finally, they noted that nursing faculty are responsible for integrating knowledge from the liberal arts and sciences into professional nursing education and practice. "Liberally educated nurses make informed and responsible ethical choices and help shape the future of society as well as the nursing profession."[13] What long-term action comes from this report remains to be seen. Since its release, there has not been as much discussion of the report as might be expected.

Most BSN graduates select hospitals as their first place of employment but then often turn to community health nursing. Those hospitals that have primary nursing, which gives nurses individual responsibility for a group of patients, seem most likely to attract and retain baccalaureate nurses. Graduates with long-term plans for teaching, administration, or clinical specialization continue into graduate study.

A baccalaureate in nursing offers many career opportunities, a fact that is widely acknowledged. Equally important is the fact that in the last 10 years, when nursing has been under particular scrutiny, the many reports and studies have agreed that what is needed to meet the nursing needs in today's complex health care environment is more baccalaureate nurses. However, this program, considered by the ANA as minimum preparation for professional nursing, is usually more expensive for students than other basic programs. This is a serious problem, as funding cuts lessen student aid.

A major phenomenon in baccalaureate nursing is the increase in the number of RNs entering these programs. In part, this is due to the fact that nurses are more eager to advance in their careers and want the greater options available with a baccalaureate degree. Since employers are aware of this and look for ways to keep their nurses, many offer tuition reimbursement as a fringe benefit. When this is added to the new flexibility offered RNs by baccalaureate educators, nurses find it less difficult to go to school, work, and maintain family responsibilities (although it's never easy). About 136 programs are designed especially for returning RNs. Other BRN or BS-RN tracks exist within regular baccalaureate programs, with the nurses mainstreamed into the basic curriculum. In most nursing programs, RNs receive some credit and/or advanced standing for their previous education through challenge examinations. Frequently, courses and clinical experiences are individualized to meet RNs' needs and goals. The degree is the same for basic and RN students. In 1992, one-third of the nursing baccalaureates were conferred on RNs.[14] Other options will be described later. It is unfortunate that some RNs, because of circumstances, desire, or lack of counseling, choose nonnursing majors, which generally precludes their acceptance into a graduate program in nursing.

Another noticeable trend, which began in the 1980s, is the increase of students with baccalaureate or advanced degrees in fields other than nursing. These students, of course, receive a second baccalaureate. Depending on how many of their previous courses satisfy the BSN requirements, their program may consist primarily of upper-division major nursing courses. A few baccalaureate programs have been especially designed for the nonnursing baccalaureate graduate. Actually, such programs may not take much more time than an AD program. Often these second-careerists do not realize, or are not told, that they will need a nursing baccalaureate for career advancement, regardless of their nonnursing degrees. More of them are looking at an accelerated master's program in which they acquire a nursing baccalaureate on the way to a nursing master's degree. These programs are described next.

OTHER PROGRAMS LEADING TO RN LICENSURE

A number of years ago, several nursing education programs, such as those at Yale and Western Reserve University, admitted only baccalaureate graduates and granted a master's degree in nursing as the basic educational credential. A variation on this theme is the accelerated masters for students with a nonnursing bachelor's degree. The bachelor of science in nursing is completed as an interim step and the student moves on to specialty preparation at the master's level. These are commonly called *articulation* programs and a student may get a license after completion of the baccalaureate degree, depending on state law, and then continue directly to the master's degree.

The first program for a professional doctorate (ND) for college graduates was established at Case-Western Reserve in 1979. It was designed for "liberally educated men and women who are gifted intellectually, willing to invest themselves in a rigorous, demanding, rewarding program of study, and committed to a sustained professional career."[15] As described, the program should be located only in universities with health science centers preparing several types of health professionals. Because such universities also offer advanced graduate education, ND students are prepared in an academic climate of scholarship and research. Faculty are prepared at the highest level of scholarship, with some engaged in teaching and research and others, jointly appointed, master's-prepared clinicians engaged in clinical practice, teaching, and some aspect of research. The curriculum prepares the ND graduates to become proficient in the delivery of primary, episodic, and long-term nursing care, and to evaluate their own practices and those of their assistants, since they are accountable for the outcomes of all nursing practice. Graduates of this program would continue graduate study in a specialization and/or a functional area such as teaching, administration or clinical practice. As is true of medical students whose professional degree is a doctorate, they may also obtain a master's or PhD concurrently with the first doctorate. This innovative approach, seen as a major step toward the emergence of nursing as a full-fledged profession, has now been adopted by several other universities, but many questions are still raised as to the functions, role, and job market for the graduates and the best organizational structure for the program.

GRADUATE EDUCATION

In 1992, about 8 percent of the nurse population had at least a master's degree. About 13,500 were estimated to have doctoral degrees. Today, the purpose of master's level education is to prepare professional nursing leaders in the areas of advanced practice, teaching, and administration. Nurses with these special skills and knowledge are desperately required now and will be for the foreseeable future. About 43 percent of RNs with master's degrees had the focus of advanced clinical practice in 1992.[16]

Perhaps because so much of the emphasis in graduate programs over the years had been on attaining functional skills in teaching and management, with little attention given to clinical knowledge and skills, a 1969 ANA statement on graduate education proclaimed that the "major purpose of graduate education should be the preparation of nurse clinicians capable of improving nursing care through the advancement of nursing service and theory."[17]

However, it soon became evident that nurses in education and management/administration did indeed need the functional skills required in these fields. Almost ten years later, a new statement focused on "the preparation of highly competent individuals who can function in diverse roles, such as clinical nurse generalists or specialists, researchers, theoreticians, teachers, administrators, consultants, public policy makers, system managers, and colleagues on multidisciplinary teams ... prepared through master's, doctoral, and postdoctoral programs in nursing that subscribe to clearly defined standards of scholarship."[18] Nontraditional approaches, such as inter-institutional exchange programs, consortium arrangements, and satellite and off-campus programs, were also seen as desirable and encouraged.

These flexible programs are increasing, with not just the "articulation" model, but also "summers only" and "Friday only" programs, programs for nurses with nonnursing degrees, a program for AD nurse-educators, various off-site programs, some with telecommunications, and a number of accelerated programs.

Graduate programs in nursing vary in admission requirements, organization of curriculum, length of program, and costs. Admission usually requires RN licensure, graduation from an approved (or accredited) baccalaureate program with an upper-division major in nursing, a satisfactory grade point average, achievement on selected tests, and sometimes nursing experience. Some programs admit a few nurses without BSNs and assist them in making up deficiencies. Part-time study is available in many, perhaps most, programs, but often certain courses must be taken in sequence, and at least some full-time study may be required. Reduced federal support and fewer traineeships have stimulated faculty to develop more part-time study options. Since 1970, when about 75 percent of students went to school full-time, there has been a total reversal of numbers. There are barely 5000 full-time students among 28,370 who are candidates for a master's degree.[19] Not all graduate programs offer all possible majors. The degrees granted are usually the MS (master of science with a nursing major); MSN (master of science in nursing); MNSc (master's in nursing science); MEd (master of education with a major in nursing); MN (master's in nursing); MA (master of arts with a nursing major); and MPH (master of public health with a nursing major). The differences are sometimes obscure.

Most NLN-accredited master's programs offer study of a clinical area, such as medical-surgical nursing, maternal-child nursing, community health nursing, or psychiatric nursing, based on a theoretical framework developed by that faculty and including relevant advanced courses in the natural and social sciences and supervised clinical experience. The depth of clinical study varies in relation to the functional role selected: teaching, management, or advanced clinical practice. A practicum (planned, guided learning experiences that allow a student to function within the role) is usual for the functional role as well as the area of clinical specialization, and often they are combined. Practice varies from program to program, from one day a week for a semester to almost a year's full-time residency. Acquisition of research methods is also considered essential. In general, master's education in nursing includes introduction to research methods. Debate continues around whether a thesis or project for the independent study of a nursing problem should be a degree requirement. As the terminal degree becomes the doctorate, the credits for the master's have decreased, and many programs have eliminated the thesis, choosing to reserve any independent research experience for the dissertation.

Although some nurses obtain graduate degrees outside the field of nursing, advanced positions in nursing, especially in nursing education, usually require a nursing degree, preferably with advanced clinical content and experience. In 1994, there were some 278 nursing master's programs in the United States, most with clinical majors. An NLN pamphlet, "Master's Education in Nursing, Route to Opportunities in Contemporary Nursing," updated frequently, presents an overview of all accredited nursing master's programs, including curricula, clinical and functional majors, admission requirements, availability of part-time study, length of program, approximate cost, and availability of housing.

Although many nurses are still enrolled in nonnursing doctoral programs, the pendulum may have swung toward doctoral degrees in nursing in the last few years. They have shown remarkable growth: 2 in 1946, 27 in 1983, and 60 in 1994. The "appropriate" doctoral degree for nurses continues to be a matter of debate. Some nursing leaders favor granting a PhD in nursing with a minor in a relevant discipline. Others have felt that although the nursing PhD is an ultimate goal, nursing science is not sufficiently developed to make this practical immediately. Instead they suggest either a PhD in some other discipline with a minor in nursing or a strictly professional degree such as the DNS (Doctor of Nursing Science). It is believed that a nurse with an academic degree (PhD) could help to generate knowledge, and the nurse with a professional degree such as the Doctor of Education or Doctor of Science in Nursing (EdD, DNSc) would apply this new knowledge. There are a variety of nursing doctorates offered today, as opinions vary. Several schools offer both the PhD and the DNS and have identified the differences.

PhDs and EdDs, not necessarily in nursing, are still the degrees most commonly held by nurses. As more doctoral programs evolve, the debate becomes more heated. Schools starting doctoral programs must consider what best suits their educational philosophy and the qualifications and interests of their faculty members. Yet, many schools choose a PhD program because it is still considered the most prestigious degree in academia. Sometimes the university denies nursing this option because of the notion that nursing science is not advanced enough; therefore the school chooses a DNS or DNSc instead. Is this important? Some think it is. Graduates of both are expected to become researchers, teachers, and administrators. (Most contemporary doctoral students are preparing primarily for education and research, not advanced clinical practice.) In actuality, the differences blur. Even nurses with a PhD employed in beginning positions in a nursing school may be teaching undergraduate students and may have little interest or time for research. In fact, a doctorate of any kind has been called a "union card" for admission to a teaching position in higher education. Whether or not the person does research of any kind depends on personal inclination or professional pressure (the publish-or-perish syndrome). It is becoming more common and even necessary to select postdoctoral fellowships to get adequate research training and experience.[20, 21]

One consistent concern is quality in doctoral programs, particularly as they proliferate, perhaps in schools that do not have an adequate number of faculty properly prepared to guide the education and research of doctoral students.[22] Monitoring of doctoral programs is usually a university prerogative, but it is not clear how well this is done. One thing that *is* made clear in all major reports is the continuing need for doctorally prepared nurses.

NURSING RESEARCH

With the growth of graduate education, nursing research has grown tremendously over the years, and it is important to have at least a basic understanding of where it is and where it's going. A more detailed discussion of nursing research is found in many sources and is useful as background.[23] It is also interesting to look at how nursing research evolved in the United States, beginning perhaps with Adelaide Nutting in 1906.[24]

Schlotfeldt's definition of the term *research* is classic: all systematic inquiry designed for the purpose of advancing knowledge.[25] Notter made a useful comparison between problem solving related to patient care (sometimes also described as the *nursing process*) and scientific inquiries.[26] Both go through such steps as (1) identifying a problem, (2) analyzing its various aspects, (3) collecting facts or data, (4) determining action on the basis of analysis of the data, and (5) evaluating the result. These steps may be relatively simple or very complex; they may involve laboratory equipment, human experimentation, or neither. Research may be designated as *basic,* the establishment of new knowledge or theory that is not immediately applicable, or *applied*, the attempt to solve a practical problem. Either way, the same steps are taken. Simply put, the questions to be studied through the research process arise from practice and the ultimate aim is to enhance our understanding of that practice so as to offer better service to the public.

Why nursing research? Practice disciplines have always needed to maintain and develop their own bodies of knowledge for survival as a profession and for the well-being of their clients. A more frustrating issue is the utilization of nursing research. After all, no matter how critical the findings of research studies may seem, if they are not tested in practice over a period of time, in a variety of settings, the results might still be questioned. If they are not used at all, practice may change, but it will not change as a result of research. The first step is communication, especially from researcher to practitioner. In the last few years, means of reporting research have increased considerably, with many more publications and conferences sponsored by organizations, universities, the government and others. Nevertheless, putting research into practice has made slow progress. Most nurses giving direct patient care do not read research journals or have contact with nurse researchers. Obstacles most frequently reported by them in relation to using research findings are reading and understanding the report, relevance of findings for practical situations, inability to find research findings, suggestions too costly or time-consuming to implement, resistance to change in the workplace, and lack of worthwhile rewards for using nursing research.[27]

Some clear trends are now emerging that may turn this situation around. First, researchers are beginning to realize that they have a responsibility for translating the research into terms and concepts understandable to the clinician and presenting their research results in places other than research conferences.[28] They must make a distinct effort to reach out to staff nurses.

Second, the interpretation of research findings and their application to practice is now a required part of basic nursing education.[29] And, perhaps most important, nursing research is being done in clinical sites, with nurse researchers and staff working together. Having organized research programs in a significant number of hospitals will take time, but the advances that have been made are impressive, especially given the interest of farsighted nurse executives.[30]

One dramatic acknowledgment is that in 1986, a National Center for Nursing Research (NCNR) was established at the National Institutes of Health (NIH). Congress not only overrode a presidential veto (and NIH objections), but key senators on both sides of the aisle spoke to the value of nursing research and the need for a visible national center. The Secretary of DHHS announced the establishment of the NCNR "for the purpose of conducting a program of grants and awards supporting nursing research and research training related to patient care, the promotion of health, the prevention of disease, and the mitigation of the effects of acute and chronic illnesses and disabilities. In support of studies on nursing interventions, procedures, delivery methods and ethics of patient care, the NCNR programs are expected to complement other biomedical research programs that are primarily concerned with the causes and treatment of disease."[31] The NCNR was awarded the full status of an institute in 1992, becoming the National Institute for Nursing Research (NINR).

The NINR supports research, research training, and career development in health promotion and disease prevention, acute and chronic illness, and nursing systems, which include such areas as innovative approaches to delivery of quality nursing services, strategies to improve patient outcomes, interventions to ensure availability of resources, and bioethics research, a special initiative. A number of research training awards exist for beginning and advanced nurse researchers through individual and institutional predoctoral, postdoctoral, and senior fellowships. Among the research priorities targeted for 1995–1999 are the following.

- Community-based nursing models (1995)
- Effectiveness of nursing interventions in HIV–AIDS (1996)
- Cognitive impairment (1997)
- Living with chronic illness (1998)
- Biobehavioral factors related to immunocompetence (1999).

EDUCATIONAL MOBILITY AND OPEN CURRICULUM PRACTICES

One of the key developments in nursing education has been the open curriculum, which began in the 1970s. The NLN defines this as a system "which incorporates an educational approach designed to accommodate the learning needs and career goals of students by providing flexible opportunities for entry into and exit from the educational program, and by capitalizing on their previous relevant education and experiences."[32] The concept emerged only gradually as nurse educators who were aware of social and economic trends and sympathetic to the goals of those struggling for upward mobility began to plan and implement programs. Soon nursing was responding to the mandate for more flexibility. Innovative faculties designed new methods for measurement of knowledge and competency or developed entirely new programs.

There are a variety of approaches for providing flexibility in nursing education. The ladder approach, which provides direct articulation between programs, is used to move from nursing assistant to practical nurse to AD or diploma nurse to baccalaureate nurse, with any combination in between.

For some, this means the ability to begin at a basic level and move one step at a time to the highest achievable level. For others, it means aiming at a particular level but being able to exit at distinct points, become licensed, and earn a living if necessary. (This exit opportunity is less common now.) An increasing number of baccalaureate programs are also being developed that enroll only RNs into the upper division, accepting past nursing education as the lower division to be built on.

There are nurses, especially nurse educators, who object to the ladder concept. They believe that each program in nursing has its own basis, content, and goals, that one cannot be based on another, and that the ladder tends to belittle the role of workers at each level, implying the necessity to move up. One solution seems to be using standardized and teacher-made tests to measure the individual's knowledge, according to clearly stated competency goals. There are a number of standardized tests available in both the liberal arts and nursing, but there is still some question as to how to test for clinical competency. Methods used include the use of videotapes, simulated experiences, practicums, and minicourses in the clinical setting. Also being used are the performance assessment centers of the Regents College Degree program, as well as their paper-and-pencil exams.[33]

Another approach is to allow students to proceed through a course at their own pace through testing, self-study, and the use of media and computers. A number of schools have been experimenting with self-pacing and self-learning, and reports indicate that students find it stimulating and satisfying, although sometimes stressful.[34]

Another version of the open curriculum concept is the external degree, sometimes called a "university without walls." This is independent study validated by testing, an approach long used in other countries (as early as 1836). In the United States the *Regents College Degree*, formerly called the *New York State Regents External Degree*, is a respected and successful example. Regents College (RC), the University of the State of New York (USNY), shares many goals and activities with conventional campus-based programs. However, it differs significantly in the ways students learn and the methods used to recognize and credential that learning. Rather than providing classroom instruction, RC provides the focus for learning through its degree requirements and related study materials. It provides a comprehensive system of objective assessment of college-level knowledge and skills, using transfer credits from regionally accredited colleges, recognized proficiency examinations, nursing performance examinations, and other specialized evaluation procedures. Sometimes referred to as "a national examining university," RC grants credits whenever college-level knowledge is validated through the use of faculty-approved, objective, academic assessment methods.

RC offers the only national total assessment nursing programs, and thus it is unique. Since 1972, RC has developed associate and baccalaureate programs in nursing through grants and federal funds. Both degrees are NLN accredited. ADN graduates, who are primarily LPNs, are eligible for licensure in 48 states; since 1975 the pass rate on licensure examinations has averaged 94 percent, with scores typically higher than the New York State and national averages.

In December 1995, there were more than 10,000 students enrolled at RC, 9458 in the ADN and 2991 in the BSN program. This represents a 100 percent increase over the past three years. Since the inception of the programs, there have been over 10,600 ADN and 3100 BSN graduates. Maintaining students in the program continues to be a problem. Only 45 percent of ADN students return each semester and 35 percent of BSN candidates.

Nearly 80 percent of the BSN candidates are RNs from diploma or associate degree programs, with an average of ten years' experience in nursing. Many BSN students have baccalaureate, master's, or doctoral degrees in other fields. Approximately 75 percent of the graduates state intentions of continuing with graduate school.

The performance examinations are conducted by some 250 nurse faculty members, all of whom have completed the extensive training developed and administered by RC. Nursing performance examinations are administered on weekends throughout the year at the national network of Regional Performance Assessment Centers created and established by RC. The written nursing examinations are administered by the American College Testing Program (ACT PEP tests) at some 160 locations throughout the country and at embassies and military bases throughout the world. Further information may be obtained by writing to Regents College Degrees, Nursing Office, Cultural Education Center, Albany, New York 12230.

Although some educators oppose the external degree on philosophical grounds and others fear the competition in the tight market for the best students, studies conducted relative to the program are providing data of significance to other states contemplating external degree programs that include nursing. Cooperative ventures with various colleges, service institutions, and service systems (such as the Air Force Nurse Corps) are part of the extensive Regents outreach.

If, as expected, the trend toward seeing baccalaureate education as the doorway to the fullest career options in nursing continues, the necessity for upward mobility becomes even more essential. However, RN students must beware of diploma mills. With nontraditional students comprising a major portion of the nursing education market, there should be plenty of options for RNs and others to continue formal education that is of good quality.

CONTINUING EDUCATION

Professional practitioners of any kind must continue to learn because they are accountable to the public for minimum safe practice. This commitment is impossible without lifelong learning and updating. For nurses, specifically, continuing education (CE) is needed primarily to keep abreast of changes in nursing roles and functions, maintain practice competency, and modify attitudes and understanding. (It is commonly accepted that the halflife of knowledge today is about five years, and less in the sciences.) To achieve these goals, various approaches to CE can be used, such as formal academic studies that might lead to a degree; short-term courses or programs given by institutions of higher learning that do not necessarily provide academic credit; and independent or informal study through opportunities made available by professional organizations and employing agencies.

In the 1970s, a number of states enacted legislation requiring evidence of CE for relicensure of nurses (and of certain other professional and occupational groups). Under the stimulus of this legislative mandate, formalized programs increased. They are given under the auspices of educational institutions, professional organizations, and commercial for-profit groups. Most now have some sort of recognition or accreditation so that their programs will be acknowledged by licensing boards as legitimate sources of continuing education. Most programs use the Continuing Education Unit (CEU), nationally accepted for unit measurement of all kinds of CE programs. (Ten contract hours equal one unit.)

Both the ANA and NLN and their constituent organizations have developed a voluntary system of CE for nurses. The ICN has also urged its members to take the lead in initiating, promoting, or further developing a national system of CE in nursing.

Now, for a variety of reasons (often related to cost), there has been somewhat of a backlash against mandatory CE, and several states have rescinded the requirement of CE for relicensure. According to a recent survey, 27 state boards of nursing now have continuing education requirements for renewal of license registration, and 42 state boards of nursing now have continuing education requirements for reentry into active practice. The requirements for renewal generally average about 10 to 15 contact hours annually. The requirements for reentry vary widely from as little as 20 hours over two years to as much as a 300-hour approved nurse refresher course.[35]

Still, more nurses seem to be attending formal programs. How much CE improves practice is still an arguable question, for measurement of direct results is seldom practical. However, it has been shown that the motivation of the learner and the opportunity to apply what is learned are key factors. Opportunities and funds to attend programs are often a benefit of employment. However, nurses, if they consider themselves professionals, should be prepared to pay for their own CE.

Although in-service programs are not always accepted for formal CE requirements, most employers make such programs available (or mandatory) for improvement of nursing practice. Because all CE programs can be quite costly, there is increased interest in providing educationally sound programs directed toward meeting specific practice goals and building in an evaluation mechanism. In some cases, evidence of CE is a job requirement or a necessity for promotion. In other cases (fire prevention and infection control), formal CE is required by the Joint Commission for the Accreditation of Healthcare Organizations (JCAHO).

Is CE readily available to most nurses? Despite some justifiable complaints that formal programs are not always available in certain geographic areas, there are many ways for nurses to continue their professional development. Examples of self-directed learning activities include self-guided, focused reading, independent learning projects, individual scientific research, informal investigation of a specific nursing problem, correspondence courses, self-contained learning packages using various media, directed reading, computer-assisted instruction, programmed instruction, study tours, and group work projects. Many nursing journals have developed self-learning programs that include evaluation, for a minimal fee. There are also other innovative ways in which nurses are offered learning opportunities, such as through mobile vans, television, telephone systems, satellites, and other forms of telecommunication, as well as increased regional programs by nursing organizations. The opportunities for CE in nursing are considerably greater than they were some years ago. What kind of CE a nurse chooses will remain, to a large extent, an individual decision. However, the need to be currently competent is both a legal and an ethical requirement for any professional.

TRENDS AND ISSUES

The 100-Year Debate

Of all the issues that create heated debate within nursing (and outside), the one that causes the strongest reactions is also the oldest. The question of how nurses should be educated to enter the nursing field, often abbreviated as "entry into practice," has been going on for almost 100 years. With the first training programs, hospital based and controlled, there were early concerns about the need to move away from the apprenticeship model. These programs had never been totally like the Nightingale model. Nightingale, for instance, advocated a better-prepared, career-oriented nurse, as well as a bedside nurse. The first baccalaureate program in 1909 added liberal arts and a degree to the nurses' education, but not much, if any, change in the nursing part of the curriculum. Nevertheless, there were now two kinds of programs. With the initiation of the AD program, there were three that produced masses of nurses; a generic master's was already in existence.

What's wrong with having choices? Confusion results from several distinctly different ways of educating nurses, which presumably produce different outcomes, yet all graduates still take the same licensing examination and have the same title, RN. Then they may hold the same kinds of jobs with the same expectations, the same responsibilities, and often the same salary. If so, what justification is there for three major educational programs, not to mention the generic masters and doctorate?

In the late 1950s and early 1960s, both ANA and NLN made a variety of statements that focused primarily on the baccalaureate as the necessary educational degree for professional nursing. Since an important function of ANA is that of setting standards and policies for nursing education, it was the ANA that made the definitive statement in 1965. A strong recommendation by the Committee on Education resulted in the ANA position that nursing education should take place within the general educational system. Reaction to the "position paper" was decidedly mixed. (This is actually correctly titled "Educational Preparation for Nurse Practitioners and Assistants to Nurses—A Position Paper.") Although the concept underlying the paper had been enunciated by leaders in nursing since the profession's inception, reiterated through the years, and accepted as a goal by the 1960 House of Delegates, many nurses misunderstood the paper's intent and considered it a threat. Probably the greatest area of misinterpretation lay in the separation of nursing education and practice into professional, technical, and assisting components. Minimum preparation for professtional nursing practice was designated at the baccalaureate level, technical nursing practice at the AD level, and education for assistants in health service occupations was to be given in short, intensive preservice programs in vocational education settings rather than in on-the-job training. An obvious omission in the position paper was the place of diploma and PN education. A large number of hospital-based diploma graduates, students, faculty, and hospital administrators were angered by this. A major source of resentment was that the term *professional nurse* was to be reserved for the baccalaureate graduate.

Even in this period of confusion, it was recognized that the largest system of nursing education at the time, the hospital school, could not be overlooked or eliminated by the writing of a position paper. Later, both the ANA and the NLN prepared statements that advocated careful community planning for phasing diploma programs into institutions of higher learning. It was also pointed out that as PN programs improved and increased their course content, their length would be close to that of the AD program. Nevertheless, the storm raged for 20 years, although repeated attempts were made to clarify the content and intent of the position paper. ANA probably suffered a membership loss due to the alienation of many diploma nurses. As expected, social and economic trends gradually brought about many of the changes suggested by the position paper, and the definitions of *professional nurse* and *technical nurse* were widely used in the literature (although there was no major indication that employers were assigning nurses according to technical or professional responsibilities).

In 1976, the New York State Nurses' Association's voting body overwhelmingly approved introduction of a "1985 Proposal" in the 1977 legislative session. Although variations of the proposal evolved over the next few years, the basic purpose of the legislation was to establish licensure for two kinds of nursing. The professional nurse would require a baccalaureate degree, and the other, whose title changed with various objections, would require an AD. The target date for full implementation was 1985; currently licensed nurses would be covered by the traditional grandfather clause, which would allow them to retain their current title and status (RN). The bill did not pass but was consistently reintroduced during each legislative session. Immediately, the 1985 Proposal became both a term symbolizing baccalaureate education as the entry level into *professional* nursing and a rallying point for nurses who opposed this change. There was, and is, considerable opposition from some diploma and AD nurses and faculty, some hospital administrators, and some physicians. Nevertheless, an increasing number of state nurses' organizations, primarily made up of diploma nurses, voted in convention to work toward the goal of baccalaureate education for professional nursing.

The NLN has played an interesting role in the entry into practice debate. In 1979, it supported all pathways (baccalaureate, associate, diploma, and practical nursing). Given the structure of the NLN and its historic position as the accrediting body for each level of nursing education, this statement is understandable. In 1982, however, the board of directors endorsed the baccalaureate degree as the criterion for professional practice. This position was affirmed when the voting body met in June 1983. (See the convention reports published in *Nursing Outlook* in the odd years during that period.)

Later reaffirmations by the board that called for two separate licensing exams infuriated the AD programs and community college presidents, who threatened to pull out of NLN agency membership.[36] There was a demand for clarification and objections that this action downgraded AD nurses for the sake of elevating BSN nurses.[37] (From all this agitation came a number of organizations whose purpose was basically to support AD nursing and to protect AD nurses and programs from ANA and NLN actions they saw as detrimental.) The LPNs were not happy either. What resulted was a compromise statement that seemed reasonably acceptable. An interesting nonaction occurred at the next convention, where the issue was tabled and other issues related to a major reorganization were given priority. In later NLN conventions, there was little, if any, focus on the "entry" issue. At the same time, where once ANA conventions were consumed with entry into practice debates, gradually the question in education became: how do we facilitate transition? (See the reports of ANA conventions in *Nursing Outlook*, and the *American Journal of Nursing* in the even years.) The 1980 Social Policy Statement,[38] which clearly stated that baccalaureate education was the basis of professional nursing practice, was accepted, and the Cabinet on Nursing Education continued to work toward this goal. In the next biennium, ANA provided grants to several SNAs to implement their plans to establish the baccalaureate as the minimum educational qualification for professional nursing and set its timetable for implementation in all states before the end of the century. The final report of the interdisciplinary National Commission for Nursing saw pursuit of the baccalaureate as an "achievable goal." A three-year project funded by the W. K. Kellogg Foundation in late 1984 to carry out selected Commission recommendations included the objective, "to outline the common body of knowledge and skills essential for basic nursing practice, the curriculum content that supports it, and a credentialing process that reinforces it." (These reports and others relating to nursing education are summarized in Appendix 1.) In later meetings, the House of Delegates became involved in trying to agree on how the two types of nurses could be accommodated as members. Eventually, this was more or less resolved by changes in the bylaws.

Entry into practice and its inevitable corollary, changes in nurse licensure, continue to be issues in nursing. Most organizations at the state and national levels have taken a stand supporting the 1985 Proposal, or its concept of baccalaureate education as the appropriate education for the professional nurse. After that, there is still disagreement as to whether the "other" nurse would be the technical nurse, with separate licensing, and whether the PN would remain the same. Some think that AD education should be required for the practical nurse, leaving only two levels of nursing for the time being. Because this means a major change in nurse licensure, which is always a political as well as a legal issue, only a few (small) states have taken that big step. As discussed in Chapter 11, the North Dakota Board of Nursing changed its administrative rules, stating that after January 1987 the appropriate educational program for those wishing to take the RN licensure exam is the baccalaureate, and that for the PN, it is the AD. While there was a legal attempt by several hospitals to prevent this ruling from going into effect, the North Dakota attorney general ruled that this decision was within the purview of the board.[39] Also in 1986, the Maine legislature stated its intent that there be two levels of nursing (AD and baccalaureate) by 1995 or as soon as possible thereafter. In 1985, a number of other state nurses' associations thought that legislation for entry-level changes was possible within a few years. This did not occur, perhaps because a more immediate concern was the nursing shortage. Opponents also seized on the shortage to maintain that this was not the time to make such changes because all types of nursing education programs were needed. Even when some of the study reports recognized the need for baccalaureate nurses, the argument to maintain the status quo continued on the rationale of educational mobility. As discussed earlier, this refers to articulation of diploma and AD programs with those programs awarding baccalaureate or higher degrees, as well as more high-quality external degree programs and flexible campus-based instructional programs for nurses who want baccalaureate education.

But are changes in licensure the inevitable corollary of entry into practice? Perhaps the time as come to divide the issues. Linking licensure to the educational differences among nurses places our internal disputes before the public and allows them to decide. There are those who see the license as no more nor less than a guarantee of basic safety in practice. The question is then whether basic safety is different for the associate degree and baccalaureate nurse. Given the assurance of basic safety, it becomes the option of the system that employs or reimburses nurses to use those with more advanced education differently, and of the profession to award certifications that will distinguish the more accomplished practitioner. This is not a novel idea. Readings in Chapter 4 describe how professions stake out their turf through licensing. Most then continue to use government to increase their visibility and take on more exclusive functions. It is not usual for professions to use government to settle their internal disputes. So choices remain: should the system stay as it is, should the baccalaureate nurse's license and title be changed, or should we wait for the time when a professional nurse doctorate, like the MD and DDS, is the entry level to the field? Several actions of the 1995 ANA House of Delegates seemed to beg if not divide the question. More than 80 percent of the delegates voted to reaffirm the baccalaureate in nursing as the educational requirement for entry into professional practice; and there was almost unanimous support for individual licensure as a means to assure the public that "registered nurses" provide safe care to the public. It does not seem that the current "oversupply" of nurses has significantly changed the argument. The shortage/surplus cycle is discussed in Chapter 6.

Yet, if we follow the trail of the entry-into-practice issue, we see a little backtracking and a lot of sidetracking, but overall, a firm path toward higher education—a historical inevitability. Step by step, nurses, the public, legislators, and even reluctant physicians and administrators have moved toward that goal. The path has been, and may continue to be, rough.

Among the obstacles is titling, with its personal and political sensitivities, especially during a transitional period. There simply is no agreement about who should be called (and licensed as) what among nurses (or anyone). Another obstacle is cost. Will costs limit access to baccalaureate education, with a resulting shortage there and an oversupply of technical nurses? Even more serious is the need for clear delineation of the differences between (or among) the various practitioners. A number of nursing groups have worked on this, and some of the outcomes are included in Appendix 3. Unfortunately, too often these studies are not coordinated, and the terms and phrases used are not consistent. Then there is the care. Some people object to separate licensure because, they say, there is no evidence that the variously educated RNs are any different in how they pass the licensure exams and practice; in fact, some insist, maybe the baccalaureate is not as good as the others. This is and has been an ongoing argument for years.

Surprisingly, the scanty research that has been done doesn't help much, since the studies are small, with different objectives, criteria, and population samples. Even nationally recorded state board results are indefinite, showing more differences among programs of the same type than among all. Finally, there is the problem of the inevitable confusion during the years of transition when nurses with a certain legal title will hold a mixture of degrees and diplomas and other qualifications among them. Even nurses' cherished easy mobility from state to state will be in jeopardy as each state changes the law at its own pace and with its own peculiarities. Only close cooperation of nursing organizations and state boards will prevent unhappy consequences.

Some natural fears of nonbaccalaureate nurses are to be expected: that they will lose status and job opportunities despite the grandfather clause and those who desire baccalaureate education will find it too expensive, unavailable, or rigidly repetitive. As to the first, there is already some probaccalaureate selectiveness; as to the second, there is slow but definite progress. These issues will not be quickly resolved, but inevitable societal and professional changes, such as the decrease in diploma schools and the expectations of professional practice, (nursing is the only health profession for which entry is less than a baccalaureate), will be major factors in the final outcome.

In the meantime, there has been a quiet revolution, one that may end the recurrence of the entry-into-practice issue. It is the steady move toward advanced education that both RNs and LPNs are making. While many RNs are not convinced that baccalaureate education necessarily equates with professionalism, others feel differently, and back to school they go.

Accelerating Change

The new crisis upon us is an old one which we have just become smart enough to recognize. In both the job market and the educational pipelines, nurses have gained very little control over cycles of shortage and surplus. Those trends related to practice are discussed in Chapter 6. In both situations, the employment market or education, it appears that need is irrelevant. The demand for nursing services is more commonly linked to the exceptional value that nurses represent. Once salaries are more equitable, fewer nurses are used. Meanwhile, nursing's educational systems have not heard the news that work is less available, and they are recruiting into educational programs on promises of a job market that does not exist.

But this is only half of the story. There are other significant social trends which have changed the face of nursing education. These include a decrease in the number of highschool graduates who were traditionally college bound or at least ready for some occupational training; multiple career options open to women who would once have chosen nursing; young people's interest in more lucrative careers; a poor image of nursing (hard work, little status, poor salary, limited opportunities for advancement, not a profession); and less financial support for nursing education. Whatever the reason, in 1986 the NLN reported as much as a 30 percent drop in enrollments in all basic RN programs. Then beginning with 1988, enrollments began to climb and continue to do so at unprecedented rates. The country's economic recession and unemployment and the fact that nursing has usually been a full-employment field (traditionally less than 1 percent unemployment) made it a good choice for the young and for those who wanted change in mid and later life.

The recruitment problems of the mid-to-late 1980s gave birth to the gigantic marketing effort of the NCNIP, discussed more fully in Chapter 4. The entire nursing community, its schools, its organizations and its service agencies came together around this campaign to alter the public image of nursing and increase recruitment to the field. Individual schools also used many new techniques to recruit students to their own particular programs. Among these were establishing relationships with liberal arts programs or schools to funnel students directly into nursing education more easily; "adopting" a high school or even middle school, or "mentoring" specific students in these schools to orient them to nursing careers; and working with unions to encourage and assist LPNs or aides to move on to RN education. One well-funded program united the forces of over 100 hospitals, long-term care facilities, and nursing programs into consortia to provide educational advancement opportunities for aides and PNs, with the expectation that since they had already chosen nursing, they would, as RNs, stay on the job. Included were accelerated training, loan/service payback programs, support services, remedial help, and counseling.[40] In addition, schools used both radio and TV spots, mail campaigns, and booths at shopping malls and health clubs. There were also much discussion and lobbying for more student financial aid from the state and national governments, since there was considerable evidence that this was needed. (Among others, NSNA has reported for years that most nursing students require financial aid.) Launching a new Cadet Nurse Corps, which had increased nursing enrollment so much during World War II, was also suggested.[41] Some hospitals provided scholarships or made arrangements with potential students to pay back funding by promising to work in that institution for a specific period of time. One diploma school even recruited students in Ireland and other foreign countries, granting them full scholarships in return for a promise to work in the hospital for three years after graduation.

As is true of colleges in general, special attention was (and is) given to recruiting the nontraditional pool of potential applicants such as second careerists and older men and women. College graduates were also seen as likely to be attracted to accelerated BSN or generic master's programs. Minorities and men, still not a large percentage of the nursing population, were also targeted for recruitment. According to the NLN, of all graduating students, about 7 percent are Blacks, 3 percent Hispanics, 2.5 percent Asians, and less than 1 percent native Americans. The largest percentage of black students (about 9 percent) are in BSN programs. Most men (11.2 percent) choose AD education, with only slightly fewer (11.0 percent) in baccalaureate programs. Almost 10 percent of all graduates are men. Attrition is a serious problem for many minority students, both for academic and financial reasons and also because they may require considerable support, for which schools are not always prepared or seem unable to provide. One interesting outcome, as described earlier, is the speed with which some rather rigid programs have managed to adjust to the need for flexibility in curriculum, class scheduling, and meeting the needs of nontraditional students as well as returning RNs.

These last years have truly changed the face of nursing education. Many students are older. They come from rich backgrounds of career success in other fields. Traditional approaches to education are counterproductive. The principles and techniques of adult education are mandatory. Many students find it necessary to combine work and career. This pattern may only increase as governmental funds for education continue to shrink. For many this means that a two- or four-year program may require more years in part-time effort. Even though admission and enrollment numbers may look good, graduations may still lag (the ultimate test is the number of nurses added to the workforce). Enrollment has already surpassed the "boom" year of 1983, but graduations have not yet rivaled the all-time high. An older student guarantees fewer productive years in the workforce, and education for the professions is costly. By 2000, two-thirds of all RNs are expected to be over age 40.[42] From a similar perspective, if attrition is a problem, when is the student lost to the program? If students leave once they have begun courses with heavy clinical requirements, the cost is high to the school.

Does Nursing Education Prepare Competent Practitioners?

There are other issues that seem to recur in nursing education. From the time that the last diploma program gave up the apprenticeship to nursing education, there have been accusations that the new graduates of modern nursing programs are not competent. Further investigation usually shows the new graduates are not as technically skillful or as able to assume responsibilities for a large group of patients as the nurses with whom they are compared—the diploma graduates of yesterday. Nevertheless, the criticisms are understandable. For the nurse executive with fiscal constraints, a lengthy orientation and in-service program is a strain on the budget; for the staff nurse and supervisor, someone who requires extra help or supervision on a usually short-staffed unit is an impediment.

Although graduates from all three types of programs are the targets of employer disapproval, the diploma graduate, whose program is focused on the hospital and who frequently stays at the hospital, may find adjustment a little easier. AD graduates who have been PNs and have had experience in caring for many patients are also somewhat immune from criticisms about slow adjustment. However, because most graduates today do not have these backgrounds, how justified are the criticisms? How differently do the graduates of the RN programs perform?

The nursing literature is full of articles on content and methods; nurse educators are certainly concerned about preparing the best possible practitioner. Everyone agrees that new graduates should be competent to give both physical and psychological/emotional care. Just how much of this is best taught in a clinical setting is a point of controversy. How much of what kind of clinical experience prepares nurses best? It has been suggested that additional emphasis be given to the physical care needed because of patients' pathophysiological problems. There is also some indication that students need practice in basic technical skills, which some schools deal with by encouraging additional self-study in labs. In others, a concentrated period of time in one or two clincial areas at the end of the program eases students into the work situation. It also allows them to integrate their clinical knowledge and skills over a continuum of time and to learn to organize the care of larger groups of patients, setting appropriate priorities. Certain programs also have cooperative arrangements with clinical facilities to allow students a paid work-study period in the summer or specific academic terms in which they work full time while being supervised in practice. Field placements, or clinical electives, are other options. There are mixed feelings about whether working as an aide or ward clerk is helpful because of the limited legal scope of practice and the possibility that students are subtly forced into assuming more responsibility than is legal.

Giving the added clinical experience in one mode or another seems to please both students and future employers. There are a number of variations of these methods. A *preceptorship* is usually a one-to-one experience for the student, with a staff nurse preceptor guiding the learning in the clinical facility. The carefully selected preceptor, who often holds a clinical faculty appointment (without pay), has an orientation and sometimes classes on clinical teaching strategies. Preceptorships seem to enhance the student's learning, if properly done, but they require careful preparation and monitoring.[43]

An *externship*, also involving preceptors, gives students full-time work experience in a real-world environment, often in the summers, for which they are paid. Since the latter involves no academic faculty if it is not part of the curriculum, both the facility and the student must be careful to adhere to the legal limitations of what the student can do. An *internship* generally occurs after the student has graduated and eases the new graduate into the work setting by providing a variety of supervised experiences. Usually the new nurse is paid less during this time, and if the internship is not carefully planned to meet both the employee's and the employer's needs, it can become nonproductive. Preceptors are often a part of this practice as well.

There is also the question as to whether the various kinds of programs actually prepare different kinds of practitioners. Nurse educators say they do, but often the statements of philosophy and objectives or the various "official" competency statements have obvious areas of overlap. Moreover, some believe that there is a lack of clarity in how heads of AD and baccalaureate programs see their type of program as different from the other. Specifically, most programs do not seem to adhere to the differences spelled out in the literature. For instance, some AD program directors think their graduates have as broad a judgment base as the baccalaureate nurse, and many prepare these nurses for management functions without the necessary educational base. On the other hand, this is probably a matter of catching up with reality, because many employers give AD nurses responsibilities for which they are not prepared. But should the teacher then educate the employer instead of reeducating the student?

If success in state boards is considered to be a criterion for competency, the results are no more definitive; as stated previously, differences within each type of program are greater than those among the programs. As to differences in practice among diploma, AD, and BSN nurses, this has been difficult to determine because studies are seldom replicated, and what is being measured is usually different from study to study. Some researchers have concluded that, if properly defined, the leadership/management role could be a viable area of differentiation.

Is faculty preparation and expertise part of the problem? There are still teachers without graduate education. Moreover, because of the kind of graduate education available at a particular time, there are nursing faculty who have learned curriculum and teaching skills but away from actual patient care because they feel inadequate. There are also clinicians with graduate degrees who have difficulty communicating their know-how or who are forced to teach in a specialty area for which they were not educated. In some areas, joint appointments of faculty and clinicians enables each to contribute to the goals of the other, but this practice is largely limited to medical centers and university programs. One trend, particularly in college and university programs, is the encouragement—sometimes the requirement—that clinical faculty maintain their clinical competence by regular practice beyond their clinical teaching. There are many versions of what is generally called *faculty practice*. (See the Bibliography for an overview of articles on faculty practice.) In some cases of faculty practice, faculty members simply give a few lectures, serve on committees, or make themselves generally helpful to a clinical facility in terms of their own expertise. In others, individual faculty may practice for set periods of time (a day, a week, in the summer, during holday breaks) in staff nurse, clinical specialist, or NP roles, either being permitted to keep the money earned or required to give it to the school toward their salaries. A number of faculty have started a faculty group practice, delivering wholistic care in the community to the poor, the homeless, the elderly, children, or even college students, faculty, and staff. Some are free, and some are fee-for-service, but almost all are nonprofit. Some are part of an established health care facility, some are independent. It may be an interdisciplinary group that also has other nurses and paid employees. Students usually have part of their clinical experience there. Clearly, such practices are not only good experience for the students but enable them to see their teachers as clinical role models. For the teachers, who may find this practice, although often stressful, stimulating and rewarding, there is one drawback: they must usually still carry a full teaching load and often find themselves pressed for time to do the necessary research and writing required for promotion. Faculty practice is not considered a scholarly activity by university promotion and tenure committees. However, the assumption is that a teacher who practices clinically on an ongoing basis prepares more competent students.

RESPONDING TO AN INEVITABLE FUTURE

The recurrent problems and issues of the profession should not distract us from taking charge of our future in an era of inevitable change. There are challenges to nursing education that must be addressed from within, even though that has not always been our tradition. Nursing has rather chosen to respond, and often simultaneously to contradictory messages. Respecting that education prepares for the future and not the past, there is clear direction that has been shaped, in part, by the National League for Nursing's *Vision for Education*.[44] It will be these qualities which distinguish the best educational programs.

1. Shift the emphasis in education to assure that graduates are prepared to function in a community-based, community-focused health care system.
2. Demand from the outset that students are accountable for their practice, including cost and quality implications.
3. Include educational experiences to prepare for practice in a multicultural society; realistically this may be no more than becoming aware of one's own biases and accepting others as they are, including their personal definition of health and wellness.
4. Establish true interdisciplinary education in the form of required courses and joint practice experiences.
5. Socialize students into the tradition of empowering consumers, making consumers the gatekeepers for their own health.
6. Realize that you can never teach everything, so make content process. Focus on critical thinking, collaboration, shared decision making, a social epidemiological viewpoint, and analyses at the systems and aggregate level.
7. Identify the databases that hold the information you need and be sure students know how to access them.
8. Remember it will be a luxury to just be responsible for your practice; students must be equipped with the skills to delegate and to evaluate the performance of assistive personnel.
9. Demand faculty-to-faculty and faculty-to-student relationships that are more egalitarian and characterized by cooperation and community building. After all, it is the people that make the difference.
10. Assure that faculty can teach for a community-based, community-focused health care system.
11. Involve employers in curriculum design, so that nursing education is truly preparing individuals suited to the realities of practice.
12. Target recruitment and retention efforts toward individuals of diverse racial, cultural, and ethnic backgrounds; especially faculty and graduate students.
13. Shift the emphasis for research toward studies concerned with health promotion and disease prevention at the aggregate and community level.
14. Seek more balance between the traditional definitions of scholarship and the "scholarship of application," so that faculty can

establish their projects within delivery systems as part of their teaching and research.

15. Become actively involved in the placement of your graduates, so that nurses will begin to claim their place in new markets.

16. Commit to increasing the numbers of advanced practice nurses, so that as a profession we can move forward to fill the primary care gap.

KEY POINTS

1. Nursing education programs share certain concerns: regulation, changes in student mix, need for clinical facilities, and educational trends.

2. Nursing education programs also differ in many ways, particularly in the expected competencies of their graduates.

3. RNs seeking baccalaureate education have more choices than they did 15 years ago, including self-learning activities and external degrees.

4. Continuing education is an ethical and professional responsibility, whether or not it is legally required.

5. Entry into practice issues center on whether baccalaureate education should be required for the professional nurse and AD education for a technical or associate nurse, how and when this should be accomplished, and whether it should be legally required.

6. Beginning with the ANA's position paper on education in 1965, the actions of the various nursing organizations have tended to support baccalaureate education for professional nursing.

7. Nursing research is a systematic inquiry into questions and problems arising from the practice of nursing.

8. Problems of translating the findings of nursing research into action are related to the lack of knowledge about nursing research held by many practicing nurses.

9. Issues in nursing education include perceived problems in student and faculty competence, desirable content in curriculum, and costs.

REFERENCES

1. Hegner BR, Caldwell E. *Nursing Assistant: A Nursing Process Approach*, 6th ed. Albany, NY: Delmar, 1995.

2. ANA. *Registered Professional Nurses and Unlicensed Assistive Personnel*. Washington, DC: ANA, 1994.

3. Rosenfeld P. *Profiles of the Newly Licensed Nurse.* New York: NLN, 1994.

4. DeLapp TD, et al. Scope of practice for beginning and experienced LPNs: The Alaska experience. *Issues* 13:6–9, 1992.

5. NLN. *Nursing Data Review.* New York: NLN, 1994, pp 74, 143.

6. Montag M. *The Education of Nursing Technicians.* New York: Putnam, 1951, p 70.

7. Ibid, p 6.

8. Ibid, p 13.

9. *Educational Outcomes of Associate Degree Nursing Programs: Roles and Competencies.* New York: NLN, 1990.

10. NLN. *Criteria and Guidelines for Accreditation of Associate Degree Programs,* 7th ed. New York: NLN, 1990.

11. *Nursing Data Review,* pp 65–66.

12. *Essentials of College and University Education for Professional Nursing.* Washington, DC: American Association of Colleges of Nursing, 1986, p 4.

13. Ibid, p 5.

14. *Nursing Data Review,* p 54.

15. Schlotfeldt R. The professional doctorate: Rationale and characteristics. *Nurs Outlook* 26:309, May, 1978.

16. Moses E. *The Registered Nurse Population.* Washington, DC: US DHHS, 1994, p 7.

17. ANA. *Statement on Graduate Education in Nursing.* New York: ANA, 1969.

18. ANA. *Statement on Graduate Education in Nursing.* Kansas City, MO: ANA, 1978, p 8.

19. *Nursing Data Review,* p 88.

20. Lev E, et al. The postdoctoral fellowship experience. *Image* 22:116–120, Spring, 1990.

21. Hinshaw AS, Lucas MD. Postdoctoral education: A new tradition for nursing research. *J Prof Nurs* 9:309, November–December, 1993.

22. Germain CP, et al. Evaluation of a PhD program: Paving the way. *Nurs Outlook* 42:117–122, May–June, 1994.

23. Kelly LS, Joel LA. *Dimensions of Professional Nursing.* New York: McGraw-Hill, 1995, pp 287–299.

24. Reilly DE. Research in nursing education: Yesterday-today-tomorrow. *Nurs Health Care* 11:138–143, March, 1990.

25. Schlotfeldt R. Research in nursing and research training for nurses: Retrospect and prospect. *Nurs Res* 24:177, May–June, 1975.

26. Notter L. *Essentials of Nursing Research,* 2nd ed. New York: Springer, 1978.

27. Weiler K, et al. Is nursing research used in practice? In McCloskey JC, Grace HK: *Current Issues in Nursing.* St. Louis: Mosby, 1994, pp 61–75.

28. Akinsanya JA. Making research useful to the practising nurse. *J Adv Nurs* 19:174–179, January, 1994.

29. Larson E, et al. Clinical application of undergraduate research skills. *Nurse Educ* 18:31–34, November–December, 1993.

30. Jairath N, Fitch M. The generic research protocol: An innovative technique to facilitate research skills development and protocol preparation. *J Cont Ed Nurs* 25:111–114, May–June, 1994.

31. Merritt D. The National Center for National Research. *Image* 18:84–85, Fall, 1986.

32. Lenburg C, Johnson W. Career mobility through nursing education. *Nurs Outlook* 22:266, April, 1974.

33. Lenburg CB, Mitchell CA. Assessment of outcomes: The design and use of real and simulation nursing performance examinations. *Nurs Health Care* 12:68–74, February, 1991.

34. Brubacker B. A faculty learns to make self-pacing work. *Nurs Health Care* 11:74–77, February, 1990.

35. Annual CE Survey. State and association/certifying boards CE requirements. *J Cont Ed Nurs* 35:5–8, January–February, 1994.

36. Two-year colleges prepare for battle over nursing programs. *Chr Higher Ed* 2, April 23, 1986.

37. Waters V. Restricting the RN license to BSN graduates could cloud nursing's future. *Nurs Health Care* 7:142–146, March, 1986.

38. ANA. *Nursing: A Social Policy Statement.* Kansas City, MO: ANA, 1980.

39. Wakefield-Fisher M, et al. A first for the nation: North Dakota and entry into nursing practice. *Nurs Health Care* 7:135–141, March, 1986.

40. Dixon A. Project LINC (Ladders in Nursing Careers): An innovative model of educational mobility. *Nurs Health Care* 10:398–402, September, 1989.

41. Kalisch P. Why not launch a new Cadet Nurse Corps? *Am J Nurs* 88:316–317, March, 1988.

42. Aiken LH, et al. The registered nurse workforce: Infrastructure for health care reform. *Statistical Bulletin* 76:2–9, 1995.

43. Williams J, et al. Collaborative preceptor training: A creative approach in tough times. *J Contin Educ Nurs* 24:153–157, July–August, 1993.

44. NLN. *Vision for Nursing Education.* New York: NLN, 1993.

6

Career Opportunities

OBJECTIVES

After studying this chapter, you will be able to:

1. Discuss the dynamics which create periodic nursing shortages and surpluses.
2. List the basic competencies most employers expect the new graduate to have.
3. Identify job opportunities available in the first years after graduation.
4. Recognize the types of positions that require advanced study.

A TIME OF UNLIMITED OPPORTUNITIES

One of the most exciting aspects of nursing is the variety of career opportunities available. Nurses, as generalists or specialists, work in almost every place where health care is given, and new types of positions or modes of practice seem to arise yearly. In part, this is in response to external social and scientific changes—for instance, shifts in the makeup of the population, new demands for health care, discovery of new treatments for disease conditions, recognition of health hazards, and health legislation. In part, these roles for nurses have emerged because nurses saw a gap in health care and stepped in (NP, nurse epidemiologist) or simply formalized a role that they had always filled (nurse thanatologist).

Usually further education is required to practice competently in specialized areas, which are expected to grow.[1] Sometimes this is part of on-the-job training, but frequently it requires formal or other continuing education. Practice in areas of clinical specialization will vary to some extent according to the site of practice and the level and degree of specialization. For instance, in a small community hospital, a nurse may work comfortably on a maternity unit, giving care to both mothers and babies; in a tertiary care setting, perinatal nurse specialists, psychiatric nurse specialists, and nurses specializing in the care of high-risk mothers may work together; in a neighborhood health center, the nurse-midwife may assume complete care of a normal mother and work with both the pediatric NP and hospital nurses.

In addition, nurses hold many positions not directly related to patient care as consultants, administrators, teachers, editors, writers, patient-care educators, executive directors of professional organizations or state boards, lobbyists, health planners, utilization review coordinators, nurse epidemiologists, sex educators, and even anatomic artists, airline attendants, and legislators.

There are few careers that can offer the diversity of nursing. Almost always, a switch to a different kind of practice or a different setting means building on your basic nursing and experience, learning some new theory, and getting some new practice. This is a good way to be stimulated and remotivated. Even if you stay in the same job, there are opportunities to try new techniques or broaden your responsibilities. The frequent crises in health care delivery present unlimited opportunities for nurses to show what they can do. With all these choices, it is difficult to find any one way to present areas of practice. In this chapter, the approach used is first to describe positions and the responsibilities and conditions of employment for each of the types of positions that a nurse can hold at graduation or shortly afterward. (You may wish to refer to Chapter 3, to review the settings in which health care is given, and Chapter 4, Exhibit 4.3, to see where nurses work.) Then an overview of other nursing opportunities is given. Exhibit 6.1 describes some of the major positions that require advanced education and experience, such as the clinical specialties. Further information is available from the specialty nursing organizations, educational programs, and career articles published in various nursing journals, some of which are listed in the Bibliography, as well as in Chapter 15 of Kelly and Joel, *Dimensions of Professional Nursing*, 7th edition (New York: McGraw-Hill, 1995). The obstacles to advanced practice are discussed in detail in *Dimensions*.

In discussing conditions of employment, specific salaries are usually not given or are presented as a range or average because there are dramatic geographic variations (highest in the West, lowest in the North Central and Southern states, but rising in the Sunbelt) and according to whether they are urban, rural, or suburban. There is agreement that nursing salaries have improved since the shortage of the late 1980s. They may level off or continue

EXHIBIT 6.1

Positions in Nursing Requiring Advanced Preparation

Position	Qualifications[a]	Practice setting	Responsibilities	Salary, benefits, working conditions[b]
Clinical Nurse Specialist (CNS): psychiatric/mental health, medical/surgical, community health, perinatal, oncology, geriatric, pediatric, and a limitless number of other highly specialized areas. May also be called nurse clinician, clinical specialist or nurse specialist.	Master's degree in clinical specialty with functional preparation as a CNS; certification for advanced practice desirable. Some institutional job descriptions for this role accept certification and experience without graduate education.	Usually hospitals, especially medical centers; increasing number in CH/PH; some ambulatory care; private practice; fewer in nursing homes.	Direct care of selected patients in specialty; consultation with nurses and other health professionals; identification of populations at risk; sometimes research; may include middle management functions. Focus on systems of care as a whole as well as care of individual patients. A heavily "mediated" role (often works through other people rather than personal "laying on of hands").	Salary usually middle manager level (anywhere from $50,000 to $80,000). Hours may be flexible. Benefits depend on setting. If position includes management, may be structured into eight-hour shifts; hours may be long. Sometimes called at home. If self-employed, must arrange own benefits.

| Nurse Practitioner (NP): clinical practice focus is broadly defined when compared to the CNS, family practice, adult and women's health, school and college health practice, geriatrics, pediatrics, to name a few. | Dramatic shift to exclusive master's preparation over the past 25 years; many NPs currently only hold certificate preparation; certification expected in most situations; experience desirable. | Community and ambulatory settings; private practice; joint practice with physicians; growing presence in nursing homes and in hospitals. | NPs assume some functions which were once the exclusive domain of the physician; prepared for the primary care role (first and continuing contact for patient in the delivery system); concerned with health promotion, disease prevention, diagnosis and treatment of minor acute illness, and management of stabilized chronic disease. Focus is overwhelmingly on the one-to-one relationship with individual clients. | May be negotiable; salary and benefits generally about same as for CN. Hours may be flexible, depending on setting. Need for significant malpractice insurance. |

(continued)

237

EXHIBIT 6.1 (*continued*)

Positions in Nursing Requiring Advanced Preparation

Position	Qualifications[a]	Practice setting	Responsibilities	Salary, benefits, working conditions[b]
Nurse anesthetist (CRNA):	Graduation from an accredited nurse anesthesia education program; national certification; 85 percent of educational programs offer a master's degree, and all are required to do so by 1998; there are clinical nursing doctorate programs in anesthesia.	Operating and delivery rooms in hospitals, surgicenters, emergency rooms, some doctor's offices.	Preanesthesia care, administration of anesthetic agents, postanesthesia care, resuscitation services, pain management, respiratory care, establishment of arterial lines. Practice in all 50 states without anesthesiologist supervision.	Salary among the highest in nursing (average above $80,000); not usually under the nursing department; day into early evening hours with frequent call; need for substantial malpractice insurance coverage.
Nurse-Midwife (CNM):	Accredited nurse-midwifery program (vary from 8 months to 2 years); a growing trend toward master's preparation; certification required.	95 percent of CNMs attend births in hospitals, 11 percent in free-standing birth centers, and 4 percent in the home. Pre- and postnatal care in ambulatory sites including clinics, physician's offices, and so on.	Require formal collaborative arrangement with an obstetrician to provide consultation and management of high-risk patients; practice includes prenatal care, labor and delivery, immediate care of newborn, postpartum, family planning, and well-woman care.	Average salary $43,600; significant malpractice insurance requirements; hours may be erratic depending on patient needs.

| School or college health nurse (student health service): | Usually baccalaureate (same as for teachers); frequently require special courses and certification as designated by state or other governmental regulations; may be a school NP with a master's degree or certificate. | Any type of school, public or private, kindergarten through high school; also colleges, universities. | Vary with requirements of board of education; may be first-aid-type care with some health teaching; routine screening for visual and hearing problems; record-keeping. For NPs, same as NP responsibilities. | Depends on types of schools—salary/benefits (health plans, retirement). Could be same as for teachers; salary often lower without master's degree or at least postbaccalaureate credits. Same holidays and vacations as teachers. Usually work only days except in higher education. |

(continued)

EXHIBIT 6.1 (*continued*)

Positions in Nursing Requiring Advanced Preparation

Position	Qualifications[a]	Practice setting	Responsibilities	Salary, benefits, working conditions[b]
Nursing faculty (formal academic setting):	Depends on educational program. Baccalaureate for LPN to doctorate for universities (usually). Nursing degree (BSN and/or MSN) preferred, sometimes required. Usually require experience, sometimes specialization.	Trade schools, hospitals, junior colleges, colleges, universities.	Develop and carry out curriculum; prepare for and teach courses in classroom, laboratory, and clinical settings; recruit, select, promote, counsel, and evaluate students; develop special projects; work on committees to meet needs of program and/or students; may be expected to do research, write, and be involved in nursing and community activities, especially in colleges and universities; may be expected to hold joint positions in the clinical setting, especially in higher education; also involved in campus activities.	In higher education, salaries vary according to rank (instructor to professor); education (doctoral/nondoctoral) and whether a 10-months or calendar year contract is given. Range, $12,600 (instructor without doctorate)–$160,000 (doctorally prepared professor in private institution). Deans to $100,000+. Hours flexible; may have evening classes; may do much work at home; may work during academic year only; may become tenured if criteria are met (emphasize scholarship, particularly research).

In-service education (staff educator):	From simply good clinical experience to a master's, the latter especially for a department director.	Hospitals, nursing homes, public health/community health.	Sees to orientation and ongoing education of nursing staff as related to job. May require similar preparation to nursing faculty for teaching classes.	May have salary and benefits somewhat in range of middle management if director; teachers usually have less. Most programs given during the day, but may also include evenings and nights for other shifts.
Nurse executive/nurse administrator (director of nursing; vice president for nursing; assistant administrator):	Preferred: baccalaureate in nursing with master's or doctorate in nursing administration. Other degrees in administration, business also acceptable. In smaller settings, baccalaureate and experience. For nursing home, varies from job experience and RN only to master's degree.	Any place that nursing services are given. Most employed in hospitals, nursing homes, public health community health agencies (PH/CH). Some corporate positions with responsibilities for nursing in several settings.	Varies with size of operation. May not include day-to-day operations. Planning, organizing, controlling, evaluating nursing services; includes personnel management, labor relations, budget, working with other administrators and public. May be limited to nursing department or include other departments. Should be part of top management.	Negotiable salary and benefits; $25,000–$200,000+. Flexible hours (may be long). Executive benefit plans and usual benefits. Lowest salaries/benefits usually in nursing homes.

(continued)

EXHIBIT 6.1 (continued)

Positions in Nursing Requiring Advanced Preparation

Position	Qualifications[a]	Practice setting	Responsibilities	Salary, benefits, working conditions[b]
Middle management (Supervisor, clinical coordinator ... various titles):	Nursing baccalaureate and master's preferred with clinical and/or administrative focus; experience. Still some acceptance of baccalaureate or no degree (especially in nursing homes) with good clinical and/or head nurse track record.	Usually hospitals, PH/CH. In nursing homes, may be the only nurse at night.	Participate in nursing policymaking and problem solving; supervising and evaluating delivery of nursing care; collaborating with other departments; coordinating staff activities, possibly scheduling staff; recruiting, selecting, evaluating personnel; sometimes facilitating research, coordinating student learning experiences.	Salary: should be higher than that of staff nurse but isn't always if nurses are unionized. May have same benefits as staff nurses plus additional managerial perks such as meeting expenses, more vacation than staff.
Nurse researcher:	Usually a doctorate; sometimes advanced research training and experience.	Any health care setting; universities; private research groups; government agencies.	Develop and carry out research; assist others in applying research findings; train nurses in research.	Negotiable, except for governmental positions. Hours flexible.

[a] All require current licensure and generally, experience in nursing.

[b] The package of benefits may vary more from place to place than among positions. Factors are location, size, and private, public, or nonprofit ownership.

to rise. Listings of current salaries are reported periodically in many nursing journals, federal statistics, ANA reports, and Appendix 2 of this text.

NURSING: SHORTAGES AND SURPLUS

Throughout the history of nursing there have been repeated shortages and, though less frequently, surpluses. Controversy has raged over the causes of these shortages, with less curiosity about how to deal with the periods of oversupply. One major incident of oversupply occurred during the Great Depression, when families could not afford private duty nurses and hospital nursing was done primarily by students. Another, more recent one, had a short life: the prospective payment system described in Chapter 3 panicked hospitals, and as they closed units and sometimes laid off nurses there was a talk of a nurse oversupply. This panic lasted for about a year, because it was soon clear that, under the new system, even more nurses were needed to care for the very ill patients. Therefore in 1986, as one nursing journal talked of layoffs another reported a surfacing shortage. Hospital admissions were rebounding, patient acuity was increasing, alternative health care facilities that required nurses were expanding, and new nonnursing opportunities were opening up for nurses. More nurses were choosing to work part-time and nursing enrollments were sagging. When these factors showed no signs of changing, the situation suddenly became a crisis. How do you define a crisis in what has always been a recurring nursing shortage? Probably not only when nurses and hospitals see a problem, but when it becomes headline news in the *New York Times*, *Time* magazine and the *Wall Street Journal*.

Nurse shortages have always been a response to either public need (as in wartime) or an economic expedient. The relatively low salaries of nurses and their readiness to take on a broad range of responsibilities have continually made them excellent value. Regardless of the cause, each shortage has prompted organized nursing to rise to the occasion, producing greater and greater numbers, but the demand has never been satisfied. Instead demand increases salaries and subsequently economic conditions force more restraint in how and when the professional nurse is used. An oversupply follows, and history repeats itself.[2]

The profession's reaction to every shortage in memory has been to respond blindly to external pressures, devising solutions with little thought about the long-term consequences. Nurses were the logical choice to provide continuity and caring as hospitals became commonplace for care of the sick. Inadequate numbers of nurses for both home care (which was the more usual site for the sick) and hospitals inspired the establishment of diploma schools. Nurses for World War I were drawn from the ranks of college-educated women and received further concentrated education for nursing at the Vassar Camp, a program that, if protected and strengthened, would have allowed nursing to resolve its perpetual struggle for educational parity. But nonnurse influentials terminated the Vassar project once wartime need was past. World War II saw the licensed practical nurse proposed as a solution to homefront shortages, and the Cadet Corps, which became the prototype for associate degree education.

The nursing community had done its work well and without question. By 1988, RN employment was at an all-time high. There was one employed nurse for every 142 Americans, most of whom were well and self-sufficient.[3] Nursing services were being offered in more varied and diverse settings, but even those new markets had not decreased the concentration of nurses in hospitals. At the peak of the most recent shortage, there were over 90 nurses per 100 hospitalized patients, as opposed to 50 in the late 1970s.[4] The optimist would say that nurses were more central than ever to the care of patients. The pessimist sees that they were an exceptional value, misused, and still unappreciated for their unique role. Nursing salaries had experienced little consistent growth over the years. Nurses willingly expanded and contracted their work, responding to the need of their patients and their employers. Nurses were the ultimate multipurpose worker, easily taking on the work of a variety of other providers. It became the mark of status in hospitals to boast of an all-RN staff. This theory of economic advantage is one explanation for the shortage that should allow us to have more control in future cycles.

The shortage of the late 1980s did provide us with some new challenges and opportunities. Organized nursing was moved to a spirit of solidarity when in 1988, the American Medical Association (AMA) proposed the creation of a new caregiver, the registered care technologist (RCT), to supplement hospital nurses. Hospitals were the hardest hit by the shortage. In some situations 22 percent of nursing positions were vacant (5 percent is considered full employment). The RCT was to follow the orders of the physician but be supervised by the nurse. The proposal was illogical and insulting, and moved nursing to a unity and assertiveness that has since come to characterize its management of issues.[5]

The shortage of the 1980s can be traced to several unique situations. In fact, in some ways it really was a different shortage, a point well established by the Secretary's Commission on Nursing.[6] An insatiable demand stemming (at least in part) from a more intensely ill hospital patient, the fact that nurses are the most versatile health care worker (and perhaps the most dedicated and docile), and increasing demands for nursing services in what had been secondary markets (home care, nursing homes, ambulatory care) set the stage. A general disenchantment among women with nursing as a career choice (about 90 percent of nurses are women) resulted in enrollment declines of more than 28 percent and 19 percent in baccalaureate and associate degree programs, respectively.[7] So, the demand was high and the future was bleak.

The National Commission on Nursing Implementation Project (NCNIP) (see Appendix 1), jointly sponsored by the leadership of organized nursing and nonnursing groups, spearheaded a major public relations campaign directed at selecting nursing as a career. This initiative, conducted with the Ad Council, in combination with a general economic recession in this country (nurses could always find work), resulted in a dramatic increase in applicants to educational programs. It was this renewed interest in nursing that put the "aging" of the field into high-gear. Nursing has become a preferred choice for the mature learner, such as those making midlife and later life career changes.

During this last nursing shortage, nursing spoke out boldly and detailed what had to be done to recruit and retain nurses. The costliness of the 20 percent annual turnover rate in nursing was graphically depicted. To attract and retain nurses, they needed fair wages and attractive benefits, emancipation from the nonnursing duties that keep them from their patients, status and prestige, and the opportunity to build a career. Salary gains have been substantial, though still not adequate to compensate for years of little or no gain. In 1988, The American Organization of Nurse Executives (AONE) proposed a 100 percent differential between starting salary and the most experienced individual in a job classification. That goal was finally realized in 1993. Nurses represented by the New York State Nurses Association and employed by a Manhattan medical center achieved a starting salary of $40,000 to $43,000 and guaranteed differentials that boost many experienced staff nurses to the $80,000 to $90,000 salary bracket. Several of the most experienced will earn nearly, or over, $100,000.[8] The growing salary range is particularly important. Salary compression, and the fact that in the late 1980s staff nurses received no increments for experience and additionally would reach their maximum earning capacity in about five years, made it impossible to realize much economic advancement over a lifetime of work. It should also be noted that there are very real salary variations between practice sites and employers; nursing homes pay 15 percent less than hospitals, with government salaries lagging behind private sector.

The health care industry (especially hospitals and nursing homes where the shortage was greatest) took additional steps to resolve their shortage problem. An increasing number recruited nurses abroad, hired contract or "traveling" nurses, employed nurses from supplementary staffing agencies (creating problems of quality and continuity of care), or formed their own pool of nurses who worked per diem (generally with no benefits). The withholding of benefits was cost-efficient. Particularly interesting was the variety of techniques used to attract and retain nurses. Most favored were increasing benefit packages, emphasizing retention, reimbursing for tuition, providing bonuses for referral and retention, seeking new hires, and paying interview expenses. Among the benefits were flexible benefits (giving choices);

dental, vision, and malpractice insurance; reimbursement for unused sick time; added vacation days (one hospital offered a nine-month year); free educational seminars; added conference days; child care programs; subsidized housing; a sabbatical after a number of years of service; differentials for shift, weekends, education, and certification; longevity bonuses; paid parking; purchasing discounts; health and fitness center discounts; nonmandatory float policies and frequent-floater bonuses; even maid service and a food purchasing co-op.

Although hospital administrators have been advised for decades, through many studies on nursing, on what it takes to retain nurses, the advice seemed to fall on deaf ears all too often. By 1990, with a drastic shortage at hand, there was at least some greater inclination to listen. Once salaries, and often benefits, were competitive in most hospitals in a particular commuting area, attention had to turn to improving the environment and the conditions of work where nurses practice.[9,10] Some changes were elementary and cost little but had been largely ignored, including better communication with access to administrators, attitude surveys, open forums, nurse-relations programs, newsletters, physician–nurse liaison committees, nurse-recognition and nursing image days, positive stories about nurses and ads praising nurses in local newspapers, employee-of-the-mouth programs, appreciation of nurses by physicians, directors' letters of commendation, and anniversary and recognition teas or receptions. There were also reward systems, including clinical ladders, clinical-excellence-in-nursing awards, promotions from within, liberal transfer policies, and perfect attendance awards.

Most important, the value of the nurse and the nurse's work was demonstrated by involving nurses in various types of planning; shared governance and nurse enpowerment,[11] as in one hospital where nurses determine their own schedules, regulate their own staffing needs and are accountable for their own productivity; employing assistive personnel under the control of nursing who do the fetching, carrying, transporting, message-taking, and other nonnursing tasks often left to nurses; and other reorganizations of staffing (with input from the nurses). Some hospitals have also installed information management systems (computers) that, while not specifically for nurses, have made their work easier.

Another important recruiting and retention factor was flexibility in scheduling. Some innovations are weekend 12-hour days for a full week's salary; 12-hour shifts and shorter work-weeks, and top pay for unpopular shifts. Some of these longer shifts have since been questioned and eliminated, because they exist for the convenience of the nurse and possibly to the detriment of the patient. There are also signs of better interprofessional relationships between nursing and medicine. Many physicians recognized the need for more collegial relationships and worked in their own settings toward this goal. The lack of such relationships is considered one aspect of nurses dissatisfaction.

Clearly, the hospital shortage received most of the publicity, but other areas of nursing such as home care also dealt with shortages. These agencies tried to match the salary and benefit packages of hospitals, as well as many of the communication and service approaches. One practice area of particular concern continues to be long-term care (LTC). Because of fiscal constraints, poor image, and the fact that the federal government mandates only a token RN presence, nurses have been less attracted to nursing homes.

By 1995, the nursing shortage was history, and in some geographic areas (but not rural America) we already have a surplus. Nursing enrollments have rebounded, and nursing is seen as a well-paying and desirable career. Nurses are aware that some hospitals are noted for their ability to attract and retain nurses, and others are beginning to emulate them. Today there are new jeopardies. Economic pressures in the health care industry have made it profitable to substitute cheaper workers for the RN.[12] Further, a flurry of activity, under the guise of restructuring systems of care, often compromises the nurses' ability to assure quality or even to guarantee the safety of patients.[13]

Renewed interest in nursing as a career, to some degree based on an assumption that jobs are plentiful, has created a challenge for new graduates. New graduates may have to compromise their choices and exhibit some patience in moving toward their eventual goals. The job market is still rich, but not precisely what you want, when and where you want it. More than ever before there is a need for information on a broad array of practice options as contained in this chapter, and for active participation in career mapping, which is discussed in Chapter 15.

WHAT EMPLOYERS EXPECT FROM A NEW GRADUATE

Although there is growing disagreement over what positions new graduates are qualified to accept, there is very little confusion over what employers expect from a new graduate. It used to be expected that the first job would be as a staff nurse in a hospital. New graduates were a little nervous over their competence, especially in the technical skills, and the acute care setting provides many opportunities to perfect techniques. There is more sensitivity today which challenges tradition. First, the need for a first position that is supportive and allows some opportunity to build confidence should not be limited to the hospital. Internships or residency programs can provide the same benefits and are offered in hospitals, nursing homes, home care and community health programs as examples.

Internships and residencies come in many forms, but basically the new nurse is gradually oriented to all aspects of nursing care, with partial assignments, good supervision, and the opportunity to get experience in specific tasks as well as in overall care of patients. While this relieves some of the pressure of feeling less than competent in what might be an understaffed, busy practice setting, the price is a lower salary for that period of time and the possibility that not all the teaching promised will be delivered. Some nurses have felt resentful because they are kept at the intern level longer than they feel necessary and still end up participating in care giving without the necessary supervision or protected status. Others have found this a good transitional period.

The internship should not be confused with the regular orientation given by almost every employer. Sometimes the orientation is almost as complete as an internship, but in other cases it can be nothing but a review of policies and a tour of the facility and the assigned patient unit. Sometimes a series of written tests and procedure check-offs are given to see what the new nurse knows or needs. A staff nurse assigned as a preceptor or someone from the in-service education staff may help supervise those practical experiences.

It is also evident that nurses become specialized very quickly after graduation. The American Nurses Credentialling Center (ANCC) first-level certifications for competence in specialized areas of practice are testimony to this fact and are discussed in Chapter 11. In short order after graduation, the scientific knowledge erodes which allowed safe practice in a variety of areas, and you become most capable in the practice area where you have chosen to start your career. This being the case, there is good reason to select the patient population or practice setting which most interests you from the very beginning.

Given that some of the issues surrounding competence and entry into the job market have been identified, it remains to describe what competence means to the employer. What is expected of you as a beginning staff nurse? You will find descriptions of competencies in Appendix 3, and statements on activities in Chapter 4. Most of these were developed through the opinion of experts. The most valid statements on the expected competencies of the new graduate come from the "role delineation" studies conducted regularly by the National Council of State Boards of Nursing (NCSBN) as the basis for developing licensing exams. A random sample of newly licensed registered nurses are surveyed within 6 months of graduation to determine what activities are critical and which are most expected by the employer.[14] In general, the newly licensed RN is expected to:

1. Practice safely and protect themselves and the patient:
   - use universal precautions
   - perform cardiopulmonary resuscitation and the Heimlich maneuver
   - recognize medical emergencies and intervene (embolus, hemorrhage, insulin shock, etc.) until a more qualified provider arrives

- monitor changes in the patient's condition and safety of equipment.
2. Coordinate care and supervise assistive personnel.
3. Communicate effectively:
    - help patient and family understand care and expected outcomes
    - document accurately, completely and in a timely fashion.
4. Be proficient in basic technical skills (no further clarification offered, specific skills depend on clinical focus).
5. Complete work assignment within the time frame of the shift (the best response to the question: how fast do I have to be?).

INSTITUTIONAL NURSING

Hospital Patient Care Positions

Hospitals may differ in size, location, ownership, and kinds of patients, but in addition, an important aspect is how nursing service is structured and the quality of nursing leadership. In an in-depth study of 16 "magnet" hospitals done between 1985 and 1986 as a follow-up to the original Magnet Hospital Study (Appendix 1), two researchers looked at the nursing departments of these hospitals in relation to the qualities of excellence described by Peters and Waterman, who cited "America's best-run companies."[15] They found a good match, because the magnet hospitals also had a bias for action; were close to the customer (had primary concern for the patient); promoted autonomy and entrepreneurship; showed true respect for the individual (a people orientation); created, instilled, and clarified a value system; had a generally simple organizational form and a management team who kept in close touch with staff; and successful coexistence of firm central direction (in terms of values) and optimum individual autonomy.[16] Although the big shortage was beginning and these hospitals had competitive but not top salaries at any level, they still enjoyed a waiting list of applicants. Head nurses chose carefully so that the new employees fit in, with a like attitude of caring and respect for quality. The nurses' statements of how they felt about their place of work are very revealing. As one said, "What is the biggest attraction here? Working someplace where your work has meaning and where you can feel good about your work."[17] These qualities subsequently provided the basis for the ANCC Magnet Recognition Program for Hospital Departments of Nursing which was initiated in 1995.[18] In 1995, the ANA's continuing concern over quality in hospital nursing resulted in the development of a *Nursing Report Card for Acute Care Settings*. This tool identifies twenty-one indicators which are strongly related to quality nursing care.[18a]

Not all hospitals are magnets; too many are far from it. However, many more are finding that, for economic if not altruistic reasons, it is good business to adopt some of the practices and attitudes of the magnet hospitals. Choosing a committed, talented, well-prepared chief nursing executive (CNE) is probably step one, for he or she sets the tone, as shown in both Magnet Hospital studies. Nurses who look for the right place to work soon learn through their networks who those CNEs are.

Another consideration is the organization of nursing care. Magnet hospitals give nurses real autonomy, but the organizational models differed, as they do in most settings. Participation in decision making is more difficult to put into action than to talk about, partly because nurses at all levels are not clear about the mechanisms. There are a number of models and sometimes an overlapping of terminology; some models differentiate between participatory management and shared governance.[19] However, it is agreed that significant participation is important, with a free flow of information in all directions.[20] Moreover, it is essential that management and staff both agree on basic principles. One proponent calls shared governance a model that offers nurses not just participation but ownership in the organization.[21] In all these models, nurses have not only autonomy but also the corollary responsibility. For instance, in one model, which the participants called *collaborative governance*, day-to-day decision making took place at the unit level. The process required special education for the head nurse, renamed the *clinical manager*, consisting of topics such as decision making, team building, group dynamics, goal development, interviewing skills, budget, discipline, and rewards.[22] Although most hospitals do not have shared governance, a nurse with choices to make needs to consider whether this is how he or she can function best. Some people prefer a more traditional structure. The mode of governance will affect the nurse's job responsibilities.

Positions described in hospital nursing include all those in which the employing agency is a hospital, whether private or voluntary, general or special, and whatever the size. The one element all hospitals have in common is that they are in existence primarily to take care of patients. The greatest differences from an employment point of view are types of responsibility, advancement opportunities, and salaries.

Many hospitals still have fewer than 100 beds, so there may be relatively little separation of specialties, with the exception of obstetrics, pediatrics, and, more frequently now, psychiatric care. Even here, when there is a declining census, hospitals in the same geographic area are beginning to cooperate by sharing such facilities: one may have the only pediatrics unit, another the only cardiac surgery. Therefore, the staff nurse is most often a generalist in these small hospitals. Positions in the emergency room and the outpatient department (which are receiving an increasing number of patient visits), operating room, rehabilitation unit, or ICU may require specialized training, but newly developed programs within the hospital, such as an outpatient surgery or "overnight" unit, or home care services, also present new challenges in nursing without necessarily mandating more formalized education.

Nursing roles are changing. In the operating room, for instance, many technical tasks are carried out by surgical technicians, whereas the RN has overall responsibility for the safety of the patient, supervision and education of auxiliary nursing personnel, and sometimes support of the patient through pre- and postoperative periods. The increased utilization of NPs and clinical specialists (see Exhibit 6.1), adds another dimension to nursing care in these specialty areas. Although students usually do not have extensive experiences in the areas noted, even limited exposure may attract the nurse to certain kinds of practice. The emergency room and ICU, where quick, life-determining decisions must be made, independent judgments are not unusual, and tension is often high, will probably not attract the same kind of individual as the geriatric or rehabilitation unit, where long-term planning, teaching, and a slower pace are the norm.

Nevertheless, in most hospitals, the variety of experiences is endless. Larger hospitals and those in medical centers may offer a greater variety of specialties, exotic surgery, and rare treatments, as well as the advantages of being in the center of hospital, medical, and nursing research. Smaller hospitals may be less impersonal, are often located in the nurse's own community, and provide the opportunity to be a generalist on smaller patient units (which does not necessarily mean a smaller patient load).

The first-level hospital position for professional nurses is that of general duty or staff nurse and is open to graduates of diploma, AD, and baccalaureate programs in nursing education. Individual assignments within this category will depend on the hospital's needs and policies and the nurse's preferences and ability. Staff nursing includes planning, implementing, and evaluating nursing care through assessment of patient needs; organizing, directing, supervising, teaching, and evaluating other nursing personnel; and coordinating patient care activities, often in the role of team leader. It involves working closely with the health team to accomplish the major goal of nursing—to give the best possible care to all patients.

To help attain this goal, the ANA, in 1973, published standards of practice applicable to all nursing situations. Additional, more specific standards were also developed for medical–surgical, maternal–child, geriatric, community health, psychiatric–mental health nursing practice, and a number of subspecialties. The general standards of practice, which can also be guidelines for practice anywhere, were revised in 1991 with the title *Standards of Clinical Nursing Practice*. Standards for advanced or specialty practice are developed by the appropriate specialty group.

The *Standards of Clinical Nursing Practice* consist of "Standards of

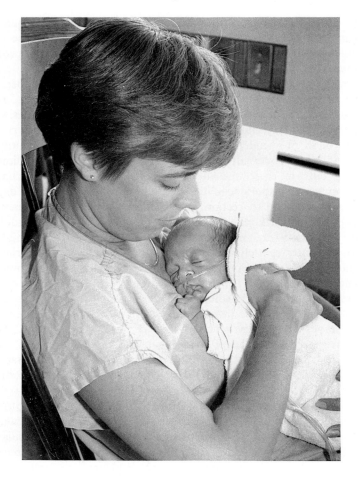

Caring for infants and children has its very special rewards. (*Courtesy of Beth Israel Hospital, Boston.*)

Care" and "Standards of Professional Performance." "Standards of Care" describe a competent level of nursing care as demonstrated by the nursing process of assessment, diagnosis, outcome identification, planning, implementation, and evaluation. "Standards of Professional Performance" describe a competent level of behavior in the professional role, including activities related to quality of care, performance appraisal, education, collegiality, ethics, collaboration, research, and resource utilization.[23] Involved in meeting these standards are literally hundreds of specific nursing tasks, some of which can be carried out by less prepared workers; it is the degree of nursing judgment needed, as well as knowledge and technical expertise, that determines who can best help any patient.

Because the goals of the various kinds of nursing education programs differ, theoretically the responsibilities of each type of nurse should also differ in the staff nurse position. Unfortunately, the tendency is to assign all nurses to the same kinds of tasks and responsibilities, so that differences are not utilized. This is so common that there is even an inclination to praise as innovative those nursing services that do delineate nursing roles and responsibilities at the staff nurse level.[24]

In an informal way, differentiating among nurses based on their competence has existed for many years. However, in the last few years, *differentiated nursing practice* has been defined as structuring of the roles and functions of nurses according to their experience, education, and competence. Although some feel that education is the best basis of such practice, others say that the model should be built on levels of demonstrated competence, that is, the clinical ladder approach. Senior practitioners are then expected to assist the less experienced and less expert to hone their practice skills (in part because middle managers are often bogged down by administrative responsibilities and cannot do so).

There are many variations of the clinical career ladder.[25] Most organizations use a committee composed of the CNE, other representatives of management, and staff nurses to develop and implement a career-ladder plan, but other approaches are also used. Criteria are set, usually including educational levels, experience, clinical competencies, certification, continuing education, peer and supervisory review, and seniority. Positions are categorized as I, II, III, and so on based on these criteria. In some settings, the nursing process is the core of the framework, with added expectations in areas such as patient and family education, leadership and coordination, and research as you progress. In others, reaching the role expectations and competencies of primary nursing is the second level, and the nurse may choose to stay there. The lateral mobility of the career ladder as opposed to vertical mobility, traditionally toward managerial positions, broadens a nurse's existing knowledge and skills and allows him or her to stay at the bedside. It may allow for a change in patient population and in job pressures and expectations. In other words, a nurse may move to another type of nursing, if qualified. Salary increases are given with each change in level. Some nurses may choose realignment (downward mobility), perhaps as they decide to go to school. There are also managerial career ladders. The guiding principle is for nurses to plan and develop their own careers. Through self-assessment, the first step, nurses identify their skills, values, and interests in the context of the practice setting. Included is an evaluation of the nurse's skills as perceived by peers and nurse managers.

As part of the review, the nurse usually prepares for the committee a portfolio that contains information demonstrating the nurse's ability to

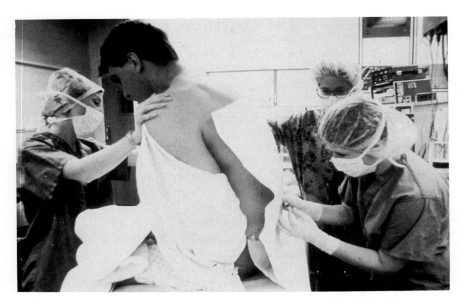

Nurse anesthetists are among the highest paid advanced practice nurses. (*Courtesy of American Association of Nurse Anesthetists.*)

meet the performance criteria of a particular level of nursing practice. Information may include a case study, a patient-teaching tool, a discharge plan, a nursing database, or other evidence of the nurse's abilities, as well as evidence of educational advancement (formal course work or CE). The review process should be objective; if it determines that the nurse does not meet the criteria, she or he should have a clear idea of what areas of behavior or practice need to be strengthened. Because both increased salary and prestige are at stake, career ladders must be carefully developed, managed, and explained.

Not everyone likes the clinical career ladder. Some nurses find it time-consuming to develop a portfolio, even with help; some do not want peer evaluation. Others think it really doesn't measure a good nurse. Still others simply don't care and want to stay where they are. However, if their salaries "top out," a number of nurses have said that they would try to "ladder" instead of "level."

Perhaps because of both staff and administrative reluctance about career ladders and other approaches to differentiated practice, even the strongest advocate says that it will not be implemented easily in most settings. However, a number of innovative models have emerged.[26] In the early 1990s the various points of view on this approach were the topic of considerable discussion, including several high-level conferences.

Regardless of how or if differentiated practice is the underlying philosophy, three basic methods of assignment for patient care in the hospital are functional, team, and case. In *functional nursing*, the emphasis is on the task; jobs are grouped for expediency, to save time, and to comply with legal requirements. For instance, one nurse might give all medications, another all treatments, aides might give all the baths. Obviously, the care of the patient is fragmented, and the nurse soon loses any sense of real nursing; patients cannot be treated as individuals or given comprehensive care. Nevertheless, there is a tendency to use this approach in many hospitals, especially on shifts that are understaffed. The work gets done but there is generally little nurse or patient satisfaction.

Team nursing involves a group of nursing personnel, usually RNs, LPNs, and aides, working together to meet patient needs. Team members are under the direction of the team leader (supposedly, but often not, a BSN), who assigns them to certain duties or patients according to their knowledge or skill. She or he has the major responsibility for planning care and coordinates all activities, acting as a resource person for the team. In addition, if there are few or no other RNs on the team, the team leader may perform nursing procedures requiring RN qualifications. Often the team leader is the only nurse directly relating to the physician, and, too often, actual patient contact is infrequent or sporadic. The original concept of the team has been diluted. Planning and evaluation are seldom a team effort; conferences to discuss patient needs are irregular; and too frequently, the team leader does mostly functional nursing, providing treatments and giving medications in an endless cycle. Most hospitals have some version of team nursing, at least to the extent that the RN supervises and directs other nursing personnel in patient care.

Instituted in the 1970s and gaining in popularity is *primary nursing*, a somewhat confusing term for the *case method*, in which total care of the patient is assigned to one nurse, the traditional caregiving pattern. A major difference between primary nursing and other methods of assignment is the accountability of the nurse. The patient has a primary nurse, just as she or he has a primary physician. A nurse is a *primary nurse* when responsible for the care of certain patients throughout their stay and an *associate nurse* when caring for the patients while the primary nurse is off duty. In most places, that nurse is responsible for a group of patients 24 hours a day, even though an associate nurse may assist or take over on other shifts. The primary nurse is in direct contact with the patient, family/significant others, and members of the health team, and plans cooperatively with them for total care and continuity. The head nurse then is chiefly in an administrative and teaching (personnel) role. Almost always the primary nurse is an RN, often with a baccalaureate. Sometimes the nursing team involved in primary nursing is made up of all RNs, with the exception of aides, who are generally limited to "hotel service," dietary tasks, and transportation. There is almost unanimous agreement that the primary pattern is much more satisfying to patients, families, physicians, and nurses and that care is of a highly improved quality.

Little agreement exists as to which of these methods of assignment is best, based on patient and nurse satisfaction, quality of patient care, cost, and administrative efficiency. Functional assignment may be the most administratively efficient form because of its division of labor according to specific tasks, but almost no one says that either the patient or the nurse finds it preferable to others. Team nursing, when done according to the original concept, may be satisfying to the team who can give their attention to a small group of patients and also develop an esprit de corps that compensates for the time expended in conference and work coordination. It is often considered expensive because of the need for this additional time spent. Primary nursing, often considered the most professional of assignments, also has its detractors: additional stress, role overload, and role ambiguity are cited. The setting and the nurses themselves may also have some effect, as there is some evidence that there are neither cost nor quality distinction between team and primary nursing.

Given functional, team and primary nursing as basic categories, there are endless variations on each theme. Modular nursing[27] and district nursing[28] both provide for continuity in provider but make more extensive use of assistive personnel. District nursing is suited to nursing homes and is not proposed for acute care. The ICON (integrated competencies of nurses) system developed at Yale–New Haven Hospital differentiates the practice role based on the educational preparation of the nurse. In this model, which would be considered a case model, the professional nurse is salaried.[29] Another variation on the case method with some unique uses of assistive personnel as environmental supports was created at the Robert Wood Johnson Hospital in New Brunswick, NJ, and is called the PROACT system.[30] The Professional Practice Model of Johns Hopkins builds on primary nursing and decentralizes management functions such as staffing and scheduling.[31] The Primm Model at Sioux Valley Hospital in Sioux Falls, SD, was one of the first systems for differentiated practice.[32] Other noteworthy variations are Manthey's Partners in Practice, which teams different skill mixes of professional, technical, and assistive personnel on a permanent basis to work in an arm's-length relationship;[33] and the New England Medical Center Case Management Model, which is driven by primary nursing but incorporates a broader view of care coordination and links each primary nurse with a case-specific physician.[34] In models that combine case management with primary nursing, the primary nurse may or may not be the case manager. New graduates should be aware of the differences and of their own comfort zone in practice.

These basic models for delivery of care differ greatly in the extent to

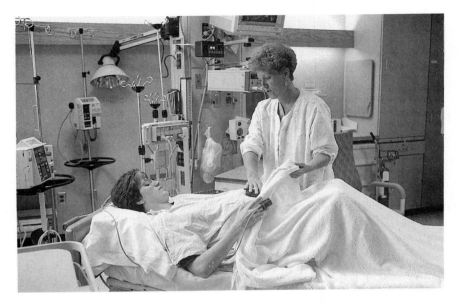

Today's labor and delivery nurses find themselves caring for more and more women with serious medical problems. (*Courtesy of Magee-Women's Hospital, Pittsburgh.*)

which they use assistive personnel. The whole assistive personnel issue has become significant and closely associated with the impending surplus of nurses. Nurses have historically complained of being burdened with work that could be as well done by other workers who were less well-educated and consequently cheaper. This point was made very strongly during the nursing shortage of the late 1980s. The intent was to access environmental support staff who would unburden nurses of much of the nonnursing activity that dominated their time. Additionally, especially in hospitals, an increasingly sicker patient made any added use of nursing assistants questionable. Apparently our reasoning was not clear enough and our message not loud enough. As cost-containment became a driving force in hospitals (not only hospitals, but hospitals drew the most attention), unlicensed assistive personnel (UAP) in a variety of forms have been participating in patient care activities. It has become rare for RNs only to be responsible for themselves; they will accomplish much of their work through others. There is potential for many legal and ethical dilemmas. UAPs must be be properly trained, assigned and supervised. Both the ANA and the American Association of Critical Care Nurses (AACN) have excellent publications to help with decisions on the delegation of nursing activities.[35] AACN advises the presenting situation be assessed for the following qualities: potential for harm, complexity of task, problem-solving and innovation required, unpredictability of outcome, level of patient interaction (where delegation reduces necessary time that the RN should spend with the patient).[36]

The basic requirement for a staff position (or any other) is graduation from an approved school of nursing and nursing licensure or eligibility for licensure. A graduate nurse (GN) must take and pass the licensure examinations within a specific period of time. A nurse is usually hired for a particular unit, but it is not uncommon to be asked to *float*—replace a nurse on any unit. Floating should not extend to units that require special knowledge and skill unless the nurse is so trained. In some hospitals, there are *float pools* or *resource teams*—highly skilled nurses who never have a regular unit. Additionally, *cross-training* has become common—preparing a nurse for practice competence in two or more specialty areas. Rather than seeing this as an expedient for management, it should be viewed as job security in times when nursing positions are harder to come by. Competence in several clinical areas is a definite asset.

In most cases, nurses are required to rotate shifts and work on holidays. For this reason, it is possible to work part time in most hospitals. Usually there are salary differentials for working evenings and nights. In recent years, flexible hours and shifts have become popular. Fringe benefits also vary greatly and may include health plans, retirement plans, arrangements for CE, holidays, sick time, and vacation time.

Another career alternative is employment by a supplemental staffing agency sometimes called a *temporary nursing service* (TNS). Nurses most commonly using TNSs are some new graduates, nurses enrolled in advanced educational programs, nurses with small children who cannot work full time or all shifts, or nurses who simply prefer the flexibility. The TNS will pay them a salary for the hours worked, with the usual legal deductions, after billing the institutions or the patient/client using the worker's services. There are local and national agencies, and selecting a reputable one is extremely important. Job assignments may be made an hour or a week ahead, but the nurse is not obligated to take them; however, a no-show is usually dismissed. As well as offering a great deal of flexibility and variety, there are also disadvantages, even with a good TNS: no job security, no benefits, sometimes only the minimum rate paid by the area hospitals with no increases, and, of course, the constant reorientation to new nursing units and patients, even to new hospitals, although some nurses limit themselves to one particular hospital. The fact that "agency nurses" are sometimes looked down on by regular staff as incompetent (although they may simply be unfamiliar with that hospital's procedure) also creates problems for these nurses.

A variation of temporary nursing is the *flying* nurse, who accepts short-term contracts directly with a hospital anywhere in the country and sometimes abroad. Arrangements are made through an agency. The hospital usually pays only the benefits required by law, but pays for the nurse's travel and sometimes arranges for or provides housing. The nurse must get a temporary license in each state where he or she is employed. Although the variety is exciting for many nurses, the place of work is seldom ideal.

Depending on the policies a hospital has regarding promotion, a nurse could become a head nurse without further education, but not without experience. *Head nurses* are in charge of the clinical nursing units of a hospital, including the operating room, outpatient department, and emergency room. They may be called *charge nurses* or, more recently, *nursing coordinators*. Head nurses are usually responsible to the next higher person on the scale, usually the supervisor, or, in a smaller hospital, the assistant director of nursing or the director. The head nurse position is the first management position most nurses achieve (or perhaps that of assistant head nurse, who may share some of the head nurse functions and substitute for the head nurse in his or her absence).

It is the head nurse's job to manage the nursing care and ensure its quality in a relatively small area of the hospital. This may or may not include supervision of ward clerks in their clerical activities. With the trend toward decentralization of nursing authority, the head nurse is expected to give more attention to acting as a consultant and teacher for staff, to following the clinical progress of the patients, and to maintaining communication with physicians and other health personnel. In most instances, the head nurse works only the day shift, but may alternate on weekends and holidays with the assistant head nurse.

Other Positions for Nurses in Hospitals

There are a number of other employment opportunities for nurses in hospitals, although they may have only a slight relationship to nursing and are often in a department other than nursing service. Nurses on the intravenous (IV) team are specially trained, and responsible for all the IV infusions given to patients (outside of the operating room and delivery room). They usually bring the appropriate solution to the patient, add ordered drugs, and start and/or restart the IV. In some institutions they are also permitted to start a blood transfusion.

The nurse-epidemiologist or infection control nurse focuses on sur-veillance, education, and research. The surveillance aspect is designed for the reporting of infections and the establishment, over a period of time, of expected levels of infections for various areas. Patients with infections are checked to see whether the infection was acquired after admission. Reports are used for epidemiologic research, and the staff are educated in the prevention of infection. Nurses have also been trained as epidemiologists in public health agencies, where they perform similar but broader duties that involve the total community. Another challenging role is that of ombudsman, or patient advocate, in which a nurse acts as an intermediary between the patient and the hospital in an attempt to prevent or resolve problems of the patient related to the hospital or hospitalization.

A new professional role is that of director or coordinator of quality assurance (QA), with a variety of titles. Although these persons may have a medical records background, most are nurses. The primary function of QA practitioners is to assess and evaluate indicators of the outcomes of care. The position arose from the increasing requirements of the JCAHO, as well as demands on the part of payers and consumers for accountability. Their numbers are estimated to be in the low thousands. QA work includes but goes beyond the boundaries of nursing. Working with the professional staff, they determine the indicators to be studied, gather and analyze data, disseminate results and recommend corrective action. Individuals in these roles may report to a variety of areas in the organization: the CNE, director of medical records or finance, the chief operating officer (COO) as examples.

It has also become common for nurses to assume roles in utilization review (UR) and coordinator of community health or community education. UR is the internal monitor to determine whether patients are being admitted and discharged appropriately and whether resources are used properly during the period of hospitalization. It is a role that is imperative to the fiscal integrity of the institution. The community health coordinator may direct the program for outpatient teaching and participate in educating the community to the needs and contributions of the hospital.

Nursing in Long-Term Care Facilities

Nursing home beds are categorized as skilled or intermediate care (and homes usually have some of each). Skilled care is reimbursed by both Medicare and Medicaid, and must include either an active medical problem on the part of the patient or a restorative regimen which is showing progress. Intermediate level care patients (or more commonly called residents in nursing homes) require care beyond room and board, but less than skilled. Intermediate care is reimbursed by Medicaid. The facilities under discussion here may be called skilled nursing, intermediate care or long-term care facilities.

Nurses may have positions in nursing homes similar to those in hospitals. In most nursing homes the pace is slower and the pressure less. (However, with earlier discharge from hospitals, patients are much sicker than they once were.) Nurses interested in nursing home care enjoy the opportunity to know the patient better in the relatively long-term stay and to help the patient maintain or attain the best possible health status. This is not the area of practice for someone impatient for quick results. Both rehabilitative and geriatric nursing require patience and understanding. In rehabilitation, nurses work closely as a team with related health disciplines—occupational therapy, physical therapy, speech therapy, and others. In geriatric nursing,

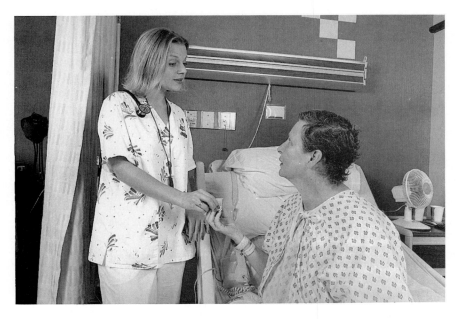

Subacute care services are being established in many hospitals and nursing homes. (*Courtesy of Robert Wood Johnson Hospital, New Brunswick, New Jersey.*)

the nurse works to a great extent with nonprofessional nursing personnel and acts as team leader, teacher, and supervisor. It may well be that there is only one professional nurse (or one licensed nurse) in a nursing home per shift, with PNs as charge nurses and aides giving much of the day-to-day care. As noted in our earlier discussion on hospital nursing, care must be exercised in delegating nursing activities.

Because the patients are relatively helpless and often have no family or friends who check on them, the nurse must, in a real sense, be a patient advocate. Physicians make infrequent visits and in some cases, where there are limited or no rehabilitative services, the nurse is the only professional with long-term patient contact. For this reason, geriatric nurse practitioners (GNPs) are considered a tremendous asset in nursing homes. The GNP may be the primary provider for these patients: monitoring their health, diagnosing and treating minor illness, and managing chronic disease. This is accomplished through a variety of practice arrangements with medicine, depending on state law. In some nursing homes, the GNP is on 24-hour call.

Requirements for employment are similar to those in hospitals for like positions, although often the need for a degree is not emphasized. Benefits and salaries have improved but are not as good as those in hospitals. Because, under Medicare, orientation and in-service education are mandatory, there is an excellent opportunity to learn about long-term care. With an aging population, there are likely to be good job opportunities for some time to come.

Subacute Care

Both hospitals and nursing homes have been recently aggressive in establishing "subacute" care units. Subacute care is for the patient who needs more clinical sophistication and professional monitoring than is possible in a nursing home, but less than is routine in a hospital. Though the rationale may be clinically sound, the motivation is often more economic than altruistic. Empty beds are better filled than standing empty. Both hospitals and nursing homes are vying for these programs. In reality, they can best service different constituencies. The nursing home has a natural capability for rehabilitation and restoration; the hospital is equipped to handle the step down from acute illness.

The premier provider in a "subacute" service is nursing. The jeopardy is that this fast developing sector will become medicalized, and that nursing will be construed as basic, but not the essential ingredient in clinical success. Should we fail in building our case, subacute care will only provide a ready occasion to cut cost by reducing the presence of professional nurses and substituting assistive personnel who will be presented as adequate to the challenge. Requirements for employment are similar to those for staff nurses in hospitals or nursing homes.

COMMUNITY HEALTH NURSING

There is an increasing tendency to refer to *public health nursing* (PHN) and *community health nursing* (CHN) interchangeably. Definitions vary. Some think of this field as focusing on population (the aggregate) and others think in terms of individuals and families. In fact, they are both right. Public health nursing (PHN) synthesizes the knowledge from the nursing and public health sciences to promote and preserve the health of individuals, families and communities. The goal is to improve the health of the community through identifying high-risk subgroups (aggregates) and directing resources towards these people.[37]

In fulfilling these responsibilities, PHN/CHN nurses practice in many settings. Most are employed by agencies that may carry the title of *public health, community health, home health,* or *visiting nurse.* They differ in both size and ownership.

PHN/CHN employment opportunities are not limited, however, to these agencies. Nurses may also be employed by hospitals to conduct home care programs or to serve as liaison between the hospital and community facilities, or by other institutions and agencies, private and governmental, in need of the kinds of services the PHN is prepared to provide in schools, industry, outpatient clinics, community health centers, free walk-in clinics for substance abuse and sexually transmitted diseases (STDs), migrant labor camps, and rural poverty areas. PHNs/CHNs may also work for various international agencies assisting less developed countries, because the need for PHN services in these countries is usually urgent.

Although situations differ, nurses in official agencies may make home visits, but their responsibilities are primarily in community health clinics focused on the needs of that agency's population. Traditionally, these have been family planning, maternal-child care, and communicable disease. These needs are increasing, especially with the escalation of TB, STDs, and drug abuse.

Visiting nurses, or home health nurses, regardless of their place of employment, also carry out these functions and may, in addition, give physical care and treatments. With the advent of much earlier discharge from hospitals, patients are quite a bit sicker when they go home, and these nurses are required to know how to care for the acutely ill.[38] If the nurse assessment indicates that such care does not require professional nurse services, home health aides/homemakers may be assigned to a patient/family, with nurse supervision and reassessment. Visiting nurses have also set up clinics that they visit periodically in senior citizen centers or apartments, as well as in the single-room occupancy (SRO) hotels commonly used for welfare clients in large cities. There are also many liaison roles with hospitals, HMOs, clinics, geriatric units, and various residences for the long-term disabled and mentally ill or retarded, primarily to assist in admission and discharge planning, as well as coordinating continuing patient care.

Besides state licensure, and for some agencies prior nursing experience, one major qualification for PHN work is graduation from a baccalaureate nursing program. Because of the shortage of nurses with the prescribed PHN preparation at the present time, however, graduates of diploma and AD programs can and do find positions in this field, working at the beginning level and under supervision. In some areas they work only in clinics and do not make home visits. Some employers encourage nurses to work toward a baccalaureate degree by providing tuition or scholarship grants.

Pay and advancement at all levels are related to educational and other qualifications. On a national level, salaries are generally competitive, except for the public agencies. Nurses may be promoted as they assume advanced or expanded role functions (NP or CNS) or administrative positions. Many official agencies operate within a civil service system. In the past, PHN/CHN nurses enjoyed standard daytime hours, with most working Monday through Friday. However, with the move toward more care in the community on a 24-hour basis, rather than in institutions,

PHN/CHN nurses are usually expected to rotate shifts and work weekends, much the same as nurses employed in institutions.

A unique and distinct aspect of PHN practice is the autonomy required when working in a setting "without walls." Clinical judgment and clinical decisions are a central part of nursing practice that demand a high level of knowledge and clinical versatility. PHNs do not generally work in the protected controlling environment of an institution, but rather in the client's setting, where the clients determine who will enter the home, and whether they follow (or even listen to) the health teaching and counseling given. If the setting is a clinic, there is no force that can make a client come to or return to a clinic, or, for that matter, follow any regimen given. Studies have indicated that the poor, especially Blacks, may reject health services because

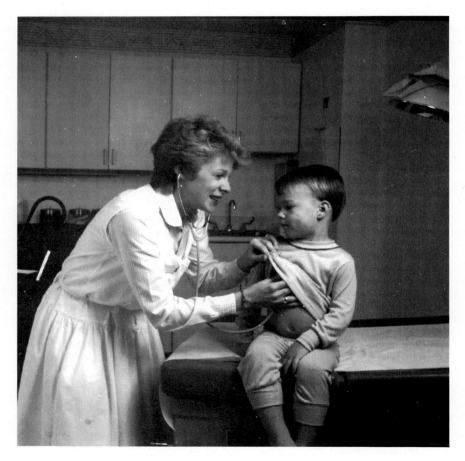

There are growing community practice opportunities for nurses who are interested in primary care. (*Courtesy of the American Nurses Association.*)

they feel a prejudicial attitude among the providers of care, whereas at the same time average middle-class white nurses hold, or feel they hold, different values concerning health care. Even with the best of intentions, nurses (and other health workers in the community) may not be able to convince their clients that certain preventive measures are necessary. Not all nurses can deal with these frustrations or have the skills and personality characteristics that enable them to work and relate effectively with clients who have a different lifestyle, culture, and value system.

Professional nurses who select PHN as a career need outstanding ability to adjust to many types of environments with a variety of living conditions, from the well-to-do in a high-rise apartment house to the most poverty-stricken in a ghetto or rural area, and to appreciate a wide range of interests, attitudes, educational backgrounds, and cultural differences. They must be able to accept these variations, to understand the differences, to communicate well so as to avoid misunderstandings and misinterpretations, and to be able to give equally good nursing care to all. PHNs in any position must use excellent judgment and are expected to use their own initiative. They have the opportunity to work with persons in other disciplines and other social agencies to help provide needed services to the clients, services that may include financial counseling, legal aid, housing problems, family planning, marital counseling, and school difficulties. In some instances, PHNs are not only case finders but case coordinators— patient advocates in every sense.

OFFICE NURSING

Office nurses are employed by physicians or dentists to see that their patients receive the nursing they need, usually in the office. Office nurses may give all of this care or assign certain duties to other personnel who work under their direction and supervision. If working for several doctors or dentists in a group practice, the nurse may supervise a staff of several employees. Nurses may be employed in a one-doctor general practitioner's office, which requires general skills, or they may be employed in a specialist's office, which requires special skills. For instance, surgeons may employ nurses who can also act as scrub nurses in surgery done at the hospital or assist them in office surgery.

What the office nurse does in terms of nursing will depend largely upon the employer's type of practice, daily schedule of appointments, and attitude about nurses' scope of practice. Tasks may be as routine as giving medications, chaperoning physical examinations, preparing equipment, and seeing that the patients' records are completed and filed at the end of the day. Better utilization would include observation, communication, teaching, and coordination with community health agencies. A few nurses make hospital patient rounds with or without the physician. Unfortunately, in too many instances the employer expects the nurse to be hostess, secretary, bookkeeper, errand girl, housekeeper, purchasing agent, public relations expert, and laboratory technician as well, tasks that a medical assistant could do. Perhaps one of the most far-reaching effects on office nursing is the development of the NP, who is often part of the physician's private practice and assumes much responsibility for patient care.

Most office nurses do not have a baccalaureate degree but do have considerable experience. Salaries and working conditions in this field are, generally speaking, both flexible and variable, representing private arrangements between the individual office nurse and the employer. Office nurses sometimes say they are willing to make some sacrifices in salary because the hours or responsibilities of office nursing fit their tastes or general life situation. Both salary and fringe benefits are likely to be lower than those for the hospital staff nurse. However, most office nurses seem to enjoy a friendly and congenial relationship with their employing physician or physicians and usually succeed in negotiating mutually satisfactory working conditions and salary. They appear to stay in the job longer than most nurses, an average of nine years.

CASE MANAGEMENT

The *case manager role* has surfaced with prominence in recent years as the health care delivery system is confronted with rising cost and increasingly complex patients. The case manager is discussed here as opposed to Exhibit 6-1 among nursing roles requiring advanced preparation because there is no consensus as to the necessary qualifications for this area of practice. The title of case manager or nursing case manager is used haphazardly for anyone who coordinates care or services. In the proper use of the term, case managers should be used very judiciously for only the most costly and complex clinical situations.[39]

Case management may occur telephonically, through paper trails or the physical presence of the client and the manager. Case managers may be employed by third-party payers (managed care systems or insurers), a health care facility, or the patient themselves (independent case managers). Regardless of who pays for the service, the manager's primary allegiance should be to the client. Case management should access the client to both the clinical sophistication and business acumen to make informed and personally acceptable decisions about the management of their health care regimen within the resources available to them. Case managers can expertly build the case for the conversion of benefits included in a policy or managed care agreement into other services which may be more suited to the client's needs and lifestyle. Where case managers are employed by the payer, they can approve such exceptions. Case managers coordinate, integrate, and negotiate all services on behalf of their clients. They challenge providers to consider options where treatment is ineffective. They advocate for the client in every sense of the word.[40]

Although you need not be a nurse to be a case manager, 85 percent are; and over 5000 nurses sat for the first case manager national certification in 1994. Because case managers are only necessary in the most complex cases, many believe that this role should be an integral part of master's preparation for advanced practice. This is not currently the case, with nurses of many skill levels filling this role.

OCCUPATIONAL HEALTH NURSING

The AAOHN states in its revised 1994 standards of occupational health nursing practice:

> Occupational health nursing is the specialty practice that provides for and delivers health care services to workers and worker populations. The practice focuses on promotion, protection, and restoration of workers' health within the context of a safe and healthy work environment. Occupational health nursing practice is autonomous, and occupational health nurses make independent nursing judgments in providing occupational health services. ...
>
> Guided by an ethical framework made explicit in the AAOHN Code of Ethics, occupational health nurses encourage and enable individuals to make informed decisions about health care concerns. Confidentiality of health information is integral and central to the practice base. Occupational health nurses are advocates for workers, fostering equitable and quality health care services and safe and healthy work environments.[41]

The occupational health unit in which an occupational health nurse (OHN) works may consist of a single room, or it may be a large department with several examining and treatment rooms, x-ray and laboratory facilities, and offices for nurses and physicians. The OHN may work in a multidisciplinary setting or multinurse unit. Physicians are often employed on a contractual basis and provide medical services as needed, but in most cases the OHN is the manager of the unit.

Whether this nurse functions in a sophisticated manner in the delivery of health care depends on his or her education and experience and the policies of the employer. As a prepared NP or nurse clinician, the nurse may assess the worker's condition through health histories, observation, physical examination, and other selected diagnostic measures; review and interpret findings to differentiate the normal from the abnormal; select appropriate action and referral; counsel; and teach. The practitioner must also be concerned with the physical and psychosocial phenomena of the workers and their families, their working environment, community, and even recreation. If the nurse is working in a more conservative environment and/or without the appropriate background, the activities may be limited to first aid and some emergency treatment, keeping records, assisting with physical examinations, and carrying out certain diagnostic procedures. Most often when the nurse does not function in an expanded role, standing orders or directions, prepared and signed by the medical director, give the necessary authority to care for conditions that develop while the employee is on the job. The nurse may refer employees with nonoccupational illnesses or injuries to their family doctor; however, this type of primary care service is being provided more and more at the work site.

A particularly interesting development that broadens the scope of the OHN's practice is an increased emphasis on workers' health problems that may or may not be directly caused by the job but affect worker performance—alcoholism, emotional problems, stress, drug addiction, and family relations. In many cases, the nurse may be involved in developing employee assistance programs and in counseling and therapy.

In a large occupational health unit in an industry that employs one or more full-time physicians, the OHN may also function as a nursing care coordinator to develop, implement, supervise, and evaluate the delivery of health care to employees, working with professional and nonprofessional staff.

The OHN must know about the laws that govern employee health. This requires interpretation of regulations and the design and implementation of standards to protect worker health. He or she should also be involved in policy decisions affecting worker health and safety. In general, OHN in a health unit of any size means much more than meeting the immediate needs of an ill or injured employee. The nurse uses interviewing, observing, and teaching skills, takes health histories, keeps health records, and is responsible for the operational management. The ability to take and recognize abnormalities in electrocardiograms and to do eye screening, audiometric testing, and certain laboratory tests and x-rays is considered useful. Health promotion and worker safety are particularly important.

Graduation from a state-approved school of professional nursing and current state registration are basic requirements for the OHN. More employers are requiring a college degree, and many find a graduate degree desirable. However, this is still not common. A career OHN will be expected to seek certification by the American Board for Occupational Health Nurses, an independent nursing specialty board authorized to certify qualified OHNs.

Salaries and fringe benefits vary according to the size of the industry or business and its location. Working hours are those of the workers; thus, in an industry with work shifts around the clock, nurses are usually there also. As a professional person, the nurse may have some of the privileges of management, such as temporary absences to attend meetings. Although some industries carry professional liability insurance that supposedly covers the OHN, it may not apply in all cases of possible litigation. It is advisable, therefore, for the nurses to carry their own professional liability insurance.

OPPORTUNITIES IN GOVERNMENT

The US government, with its various departments and agencies including the armed forces, offers excellent career opportunities. Positions range from staff nurse to top executive positions. The settings include hospitals, clinics, classrooms, and administrative offices, with responsibilities similar to those in civilian practice, except, of course, in wartime, when the sites are quite different. There are many benefits not otherwise available.

US Public Health Service (PHS)

The graduate nurse may enter the PHS by appointment to either the Commissioned Corps or the Federal Civil Service. Minimum requirements are US citizenship, at least (generally) 18 and less than 44 years of age, graduation from an approved school of nursing, and physical eligibility. The nurse must have earned a baccalaureate in nursing or a first professional nursing degree from a program NLN accredited at the time of graduation. AD graduates are not eligible for the Commissioned Corps.

The Commissioned Corps is a uniformed service composed of professionals in medical and health-related fields. Pay, allowances, and other privileges are comparable to those of officers of the armed forces. Appointments are generally made at the senior assistant grade, equivalent to lieutenant junior grade in the navy or first lieutenant in the army. The top rank is surgeon general, equivalent to vice admiral and lieutenant general.

Opportunities for collegiate nursing students to become familiar with the careers in the PHS, as well as to further their professional knowledge, are offered through the Commissioned Officer Student Training and Extern Program (COSTEP). In the junior COSTEP, a limited number of carefully selected students are commissioned as reserve officers in the corps and called to active duty for training during "free periods" of the academic year.

The civil service system is considered the basic mode of federal employment and comprises a range of professional and nonprofessional personnel. A civil service examination is not required for RNs before appointment. There is opportunity for advancement through a well-defined merit system.

Included in the areas of employment are the Indian Health Service and the Clinical Center at NIH. For information about job opportunities with the DHHS or the PHS, contact the Federal Job Information Center in your area listed in the telephone directory under "US Government."

Department of Veterans Affairs

The Department of Veterans Affairs (VA) was established in 1930 as a civilian agency of the federal government. Its purpose is to administer national programs that provide benefits for veterans of this country's armed forces. It is the nation's largest organized health care system, with hospitals, clinics, nursing home units, and domiciliaries throughout the United States.

To qualify for an appointment in the VA, a nurse must be a US citizen, a graduate of a state-approved school of professional nursing, currently registered to practice, and must meet required physical standards. Graduates from a professional school of nursing may be appointed pending passing of state board examinations.

There are several salary grades for VA nurses, ranging from junior grade through associate, full, intermediate, senior, chief, assistant director, director, and the executive grade of director, the last reserved for the national leader of the VA Nursing Service. Qualification standards relating to education, experience, and competencies are specified for appointment or promotion to each grade. The VA salary system recognizes excellence in clinical practice, administration, research, and education. Applications and inquiries for full- or part-time employment should be directed to the Personnel Office at the VA Medical Center at the location of interest. A toll-free telephone number (800-368-5629) is available for information about nationwide employment opportunities.

Armed Services

Despite similarities, there are specific differences among the Army Nurse Corps, Navy Nurse Corps, and Air Force Nurse Corps. In recent years there have been a number of changes in qualifications and assignments to meet the changes in society and in the health field. All the armed services have a reserve corps of nurses to provide the additional nurses needed to care for members of the services and their families in time of war or other national emergency. Nurses may join the reserve without

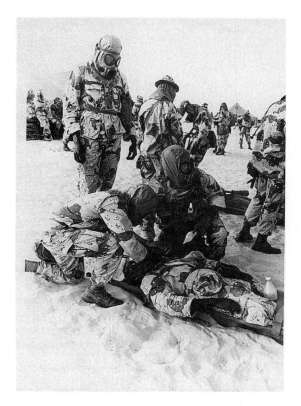

The 31st Combat Support Hospital prepares for Desert Storm. (*Courtesy of the US Army Nurse Corps.*)

having joined the regular service; the requirements are similar. A certain amount of training (which is paid) is required, usually one weekend a month and two consecutive weeks a year, at local medical units related to that particular service. There are opportunities for promotion, CE, and fringe benefits such as low-cost insurance, retirement pay, and PX shopping.[42] More information is available from the reserve recruiter of the particular service. In all the services, nurses have the economic, social, and health care benefits of all officers, as well as the opportunity for personal travel. After discharge (or retirement, which is possible in 20 years), veterans' benefits are available.

In all the armed services, nurses are commissioned at an officer rank and may advance to a top rank. The basic requirements for a commission

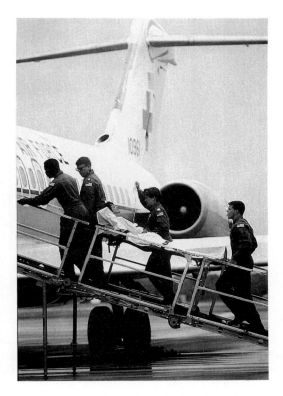

Air Force nurses not only care for patients in hospitals, but provide expert care during air evacuation. (*Courtesy of the US Air Force Nurse Corps.*)

are similar: physically qualified, licensed, US citizen (usually), and educationally qualified. However, because of other differences and the fact that these criteria change, it is best to contact the local recruiting stations of the various services for specific information. All three generally send recruiters to nursing conventions, advertise in nursing journals, and are available to speak at schools of nursing. Nurses in the armed services have outstanding opportunities for advancement, further education, and professional nursing experiences throughout the United States and often overseas.

NURSE ENTREPRENEURS AND INTRAPRENEURS

While private duty nurses can be considered one of the first of the entrepreneurs, nurses in private practice seem to be a growing phenomenon.

It is estimated that some 250,000 nurses have their own businesses. An *entrepreneur* is defined as one who organizes and manages a business undertaking, assuming risk for the sake of profit.

A private practice is a business, and setting it up and running it must be a businesslike process or it will not survive.[43] There are basic decisions to be made: what kind of organization should be created (corporation, partnership, for-profit, nonprofit); by whom (nurses and other professionals); for whom; at what fees; what kind and how many employees will be needed; how to get clients (marketing); types of advertising; how to relate to other health professions; where the services will be offered; at what hours; and policies about telephone counseling and/or home visits (house calls).

What kinds of services would these entrepreneurs offer in private practice? If nurses do not have NP training, the usual services offered are any combination of health teaching and health promotion, counseling, home health, professional education (CE programs), and consulting. Some own health-related businesses such as dialysis centers, home health agencies, and equipment rental.

NPs in private practice may have a backup physician, or they may have developed relationships with physicians from whom and to whom referrals are made. (Some NPs are in full partnership in a group practice of physicians.) These NPs do all the things NPs are legally permitted to do in their state, which may or may not include writing prescriptions. Sometimes their practices are in an urban/suburban area, but frequently they are in rural areas with few physicians available, and the nurse is the only health care provider.

Assuming that the nurse does not have legal problems about the scope of practice, a major problem is getting enough patients and reimbursement to earn a living. Many nurses can afford to give only part of their time to the practice because of limited reimbursement, and perhaps hold university teaching positions or are subsidized by some organization.

Another problem has been individual practice privileges in health care institutions, especially hospitals and nursing homes. What this means basically is the privilege of a nurse not employed by that institution to admit patients and/or write orders for their care or participate in any part of his or her patients' care. Some good progress is being made.

In rural areas where there is no source of health care, the NP may have the same physical, professional, and psychological problems as physicians—isolation, overwork, and some lack of stimulation. Nevertheless, independent practice provides a degree of professional autonomy that many nurses crave.

Intrapreneur is a term coined to describe a person who takes hands-on responsibility for creating innovation of any kind within an organization. As opposed to entrepreneurs, who leave a place of employment to start their own business, intrapreneurs work within the system to create exciting new things.[44]

The reader is referred to Pinchot's early work on intrapreneuring. In analyzing both the system and personal characteristics for the successful intrapreneur, he used the case study technique, interviewing pioneer intrapreneurs from a variety of backgrounds.[45] He calls the intrapreneur the hedge against the "dead wood" syndrome in corporate America. Neither the entrepreneur nor the intrapreneur is taking the safer route; they are not better or worse, just different.

Examples of successful intrapreneurial activities are a new type of Kardex, an educational program for certain types of patients, educational materials for community use, and a community nursing center. Depending on the arrangements made, the nurse may receive royalties, direct payments, profits shared with the institution, income for the nursing department to be used in a variety of ways, or nothing extra financially at all, just freedom and excitement. An interesting approach is that of a self-managed group running a unit and being paid by the hospital.[46]

Private Duty Nursing

Private duty nursing goes back to the beginning of nursing schools, when students were sent to homes to give patient care and upon graduation continued to do this kind of nursing because there were almost no positions for graduate nurses in hospitals.

Until the last 20 years or so, private duty nursing still attracted many nurses, because they could set their own schedule, often their preferred place of work, and, best of all, could devote their time and nursing skills to one patient. Most now give care in hospitals in 8- or 12-hour shifts, but they are private practitioners, employed by the patient or family. Obviously, this means that they are on their own in terms of retirement plans, Social Security payments, and taxes. They have no paid sick leave, vacation, or other benefits. If they want a day off, they must find a relief nurse. Fees vary but may be quite good. Sometimes nurses going on to school for degrees choose private duty as a way of earning extra money, either by relieving another nurse or by taking short cases. Most private duty nurses are listed in a hospital or other registry where their preferences are noted. Because more LPNs are being employed for less complex cases and the very ill may be in ICUs, there may be times when the private duty nurse cannot get the kind of work he or she prefers.

OTHER CAREER OPPORTUNITIES

It would probably be impossible, or at least extraordinarily lengthy, to give information about every career possibility available for nurses. A list of specific *positions* directly related to nursing, not even including the specialization or subspecialization, runs into the hundreds when the diverse settings in which nursing is practiced are considered. Overall, these are clinical nursing, administration, education, or research (or a combination of all), but the specific setting brings its own particular challenges. Each may require knowledge of another culture and the physical and psychosocial needs of these people, such as nursing in an Indian reservation, or a new orientation to practice such as working in an HMO, or in juvenile court, or the prison system, or even camp nursing. Almost all types of nursing are practiced in international settings for WHO, the Peace Corps, or Project Hope—not easy jobs, but rewarding and often exciting. Some require a baccalaureate.

In some cases, specialization or subspecialization, usually demanding additional education and training, becomes a new career path. There are any number of these, and as each becomes recognized as a distinct subspecialty, involved nurses tend to form a new organization or a subgroup within ANA or some related organization to develop standards of practice.

This is not really new; operating room nurses have been practicing since the beginning of American nursing, and coronary care nurses or enterostomal therapists are in their third decade. More recently, there is new emphasis and, consequently, a number of new educational programs in such areas as women's health care, men's health care, family planning, thanatology, and sex education, all of which have an interdisciplinary context that brings additional dimensions to the practice.

When nurses assume positions such as editors of nursing journals or nursing editors in publishing companies, they not only draw on their nursing background but must learn about the publishing field and acquire the necessary skills. In the same way, nurses employed as lobbyists, labor relations specialists, executive directors or staff of nursing associations, nurse consultants for drug or supply companies, or administrative consulting firms and staff for legislators or governmental committees, all use their nursing but must learn from other disciplines not related to nursing and develop new role concepts.

As health care and nursing expand, some nurses will develop new positions themselves. It seems safe to say that opportunities and challenges in nursing today are practically unlimited.

KEY POINTS

1. Nurses have unlimited opportunities within the profession if they continue to develop through formal or continuing education.
2. Nursing positions are available or can be developed in every setting where health care is given.

3. Because of social and economic factors that can create rapid and unexpected demands in health care, it is difficult to predict the number of nurses that would provide a balance of supply and demand.

4. Employers expect new graduates to have at least basic nursing skills, the ability to become proficient in the skills that are more complex, and to apply these by using the nursing process.

5. Employers expect new graduates to be responsible in the employment setting and to practice ethically.

6. Nursing positions that currently do not require advanced education are primarily at the staff level.

7. Nursing positions that generally require further formal education include the CNS, CNM, CRNA, NP, student health services, teaching, and administration.

REFERENCES

1. American Nurses Association. *Nursing's Social Policy Statement.* Washington, DC: ANA, 1995.

2. Aiken L. Charting the future of hospital nursing. In Lee PR, Estes CL (eds): *The Nation's Health*, 4th ed. Boston: Jones & Bartlett, 1994, pp 177–187.

3. Ibid.

4. Aiken L. The hospital nursing shortage: A paradox of increasing supply and increasing vacancy rates. In Harrington C, Estes CL (eds): *Health Policy and Nursing.* Boston: Jones & Bartlett, 1994, pp 300–312.

5. Leavitt JK, Herbert-Davis M. Collective strategies for action. In Mason DJ, et al (eds): *Policy and Politics for Nurses*, 2nd ed. Philadelphia: W.B. Saunders, 1993, pp 166–183.

6. *Secretary's Commission on Nursing: Final Report*, vol I. Washington, DC: Government Printing Office, 1988.

7. McKibbon RC, Boston C. An overview: Characteristic impact and solutions. Monograph 1 in *The Nursing Shortage: Opportunities and Solutions.* Chicago: American Hospital Association/American Nurses Association, 1990.

8. Pay levels rise to record highs at NYC hospitals. *Am J Nurs* 93:71, July, 1993.

9. Klem, R, Schreiber EJ. Paid and unpaid benefits: Strategies for nurse recruitment and retention. *J Nurs Ad* 22:52–56, March, 1992.

10. Havens DS, Mills ME. Professional recognition and compensation for staff RNs: 1990 and 1995. *Nurs Econ* 10:15–20, January–February, 1995.

11. Klinefelter G. Role efficacy and job satisfaction of hospital nurses. *J Nurs Staff Dev* 9:179–183, July–August, 1993.

12. Begany T. Layoffs: Targeting RNs. *RN* 57:37–38, July, 1994.

13. Healthcare consulting boom fuels cutbacks in RN staff. *Am J Nurs* 94:75, 78–80, April, 1994.

14. Chornick N, et al. *Job Analysis of Newly Licensed, Entry-Level Registered Nurses.* Chicago: National Council of State Boards of Nursing, 1993.

15. Peters T, Waterman R Jr. *In Search of Excellence.* New York: Harper & Row, 1982.

16. Kramer M, Schmalenberg C. Magnet hospitals: Institutions of excellence. Part I. *J Nurs Admin* 18:13–24, January, 1988.

17. Kramer M, Schmalenberg C. Magnet hospitals: Institutions of excellence. Part II. *J Nurs Admin* 19:11–19, February, 1988.

18. Magnet program concludes pilot study. *American Nurse* 26:28, November–December, 1994.

18a. ANA. *Nursing Report Card for Acute Care Settings.* Washington, DC: ANA, 1995.

19. Porter-O'Grady T. Working with consultants on redesign. *Am J Nurs* 9:33–37, October, 1994.

20. Joel LA. Restructuring: Under what conditions? *Am J Nurs* 94:7, March, 1994.

21. Porter-O'Grady T. Autonomy in nursing practice. Monograph 6 in *The Nursing Shortage: Opportunities and Solutions.* Chicago: American Hospital Association/American Nurses Association, 1990.

22. Jacoby J, Terpstra M. Collaborative governance: Model for professional autonomy. *Nurs Mgmt* 21:42–44, February, 1990.

23. American Nurses Association. *Standards of Clinical Nursing Practice.* Kansas City, MO: ANA, 1991.

24. Koerner JG, et al. Implementing differentiated practice: The Sioux Valley Hospital experience. *Nurs Admin* 19:13–20, February, 1989.

25. Sigmon P. Clinical ladders and primary nursing: The wedding of the two. In Brown B (ed): *Operations and the Working Environment.* Gaithersburg, MD: Aspen, 1994, pp 191–194.

26. Moritz P. Innovative nursing practice models and patient outcomes. *Nurs Outlook* 39:111–114, May–June, 1991.

27. Abts D, et al. Redefining care delivery: A modular system. *Nurs Mgmt* 25:40–43, 46, February, 1994.

28. Joel, LA, Patterson JE. Nursing homes can't afford cheap nursing care. *RN* 53:57–59, April, 1990.

29. Lenkman S. *Work Re-design on Nursing Units*, Part I. Hazelwood, MO: Lenkman & Associates, 1994.

30. Brett JL, Tonges MC. Restructuring patient care delivery: Evaluation of the PROACT model. *Nurs Econ* 8:36–41, January, 1990.

31. Rowland HS, Rowland BL. *Nursing Administration Handbook*, 3rd ed. Gaithersburg, MD: Aspen, 1992, pp 206–216.
32. Brubakken KM, et al. CNS roles in implementation of a differentiated case management model—Primm's model of differentiated case management. *Clin Nurs Spec* 8:69–73, March, 1994.
33. Lenkman, loc cit.
34. Zander K. Managed care and nursing case management. In Mayer GG, et al (eds): *Patient Care Delivery Models*. Gaithersburg, MD: Aspen, 1990.
35. American Nurses Association. *Registered Professional Nurses and Unlicensed Assistive Personnel*. Washington, DC: ANA, 1994.
36. American Association of Critical Care Nurses: *Delegation: A Tool for Success in the Changing Workplace*. Aliso Viejo, CA: AACN, 1995.
37. Colbourn V. Community health nursing as a career. *Imprint* 41:59–60, September–October, 1994.
38. Mignor DM. Home health nursing. *Imprint* 42:53–54, April–May, 1995.
39. Michaels C. A nursing HMO—ten months with Carondelet St. Mary's hospital-based case management. *Aspen Advs Nurse Exec* 6:3–4, January, 1991.
40. Bower KA. *Case Management by Nurses*. Washington, DC: American Nurses Publishing, 1992.
41. American Association of Occupational Health Nurses. *Standards of Occupational Health Nursing Practice*. Atlanta, GA: AAOHN, 1994.
42. A star-spangled career. *Am J Nurs Career Guide*, 1994, pp 238, 240, 242.
43. Carpenito LJ, Neal MC. Nurse entrepreneurs. In McCloskey JC, Grace HK (eds): *Current Issues in Nursing*, 4th ed. St. Louis, MO: Mosby, 1994, pp 43–48.
44. Manion J. *Change from Within: Nurse Intrapreneurs as Health Care Innovators*. Washington, DC: American Nurses Publishing, 1990.
45. Pinchot G. *Intrapreneuring*. New York: Harper & Row, 1985.
46. Boyar D, Martinson D. Intrapreneurial group practice. *Nurs Health Care* 11:28–33, January, 1990.

7

Leadership for an Era of Change

OBJECTIVES

After studying this chapter, you will be able to:

1. Define autonomy and describe how a nurse functions autonomously in patient care.
2. Discuss three theories of leadership.
3. Compare two different approaches to leadership.
4. Identify five sources of power.
5. Describe how mentorship works.
6. Identify the relationship of nursing to feminism now and in the future.
7. Describe how nurses can prepare to influence health policy in their community.
8. Explain how you can market a positive nursing image.

Why bother to concern yourself with issues of power, autonomy, and influence? Maybe you don't care whether nursing is considered a profession. Maybe, right now, you plan to do your nursing job, do it well, and not get involved in issues of politics and power. Leave that to those who enjoy it. It's not as easy as that. "Right now" will become the future, and unless you're unlike most people, you'll want a part in deciding the future. Chances are that you will be in the workforce for as long as 45 years. (Even if you started your nursing program late in life, you probably expect to work for at least 15 or 20 years.) Chances are also that you will be an employee most of that time, with all the constraints a bureaucracy can put on you. Without doubt you're going to want, at the least, some say about how you do your job, how best to care for your patients or clients. You won't be alone. Every survey and study done about nurses' job satisfaction comes up with autonomy as a major factor. And with autonomy, there is accountability—to the public.

If nurses do have the ability and responsibility to control their practice so that they can give the best possible care, then they have to use their knowledge, talents, and numbers to influence health care, either directly through personal leadership, or through leaders they choose. They need to develop collegial relations that provide a support system; they need to help one another. Too often nurses have discovered this too late and have had to scramble to catch up in a health care system where the power figures started their influence training early. As a nurse, you can't divorce yourself from what your profession is; its influence or lack thereof will affect your working life in every way. A strong profession can make your practice more rewarding. Whether or not you choose to be an activist now or see that role only as part of the dim future, it's not too early to know where nursing is in the power game and who the players are.

NURSING AUTONOMY

Professional *autonomy* has been defined as the right of self-determination and governance without external control. Identified as components of autonomy are control of the profession's education, legal recognition (licensure), and a code of ethics that persuades the public to grant autonomy. A distinction has been made between "job content" autonomy, the freedom to determine the methods and procedures to be used to deal with a given problem, and "job context" autonomy, the freedom to name and define the boundaries of the problem, the role relationships with other providers, and the price to be paid for our service. The keys to autonomy as applied to nursing are that no other profession or administrative force can control nursing practice, and that the nurse has freedom of action in making judgments in patient care within the scope of nursing practice as defined by the profession.

The issue of nursing's autonomy as a profession was discussed in Chapter 4. By admission, nursing does not have full autonomy, but we have made significant progress. Current restrictions on autonomy are experienced in both one's personal practice and with the discipline as a whole. The most blatant insult to nursing's autonomy in recent years was the American Medical Association's plan to remedy the nursing shortage of the late 1980s by the creation of a new caregiver called the registered care technologist (RCT), who would do the work of nurses under the direction of physicians. The common practice for government to consult with the AMA on health care legislation has often been presented as proof of the autonomy of American medicine. We can debate whether the interpretation is correct; but given that it is, American nursing has moved closer to that standard through the American Nurses Association's prominence on Capitol Hill.

There are other indicators of progress toward autonomy for nurses. Shared governance models that bring staff nurses and nursing service managers together to achieve consensus on clinical management; peer review as a mechanism in retention and promotion; nursing staff organizations and the right to professional staff privileges when JCAHO or Medicare guidelines are applied as they are written; are all intermediate steps toward full autonomy.

Most nurses do not identify with the issues of autonomy as they are played out in the profession. They are more concerned with their personal practice. Nurses have gravitated toward roles that hold the promise of autonomy. For the staff nurse this has been primary nursing. Primary nursing in its distinguishing features holds promise of autonomy but will depend on how these qualities are played out given the presence of an administrative hierarchy. It is consistently agreed that the primary nurse:

1. Is responsible for comprehensive and continuous care of the patient from admission to discharge.
2. Makes independent decisions that need not be ratified by any other provider.
3. Consults with patients and their support systems to allow informed and acceptable decisions.
4. Accesses others to the information they need to participate intelligently in care of the patient.
5. Decides how nursing care will be delivered, and communicates this to those who will share in implementing the plan.
6. Participates in a communication triad with the physician and patient.
7. Participates as an equal and fully accountable member of the health care team.
8. Has ready access to peer support and participates in peer review.
9. Incorporates consultation, continuing education, and research into their practice.

A LEADER AMONG LEADERS

Hein and Nicholson propose that leadership is "every nurse's domain." Leadership is about influencing the behavior of others. Registered nurses influence the behavior of their patients, provide leadership to the nursing care team, and are often called as individuals to be the leader among leaders as the professions speaks out on behalf of the public welfare.

Successful leadership depends on the artful blending of four forces: the leader, the followers (for without followers there are no leaders), the immediate organization, and the environment or context within which the goal is to be accomplished (see Exhibit 7.1). Early writings on leadership focus on the style and theoretical orientation of the leader. Most models assume that there is a basic instability in human relations and that leaders must control the behavior of their followers to assure the desired results. Freedom and independence is only meted out to followers once they have proved their motivation, readiness, capability and so on. One classic model proposes leadership styles which are autocratic, democratic or laissez-faire. Each style depicts the degree of control exerted by the leader with a complementary restriction on the freedom allowed subordinates. Maximum control by the leader and maximum freedom by the followers are mutually exclusive. Regardless of the labels, the qualities of control of behavior and freedom to act are central to the process of leadership. Democratic leadership assumes that some degree of autonomy (the ability to act without permission) has been voluntarily relinquished by all participants for the common good.

Aspiring leaders have been encouraged to select an approach most suitable to themselves or the situation at hand. Finding no suitable match, one could always create an eclectic style, borrowing from a variety of orientations. The best advice is that there must be a good fit between a situation, the qualities of the leader and the traits of the followers.[1] There is no one combination that is right all of the time, and many combinations are possible. Leadership theories help us to see the options:

1. *The great man theory.* Select people are born to leadership. The greatest of leaders are both expert managers and personally supportive.
2. *Charismatic theory.* The ability to lead is dependent on an emotional commitment from followers. Followers feel secure in the presence of a specific leader, which is particularly helpful when sacrifices are asked of followers that could only be expected based on personal loyalties.
3. *Trait theory.* Leadership ability can be acquired (or talent identified) given the fact that certain traits have been proved to be most commonly associated with leadership talent: intelligent, emotionally mature, creative and able to see novel solutions for problems, possessing initiative, speaks and writes clearly, listens carefully, able to derive meaning from even clouded communications, skilled at persuasion, a good judge of people, social and socially adaptable.

EXHIBIT 7.1

The Interplay of Forces in Leadership

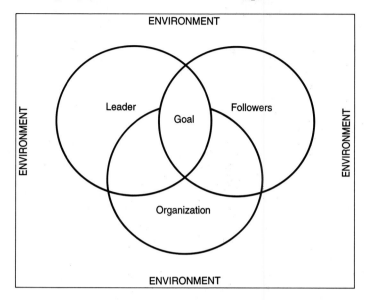

4. *Situational theories.* Leadership depends on the situation. Who will be the most successful leader at any one point in time is relative, depending on the best match with the circumstances: amount of pressure, task at hand, technical demands, closeness of the working relationship, and on and on.

5. *Contingency theory.* A three-dimensional model that aims to create the best fit between leader–follower relations, the task at hand, and the resources or support that can be accessed by the leader due to their position or status.

6. *Path–goal theory.* The leader structures work for subordinates and removes obstacles so that they can be successful. Caring and consideration is added to the leadership prescription based on the needs of the group.

7. *Life cycle theory.* The most appropriate leadership style is based on the maturity of the followers. With growing maturity there is less need for structure, and greater need for the leader to assume an active role in the work at hand.

Whereas these varied perspectives on leadership are interesting and provide a useful orientation, most emphasize control, power-wielding and

EXHIBIT 7.2

Qualities of Transactional and Transformational Leadership

Quality	Transactional	Transformational
General orientation	Technical	Philosophical
Assumptions	Instability in human relations; stability in the environment and organizations	Instability in the environment; stability in human relations and relative permanence in organizations
Response to goal	Reactive	Proactive, visionary
Plan for action	Predetermined by vision of the leader	Creation of shared vision
Prevailing focus	Content	Process
Roles	Division of labor	Group unified by goal; roles emerge over time and in response to work plan
Group dynamics	Competitive	Collaborative
Emotions	Work to distance feelings	Accept and recognize feelings and work them through
Cognitive qualities	Rational, objective, strive to decrease complexity and ambiguity	Acknowledge complexity and ambiguity; value intuition
Decision-making	Directive	Participative
Governance	Managerial	Self-governance
Human relations	Work to ensure stability	Assume and exploit stability
Leadership style	Command/control	Facilitate/protect/empower
Distribution of power	Centralized	Decentralized
Structure	Hierarchy	Networking

rationality and infer a hierarchy. They are limited in their usefulness for times where there is greater stability in human relationships than in the environment.

A body of knowledge has begun to take shape around the dynamic of *transformational* leadership. A transformational model assumes situational instability. In most earlier models, which are *transactional*, differences between the leader and the follower are seen as the major point for planning and analysis. In a transformational context, the goal is for the leader and the followers to fuse and evolve toward a shared agenda. All parties grow and develop through the process.[2] (See Exhibit 7.2 for a comparison of transactional and transformational models of leadership.)

In his discussion of organizations that will thrive in our age of uncertainty (and sometimes chaos), Senge proposes the following strategies[3] (the leadership counterpart is obvious):

1. *The whole is greater than the sum of its parts.* You cannot think of your work in isolation. Whereas earlier studies of leadership expected only the designated leader to focus on external events, newer thinking expects that all participants will have this broadened view.

2. *Look internally for solutions to problems.* It is more comfortable to blame our misfortunes on external circumstances or personalities. They are often beyond our control, so failure is less personal. From a position of strength, the first step in problem-solving should be to straighten your own thinking or behavior.

3. The voguish strategy is to become proactive or to *rise to address difficult issues before we are faced with crisis management* and forced into a reactive mode. All too often, we are still reacting, though at an earlier stage in the development of the issue. In other words, "the illusion of taking charge" is just that, an illusion.

4. We are hampered by our preoccupation with events and short-term planning. Survival in today's environment of rapid change demands a *search for themes, and the identification of trends over time.* Dig under events for the real theme. The consumer demand for "final directives" is more than that; it is the public outcry for more personal control over decisions in the health care delivery system.

5. *We tend to adjust to a bad situation* and learn to live with it, focusing on the reality of the moment. The deep penetration of the Japanese into the US car market occurred over a period of many years. Seeing threats for what they are requires us to slow down, compare situations across time, and attempt to forecast.

6. Even given the rapid pace of change, it is *difficult or impossible today to learn from your mistakes.* Decisions made at one time and place will impact people and events in a distant time and place, often generations away. The best hedge against doing harm is to assure

that leadership for the far-reaching issues is a blend of people from many perspectives. Examples of the application of this strategy can be seen in the Robert Wood Johnson Teaching Nursing Home Program of the 1980s and the current Pew Charitable Trust's project to strengthen hospital nursing.[4,5] In each of these instances, the active participation of the entire executive team from each funded site was required.

7. The traditional image of *the team is useless for today's problems.* Over time most teams invest more effort maintaining their image of cohesiveness than participating in the process of change. Better suited to the times is a model where everyone has something to contribute and no proposal is dismissed. This decidedly transformational style is inconsistent with the inevitable hierarchy in transactional leadership models. The role of the leader evolves into one of developing people, actually instigating openness and honesty while removing the threat of reprisals. The leader often assumes the position of consultant on process and facilitator, as opposed to expert and controller ... a very difficult transition for those socialized into the traditional mode of leadership.

Transformational leadership focuses on creating the social architecture to sustain a vision, and the attitudes and behaviors that allow progress in these uncertain times. This brand of leadership builds on organizational trust first, because of the organization's likelihood of greater permanence, and then on leaders with positive self-regard and a capacity for humanism.[6] The trick is to bridge the gap between transactional and transformational leadership. The insights generated by the transactional school of thinking are not to be dismissed but should be enhanced with new assumptions and ways of operating.

The literature supports an additional variation on leadership, perhaps best suited where both the environment and the organization are unstable (a very likely picture in the health care industry today). The dynamics here may require a very narrowly defined goal and a very special group of participants. A collegial style is proposed as the natural complement for leadership. In this context, leadership is relative and functional only once it is legitimized by the group. In other words, the claim to leadership must be achieved. Collegial leaders are catalytic, not merely consultative or facilitative. They don't build teams but integrate the assets of the group. Although the "buck" does stop somewhere, leadership is shared, as is the responsibility and recognition for success. Communication is authentic and genuine, with emphasis on precision in communicating the message, whatever the form may be. Supervision and motivational techniques are nonexistent because these qualities reside in the individual.[7] Shared vision, responsibility, and accountability are more then rhetoric. The narrowly defined goal is another concession to today's instability. Once the work of the group is done, the participants disband. This is called "ad hocracy." It removes the pressure of long-term commitment from the participants and recognizes that each challenge is new and different.

During the late 1970s and 1980s, there was a series of studies of leadership in nursing. In chronological order the investigators or authors were Safier, Vance, Kinsey, and Schorr and Zimmerman.[8-12] Each of the influentials who were studied had demonstrated their leadership acumen. They ranked the following qualities as most important to their success:

- Communication skills
- Intellectual ability
- Drive
- Integrity
- Willingness to take risks
- Interpersonal skills
- Creativity
- Ability to mobilize people
- Recognition in the profession
- Charisma

Much is written, in these studies and elsewhere, about the price of leadership: the loneliness at the top, for instance, and it has been said that a good leader must get over the need to be loved and must learn to function without the need for approval of others. No leader can please all of his or her constituents all the time. To lead inevitably requires commitment; at times the leader must sacrific personal desires, interest, time. The rewards, of course, are to see goals that one believes in met and to know that this might not have happened without you.

PERSPECTIVES ON POWER

Leadership involves power, the power to move people to a desired effect, the power to secure and retain resources. The first step towards personal empowerment (the ability to act) is to recognize that you have power. Power may be associated with your position, awarded by a system, given to the leader by the followers, or shared with the followers by the leader. Most basically, power is the by-product of a social relationship, and is given or it does not exist. Individuals derive their power from specific sources, and then use that power according to their personal power orientation. A typology of power bases deriving from the work of many authors is as follows:

1. *Coercive power*—real or perceived fear of one person by another.
2. *Reward power*—perception of the potential for rewards or favors by honoring the wishes of a powerful person.
3. *Legitimate power*—derives from an organizational position rather than personal qualities.
4. *Expert power*—knowledge, special talents, or skills held by the person.
5. *Reputational power*—known for being influential.
6. *Referent power*—power flowing from admiration, or charisma, usually rooted in similar backgrounds or some other mutual identification.
7. *Information power*—exclusive access to information needed by others.
8. *Connection power*—privileged connections with powerful individuals or organizations.
9. *Collective power*—ability to mobilize a critical mass or a system on your behalf.

One's power orientation indicates how an individual perceives or values power. Is power an essential part of one's identity, even if it is never used constructively? "He could do so much good if he only wanted to." Is power interpreted as the exclusive possession, something that is not shared? "You never quite feel that she is telling you everything." Power orientation may be seen exclusively or in combination as:[13]

1. *Good*—power as natural and desirable and used in an open and honest manner. Would probably build on expert, reward, and legitimate power bases.
2. *Resource-dependent*—power depending on possession of things, including information, property, wealth. Associated with withholding patterns in the information power base. Greatly diminished in a computer age and the growing presence of transformational leadership.
3. *Instinctive drive*—power as a personality attribute, and usually associated with referent power.
4. *Charisma*—influence over people through personal magnetism. Power often given to people who are ill prepared or even destructive, and could stifle the growth of those who do the giving.
5. *Political*—drawing heavily on referent, connection, and collective bases, power is linked to an ability to negotiate the system.
6. *Control and autonomy*—the power broker always calls the shots operating from a base of coercion, information, and connection.

The power base of individuals in combination with their power orientation allows prediction on how they will function and provides you with a

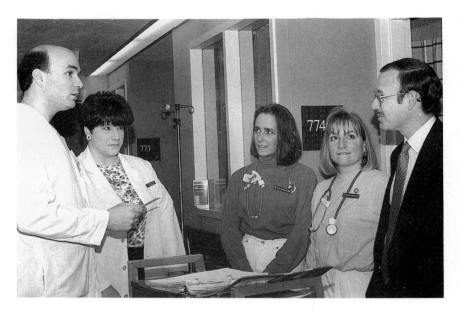

The power for nurses is in their practice, which allows them to make a rich contribution to interdisciplinary patient care rounds. (*Courtesy of Beth Israel Hospital, Boston.*)

model to identify your own capacity and style. It can also provide direction for what people expect before they will *give* power.

Power and influence are sometimes equated, because both affect or change the behavior of others; however, when they are separated, it is on the theory that power is the potential that must be tapped and converted to the dynamic thrust of influence.[14] Almost all authorities agree that a person or group must be valued on some level in order to have power or influence, again reinforcing the interpersonal dimension of the concept.

Does nursing have power? Considering these concepts, it is clear that nursing has the *potential* for power with its overwhelming numbers, its special knowledge and skill, and its place in public trust. Nursing leaders also have power of various kinds, including positional power in high government policy-making positions. But what of nurses as individuals? They are still complaining of lack of power on the job—the lack of autonomy and of involvement in budget setting and in policy making. Yet nurses do not seem to mobilize their constituency, or capitalize on their position at the center of health care information networks. Is it a historical pattern of obedience to authority, which has been transmitted by education and practice? Is it their social, cultural, or economic background? Is it because, according to personality tests, nurses have a low power-motive? Is it that they think they don't have what it takes to be powerful and influential—for whatever reason? Groups or individuals "choose" to obey for a number of reasons: habit, fear of sanctions, moral obligation, self-interest, psychological identification with someone in charge, indifference, and lack of self-confidence.[15] No doubt there are nurses who fall into one or more of these categories.

However, those who maintain that lack of self-confidence is the root cause for nurses' apparent lack of interest in gaining power should remember that "both the powerful and the powerless tend to take existing social systems for granted and rarely recognize that it is not *talent*, but rather laws, customs, policies and institutions that, in reality, keep the powerless ... powerless."[16]

THE CONSTANCY OF CHANGE

Change will be your constant companion throughout the course of life. You will be able to feel it, see it, smell it, hear it and taste it. You have a responsibility to change with the times, and to move the whole of nursing to action if you see indifference and too much comfort with the status quo. Your practice must change, as must the systems that support that practice. Patients must be helped to adjust to change, or to change so that they can adjust. Whether it is changing the health care practices of the newly diagnosed diabetic, or the body image of the traumatic amputee, a transition from team to primary nursing, or the decentralization of all management decisions to the unit level, the theoretical constructs and strategies are much the same.

Change is any significant departure from the status quo. Change may be planned or accidental. Planned change is a deliberate, conscious effort intended to improve a situation and make those improvements acceptable to the parties involved. In comparison, accidental change is a shift that occurs to maintain balance between a system and its environment.[17] Planned change allows a degree of control, where accidental change happens despite us, and we are more or less swept along. Another way of describing change is as first-order and second-order. First-order change may happen, but the larger system remains unaltered. In second-order change, the system itself changes. One common example may be the requirement to maintain current care plans on every patient, but are those plans merely tokenism (first-order), or do they become an essential tool in the operation of the unit, including staffing (second-order).[18]

Lewin's theory of change is probably the basis for the adaptations of most other theorists. He identifies three basic stages: *unfreezing*, in which the motivation to create change occurs; *moving*, the actual changing, when new responses are developed and initiated; and *refreezing*, in which the change is integrated and stabilized. A further notion is that in all changes there are *driving forces* that facilitate action and *restraining forces* that impede it. Each must be identified—the first so that they can be capitalized on, and the second so that they can be avoided or modified.[19]

Lippit's theory includes seven phases within Lewin's stages, a delineation that is useful in thinking through action and introduces the role of the change agent, the architect of the change process:[20]

Unfreezing:
1. Diagnosis of the problem.
2. Assessment of the motivation and capacity for change.
3. Assessment of the change agent's motivation and resources.

Moving:
4. Selecting progressive change objectives.
5. Choosing the appropriate role of the change agent.

Refreezing:
6. Maintenance of the change once it has been started.
7. Termination of a helping relationship between the change agent and the changed system.

The Lewin and Lippit models paint a very simplistic picture of the change process. On the contrary, even the most adventuresome participants have trepidation because human nature fears the unknown. The test will be in the day-to-day arduous implementation process. A review of the numerous change strategies and tactics reported in the literature urges the following conditions to make change more acceptable:[21]

1. Assure that the need for change is justified, even if there is not agreement. This requires total honesty, exquisite communication, and sensitivity to the cues that you have been heard. Change for the sake of change is never justified.
2. Try to safeguard the future security of those who are involved in change.
3. Diffuse anxiety by having those involved create the vision for change.
4. It is helpful to work from a previously established set of impersonal principles.

5. Change is best received when it follows other successes rather than failures.
6. It is better to space events so that there is adjustment to one change before another is introduced.
7. People new to the organization react more comfortably to change than people with longevity in the system targeted for change (vested interest).
8. Try to guarantee that there will be personal benefits to those who participate. Things should be better, not worse, after the fact.
9. Establish a venturesome environment by making change and improvement a priority.
10. Choose the change agent with psychological sensitivity and to serve as a bridge to other participants.
11. Focus attention on the future, not the past.
12. Allow for failure. Nothing is forever. Be ready to compromise once everyone is clear on the things that are nonnegotiable.
13. Provide assurance of administrative support and freedom to act without the constant need for approvals.
14. Encourage open expression of concerns.
15. Avoid experimentation and never withhold information; be sure people see "the big picture" and know what they are doing.

The skills necessary to participate in change and even initiate change projects are an integral part of the curriculum for entry into practice. The role of change agent is more demanding. The change agent is the architect of change and participates with the intent of disengaging when the process is complete.

OBSTACLES TO THE EXERCISE OF POWER

Based on our analysis of leadership, autonomy and change, it becomes obvious that the single most important ingredient to advancement of the profession and protection of the public welfare is power and its conversion into strategic influence. The fact that nursing is a "sleeping giant" holds little comfort when the health care delivery system grows in instability and decisions are made which promise a less than preferred future for nurses and nursing. Though there are many situations which have minimized the influence of nursing, there are just a few which have persisted over the years and deserve special consideration.

Nursing and Feminism

A point frequently made, when it is asked why nurses, with so much potential for influence, do not seem to be able to or want to use it, is that nursing is still 96.7 percent a woman's profession, and, even with changing legislation and attitudes, women as a whole are still subject to discrimination and harassment and still often victims of female socialization.

For many years, most women nurses looked at nursing as a useful way to earn a living until they were married, a job to which they could return if circumstances required. Most nurses did marry and most married nurses did drop out to raise families, working only part-time, if at all. Unmarried nurses (like male nurses) were more inclined to stay in nursing but, unlike men, frequently did not plot an orderly path to positions of authority and influence. This is similar to the career patterns of other women. In business, most women have traditionally been in their thirties or forties before they realized that they either wanted to or would be forced to continue working, and by then they were often frozen in dead-end, low-prestige (but productive) jobs. When they decided to compete for power positions in management, they were up against an "old boy" network that prevented or deterred their progress. Moreover, they had to overcome their own reluctance to be aggressive and to reject traditional female social goals.

Has the women's movement had an impact on this situation? As noted in Chapter 3, despite many obstacles still in the path of women on the way up (and even of those who aren't interested in this path) the women's movement has had a tremendous influence in improving many aspects of women's lives. Yet, nurses have had an uneasy relationship with feminists as a group, in part because many feminists have incorrect knowledge about nursing and were more interested early on in encouraging women to move into the powerful male bastions of law, medicine, and business. On the other hand, many of the issues concerning nurses such as comparable worth and child care are also feminist issues.

Feminism can be defined as a world view that values women and confronts systematic injustices based on gender. There are a number of feminist theories and ideologies, but none are antimale, they are simply opposed to the male-defined systems and ideologies that oppress women. These feminists point out that, even now, women believe that they must choose between the male-defined feminine role and the more interesting male role. Overall, they feel that nursing, with its largely female component, follows oppressed group behavior and also tries to emulate what they see as powerful, that is, male.[22]

Shea agrees that nursing tends to identify with the oppressor (administration? medicine?) and is sometimes self-aggressive. An example of this self-aggression is given in relation to the long-standing entry-into-practice battle. It is pointed out that the debate is largely taking place on the professional organization level, to which most nurses don't belong, ignoring the fears of those without a baccalaureate and the means or motivation to get one. The fact that nurses blame themselves and each other for failure to solve the complex dilemmas of the profession is seen as another form of antifeminist self-aggression.[23]

The winds of change blow constantly. As we approach the turn of the century, there is a decided change in the feminist perspective. Feminists today choose a more low-key and gentler approach to their issues. They emphasize the differences between men and women as opposed to their similarities. This shift in ideology comes on the scene as nursing is more influenced to define its own uniqueness as caring. The emergent "soft feminism" is comfortable and persuasive to nursing. You could well see these constituencies converge on the issue of women's health.[24]

Physician–Nurse Relationships

Physician–nurse relationships are a large, if not major, factor in nurse autonomy. There is necessarily a fine line between overstating and understating the problems, or, as some would have it, between paranoia and servility. Physicians' recognition of nurses as coprofessionals and colleagues has been present almost since the beginning of nursing. But a hard core of physicians who see and prefer a nurse-handmaiden role, although less common than even a decade ago, still exists.

Some physicians and, to some extent, a part of organized medicine seem to have limited, stereotypic images of nurses and resist nurse autonomy— either because they honestly doubt nurses' ability to cope with certain problems (bolstered, unfortunately, by the behavior of some nurses they work with) or because they are threatened by the expansion of nursing roles. The latter is demonstrated by the periodic action of certain medical societies and boards to restrict expanded nursing practice by lobbying against the newer expanded definitions of practice in nurse practice acts, by opposing reimbursement for nursing services unless there is physician supervision, or by using their power to limit nursing practice in a particular community or health care setting.

The reasons for problems in nurse–physician relationships have been examined repeatedly. One reason given is that physician education tends to impress on the medical student a captain-of-the-ship mentality and a need for both omniscience and omnipotence (Aesculapian authority), whereas nursing education often does not develop nurses as independent and fearless thinkers. This is also seen as one cause of the doctor–nurse game in which the nurse must communicate information and advice to the physician without seeming to do so, and the physician acts on it without acknowledging the source.[25]

Other reasons include the different socio-economic and educational status of doctors and nurses; the physicians' lack of accurate knowledge about nursing education and practice, and vice versa, which enables them to work side by side without really understanding each other or communicating adequately; different orientations to practice; nurses' lack of control over their practice, particularly in hospitals; and physicians' exploitation of nurses.

With more nurses looking toward expanded practice, the fact that many physicians surveyed do not seem comfortable with having nurses carry out responsibilities that were traditionally medicine has caused considerable misunderstanding. This is particularly true when nurses feel that they must prove themselves to be accepted in new roles and that a "role challenge" has been thrown out by physicians.

On the other hand, an increasing number of physicians encourage and promote nurse–physician collegial relationships and see them as inevitable and necessary for good health care. Joint practice and other collaboration, both at the unit level and in various manifestations of physician–nurse practitioner practice, are evidence of this cooperation.[26]

That doctors and nurses are willing to work together—that is, to collaborate—has a more serious meaning than symbolism. Over the years, impressive amounts of data have been gathered to show that nurse–physician collaboration has a significant outcome for patient well-being. The critical attributes of collaboration are shared planning and decision making, joint problem solving and goal setting, and genuine and open responsibility and accountability to one another and to the patient.

In a number of studies, it was shown that this kind of collaboration had positive results by improving the conditions of geriatric patients in several settings, including lowering mortality; lowering costs; increasing patient satisfaction; improving professional nurse–physician relationships; decreasing the hospital stay of patients; and, most dramatic, being the key factor in the life or death of ICU patients.[27]

Does the doctor–nurse game still exist? Stein is convinced that there have been major changes in the two decades since his first observations. He admits that in some places the game still functions as described in 1967, but he predicts that the changes visible elsewhere will spread. One factor is that "the image of nurses as handmaidens is giving way to that of specialty-trained and certified advanced practitioners with independent duties and responsibilities to their patients."[28] Physicians depend on this special expertise. Interdisciplinary models have also been shown to improve care in specialty areas. Stein adds that the many other influential roles nurses take in utilization review and quality assurance may threaten doctors' authority in clinical decision making. In explaining how and why the physician–nurse interaction has changed, he stresses the nurses' goal of becoming autonomous practitioners; changes such as the civil rights and women's movements and the nursing shortage; nurses' education, in terms of both content and socialization of nursing students to relate to physicians differently than in the past; the success of the National Joint Practice Commission; and the improved environment of some hospitals.

Is Stein too optimistic? Given his caveat that the doctor–nurse game still exists and realizing that everything takes time, probably not. In recent years, there have been many more reports of health care settings where the new interdependent mode prevails. Resolving the overall issue is a part of the challenge that both medicine and nursing must face.[29]

Nurses as Employees in a Bureaucracy

Nursing leadership has frequently blamed the employee status of nurses for our lack of empowerment. Even more telling is the fact that nursing has been buried in a department within the institutional hierarchy. Most decisions occurred at the top of the bureaucracy and few if any choices filtered down to those who gave the direct care. If, in the course of implementing those decisions, the nurse's ethics were challenged or professional goals for the patient jeopardized, any assertive action on the nurse's behalf may have resulted in the loss of a job. The rights of nurses as employees are discussed more fully in Chapter 15.

Though in many places the oppression of nurses has not changed considerably, the world of health care has changed around us. We are moving toward an era where most provider professionals will be employees in some fashion. This fact has created legal sensitivity to the fact that there are those things we do as employees, and there are other areas of accountability to the public which cannot be compromised by the demands of any employer. Relevant court decisions and public policy which recognizes these distinctions enable us to speak out.

Neither has the organizational structure remained the same after some very tumultuous years of nursing shortage and an increased acuity of hospital patients (hospitals still being the major employer of nurses). The much publicized shortage of the late 1980s created a new appreciation for the long-term employee, and dollars once invested in recruitment were redirected to retention. As part of this changed philosophy, a series of studies and programs were initiated which explored the disillusionment of new graduates with their work,[30, 31] and the qualities of hospitals which were successful in recruiting and retaining the best and the brightest nurses.[32] One significant factor was the powerful positioning of the chief nurse executive in the structure of the organization. Not that this realignment has occurred everywhere, but it has been frequent enough to allow nursing to surface as an institutional force. And the most successful nurse executives have rejected the idea that shared power is loss of power. Sharing power with staff who are experts in what they do actually enhances the positions of all the shareholders.

The mid 1990s brought us to a new and different era in the battle between nurses and the bureaucracy. The salary gains made by nurses during the recent shortage and institutional pressures to cut costs (mostly hospital costs) have initiated a period of restructuring or reorganization. Nursing is always prominent in these decisions because of the magnitude of dollars involved. It has become common practice to reduce the number of professional nurses on staff, substitute unlicensed assistive personnel, meet patient care needs through part-time and agency nurses, or any combination of the above.[33] Possessed with a new militancy, nurses have taken their case to the courts, pushed their issues in public policy and brought their concerns to the consumer.[34] All of these strategies intend to build new sources of power.

STRATEGIES FOR ACTION

And the "sleeping giant" that is nursing has begun to awaken. It is evident in the increased status of nursing and in the expansion of nursing practice to every possible setting. It is probably a healthy sign that so many nurses are saying, "But compared to what we can do and should do, it's not enough." And they're right. The major problems within nursing are caused by the lack of cohesiveness, the lack of agreement on professional goals, the lack of planned leadership development, the diversity of nurses in background, education, and position, the lack of internal support systems, and the divisiveness of nursing subcultures, all coping with a rapidly changing society. If nursing is to have the full autonomy of a profession, there must be unity of purpose and action on major issues. Leadership is vital, but grassroots nurses must be a part of the final decision, or achievement of the goals will continue to be an uphill struggle. Therefore, strategies (and they are not all inclusive) are suggested in the following sections that are the responsibility not just of nursing leaders but of all nurses.

Mentors, Networks, Collegiality: The Great Potential

The term *mentoring* is usually defined as a formal or informal relationship between an established older person and a younger one, wherein the older guides, counsels, and critiques the younger, teaching him or her (the protégé) survival and advancement in a particular field. The system has been described as the *patron system*, a continuum of advisory support relationships that make access to positions of leadership, authority, or power easier.

At the far end of the continuum is the *mentor*, a very powerful, influential individual. Here the relationship with the protégé is the most intense (and perhaps the most stressful). A mentor supports a younger adult's dreams and helps him or her to make them a reality, and is a protector and supporter who provides the extra confidence needed to take on new responsibilities, new tests of competence, and new positions. Emphasis on competence is of paramount importance; the mentor teaches, supports, advises, and criticizes.

Protégés are carefully selected. True, someone who wants another for a mentor can bring himself or herself to that person's attention, but the protégé must be seen as worthy. One group of executives cited certain qualities that they looked for in potential protégés: has depth, integrity, a curious mind, good interpersonal skills; wants to impress; has an extra dose of commitment; has a capacity to care; can communicate; understands ideas; can identify problems and help find solutions; ambitious; hard-working; willing to do things beyond the call of duty; someone looking for new avenues and new challenges; someone dedicated to a purpose; and always—someone who would be a good representative of the profession. Usually the individual is also expected to be well groomed and appropriately dressed.

Interest in mentoring in nursing has been rising in terms of preparation for scholarliness, development of minority nurses, and leadership in general. However, although almost everyone says that being mentored is a key to success, even quick success, others disagree.[34a] After all, there are not enough true mentors for every ambitious person, and many succeed with no mentor at all.

There is now much literature on mentoring in business and education, and a growing body of knowledge in regard to the development of today's nursing leaders. In Vance's study, 83 percent of the nursing leaders surveyed reported having mentors, and 93 percent were mentors to others.[35] In Kinsey's replication, the percentages were about the same.[36] In both studies, the mentors were primarily women nurse educators (teachers) or teacher colleagues, advisors, and educational administrators. A more extensive study of 500 women graduates of doctoral programs also showed the importance of mentoring.[37] Those mentored attributed much of their success to their mentors, and those not mentored expressed deprivation. The mentored were slightly more satisfied and productive in their work and with nursing as a career than were the nonmentored. With the exception of a very few of the subjects, the mentors and protégés parted amicably and have continued to be friends.

A 1995 study focused on mentoring in the career development of hospital staff nurses.[38] Regardless of their age or experience in nursing, mentorship seemed to continue to be an important resource in their professional lives.

Although the term mentoring was loosely defined, participants agreed that what they had experienced was a dynamic, interactive process in which influentials had moved them toward crucial career decisions or adjustments. The most influential patrons or mentors to the hospital staff nurse were select peers and nurse managers. Staff nurse peers enabled development of their clinical problem solving, and nurse managers helped with career advancement opportunities.

The *sponsor*—a strong patron, but less powerful than a mentor in shaping or promoting the protégé's career—is seen as next in the patron continuum, followed by the *guide*, less able than either of the other two to serve as benefactor or champion, but capable of providing invaluable intelligence and explaining the system, the shortcuts, and the pitfalls. (Any of these can also act as role models, although role models may also be more distant figures that are admired.) At the beginning of the continuum are the *peer pals*, peers who help each other to succeed and progress. The first step is seen as being more like the feminist concept of women helping women, less intense and exclusionary, and therefore more democratic, by allowing access to a large number of young professionals.

Peer pals can create their own networks. There is a male corollary—the "good old boy" networks—which, through an informal system of relationships, provide advice, information, guidance, contact, protection, and any other support that helps a member of the group, an insider, to achieve his goals, goals obviously not in conflict with those of the group. The good old boys frequently share the same educational, cultural, or geographic background, but whatever the basis of their commonalities, mutual support is the name of the game. It could be group pressure; it could be a word to the right person at the right time; it could be simply access to information sources, but it exists. You can count on it; you can take risks; you won't be alone. (And you don't necessarily have to like each other or agree on everything.) Could this work for nurses? Why not? What is needed is a network that promotes support *of* nurses *for* nurses, men or women. A network that provides backup for the risk takers until all can become risk-takers for a purpose. A network that shows unified strength on issues that can be generally agreed upon, so that the profession as well as the individual practitioner can put into practice the principles of care to which both voice commitment. A network that avoids destructive competition and instead develops new leaders at all levels through peer pals, mentors, and role models. A network that encourages differences of opinion but provides an atmosphere for reasonable compromise. In essence, a network that develops and uses the essential abilities of nurses to share, to trust, to depend on one another.

Puetz describes how to start a network in a formal sense, almost like a new organization, and offers a number of practical tips on networking:[39]

- Learn how to ask questions.
- Try to give as much as you get.
- Follow up on contacts.
- Keep in touch with contacts.
- Report back to contacts.
- Be businesslike as you network.
- Don't be afraid to ask for what you need.
- Don't pass up any opportunities.

Because networking is "in" and is sometimes seen as what one writer called a "quick fix for moving up," and because it is also new to many women, it is being abused by some. Besides the warnings noted above, networkers are advised to observe both common and uncommon courtesies: don't make excessive requests; be appreciative; be sensitive to your contacts' situation; and be helpful to others.[40]

There are already formal nurse networks in operation, often initiated by a nursing organization or subgroup made up of nurses with common interests, clinical or otherwise. The participants help each other make contacts when they relocate, or they supply needed information or suggest someone else who would know. They alert one another to job opportunities and suggest their colleagues for appointments, presentations, or awards. They give visibility to nurses and boost and praise one another, instead of being unnecessarily critical.

Could this also be called collegiality? In a sense, yes. A *colleague* is usually defined as an associate, particularly in a profession. In a thesaurus, we also find ally, aider, collaborator, helper, partner, peer, friend, cooperator, coworker, cohelper, fellow worker, teammate, or even right-hand man and buddy. The implications are great. Colleagues may be called upon confidently for advice and assistance, and will give it. Colleagues share knowledge with one another, together rounding out the necessary information to improve patient care. Colleagues challenge one another to think in new ways and to try new ideas. Colleagues encourage risk-taking when the situation requires daring. Colleagues provide a support system when the risk-taker needs it. Colleagues are equal, yet different—that is, they may have varying educational preparation, experience, and positions, perhaps even belong to another profession, but when they work together for a particular purpose, that work is bettered by their cooperation.

Political Action

Politics may be defined as the art or science of influencing policy. There is a legitimate tendency to think of politics in the context of government, but affecting policy and operations at the institutional level is often just as important in the work life of a nurse. The term *inhouse law* has been used to describe the power nurses can have if they can determine policies and procedures that affect daily practice. An example is a policy stating that nurses may (or should or must) develop and implement teaching plans for patients or arrange for referrals to the visiting nurse, all of which have been blocked by physicians or administrators in some hospitals.

It is vital that nurses participate actively in the agencies or community groups where decisions are being made, such as local or state planning agencies. The strategy used to gain input may vary. A basic principle is applicable: before, during, and after gaining entrée, nurses must show that they are knowledgeable, that they have something to offer, and that they can put it all together into an action package. There are many places to start, for most community groups are looking for members who work and are willing to hold office (for example, church groups, charity groups, and PTAs). These activities may be seen as (1) a way of getting experience on boards, using parliamentary procedure to advantage, politicking, gaining some sophistication in influencing decisions, and (2) being visible to other groups and the public. Many community groups interlock, and by being active in some, nurses come in contact with others. It also helps to gain the support of women other than nurses. Organized women are becoming more successful in getting representation on policy-making groups. It pays for them to have someone who is ready and able to assume such responsibilities. But participating nurses must be capable; there is nothing worse than having an incompetent as the first nurse on a major board or committee. That could do the profession more damage than having a nonnurse, for it appears that women (and nurses) still have to be better than those already in power to gain initial respect.

Another aspect to consider and use is the potential economic power of nurses. A nurse executive who controls a multimillion-dollar budget wields power in determining how that money is spent. This kind of status enables these nurses to move in power circles where they can cultivate individuals who influence public and private decision making. Community nurses are also particularly good resources, because most make strong community contacts. Today the participation of the consumer in health care decisions is increasing. An activated consumer who supports nursing has impact on local decision making, as well as on state and national legislation. A legislator is more inclined to hear the consumer who presumably is a neutral participant, as opposed to an obvious interest group. But nursing must sell that consumer the profession's point of view, and must balance consumer needs and nursing goals.

Although it is often through the influence of consumer groups and the community's traditional power figures that nurses get on decision-making committees, boards, and similar groups, after that, they're on their own and must be prepared, perceptive, articulate, and under control. In meetings and at coffee breaks, the politicking and the formation of coalitions may well influence which way a decision goes. Nurses who haven't learned to play that game had better take lessons: using role play, assertiveness training, group therapy, group process, speech lessons—whatever is necessary.

On the level of governmental politics, nurses not only can and have influenced such issues as Social Security, quality assurance, patients' rights, and care of the long-term patient, but have a vital interest in such issues as reimbursement for nursing services, use of technology, children's services, nurse licensure, funds for nursing education, and a national health plan. The specifics of the legislative process and political action in the governmental arena are described in Chapter 10. However, in addition, there is no reason that nurses should not run for office. They are intelligent, frequently well educated, and know a lot about human relations. Those who have won office are not only effective, but often offer extraordinary insight into health issues. Some have been responsible for major legislative breakthroughs for nursing and health care. This is equally true of the dynamic group of nurses in regulatory agencies and congressional offices.

Regardless of the setting, there are some basic guidelines for effective political action. The first is to know the social and technical aspects of professional practice; second, to know the current professional issues and the implications for various alternative actions; third, to be aware of emerging social and political issues and trends that will affect health care and nursing; fourth, to learn others' points of view (those of potential supporters or opponents) and come to terms with what policy changes are possible, as well as desirable; and fifth, to seek allies who can espouse or at least see the desirability of a particular course of action.

Professional Unity, Professional Pride

It is a political fact that the most powerful groups are those that are united. Almost always this means that an organization speaks for that group, and that is one of the purposes of a professional organization. Nursing has many organizations representing various interest groups (see Chapter 13). At times they cooperate, but too often they are at odds or simply act separately. Fortunately, more serious efforts are being made by most groups to form coalitions in relation to important issues for nurses. This trend may or may not overcome the fact that only about 10 percent of nurses belong to the largest nursing organization, ANA. Yet almost everyone agrees that support of the professional organization, where unity and a resolution of internal problems must occur, is crucial if nursing is to be an autonomous, influential power group.

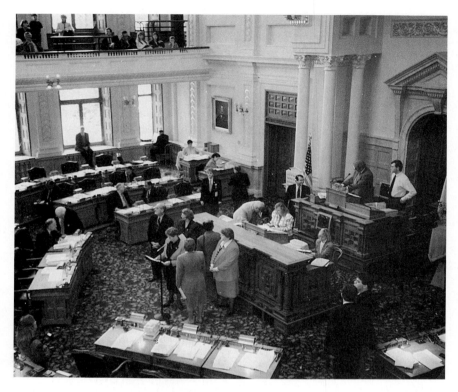

Nurses are exceptional candidates for public office. Here a nurse member of the State Assembly addresses the legislature. (*Courtesy of the New Jersey State Nurses Association.*)

Unity is hard to achieve, however, if you're not proud of yourself and your profession and what it stands for; if you're embarrassed by nursing's image or if, worse yet, you believe it. Because then, nurses are not a group with whom you want to be identified. Unity is not important because it doesn't seem worth the effort. The feeling of powerlessness is a comfort, in a sense, because it excuses you from taking action. That action *can* be taken is illustrated in the preceding pages. To look at the image of nursing is to see what you want to see. A nurse is not one kind of person, good or bad, handmaiden or entrepreneur. Nursing, like its components, has various images at various times. When you are that reflection, it should be what you want nursing to be.

A small point—or, perhaps, a large one: the fashionable image might be woman as slob, but nurse as slob is not attractive. Thirty years ago, how to dress was taught in nursing schools to young working-class women. A sloppy uniform was cause for a reprimand. The same was true for the RN. Then that was no longer considered appropriate; modern women knew how to dress and behave in a socially correct manner without needing lessons. Are the results evident today? But perhaps we've come full circle. The business literature aimed at men and women is full of advice on "dressing for success," and now it might be nursing's turn. What is nursing's image when a patient is cared for by an unkempt nurse in nondescript clothes with long hair sweeping across the patient's body? Yes, the public does notice. One individual being treated in a college health clinic reported, "I wondered who that person was in blue jeans and a top like men's underwear." A noted editor said at a meeting, "If you nurses are so worried about your image, you'd better clean up your nurses." Not you? Then perhaps a little peer pressure would help—a little direct or indirect action. Personal image and nonverbal behavior do convey a message—possibly a message of "no pride, no interest." Now, both nurses and their employees are taking a second look at this state of affairs and making changes. So are students. A positive image creates power. Who better than the nurses can shape that image?

It is time to look at what nursing has accomplished and is continuing to accomplish. It is a career of unlimited opportunities. It has produced documented evidence that its practitioners make major contributions to health care. And they are reaping some recognition and rewards. But there is unfinished business. Power and autonomy do not come to the spineless, the indifferent or downtrodden, or those who think they are.

Everyone has his or her own concerns, but individuals acting in isolation are vulnerable. In this era of social revolution, more and more individuals are uniting to secure their legitimate rights and privileges. Why would nursing want less? As Edith Draper, one of nursing's leaders, said in 1893, "To advance, we must unite."

KEY POINTS

1. Practice autonomy is one of the most crucial qualities of a profession.
2. The requirement to change and to lead others to personally meaningful change will be a constant characteristic of your practice.
3. Today's successful leaders bring out the best in their followers and involve them in defining the problem and inventing the solution.
4. Power can be coercive, but a more effective approach is shared power that strengthens both leader and follower.
5. Staff nurses have real power that can be used positively.

6. Nurses who are women must overcome some of the stereotypes others have of what women can and can't do.
7. Physician–nurse relationships can be problems or assets, depending on how the two professions understand each other and whether each sees the other as rival or colleague.
8. Peers as colleagues enhance one another's practice.
9. Networking is an effective way to broaden professional opportunities.
10. Nurses can have a strong impact on health policymaking by their effective participation in community groups.
11. Nurses who have pride in nursing, themselves and one another, can move nursing forward toward a preferred future.

REFERENCES

1. Marriner A. Theories of leadership. In Hein EC, Nicholson MJ (eds): *Contemporary Leadership Behavior*, 4th ed. Philadelphia: Lippincott, 1994, pp 55–61.
2. Porter-O'Grady TP. Transformational leadership in an age of chaos. *Nurs Admin Quart* 17:17–24, January, 1992.
3. Senge P. *The Fifth Discipline*. New York: Doubleday, 1990, pp 17–26.
4. Small N, Walsh M. *Teaching Nursing Homes: The Nursing Perspective*. Maryland: National Health Publishing, 1988.
5. Pew Charitable Trusts and Robert Wood Johnson Foundation. *Strengthening Hospital Nursing: A Progress Report*. St. Petersburg, FL: the authors, 1992.
6. Barker AM. An emerging leadership paradigm: Transformational leadership. *Nurs Health Care* 12:81–86, April, 1991.
7. Block P. *The Empowering Manager*. San Francisco: Jossey-Bass, 1991.
8. Safier G. Leaders among contemporary US nurses: An oral history. In Chaska N: *The Nursing Profession: Views Through the Mist*. New York: McGraw-Hill, 1978.
9. Safier G. *Contemporary American Leaders in Nursing: An Oral History*. New York: McGraw-Hill, 1977.
10. Schorr T, Zimmerman A. *Making Choices, Taking Chances*. St. Louis: Mosby, 1988.
11. Vance C. *A Group Profile of Contemporary Influentials in American Nursing*. Unpublished EdD Dissertation, Teachers College, Columbia University, 1977.

12. Kinsey D. The new nurse influentials. *Nurs Outlook* 34:238–240, September–October, 1986.
13. Ferguson VD. Perspectives on power. In Mason DJ, et al (eds): *Power, Politics and Policy in Nursing.* New York: Springer, 1993, pp 118–128.
14. Syrett M, Hogg C. *Frontiers of Leadership.* Cambridge: Blackwell, 1992.
15. Sweeney S. Traditions, transitions and transformations of power in nursing. In McCloskey JC, Grace HK (eds): *Current Issues in Nursing*, 3rd ed. St. Louis: Mosby, 1990, pp 460–464.
16. Ibid.
17. Gillies DA. *Nursing Management: A Systems Approach*, 2nd ed. Philadelphia: W.B. Saunders, 1994, pp 457–478.
18. Watzlawick P, et al. *Change.* New York: Norton, 1974.
19. Welch LB. Planned change in nursing: The theory. In Hein EC, Nicholson MJ (eds): *Contemporary Leadership Behavior.* Philadelphia: J.B. Lippincott, 1994, pp 313–324.
20. Ibid.
21. Rowland HS, Rowland BL. *Nursing Administration Handbook*, 3rd ed. Gaithersburg, MD: Aspen, 1992, pp 34–35.
22. Reverby SM. Other tales of the nursing–feminism connection. *Nurs Health Care* 14:295–301, June, 1993.
23. Shea CA. Feminism. In McCloskey JC, Grace HK (eds): *Current Issues in Nursing*, 4th ed. St. Louis: Mosby, 1994, pp 572–579.
24. Ibid.
25. Pillitteri A, Ackerman M. The "doctor–nurse" game: A comparison of 100 years, 1888–1990. *Nurs Outlook* 41:113–116, May–June, 1993.
26. Williamson AM, Kives AA. Nurse–physician collaboration in emergency services. *Top Emer Med* 13:1–12, March, 1991.
27. Knaus WA, et al. An evaluation of outcomes from intensive care in major medical centers. *Ann Inter Med* 104:410–418, March, 1986.
28. Stein L, et al. The doctor–nurse game revisited. *New Engl J Med* 322:546–549, February 22, 1990.
29. Jones RAP. Conceptual development of nurse–physician collaboration. *Holistic Nurs Pract* 8:1–11, March, 1994.
30. Kramer M. *Reality Shock.* St. Louis: Mosby, 1979.
31. Bradby M. Status passage into nursing: Another view of the process of socialization into nursing. *J Adv Nurs* 15:1220–1225, October, 1990.
32. Kelly LY, Joel LA. *Dimensions of Professional Nursing*, 7th ed. New York: McGraw-Hill, 1995, p 594.
33. American Nurses Association. *Testimony Before the Institute of*

Medicine, Commission on the Adequacy of Nurse Staffing. Washington, DC: ANA, September 21, 1994.

34. American Nurses Association and New York State Nurses Association. *Testimony Before the New York State Assembly Standing Committees on Labor, Health, Higher Education and Social Services.* Washington, DC: the authors, May 9, 1995.

34a. Yoder L. Mentoring: A concept analysis. In Hein EC, Nicholson MJ (eds): *Contemporary Leadership Behavior*, 4th ed. Philadelphia: Lippincott, 1994, pp 187–196.

35. Vance, loc cit.

36. Kinsey, loc cit.

37. Spengler C. *Mentor–Protégé Relationships: A Study of Career Development Among Female Nurse Doctorates.* Unpublished PhD Dissertation, University of Missouri–Columbia, 1982.

38. Angelini DJ. Mentoring in the career development of hospital staff nurses: Models and strategies. *J Prof Nurs* 11:89–97, March–April, 1995.

39. Puetz BE. Networking: Making it work for you. *Healthcare Trends Trans* 3:20–28, November–December, 1991.

40. Darling LAW. What to do about toxic mentors. In Hein EC, Nicholson MJ (eds): *Contemporary Leadership Behavior*, 4th ed. Philadelphia: Lippincott, 1994, pp 205–207.

Nursing Ethics
and Law

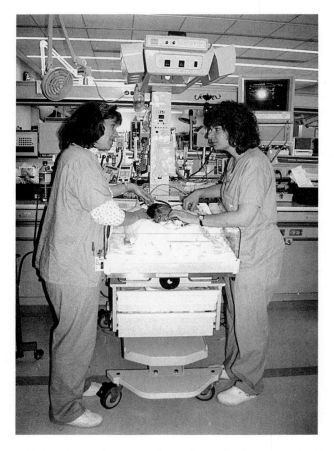

Complex high-tech care has created new issues in the areas of ethics and
patients' rights. (*Courtesy of Beth Israel Hospital, Boston*)

8

Ethical Issues in Nursing and Health Care

OBJECTIVES

After studying this chapter, you will be able to:

1. Differentiate between the concepts of morals and ethics.
2. Recognize the kinds of dilemmas nurses and others face in health care.
3. List factors that create these dilemmas.
4. List factors that influence the way you react to ethical problems.
5. Develop a way of assessing and dealing with ethical concerns.
6. Relate and apply the ANA Code for Nursing to your professional life.
7. Identify principles that underlie DNR procedures.
8. Recognize some of the major issues related to assisted suicide.
9. Understand the issues of access to care.
10. Identify actions you can take in relation to chemically impaired or incompetent colleagues.

Most people who decide to enter nursing are aware that there are times that they will be dealing with life and death. If they think about it to any extent, they probably assume that they would do their best to help the patient to live or keep him or her comfortable until death. Asked whether they expected to have a conflict with the law or with other colleagues or even a conflict within themselves at such a time, they would probably react with astonishment. How could this happen? If you asked whether they expected to have any trouble behaving ethically in these situations, the reply might well be, "Why would I?"

Is that the way you felt? Is that the way you feel now? It's quite possible that the shock of dealing with ethical questions is not as great now as it might have been even a few years ago. Movies, plays, television, books, magazines, and even newspaper reports are beginning to recognize that the ethical dilemmas in health care faced every day by those in the field must also be faced by the public.

WHAT CREATES ETHICAL DILEMMAS?

Why are things different now? One simple answer is that it is a much more complex world, with many conflicting pressures on both consumers and providers. For instance:

1. Technology in the form of transplants, artificial parts, and machinery, as well as new drugs, can keep alive young and old patients who would once have died, *but* the cost of surviving after such intervention may be so high financially that either the government must pay for both the treatment and lifelong care, or only the rich can afford it. An average family would become impoverished. In some cases, the public pays to keep alive a nonfunctioning human being and then has to deny resources to someone with the possibility of a productive life. And people's notions are changing about whether the quality of life made possible by technology, or its sanctity, is most important.

2. New knowledge and techniques involving alteration of genes in a human being, and the ability to identify genes causing serious disorders, now exist, *but* this also raises questions of commercialization, cost, safety, and confidentiality.

3. People are beginning to recognize their right to make decisions about their medical treatment even if the decision would lead to death; *but* even though family and significant others agree with the individual, his or her wish may be thwarted after the individual becomes technically "incompetent," because the health professionals and/or institutions are afraid of lawsuits, and the law does not always clearly define how or whether such wishes can be carried out.

4. The law does cover certain rights, such as abortion; *but* groups with their own religious or moral agendas try to prevent people from exercising those rights.

5. In general, the public accepts the idea that everyone has a right to health care; *but* there are limited resources and no one wants to pay for the reality of equal access.

These situations may not only create conflict between professionals and family but pit colleague against colleague, health professional against administration, family against courts, lawyer against lawyer, church against individuals, and any variation of these. Yet, almost everyone wants to do what is right. What is "right"? It's not easy to decide. Look at these not uncommon ethical dilemmas.

- A fragile man in his eighties, riddled with cancer, is admitted to the hospital. When his heart stops, he is resuscitated and awakens with tubes in every orifice. He begs to be allowed to die but is repeatedly resuscitated.
- A 26-year-old quadriplegic woman with cerebral palsy has herself admitted to a hospital and then asks to be kept comfortable, but allowed to die by starvation because she finds life unbearable. The hospital force-feeds her.
- An 85-year-old man with many illnesses has been fasting in a nursing home to hasten his death. His daughter supports his decision, and he dies in a few days.
- Two physicians terminate intravenous feeding of a comatose man, with the consent of the family. They are reported by nurses and criminally prosecuted.
- A baby is born with Down's syndrome and various other congenital defects, one of which requires immediate surgery in order to save the infant's life. The parents refuse permission because they believe that the child, if she survives, will not have a reasonable quality of life and they will not be able to care for her.
- Another baby with similar defects undergoes surgery, but the mother, an unwed teenager, cannot keep the child. It is in a public institution, requiring total care for all of its five years of life.
- A depressed patient admitted to a mental hospital refuses electroshock therapy after several treatments because he thinks it will kill him even though he is improving with treatment. He cannot care for himself at home, and his wife cannot manage his erratic behavior. He is committed, under the state's laws, given the treatment, and recovers.
- A retarded 15-year-old boy in the county home refuses kidney dialysis because he fears it. No effort is made to relieve his anxiety, and others on the hospital's waiting list are moved forward into therapy. The boy dies.
- Two men on the same hospital unit have a cardiac arrest within several minutes of each other. The first to arrest is an alcoholic street person with various other conditions; the other is a businessman with a wife and four children. There is one cardiopulmonary resuscitation cart. The resident says, "First come, first served" and resuscitates the alcoholic; the businessman dies.

- A young couple with two boys decides that they can afford only one more child and want a girl. If amniocentesis indicates a boy, the mother wants an abortion.
- After genetic screening, a couple has been advised that they are carriers of a hereditary disease. Two of their teenage children have it, and one does not. When the mother becomes pregnant again, she decides on an abortion, but both parents decide not to "spoil the children's lives" by telling them they may later manifest the disease or carry the gene that might condemn their children to that disease.
- A patient about to undergo surgery clearly does not understand the risks or the available alternatives. The nurse tells the physician, but he replies that he did explain, that patients seldom understand these explanations, and that the patient should be prepared for surgery.
- A patient with cancer is on an experimental drug. Although hospital policy states that the physician must get an informed consent before the drug is administered, the patient's very prestigious physician calls in and tells the nurse to start the drug because it is important to begin at once; he will be in later to get the consent. When the nurse hesitates, her supervisor tells her to go ahead.
- A colleague in the OR confesses to his friend that he has AIDS and that he is afraid to let management know. The nurse friend is concerned because the individual assists in surgery every day.
- An older respected physician in a renowned hospital has been making mistakes in surgery. The residents have been able to catch and/or repair them thus far, but the scrub nurse thinks that he ought to be prevented from operating. No physician will report him officially.

If you were the nurse involved in any of these situations, what would you do? How would you react? Whose rights are or might be violated? The patient's? The family's? The nurse's? The doctor's? Society's? Nobody's? How much would you be affected by your own moral beliefs? If your action was contrary to what the hospital administrators, the physicians involved, or even some of your colleagues thought best (for whatever reason), would you be willing to face the consequences? What if your concept of "right" collided with a legal ruling? What if the patient or family asked you to help them?

All of these cases cited are real, but not always made public. A nurse somewhere faced one of these difficult situations (and probably others) and had to make the decision to act or not to act. How that decision was arrived at is the essence of ethics.

Almost every day, some situation that has presented an ethical dilemma to family, friends, health care professionals, and health care institutions is reported in the media, often because it is no longer in the arena of unofficial voluntary action but has become a legal battle. One that got months of attention is the case of Nancy Cruzan, who after a car accident remained in a permanent vegetative state (PVS) for years. When her parents wanted her gastric tube feeding discontinued so that she could die peaceably, objections by others eventually took the case to the US Supreme Court.[1] (This and similar ethical–legal issues are discussed in Chapter 9.) The aftermath of this decision had legal implications for what might once have been a private matter, decided according to the ethical beliefs of the family and the quiet cooperation of like-minded health professionals. In fact, it has been estimated that a large percentage of those who die in hospitals die because some potential life-prolonging treatment is willingly withheld. Once, these issues would not have come up at all. People got sick and died, probably at home. Grossly malformed infants were quietly allowed to die. There was no technology to keep these people alive, and except in very rare circumstances, available life-prolonging techniques like feeding tubes were not used. Dying was a natural act—sad, perhaps, but inevitable.

There was also a quiet understanding that a dying patient in pain could be helped to die, perhaps by giving a larger dose of a narcotic than usual. Doctors ordered it; nurses gave it. Yet, one of the big ethical issues evolving is *physician- or professionally-assisted suicide*. An opinion piece by a physician was published in a respected medical journal, describing how he had prescribed barbiturates for a patient dying of cancer, at her request. He knew her well and knew she had asked because this was an essential ingredient in Hemlock Society (a right-to-die group) suicide.[2] The article created some furor but no legal prosecution, as opposed to the reaction to another physician who helped a women with early Alzheimer's disease to commit suicide with a "death machine." Even that case was eventually dismissed, and he helped others to die later (for which prosecution was always threatened). Just how many dying or PVS patients are helped to die will never be known. But to some nurses and others, *not* to help them would be unethical; to others, to do so would be both unethical and worthy of legal action. This is discussed in more detail later.

On a much larger scale is the ethical question of access to care when limited access could well result in death. Not a nursing problem? But it is: every time a nursing unit is short-staffed and a nurse must make continuous decisions on priorities, the possibility of some patients being neglected and even dying becomes a reality. In fact, nurses have admitted that this is exactly what happens, because they have no other choice. Moreover, the very fact that nurses are the largest group of health professionals makes them important players in resolving issues of access to care, difficult though this is. An example is the national health plan developed by the Tri-Council (ANA, NLN, AACN, AONE), which represented many other nursing organizations on this issue.

Nurses are well aware that ethical issues arise constantly in their professional practice. A survey was conducted by the ANA Center for Ethics and Human Rights at the ANA convention in June 1994. The 934 valid returns represented nurses from all states except Alaska and the District of Columbia, with 31 percent being staff nurses, 23 percent educators, and the next largest number consisting of nurse managers, administrators and advanced practice nurses. Most worked in hospitals. Fewer than 1 percent indicated that they had never been confronted with an ethical issue, and 43 percent said that they faced ethical dilemmas daily, 36 percent weekly. The four issues most frequently encountered were: cost containment issues that jeopardize patient welfare; end-of-life decisions; breaches of patient confidentiality; and incompetent, unethical, or illegal practices of colleagues. Others noted were pain management, use of advance directives, informed consent for procedures, access to health care, issues in the care of HIV/AIDS persons, and providing "futile" care.[3]

This survey reinforced an earlier national ANA survey in which the respondents cited rationing of health care and end-of-life decisions as the top two "most pressing" ethical issues faced by nurses, followed by abortion, advanced directives, assisted suicide and euthanasia.[4] There were some differences in relation to position and length of time since licensure. Some

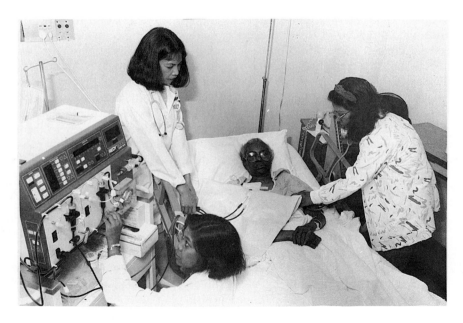

What has become the new standard of care may present significant ethical dilemmas. (*Courtesy of Beth Israel Hospital, Medical Center, Newark, New Jersey.*)

interesting aspects of this survey will be mentioned as various ethical topics are discussed later.

One inevitable result of the increasing concern about ethics in health care by both the health professions and the public is legal action. Such actions range from court decisions to legislation on both the state and federal level. Sometimes the trail from ethical problem to legal action is very clear. Unfortunately, what becomes law is not always seen as ethical by individuals and groups, and this creates problems for both practitioners and the public. The reality is that resolving ethical concerns is not easy and probably never will be. Sometimes it is also difficult to disentangle just how and where law and ethics interact. To attempt as rational an approach as possible, this chapter will focus primarily on ethical theories, codes of ethics, approaches to ethical decision making, clarification of common misunderstandings related to end-of-life care, assisted suicide, an overview of access to care issues, and collegial relationships. Ethical issues that have seen considerable legal action will be discussed in Chapter 9.

As you read the sections on morality and the various theories of ethics, as well as the nursing code of ethics, consider the ethical problems given as examples and note how your decisions depend on your ethical or, perhaps, moral beliefs. Even if you are not in a position to make a direct decision, inevitably you will be in an environment where such dilemmas will continue to occur, and you will have to come to some understanding about how you can deal with them, directly or indirectly. There is no such thing as "no decision."

FACTORS THAT INFLUENCE ETHICAL DECISION MAKING

Morals and Ethics

There is a tendency to use the words *moral* and *ethical* interchangeably in the literature of health professions. However, in the last few years, the need to differentiate between the two terms has become more evident. One simple explanation is:

> Morality is generally defined as behavior according to custom or tradition. Ethics, by contrast, is the free, rational assessment of courses of actions in relation to precepts, rules, conduct. ... To be ethical a person must take the additional step of exercising critical, rational judgment in his decisions.[5]

Kohlberg, structuring a theory of moral development, used the term *stages* for individual phases of moral thinking.[6] Although his theory is

still widely used when discussing moral development, there is some disagreement with his approach, in part because of certain limitations in his study,
including the fact that he had only male subjects.

Gilligan[7] was particularly disturbed that Kohlberg did not acknowledge
the concerns and experience of women in moral development. She carried
out a study designed to clarify the nature of women's moral judgment as
they faced the moral dilemma of whether to continue or abort a pregnancy.
Results showed that women's moral judgment differs from that of men.
For women, the worst problem was defined in terms of exercising care and
avoiding hurt. The infliction of hurt was seen as selfish and immoral.
"Women's moral judgment proceeded from initial concern for survival, to
focus on goodness, to a principled understanding of care."[8]

Noddings' model,[9] building on the work of Gilligan, is more recent,
and has been given considerable attention in nursing. She centers her
ideas on the value of care and caring, stressing that caring is a relationship,
not a unilateral activity. "The choice to enter a relationship as one caring
... is grounded in a vision that we hold of our best selves," our "ethical
ideal."[10] In an effort to see whether "caring" uniquely reflects the moral
orientation of nursing students as opposed to medical students, the research
results indicated that while there were such differences, the *female* medical
students had the same caring ethical orientation as the nurses, all female.[11]

The whole issue of ethics versus morals may seem to be purely philosophical; however, given the differentiation described, the code of ethics of
professional nurses may require action that goes beyond what their immediate
associates see as necessary. It is also possible that individuals must struggle
with what seems to be a conflict between ethical behavior and personal
religious beliefs. However, in another study consisting of in-depth interviews
about moral beliefs, the nurses had a very clear concept: a moral right was
anything that benefited the patient and a moral wrong was anything that
did not.[12]

Theories

There are a number of theories on which ethical decision making is
based. Using the cases mentioned earlier as examples, some of these theories,
which are more or less classic, will now be described. There are other themes,
some newer, some developed by "experts" in the field. Just about all nursing
books on ethics include the authors' interpretation of these theories. Several
ethics books are cited in the Bibliography; even earlier books, listed in the
last two editions of this book, are valuable for studying ethics theories.

The *egoism* theory says that a decision is right because the doer or
"agent," in this case the nurse, desires it; it is the most comfortable one for
that person, without consideration for how the decision might affect others.

For example, the nurse may simply prepare the patient for surgery, accepting the doctor's statement that the patient was given an adequate explanation.

The theory of *deontology* (formalism) asserts that rightness or wrongness must be considered in terms of its moral significance. *Act deontology* considers the agent's own moral values. *Rule deontology* suggests that there are rules or standards for judging morally, often a command by God. Thus, a nurse may oppose abortion because of either personal moral beliefs or religious beliefs.

Utilitarianism defines right as the greatest good and the least amount of harm for the greatest number of people. For instance, severely congenitally deformed babies might be allowed to die rather than be a burden on society for many years.

Justice as fairness—the distribution of benefits (good) or harm (evil) to society—is Rawls's theory. The two principles of justice are equal rights for everyone and the greatest benefit given to the least advantaged. With this reasoning, the retarded boy would take precedence over others for the kidney dialysis, and efforts would be made to persuade him into therapy.

More contemporary views have been offered by modern philosophers dissatisfied with the traditional choices. Frankena's *theory of obligation* focuses on the principle of beneficence and the principle of justice as equal treatment. However, the definition of these principles leads to some confusion. For instance, distributive justice is seen as treating people according to their needs. The difficulty of deciding which criterion to use can be illustrated by considering this theory in the case of the two men with cardiac arrest.

The *ideal observer* theory proposed by Firth requires that a decision be made from a disinterested, dispassionate, consistent viewpoint, with full information available and consideration of future consequences. While this approach can theoretically be applied to any ethical situation, the probable impossibility of any one person being able to do so might necessitate the involvement of other people, perhaps an ethics committee.

These theories, which have been presented very briefly, and others, are often complex and sometimes appear more philosophical than practical. However, they provide an interesting framework for ethical decision making.

Codes of Ethics

Another guide to ethical behavior is a professional code of ethics. In the last several years, ethical behavior has been increasingly a topic of discussion in almost every field—business, politics, law, and, perhaps most of all, health. One sign of this focus is the new interest in codes of ethics. Codes of ethics, by whatever name, have been common in professions for some time. It is generally conceded that medicine was the first profession in the United States to adopt a code of ethics, but law, pharmacy, and veterinary medicine were also early comers. However, in the last decade or so, an interesting phenomenon has occurred: ethics has become fashionable, and codes have been newly adopted by organizations representing business and industry.

A code of ethics is considered an essential characteristic of a profession, providing one means whereby professional standards may be established, maintained, and improved. It indicates the profession's acceptance of the trust and responsibility with which society has invested it. The public has granted the professionals certain privileges, with certain expectations in return. Nevertheless, one ethicist stated, "There is a fair degree of public and professional cynicism about codes and a wide range of complaints about them—that they are self-serving, pious, or public relations devices."[13] Unfortunately, not only is this attitude still somewhat prevalent, but in some cases also accurate, as seen in recent political scandals. Yet perhaps because of the influence of changing times, the self-serving aspects of ethical codes have diminished considerably over the last few years, and recent revisions of most codes are beginning to show more concern for protecting society than for protecting the profession. An interesting example is the AMA's detailed *Code of Medical Ethics: Current Opinions with Annotations* (1994).

Nursing's code of ethics has also changed over the years.[14] The 1976 version of the code, with interpretive statements, was developed by an ad hoc committee of the ANA's Congress for Nursing Practice and is available from the American Nurses Association (Exhibit 8.1). The interpretive statements are especially valuable because they not only enlarge upon and explain the code in more detail, but also provide more focus and direction on how the nurse can carry out the code. Particularly important is the first statement, which sets the tone of the nurse–client relationship as partners:

> Whenever possible, clients should be fully involved in the planning and implementation of their own health care. Each client has the moral right to determine what will be done with his/her person.

Key areas in the interpretations deal with the nurse as patient advocate, nurse participation in political decision making and public affairs, and nurse involvement in advertising of products. Nurse accountability is a major issue and is considered important enough to require a separate statement; the code now has 11 instead of 10 statements.

Overall, the code was intended to express nursing's moral concerns, goals, and values, rather than announcing a set of laws dictating nurses' behavior. However, in 1988, the ANA published *Ethics in Nursing: Position Statements and Guidelines* because of nurses' stated need for help in applying the code to newly complex situations. Most relate to relatively new or emerging issues. For instance, in a statement examining at what point it ceases to be a nurse's duty to undergo risk for the benefit of the patient,

EXHIBIT 8.1

American Nurses Association Code for Nurses (1976)

PREAMBLE

The Code for Nurses is based on beliefs about the nature of individuals, nursing, health, and society. Recipients and providers of nursing services are viewed as individuals and groups who possess basic rights and responsibilities, and whose values and circumstances command respect at all times. Nursing encompasses the promotion and restoration of health, the prevention of illness, and the alleviation of suffering. The statements of the Code and their interpretation provide guidance for conduct and relationships in carrying out nursing responsibilities consistent with the ethical obligations of the profession and quality in nursing care.

1. The nurse provides services with respect for human dignity and the uniqueness of the client unrestricted by considerations of social or economic status, personal attributes, or the nature of health problems.

2. The nurse safeguards the client's right to privacy by judiciously protecting information of a confidential nature.

3. The nurse acts to safeguard the client and the public when health care and safety are affected by the incompetent, unethical, or illegal practice of any person.

4. The nurse assumes responsibility and accountability for individual nursing judgments and actions.

5. The nurse maintains competence in nursing.

6. The nurse exercises informed judgment and uses individual competence and qualifications as criteria in seeking consultation, accepting responsibilities, and delegating nursing activities to others.

7. The nurse participates in activities that contribute to the ongoing development of the profession's body of knowledge.

8. The nurse participates in the profession's efforts to implement and improve standards of nursing.

9. The nurse participates in the profession's efforts to establish and maintain conditions of employment conducive to high quality nursing care.

10. The nurse participates in the profession's effort to protect the public from misinformation and misrepresentation and to maintain the integrity of nursing.

11. The nurse collaborates with members of the health professions and other citizens in promoting community and national efforts to meet the health needs of the public.

Source: Reprinted with permission of the American Nurses Association.

probably in response to the care of AIDS patients, responsibility to the patient is stressed, but the conclusion is that there are limits to the moral obligation of the nurse to benefit patients. Examples are given. Other statements emphasize the importance of nurses' participation in institutional ethics committees, a prohibition of nurses' participation in capital punishment, and the "nonnegotiable nature" of the Code. A number of ANA resources on ethics are also listed.

As nurses became more involved in research activities, especially nurse-initiated research, the ANA published, in 1968, *The Nurse in Research: ANA Guidelines on Ethical Values.* Among the points made, which are still pertinent, are that the nurse is expected to participate in a research or experimental activity only with assurance that the project has the official sanction of a legally constituted research committee or other appropriate authority within the institutional or agency settings, and he or she must have sufficient knowledge of the research design to allow participation in an informed, effective, and ethical fashion. If the nurse sees conflicts or questions related to the well-being and safety of the patient, this concern must be voiced to the appropriate person in the institution. At all times, nurses remain responsible for their own acts and judgments. Since then, there have been updates on ethical guidelines for nurses involved in research. The latest (1995) is quite detailed and is accompanied by an excellent annotated bibliography. Both are listed in this chapter's bibliography. Legal/ethical rights of patients in research are discussed in Chapter 9.

The International Council of Nursing (ICN) also has a code of ethics. The 1973 version was presented as "useful to nurses in many cultures but able to stand the tests of time and social change." (Exhibit 8.2.) A striking change from the 1965 code is one that makes explicit the nurse's responsibility and accountability for nursing care, deleting statements in the 1965 code that had ignored the nurse's judgment and personal responsibility and showed dependency on the physician that nurses worldwide no longer see as appropriate. This code was reaffirmed in 1989.

Using the ANA Code

The ANA Code of Ethics, like other professional codes, has no legal force, as opposed to the licensure laws, enforced by state boards of nursing (not the nurses' associations). However, the requirements of the Code often exceed, but are never less than, the requirements of the law. Violations of the Code should be reported to constituent associations of ANA, which may reprimand, censure, suspend, or expel members. Most state nurses' associations (SNAs) have a procedure for considering reported violations that also gives the accused due process. Even if the nurse is not an SNA member, an ethical violation, at the least, results in the loss of respect of colleagues and

EXHIBIT 8.2

International Council of Nurses' Code for Nurses (1973) Ethical Concepts Applied to Nursing

The fundamental responsibility of the nurse is fourfold: to promote health, to prevent illness, to restore health, and to alleviate suffering.

The need for nursing is universal. Inherent in nursing is respect for life, dignity, and rights of man. It is unrestricted by considerations of nationality, race, creed, colour, age, sex, politics, or social status.

Nurses render health services to the individual, the family, and the community and coordinate their services with those of related groups.

NURSES AND PEOPLE

The nurse's primary responsibility is to those people who require nursing care.

The nurse, in providing care, promotes an environment in which the values, customs, and spiritual beliefs of the individual are respected.

The nurse holds in confidence personal information and uses judgment in sharing this information.

NURSES AND PRACTICE

The nurse carries personal responsibility for nursing practice and for maintaining competence by continual learning.

The nurse maintains the highest standards of nursing care possible within the reality of a specific situation.

The nurse uses judgment in relation to individual competence when accepting and delegating responsibilities.

The nurse when acting in a professional capacity should at all times maintain standards of personal conduct that would reflect credit upon the profession.

NURSES AND SOCIETY

The nurse shares with other citizens the responsibility for initiating and supporting action to meet the health and social needs of the public.

NURSES AND CO-WORKERS

The nurse sustains a cooperative relationship with co-workers in nursing and other fields.

The nurse takes appropriate action to safeguard the individual when his care is endangered by a co-worker or any other person.

(continued)

EXHIBIT 8.2 *(continued)*

NURSES AND THE PROFESSION
The nurse plays the major role in determining and implementing desirable standards of nursing practice and nursing education.

The nurse is active in developing a core of professional knowledge.

The nurse, acting through the professional organization, participates in establishing and maintaining equitable social and economic working conditions in nursing.

Source: Reprinted with permission of the International Council of Nurses.

the public, which is a serious sanction. All nurses should be familiar with the profession's ethical code. It is a professional obligation to uphold and abide by the code and ensure that nursing colleagues do likewise. (Not all ethical problems deal with patient care; some relate to the behavior and actions of nursing and other colleagues.)

Implementation of the code is at two levels. The nurse may be involved in resolving ethical issues on a broad policy level, participating with other groups in decision making to formulate guidelines or laws. But the more common situation is ethical decision making in daily practice, on a one-to-one basis, on issues that are probably not a matter of life and death but must be resolved on the spot. Still, in clinical areas, such as intensive care units, there *are* life-and-death ethical issues that require decisions.[15] The Code, and particularly its interpretations, are useful as a guideline here, but more than likely in specific incidents, personal reactions will be both intellectual and emotional and strongly influenced by the nurse's own cultural background, education, and experience.

GUIDELINES FOR ETHICAL DECISION MAKING

How can you tell if you're facing an ethical issue? Some ethicists maintain that all decisions made with, for, or about patients or clients or other human beings have an ethical dimension.[16] Theoretically, then, there are ethical decisions that do not create a problem. However, in reality, everyone involved may agree on an action, but it could still be considered unethical by someone's standards. What creates most crises is the ethical dilemma—a situation involving a choice between equally satisfactory (good) or unsatisfactory (bad) alternatives or a problem that seems to have no satisfactory solution. Curtin argues that a true dilemma is relatively rare because often, if there is adequate information and time, there are clear guidelines for action. But, she says:

> A dilemma may not be solvable, but it is resolvable. Even though there is no right or wrong between two *equally* unfavorable actions, taking no action may be even worse than making the choice.[17]

Models and Ethics Rounds

Making that choice, whether or not it can be made by the nurse as an individual or as part of a group, is not easy. To make ethical decisions, it is sometimes useful to use a structured format. A number of bioethical decision models have been presented over the years;[18,19] most include the steps found in Exhibit 8.3 or variations of them. Having some educational background on the issues, including a course in which these frameworks are explained and used, is also helpful.

While going through these steps does not permit snap decisions, there are many ethical dilemmas in which the nurse can take time for thought

---

EXHIBIT 8.3

A Bioethical Decision Model

1. Identify the health problem.
2. List the relevant facts needed to understand the situation.
3. Identify the ethical problem or issues.
4. Determine who's involved in making the decision (the nurse, the doctor, the patient, the patient's family).
5. Identify your own role. (Quite possibly, your role may not require a decision at all.)
6. Define your own moral/ethical position, the profession's (code of ethics), and, as much as possible, that of the key individuals involved.
7. Consider as many possible alternative decisions as you can.
8. Try to identify value conflicts.
9. Consider the long- and short-range consequences of each alternative decision.
10. Reach your decision and act on it.
11. Follow the situation until you can see the actual results of your decision, and evaluate it.
12. Use this information to help in making future decisions.

and discussion with others. Even if the situation does not allow this kind of thoughtful decision making (such as the case in which the doctor made an instant decision as to whom he would resuscitate), later analysis can help in future situations. The nurse can also gain insight into others' thinking and reasoning.

Some health care institutions have an ethics consultant, who helps staff and families clarify and resolve ethical issues (particularly if there is some confusion about what is possible).[20] In many ways, such an individual assumes some of the role of the hospital ethics committee.

Nursing ethics committees (NECs) can also be helpful and supportive to nurses. However, although the value seems to be clear, there are relatively few. The June ANA survey, cited earlier, reported that only 27 percent of the settings had NECs, although 51 percent had interdisciplinary committees. The purposes are somewhat but not totally different. NEC's functions include: identifying, exploring, and resolving ethical issues in nursing practice; educating nurses in bioethics and nursing ethics; preparing nurses for interdisciplinary decision making regarding ethical issues; serving as a resource group; reviewing nursing ethics materials; reviewing departmental policies related to ethics; encouraging nursing ethics research; and preparing nurses to serve on institutional ethics committees.[21]

Another useful way to learn to make ethical decisions is to initiate or participate in "ethics rounds." The format is the same as that of most rounds—discussing a case in an organized fashion—but this time the clinical aspects are background. The case could be hypothetical, a recently discharged or deceased patient, or a current patient. The key is open and free discussion with no blame-laying.

Sources of Information

Learning as much as possible about ethical issues in health care is useful because then the nurse can be somewhat prepared when dealing with them personally. There are, of course, many books, journals, articles, and even videotapes and movies, on ethics in health care and nursing. A particularly interesting series of reports came out of the President's Commission for the Study of Ethical Problems in Medicine and Biomedical Behavioral Research, which is still quite pertinent. The Commission's 1983 reports covered such issues as informed consent, the right to die, whistle blowing in biomedical research, protecting human subjects, implementing human research regulations, genetic engineering, and access to health care. The reports were decidedly pro-public and pro-patient. Among other things, they included results of polls and surveys taken on crucial ethical issues and extensive searches of literature, which resulted in quite valuable and otherwise unavailable information. The reports should be available at most libraries.

Other good resources are organizations with an ethical focus. Their publications and meetings are usually directed at both the public and the professional. Among these are the Hastings Center (Institute of Society, Ethics, and the Life Sciences) in Hastings-on-the-Hudson, New York, and Choice in Dying, the merged Concern for Dying and Society for the Right to Die, in New York City. The latter is particularly involved with the living will, a voluntary statement of a person's wishes in the event of incapacity. (See Chapter 9.)

A particularly important source for nurses is ANA's Center for Ethics and Human Rights. One of its most important functions is to develop and disseminate information on ethics and human rights issues facing nurses. Through consultation and resources, the Center provides both theoretical and practical guidance. They answer queries from many nursing and nonnursing groups. They can be reached at ANA headquarters. NLN and other nursing organizations, although not as extensively involved, offer publications and position papers on ethics.

Interdisciplinary Ethics Committees

Ethics committees in one form or another have been in existence for about 20 years. In 1976, a New Jersey Supreme Court judge ordered a sort of internal ethics committee (actually more of a prognosis committee) to help institutions and physicians make decisions about situations such as the Karen Quinlan case, over which he presided. Karen had been in a permanent vegetative state for some years and her family wanted to remove her respirator. Although it was thought that such a mechanism would be quickly adopted, in 1983 a survey showed that less than 1 percent of all hospitals had established an ethics committee. Today, the majority have one, as well as do an increasing number of long-term-care facilities. In 1991, the Joint Commission on the Accreditation of Health-care Organizations (JCAHO) began to require that institutions have "a mechanism for the consideration of ethical issues arising in the care of patients and to provide education to caregivers and patients on ethical issues in health care." In 1993, JCAHO mandated the same for home health agencies.

The ethics committee may or may not be integrated into the hospital's administrative structure, but the members usually include one or more nurse managers and staff nurses, one or more physicians, a therapist, a social worker, a member of the clergy, an attorney, an ethicist, and one or more representatives from the community. This multidisciplinary group, usually volunteers, form a "community of concern" defined as "that group of persons necessary to grasp all of the essential dimensions of a given issue."[22] The functions of most committees are generally within the framework of those suggested by the President's Commission for the Study of Ethical Problems in Medicine and Biomedical and Behavioral Research in 1983. These are as follows:

1. They can review the case to confirm the responsible physician's diagnosis and prognosis of a patient's medical condition.
2. They can provide a forum for discussing broader social and ethical concerns raised by a particular case; such bodies may also have an educational role, especially by teaching all professional staff how to identify, frame, and resolve ethical problems.
3. They can be a means for formulating policy and guidelines regarding such decisions.
4. Finally, they can review decisions made by others (such as physicians and surrogates) about the treatment of specific patients or make such decisions themselves.[23]

The commission noted that ethics committees have an important role in educating professionals about issues relevant to life support, but heads of these committees have reported that this was not a particularly successful activity, perhaps because of the difficulty in getting staff, especially physicians, to attend lectures on this topic. The committees were also seen as providing a setting for people within medical institutions to become knowledgeable and comfortable about relating specific ethical principles to specific decisions, especially when real cases in the hospital were used as examples. There was also some concern that the case review function, that is, reviewing certain decisions made by the family of an incapacitated person and his or her practitioner, would be overutilized.[24] However, in 1992, one expert reported that just the opposite had occurred.[25] The reasons were political (infringing upon the authority of the physician), psychological (the difficulty a group might have in making life and death decisions), and cultural or intellectual (the differences in attitudes about certain ethical dilemmas).[26]

From a practical point of view, the members of the committee, most of whom do not have training in ethics, should be educated themselves, perhaps by the ethicist or external experts. They are then in a better position to recommend or set policies for the institution (depending on what authority the committee is given). They will also be more knowledgeable when called upon for consultation. One role that seems to be helpful is to provide a neutral forum for discussion of difficult cases in which the nurses and others involved, including families, can talk out their concerns. The emotional support provided seems to be very helpful in alleviating the stress that usually accompanies difficult ethical situations. One important point is that staff nurses should be on the committee, since they are on the firing line. Unfortunately, there is some indication that this is not a given, and consequently there may be major disagreement between nurses and the committee about issues considered important. Some committees are seen as inadequate to address ethical issues. "Too medically oriented, too theoretical, not knowledgeable, and too inactive" are some of the complaints about them. Nevertheless, nurses are becoming more aggressive about their right to be on ethics committees, and their value as participants is quickly acknowledged when they are members. A good ethics committee has an important role in working out ethical problems. Their importance is recognized by the formation of a Multi-Facility Bioethics Committee (MFBC). Founded by several health care institutions in New Jersey, it is composed of an ethicist and a maximum of four people from each facility. It functions much the same way as any single institutional committee, but, for instance, is developing forms to flag DNR orders, which would be valid in each facility.

DEALING WITH ETHICAL CONCERNS

The major ethical issues for those in the health professions today have been identified as the quality of life versus the sanctity of life; the right to live versus the right to die; informed consent; confidentiality; rights of children; unethical behavior of other practitioners; role conflict (who's responsible?); and the allocation of scarce resources (who shall live?). Increasingly, these issues have become subjects of legislation or court decisions (as discussed in later chapters), but even this does not lessen your potential conflicts. Not only must you confront the distinct possibility that your personal value systems may be different from that of the profession, but you may also be caught in the value system of your employing institution.

In the first situation, you must come to terms with your responsibility to the patient or client, regardless of your personal beliefs. For instance, nurses today are faced constantly with the need to make decisions about their roles in end-of-life decisions or abortion. The decision for action may not be easy. When it comes to ending the life of a terminally ill patient or participating in an abortion, you may choose not to participate if the action is against your moral principles. Your responsibility, however, is not to abandon your patient, but to speak to your manager early enough to allow another nurse to take over. Physicians have the same responsibility. But what about caring for responding, reacting patients? There have been reports of health professionals neglecting or even abusing (mentally if not physically) patients about whom they have moral reservations, such as homosexuals, criminals, alcoholics, or women having abortions. Clearly, this situation is intolerable and violates any professional code of ethics.[27]

Still, there is no question that nurses may experience what has been termed *moral distress*, painful feelings that occur because they or someone else performs an action they believe to be immoral but are powerless to stop.

If the action is by someone else, the feeling escalates to one of *moral outrage*. An example is the repeated resuscitation of an elderly patient with a terminal illness who does not want to be resuscitated. Fear of sanctions often restrains the nurse from acting, even though the threatened sanction is an unlikely one, such as loss of the license. The results are often a feeling of loss of self-worth, a negative effect on personal relationships, psychological effects (depression), behavior manifestations (nightmares), and even physical symptoms (headache, diarrhea). Some nurses even leave the workplace or nursing altogether because they feel that they "can't fight the system." The ones who are not upset are generally those who hold the same values as the institution and the physician. Moral distress and moral outrage are felt by nurses across the age range. An interesting sidelight is that many nurses see the nurse administrator as an enemy in these situations and feel that they have no support.[28]

There are many specific patient-related ethical issues that may cause the nurse distress, anxiety, or confusion beyond the classic right-to-die/right-to-live issues involving both newborns,[29,30] and at the other end of the life cycle, the chronically ill and the elderly.[31,32] One is the questionable use of invasive technology, which nurses at the bedside 24 hours a day certainly recognize. Yet they often find themselves at a disadvantage in arguing with a physician.[33] The use of mechanical restraints when there is uncertainty about their safety or effectiveness is another.[34] As in a number of other situations, the law is becoming involved in the latter issue, particularly in relation to the elderly. Unfortunately, as described in Chapter 12, a nurse may be sued if a patient is hurt with or without such restraints. At times, it is difficult to untangle ethical and legal responsibilities; indeed, there are times when the law or the legal decision in a case does not seem ethical in itself.

At the End of Life: What is Ethical?

Both nurses and physicians are sometimes unclear as to whether certain of their actions are illegal, even if they themselves believe that the actions are ethical. Sometimes they are also not clear as to whether such actions might be seen as unethical by their own profession or the public. Therefore, they may choose the more conservative path. This is particularly true in so-called right-to-die issues. Vladeck, then head of the Health Care Financing Administration, pointed out that contemporary American hospitals are complex institutions and decisions are rarely made by one person. The problem is not that health care professionals are insensitive, unfeeling, or driven by a "technological imperative," at least not most of them. "Rather, those professionals work—perhaps increasingly—in large complex systems that frustrate their ability to be as sensitive and compassionate as they would like to be."[35]

The confusion and difficulties concerning what is "right" and what is legal was illustrated in a survey of 687 physicians and 759 nurses in 5 hospitals.[36] Most reported that they were aware of guidelines at their institutions about obtaining informed consent, issuing do-not-resuscitate orders, documenting the reasons for such orders, recording patients' wishes, and determining patients' capacity to make decisions. Yet the majority reported substantial dissatisfaction with the way their patients were actually involved in treatment decisions. Attending physicians seemed most satisfied, but nurses expressed great dissatisfaction, with only 25 percent satisfied that patients' wishes were recorded on the patient chart. The concerns of the house officers were much closer to those of the nurses than to those of the attending physician. Almost half of all the providers reported that they had sometimes acted against their conscience in providing care to the terminally ill. Many more were troubled about providing overly burdensome treatment than about undertreatment. Eighty-seven percent of the total sample agreed that "all competent patients, even if they are not considered terminally ill have the right to refuse life support, even if that refusal may lead to death." (This principle of informed consent is discussed in considerable detail in Chapter 9.) A like number agreed that "to allow patients to die by for-going or stopping treatment is ethically different from assisting in their suicide."

Some disparities were clear in relation to specific beliefs. One of the most common was that while it was ethical and legal to withhold treatment, once started it could not be withdrawn. However, both medical and nursing guidelines as well as the opinions of ethicists agree that there is *no ethical difference*. Another involved delineating the difference between "extra-ordinary" and "ordinary" treatment, which the respondents thought was useful in making termination-of-treatment decisions. In fact, major national ethical guidelines argue that treatment should not hinge on whether it is technologically simple or complex but rather on its potential benefits and burdens to the patient as perceived by the patient or surrogate. A sizable portion of the respondents also felt that "even if life supports such as mechanical ventilation and dialysis are stopped, food and water should always be continued." Yet again, most national and legal guidelines agree that decisions about nutritional support and hydration should be governed by the same principles that guide other kinds of life-sustaining treatments. (See Chapter 9.) Nurses and attending physicians were most likely to believe food and water should be continued than house officers. Part of the reason for the hesitation to stop food and fluid may be related to the belief that the patient deprived of fluids and nutrition suffers. Possibly because of this, this issue was studied to determine whether symptoms of hunger and thirst could be palliated without forced feeding or hydration or parenteral alimentation. It was concluded that the patients studied, who were terminally ill with cancer, generally did not experience hunger and needed only small sips of water. The lack of food and fluid did not substantially contribute to their suffering. Caregiver time could better be devoted to providing comfort care.[37] "Aggressive comfort treatment" is seen as ensuring a peaceful death.[38] Nurses in long-term-care facilities (not included in this study) are particularly concerned about the ethical dimension of long-term tube feeding, since they see daily the discomfort patients endure with this treatment.[39]

In relation to pain control, the vast majority of participants in the Solomon study believed "sometimes it is appropriate to give pain medication to relieve the patient's suffering even if it may hasten a patient's death" and that large quantities of narcotic analgesics may be given when the purpose is not to shorten patients' lives but to alleviate their suffering. Yet 44 percent of nurses felt clinicians gave inadequate pain medications because they feared hastening the patient's death; only one-third of all the physicians thought that. Actually both the medical and nursing literature find that inadequate pain management is a major issue in the care of patients, often because of insufficient knowledge about appropriate pain management and poor communication about pain between patients and providers.[40,41] A Canadian study of potentially eligible ICU attending staff, ICU residents, and ICU nurses presents another interesting perspective on withdrawing life support. The most important factors influencing choice of levels of care to be given, from comfort measures to intensive care, were: likelihood of surviving the current episode; likelihood of long-term survival; patient advance directives; premorbid cognitive function; family directives, premorbid physical function; and age.[42]

Some of the issues that seem to be creating confusion can be clarified when the patient makes a "living will," or as it is more commonly called now, an advance directive, which has legal approval in every state. (See Chapter 9.) However, most people, including health care providers, still do not have a living will, so if they are not able to speak for themselves, their unwritten wishes about terminating treatment, whatever that may be, could become a legal case, as the institution or physician attempts to get court permission to give the treatment that *they* think is necessary. It's true that sometimes the care provider or institution fears a lawsuit from family or even the patient, if the patient changes his or her mind; but more often, it is simply that years of medical education have trained physicians more to save lives than to consider the quality of life. Physicians, nurses, judges, and others may also have a moral belief that life is sacred, no matter what kind of life, so that fatally deformed newborns, the very old, and those with illnesses or accidents that are totally devastating to them are victims of someone else's moral beliefs. It's possible that, once more, the sheer visibility of such situations, often through the media, is making people more aware of the problems and forcing them to think through the issue for themselves and their loved ones. This is equally true of health professionals.

The Do-Not-Resuscitate Order

DNR (do-not-resuscitate) means that "in event of cardiac or respiratory failure, no resuscitative efforts should be instituted,"[43] but that does not mean that any other care or interventions should be lessened. Presumably, the DNR order should be a shared decision by the patient or surrogate and the physician, with the patient's decision being the ultimate determinant. The order should be written clearly and promptly by the physician, supported in the progress notes, and reviewed as needed.

While this should be clearly understood, nurses cite DNR as a major problem for them. Why? Physicians and others do not like to speak about negative truths, and after all, DNR implies that death will follow. Some patients and families also avoid the topic, although fewer than health providers think. Therefore, a variety of subterfuges are used.

Unwritten orders are a special problem for the nurse. Some physicians believe, wrongly, that their liability is dispelled by not writing a do not resuscitate (DNR) order, or cloaking the intent with words such as "comfort nursing measures only." Sometimes a *slow code* is understood or carried out by nurses when a terminally ill patient is not put on DNR. This means that they do not hurry to alert the emergency team. Again, the fear is that the doctor or hospital would be sued. Yet this is completely unreasonable, since guidelines published by the American Medical Association, the AHA, the Hastings Center, which deals with ethical issues, and the ANA are clear about what is involved, including the fact that the patient's choices must be given priority (or if the patient is not competent, that of the surrogate); that the DNR must be clearly documented, reviewed, and updated periodically (also a JCAHO requirement); that other necessary care must continue to be given; and that there be mechanisms in place, preferably the ethics committee, for resolution of disputes among health care professionals, patients, and/or families. It is also recommended by ethicists and others that nurses be educated about various advance directives, that they then can educate the family and that they should be involved in developing DNR policies. Nurses who are morally opposed to carrying out DNRs should see about transferring the responsibility for that patient to another nurse.

An important AHA publication makes a similar statement and reiterates that having nurses or other staff solely responsible for making DNR decisions is inappropriate and probably illegal.[44] DNR orders are legally valid, provided that they are in accordance with accepted medical standards. Development of hospital policy on the matter is recommended, including review mechanisms. If there is continuing disagreement about resuscitation, the statement says, the case should be brought to court.

One issue that is receiving considerable attention is the implementation of DNR orders in the operating room. Because CPR was originally developed for the OR, carrying out a DNR order there may present an ethical difficulty. Undergoing surgery may be compatible with having a DNR order when its purpose is the amelioration or palliation of symptoms (for example, treating a pathologic fracture or curing a lesion unrelated to the basic disease). If surgery cannot achieve a beneficial objective, it should not be undertaken. The usual recommendation is that the DNR orders should be suspended during the perioperative period, but reinstated if cardiac arrest occurs during surgery and it is clear that the arrest is due to the underlying condition. Of course, this should be discussed with the patient or surrogate before surgery.[45] Perioperative nurses are urged to review policies related to DNR and to support the surgeon and anesthesia provider in the decisions made in the OR. Again, participation is not required if against the nurse's moral and religious beliefs.[46]

One point that is made consistently is that nurses have a responsibility for reforming deficient DNR policies, putting forth the necessary efforts "to effect improvement in DNR policies and practices in terms of putting the patient first."[47]

Because DNRs are usually intended for direction when an individual is in an institution, problems have arisen when, for instance, an emergency medical team has been called to a home because a person has stopped breathing. It is generally understood that these medics must make an attempt to resuscitate. Therefore, *Choice in Dying* reports that a nonhospital DNR has been developed. A physician must complete a form indicating that the person does not want to be resuscitated. Presumably, that person wears a bracelet or carries some sort of card that gives the DNR information. A few states have enacted laws to provide for nonhospital DNR orders.

Assisted Suicide

An ethical and legal issue that has received considerable public attention in recent years is euthanasia—literally, "good death." The term, which has many meanings,[48] is now related more commonly to *assisted suicide*, when someone either directly kills another (who may want to die), or who assists that person to die. There are many legal ramifications to this, such as an accusation of murder, but from an ethical point of view the question is, "Is it right?" Physicians and others were upset at a published essay written by a "gynecology resident," who related how he helped a suffering young woman with terminal ovarian cancer to die by giving her a large dose of morphine (mentioned earlier in this chapter). Many agreed that it was a merciful thing to do, while others maintained that if a doctor (or nurse) was seen as "killing" patients, based on his or her own judgment, people would be terrified. The topic is, and has been, hotly debated. On the other hand, right or wrong, this kind of situation has happened before, and is still happening, from the highly visible Dr. Kevorkian who is willing to help nonterminal patients to die, to the deaths in hospitals that are reported to be quietly assisted by physicians and nurses (but considered murder if reported). The AHA has estimated that 70 percent of the 6000 deaths that occur in the United States each day are somehow timed or negotiated by patients, families, and doctors, who decide not to do all they can do and to let a dying patient die. There are also other publicized (and many quiet) incidents in which family or friends helped an ill person to commit suicide. Doctors admit that the known elderly suicide rate is twice that of younger groups, and many other deaths may well come from the mixed array of very powerful drugs the elderly have at hand. In fact, many people feel that, under certain circumstances, assisted suicide is morally acceptable. In 1990, after a Kevorkian incident, 53 percent of those polled thought that a doctor should be able to assist a patient who wants to die. More recent polls suggest that this figure is rising. In 1993, *Choice in Dying* queried readers of their newsletter, receiving over 8000 returns. Over 75 percent said physician assistance was acceptable if the person was in severe pain, or dying, or couldn't commit suicide without help.[49] A number of physicians and ethicists disagree.[50]

Nurses in the March ANA survey mentioned previously had mixed opinions about assisted suicide. While 57 percent said that *physician-assisted suicide* should be legalized, 49 percent did not want to see euthanasia legalized. Does that mean that they themselves did not want to participate? The argument that active euthanasia—that is, performing an intervention that directly causes a person's death—is against nursing's code of ethics and morally wrong, is strongly defended,[51,52] but since other nurses clearly disagree, the issue is far from closed. However, in 1995 the ANA released a position statement on assisted suicide. In essence, it stated that there is a continuum of choices that encompass a broad spectrum of interventions for end-of-life care, and nurses can respond with "compassion, faithfulness and support," but not assistance in ending life.[53] Some SNAs agreed; some did not.

Meanwhile, Oregon voters passed the Oregon Death with Dignity Act in November 1994, the first jurisdiction in the world to make physician-assisted suicide legal. (In the Netherlands it is not legal, but is permitted under certain circumstances and with specific restraints.) The Oregon law never went into effect because it was immediately challenged in the courts. In August 1995, a federal court called it unconstitutional; no doubt it will head for the Supreme Court. However, 14 states had, by 1995, introduced similar legislation.[54]

Other Ethical Dilemmas

New technology, scientific discoveries and the enemy, disease, all present ethical dilemmas that nurses must think about, if not deal with. Transplants, a life-saving blessing to many, have raised questions about access and availability which will be discussed in the next section. But there are other concerns. Should organs be "harvested" from irrevocably damaged newborns, specifically anencephalic babies?[55] Recently, the AMA Council on Ethical and Judicial Affairs concluded that such neonates could ethically be considered potential organ donors,[56] but some religious and other groups angrily disagree. There is similar hot disagreement as to whether the tissues of aborted fetuses may be used for research[57] and for transplants, as has been done experimentally to improve the deteriorating condition of patients with Parkinson's disease. The Bush administration forbade it, President Clinton lifted the ban, and a Republican Congress opposed it. Who's right?

Gene research has been greeted with much excitement as genes are being identified with certain clinical disorders, which would enable individuals carrying those genes to decide about the risk of passing them on to descendants. Yet, what if the person chooses not to tell children or family members about their susceptibility? Should the genetic counselor, doctor or nurse do so? What about the patient's right to privacy and protection from coercion?[58] What about gene modification, which could shape future generations? Will this expensive intervention be used to enhance future generations? Does a person have a right to any available technology for purposes of having a healthy child? Ethicists are wary about the consequences of new gene techniques.[59] Indeed, is gene therapy too risky and expensive, whatever its potential good?

AIDS, the modern world's new plague, has brought on new ethical dilemmas. One survey showed that AIDS patients were much more likely to have "do not resuscitate" (DNR) orders than other patients with equally serious diseases. Some health professionals refuse to treat them or even interact with them. Although nurses have been applauded for the quality of personalized care they have given to AIDS patients, a number of studies have shown that the majority of nurses feel that nurses should have a right to refuse to care for AIDS patients, especially if the nurse is pregnant. The majority, also given the choice, would prefer not to care for AIDS patients.[60] However, the reason appears to be fear of infection, not matters of morality or prejudice. This raises the question of whether all patients should be tested for AIDS. Should health professionals be tested? (They think not.) Should they be allowed to care for patients? If so, where? What protection should patients and colleagues have? (Generally, use of universal precautions is considered appropriate and safe.) In addition, the issue of confidentiality is at the forefront. Do families or lovers of AIDS patients have the right to know the patient's diagnosis, if the patient doesn't want them to know?[61] Should all newborns be tested for the HIV virus, and if so, should the mother be told if the test is positive? And, of course, the question of assisted suicide is of major concern to many AIDS infected people.

ACCESS TO CARE: ETHICS AND REALITY

Experts in health care and health policy generally agree that ethical decision making will be of increasing concern in the coming years, and access to health care is already a major problem. Most of these experts may look with pride at the new technology, surgery, and drugs that can prolong life, but they are also forced to look at the cost and, sometimes, simple unavailability. For instance, new technology has made possible heart, liver, and kidney transplants and new drugs that fight against organ rejection, but the organs are not readily available and surgery, aftercare, and drugs may run into the hundreds of thousands of dollars during a lifetime, if there even is an extended lifetime. Some people can afford it; health insurance covers others, at least partially, and still others get the attention of the media or powerful figures and receive donations and priority. What of the person who can do none of this? Should the public, through some sort of governmental funding pay for extraordinary treatment an individual can't afford? Or *is* it extraordinary? Under what circumstances should it be paid? Should age, potential quality of life, possibility of good outcome, ability of the individual and significant others

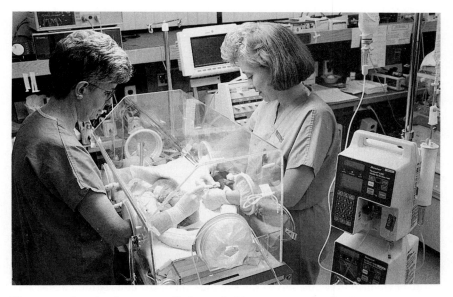

The cost of technology may limit equitable resource distribution. (*Courtesy of Magee-Women's Hospital, Pittsburgh.*)

to give proper follow-through care, or "worthiness" be considered? What of the simple primary care or any care that vast numbers of Americans cannot access? If we say everyone should have equal access in an era of limited resources that will probably never change, what other funding should be cut? Education? Environment? Housing? Social service? Transportation? Civil rights enforcement? Drug enforcement? Police? Defense? Not only is the decision not a simple one, it is highly political. Every one of the other areas that exists primarily through public funding is important one way or another to the public's well-being. Every legislator has one or more constituencies that demand attention to their needs or wishes. Therefore, it's not surprising that legislative action is slow in coming, seldom satisfactory, and, unfortunately, hardly in effect before it is evident that the action taken is not enough, too much, or already out of date. Moreover, the cost factor will undoubtedly increase, not decrease, and new, expensive technology continues to develop.

So what happens? Except in rare instances, limits are set by default. In the case of health care, silent or not so silent, rationing is, and has been, in effect. Unequal access to health care is not a new phenomenon, so its current visibility may be due to the unrelenting voices of advocates for the have-nots, the slight possibility of the public having more of a social conscience, or the simple fact that it is quite evident that there are many who do not receive even basic care, particularly children. Nevertheless visibility does not guarantee solutions. What standards should be used to determine who gets what?

There has been considerable discussion about age as a criterion, especially in terms of prolonging the life of an elderly patient. In part, this is because a large percentage of Medicare funds is used for life-prolonging care in the last few months of an elderly patient's life. The fact that such a person may not wish such care, but is given no choice, is another issue. Moreover, there is some disagreement about whether the long-living "old-old" really are so costly to Medicare; the increased cost, some researchers say, will be due to the increase in absolute numbers of elderly people.[62] Statements by some ethicists and others that, with persons having lived out a natural life, medical care should be limited to relief of suffering,[63] have created a furor, but Callahan, then head of the Hastings Center, argued that the moral problem was to "devise a plan to limit health care for the aged that is fair, humane, and sensitive to the special requirements and dignity of the aged."[64] (No one extended that argument to those who could pay with their own funds.) There were some arguments that probably the majority of the aged preferred such a plan; what they feared was helplessness, pain, disability, and loss of mental alertness—that is, a deteriorating quality of life. Actually, there is some evidence that not only is the suicide rate of the elderly increasing; but also that this kind of rationing is already silently in effect as technology expands.

As noted earlier, the entire issue of transplants is another ethical dilemma, even beyond the issue of access and cost. There are many questions, seldom a clear-cut answer, and never an easy answer. Overall, putting aside legal ramifications, the health care provider simply acts according to his or her own moral beliefs, or sometimes, the needs or attitude of the health care institution. For instance, in a study on how people were selected for kidney transplants, the most important criteria were reported as medical benefit, prognosis, psychological stability, age, and willingness. Also considered were social value, unique moral duties (whether the life of another person or something equally important depends on the patient's survival), and disproportionate resources (whether the patient would require long or expensive treatment and support of patient's family, friends, and community). A large minority would consider ability to pay, and restrictions would be tighter if resources became scarcer. Neither race nor age was reported as a factor.[65] However, other studies of over 6000 kidney transplant patients showed that white men were disproportionately receiving kidneys, twice as likely as Blacks of either sex and a third more likely than white women. A number of explanations were offered, but physician attitude and cost factors were seen as major reasons for the discrepancy. As is often the case, what is said and what is done is not always the same. Reports in 1993 also indicated that blacks and women had fewer heart bypasses, and that the death rate was higher for poor and poorly educated people regardless of race.[66] One study reported that many US residents—most of whom have insurance—are unable to obtain needed care, usually because of high costs.[67] There is also increasing concern about rationing care to the mentally ill,[68,69] as well as the handicapped (who may or may not be protected by the Americans with Disabilities Act).[70]

What to do about these access issues? Many suggestions are made, and little agreement is reached. Some ask, "Can we any longer afford the moral price of inequity in health care?"[71] and maintain that although it might prove costly, a universal system of health insurance and government- and employer-based programs is the only answer. Others say we must set limits on new technology, if too costly.[72] Still others have simply concluded that overt, orderly rationing of health care is inevitable. A consumer poll by the Yankelovich group showed 91 percent felt that *they* should get *maximum* care, but really were not knowledgeable about costs, what contributed to costs, or how maximum care for all could be achieved. In fact, most people now recognize that this would be impossible.

Oregon was probably the first to get federal approval for a plan[73] that involved some rationing of care. With the input of the public as well as health professionals, a priority list of conditions that would be paid for by Medicaid and the state was developed. The purpose was to "insure equitable access, without excessive burdens, to an adequate level of health care for all ..."[74] Needless to say, not everyone agreed; sometimes silent rationing is preferred o overt rationing. The outcome of the plan over the years is being followed closely. Politicians on both the state and national level have indicated that managed care (see Chapter 5) is the answer to high health care costs, but when denying care makes money for the organization and their physicians, ethical questions inevitably arise. The AMA has published guidelines for physicians concerning such conflicts, with the emphasis on placing the interests of the patient first.[75] The strong possibility of some kind of national health care reform will, over the period of its implementation, raise more ethical issues. As one nurse ethicist noted, "The real challenge is to design a reformed health care system that will protect and possibly enhance our most important health values while not ignoring other values important to human dignity and privacy."[76]

Nurses certainly are concerned, as indicated by the two ANA polls mentioned earlier, and nurse executives have indicated that their most pressing ethical concern is allocation of scarce resources, including use of staff inappropriate to levels of patient acuity.[77] Nurses, too, feel that the interests of the patient should come first—all the more reason for participating in legislative decision making (see Chapter 10).

NURSES AS PATIENT ADVOCATES

Over time it appears that, more and more often, nurses themselves, and others, have come to see nurses as natural patient advocates. "Patient advocate" could be an employment position or simply individual action. Just what does it mean to be an advocate on an individual basis, officially or unofficially? In general, it means acting on behalf of a patient/client. It also includes the role of mediator, coordinating services and clarifying communication, trying to resolve conflicting interests of patient and provider. The nurse advocate is also a protector of the patient's right to be actively involved in decision making related to his or her health. This means informing clients adequately so that they can make knowledgeable decisions and supporting their decisions, even if you don't agree. To do this job well, nurses need to understand their role and competing loyalties (the doctor and the employer), be recognized by others as an advocate (including the patient), have sufficient power, and recognize and be willing to deal with the fact that advocacy in a bureaucracy is bound to be controversial.

A serious issue, listed in the June 1994 ANA poll as one of the top four ethical problems confronting nurses in practice, is the "incompetent, unethical, or illegal practices of colleagues." This appears to be reinforced by the kind of ethical problems about which nurses ask for help. In less than a year, ethics columnists in two major journals dealt with concerns that included: unprofessional intimacy with patients by a nurse; a nurse requesting from a nurse friend access to a neighbor's chart (no: tell her to talk with the family); nurses and physicians who appear to be under the influence of some drug (including alcohol); incompetent nurses and physicians (many times); colleagues confessing to testing HIV–AIDS positive and wanting to keep it a secret (assist in getting help; support, but don't report unless endangering others); a nurse who leaves a unit at night to visit with her boyfriend; an administration that requires that all patients being admitted be treated, unnecessarily, with a delousing drug; a manager insisting that a nurse rotate to a unit for which she is not clinically prepared (see nurses' rights); a physician who secretly tapes conversations with patients and colleagues; medical students practicing invasive procedures on a patient who has just died.

Often, the advice was more or less to speak with the individual, and if that were not successful, to report the situation to the appropriate administrative person. If the problem is one caused by a manager or administrator and the situation cannot be resolved, the reality is that the nurse may need to resign if he or she cannot live with it. Obviously, those who pursue resolution with an ethical problem involving colleagues become "whistle-blowers." While this should be seen as the right thing to do, as it is, whistle-blowers in a work setting often have a very difficult time—reviled, ignored, harassed, sometimes fired. The "informal, often invisible coercion of the group" is seen as a serious inhibition to whistle-blowing that the nurse or other employee faces. Whistle-blower is not likely to be an easy role.[78] Sometimes a nurse chooses to leave a position voluntarily because it seems impossible to deal with resolving unethical situations; sometimes he or she, even when not fired, cannot tolerate being mistreated by colleagues for doing what is the right thing, and feels compelled to leave. Not a very encouraging outlook? No, it isn't, but one positive aspect is that there are also places where a bad situation is dealt with ethically and effectively, with an effort made to help the person guilty of unethical behavior, while the patients and others involved are protected from damage by that behavior.

Just such a situation seems to be occurring more often in the case of impaired, or chemically dependent nurses and students. Institutions have set up policies, so that the individual can get treatment and support through employee assistance programs and involvement with the state nurses' associations.[79] Although nurse executives appear to be more willing to help alcohol-dependent nurses than drug-dependent nurses,[80] both state nurses' associations and individual employers have developed plans for helping these nurses, but also for protecting the public from them.[81] Peers of the troubled nurse are being alerted to warning signs of chemical dependency and advised on what to do: don't cover for her, and don't make excuses for her, which prevents her from getting help; report to her supervisor and follow through to get her the appropriate help. A list of resources is available.[82] Nurses surveyed on this issue seemed to agree that they should not turn their backs on colleagues whose performance was deteriorating, for whatever reason, perhaps problems that were family-related or otherwise personal. But "putting patients first is our duty, but being compassionate to colleagues is our honor," seemed to be a common sentiment.[83]

Students also face ethical dilemmas, both in terms of chemical dependency themselves or observed in a fellow student. Similar guidelines for action are applicable to students, and more schools are developing policies.[84] Students may also find themselves in the kinds of clinical situations noted above, but they should be able to turn to their faculty for help. Within the academic setting, one study pinpointed students covering up for the incomplete nursing care by a classmate as a problem. Faculty-proposed actions for some problems cited seemed fairly rigid and rule-bound.[85]

Most nurses work in institutions, and the environment in which they function has a major effect on how ethical dilemmas are perceived and resolved. It has been recommended that in this rapidly changing health care scene, the health care organization (and this clearly means the people) explore the values determining their actions, just as the professionals need to reappraise the ethics governing their practice. "Health care organizations should educate their personnel to perform their tasks in an ethical context, to assure that they use their powers for humane purposes."[86] Nursing is certainly an important part of that effort.

KEY POINTS

1. Ethics requires a degree of decision making beyond morality, which relates to custom, tradition, and religion.
2. Technology, the economy, and changes in attitudes about life and death have helped to create some of the ethical dilemmas in health care.
3. A code of ethics is an essential element in professionalism, but if the practitioners violate it, society may take away their special status and privileges.
4. Nurses can use the ANA Code as guidelines for ethical practice, in conjunction with decision-making models.
5. Other useful ways to learn to deal with ethical concerns are ethics rounds, ethics committees, and self-study to become familiar with the issues.
6. It is important that nurses become knowledgeable about major ethical issues, such as access to care, use of DNR orders, end-of-life decisions, and professionally assisted suicide.
7. As patient advocates, nurses have a responsibility to see that patients

are not endangered by the practice of impaired health professionals or by other unethical behavior of their caretakers.

REFERENCES

1. Aroskar M. The aftermath of the Cruzan decision: Dying in a twilight zone. *Nurs Outlook* 38:256–257, November–December, 1991.
2. Quill T. Death and dignity: A case of individualized decision making. *New Engl J Med* 324:691–694, March 7, 1991.
3. Scanlon C. Survey yields significant results. *Communique* 3:1–3, Winter, 1994.
4. Health care rationing tops list of pressing ethical issues. *Am Nurse* 26:11, March, 1994.
5. Churchill L. Ethical issues of a profession in transition. *Am J Nurs* 77:873, May, 1977.
6. Chally P. Theory derivation in moral development. *Nurs and Health Care* 11:302–306, June, 1990.
7. Gilligan C. *In a Different Voice*. Cambridge, MA: Harvard University Press, 1982.
8. Chally, op cit.
9. Noddings N. *Caring: A Feminine Approach to Ethics and Moral Development*. Berkeley: University of California Press, 1984.
10. Crowley M. The relevance of Noddings' ethics of care to the moral education of nurses. *J Nurs Ed* 33:74–86, February, 1994.
11. Peter E, Gallop R. The ethic of care: A comparison of nursing and medical students. *Image* 26:47–51, Spring, 1994.
12. Gournic J. Responses of clinical nurses about what is moral in nursing. *Nurs Connections* 7:33–37, Winter, 1994.
13. Revising the United States Senate code of ethics. *Special Supplement, Hastings Center Rep* 11:1–28, February, 1981.
14. Kelly L, Joel L. *Dimensions of Professional Nursing*, 7th ed. New York: McGraw-Hill, 1995.
15. Baggs J. Collaborative interdisciplinary bioethical decision-making in intensive care units. *Nurs Outlook* 41:108–112, May–June, 1993.
16. Thompson J, Thompson H. *Bioethical Decision Making for Nurses*. Norwalk, CT: Appleton–Century–Crofts, 1985.
17. Curtin L, Flaherty MJ (eds). *Nursing Ethics: Theories and Pragmatics*. Bowie, MD: Robert J. Brady Co., 1982, p 39.
18. Thompson, op cit.
19. Fry S. *Ethics in Nursing Practice: A Guide to Ethical Decision Making*. Geneva, Switzerland: International Council of Nurses, 1994.

20. Bosek M. What does an ethics consultant do? *Med Surg Nurs* 4:55–57, February, 1995.

21. Zink M, Titus L. Nursing ethics committees—where are they? *Nurs Mgmt* 25:70–76, June, 1994.

22. Haddad A. Developing an organizational ethos. *Caring* 5:10, June, 1992.

23. President's Commission for the Study of Ethical Problems in Medicine and Biomedical and Behavioral Research. *Deciding to Forgo Life-Sustaining Treatment.* Washington, DC: the Commission, 1983, pp 160–161.

24. Ibid, pp 162–168.

25. Blake D. The hospital ethics committee: Health care's moral conscience or white elephant? *Hastings Center Rep* 22:6–11, January–February, 1992.

26. Fry-Revere S. Ethics consultation: An update on accountability issues. *Pediatr Nurs* 20:95–98, January–February, 1994.

27. Davis AJ. Professional obligations, personal values in conflict. *Am Nurse* 22:7, May, 1990.

28. Wilkenson JM. Moral distress in nursing practice: Experience and effect. *Nurs Forum*, 23(1):17–29, 1987/1988.

29. Erlen J. Ethical dilemmas in the high-risk nursery; wilderness experiences. *J Pediatr Nurs* 9:21–25, February, 1994.

30. Pearson C. Facing ethical dilemmas in the neonatal intensive care unit. *J Pediatr Nurs* 9:131–132, April, 1994.

31. Carter M. Ethical framework for care of the chronically ill. *Holistic Nurs Pract* 8:67–77, October, 1993.

32. Wilson VC. How can we dignify death in the ICU? *Am J Nurs* 90:38–42, May, 1990.

33. Pauly-O'Neill S. Questioning the use of invasive technology. *Am J Nurs* 91:19–20, January, 1991.

34. Moss RJ, La Puma J. The ethics of mechanical restraints. *Hastings Center Rep* 21:22–24, January–February, 1991.

35. Vladeck B. Editorial: Beliefs versus behavior in healthcare decision making. *Am J Public Health* 83:13, January, 1993.

36. Solomon M, et al. Decisions near the end of life: Professional views on life-sustaining treatments. *Am J Public Health* 83:14–23, January, 1993.

37. McCann R, et al. Comfort care for terminally ill patients: The appropriate use of nutrition and hydration. *JAMA* 272:1263–1266, October 26, 1994.

38. Murphy P, Price D. "ACT": Taking a positive approach to end-of-life care. *Am J Nurs* 95:42–43, March, 1995.

39. Wilson D. Ethical concerns in a long-term tube feeding study. *Image* 24:195–199, Fall, 1992.

40. Mitchell J. Administering mercy: The ethics of pain management. *Cancer Invest* 12:343–349, May–June, 1994.
41. Henkelman W. Inadequate pain management: Ethical considerations. *Nurs Mgmt* 25:48A–48D, January, 1994.
42. Cook D, et al. Determinants in Canadian health care workers of the decision to withdraw life support from the critically ill. *JAMA* 273:703–708, March 1, 1995.
43. Price D, Murphy P. DNR: Still crazy after all these years. *J Nurs Law* 1:1, Spring, 1994.
44. Read W. *Hospital's Role in Resuscitation Decisions.* Chicago: Hospital Research and Educational Fund, 1983.
45. Cohen C, Cohen P. Do-not-resuscitate orders in the operating room. *New Engl J Med* 325:1879–1882, December 21, 1991.
46. The do-not-resuscitate order: Moral responsibilities of the perioperative nurse. *AORN J* 59:641–650, March, 1994.
47. Price, Murphy, op cit, p 5.
48. Curtin L. Euthanasia: a clarification. *Nurs Mgmt* 26:64–67, June, 1995.
49. How do Choice in Dying members stand in the debate over assisted suicide? *Choices* 4:1, Summer, 1995.
50. Almost all the articles in the March–April 1992 and May–June 1995 issues of the *Hastings Center Report* are on professionally assisted suicide.
51. Kowalski S. Assisted suicide: Where do nurses draw the line? *Nurs Health Care* 14:70–76, February, 1993.
52. Valko N. The ethics of death: selling euthanasia to nurses and doctors. *Revolution* 5:47–49, Summer, 1995.
53. Curtin L. Nurses take a stand on assisted suicide. *Nurs Mgmt* 26:71–76, May, 1995.
54. The uncharted waters of Oregon's assisted suicide law. *Choices* 4:1, 6–7, Summer, 1995.
55. Fry S. Brave new world: Removing body parts from infants. *Nurs Outlook* 38:152, May–June, 1990.
56. Council on Ethical and Judicial affairs: AMA. The use of anencephalic neonates as organ donors. *JAMA* 273:1614–1617, May 24/31, 1995.
57. Robertson J. Symbolic issues in embryo research. *Hastings Center Rep* 25:37–38, January–February, 1995.
58. Williams J, Halsey D. Applying new genetic technologies: assessment and ethical considerations. *Nurse Pract* 20:16–26, July, 1995.
59. Kolata G. Gene technique could shape future generations. *New York Times* November 22, 1994, pp A1, C10.
60. Wiley K, et al. Care of HIV-infected patients: Nurses' concerns, opinions, and precautions. *Appl Nurs Res* 3:27–33, February, 1990.

61. Laufman J. AIDS, ethics and the truth. *Am J Nurs* 89:924–925, July, 1989.

62. Lubitz J, et al. Longevity and medical care expenditures. *New Engl J Med* 332:999–1003, April 13, 1995.

63. Callahan D. Terminating treatment: Age as a standard. *Hastings Center Rep* 17:21–25, October–November, 1987.

64. Callahan D. *Setting Limits: Medical Goals in an Aging Society.* New York: Simon & Schuster, 1987.

65. Kilner J. Selecting patients when resources are limited: A study of US medical directors of kidney dialysis and transplantation facilities. *Am J Pub Health* 78:144–147, February, 1988.

66. Blakeslee S. Studies find unequal access to kidney transplants. *New York Times*, January 24, 1989, pp C1, C9.

67. Himmelstein D, Woolhandler S. Care denied: US residents who are unable to obtain needed medical services. *Am J Pub Health* 85:341–344, March, 1995.

68. Minds and Hearts: Priorities in Mental Health Services. Special supplement of articles, *Hastings Center Rep*, September–October, 1993.

69. Olsen E, et al. *Controversies in Ethics in Long-Term Care.* New York: Springer, 1995.

70. Orentlicker D. Rationing and the Americans with Disabilities Act. *JAMA* 271:308–314, January 26, 1994.

71. Bayer R, et al. Toward justice in health care. *Am J Pub Health* 78:583–588, May, 1988.

72. Callahan D. Rationing medical progress. *New Engl J Med* 322:1810–1813, June 21, 1990.

73. Rooks J. Let's admit we ration health care—then set priorities. *Am J Nurs* 90:38–43, June, 1990.

74. Capuzzi C, Garland M. The Oregon plan: Increasing access to health care. *Nurs Outlook* 38:260–263, 286, November–December, 1990.

75. Council on Ethical and Judicial Affairs: AMA. Ethical issues in managed care. *JAMA* 273:330–335, January 25, 1995.

76. Fry S. Ethical implications of health care reform. *Am Nurs* 26:25, March, 1994.

77. Silva M. Nurse executives' responses to ethical concerns and policy formulation for allocation of scarce resources. *Nurs Connect* 7:59–64, Spring, 1994.

78. Curtin L. Damage control and the whistle-blower. *Nurs Mgmt* 24:33–34, May, 1993.

79. Peery B, Rimler G. Chemical dependency among nurses: Are policies adequate? *Nurs Mgmt* 26:52–56, May, 1995.

80. Hughes T. Chief nurse executives' response to chemically dependent nurses, *Nurs Mgmt* 26:37–40, March, 1995.
81. Miller H. Addiction in a coworker—getting past the denial. *Am J Nurs* 90:72–75, May, 1990.
82. Hughes T, Smith L. Is your colleague chemically dependent? *Am J Nurs* 94:31–35, September, 1994.
83. Haddad A. Acute care decisions: Ethics in action. *RN* 57:22–25, May, 1994.
84. Polk D, et al. The chemically dependent student: Guidelines for policy development. *Nurs Outlook* 41:166–170, July–August, 1993.
85. Schmitz K, Schaffer M. Ethical problems encountered in the teaching of nursing: student and faculty perceptions. *J Nurs Ed* 34:42–44, January, 1995.
86. Reiser S. The ethical life of health care organizations. *Hastings Center Rep* 24:28–35, November–December, 1994.

9

Patients' Rights;
Students' Rights

OBJECTIVES

After you have studied this chapter, you will be able to:

1. Identify trends in patients' rights.
2. List the elements of informed consent.
3. Describe the nurse's responsibilities in informed consent.
4. Explain briefly the major legal actions that have affected the patient's right to die.
5. Discuss how a living will or advance directive can be used.
6. Explain the role of the nurse in protecting a patient's legal rights when research is being carried out.
7. Give two examples of legal problems related to reproduction.
8. Explain what specific kinds of acts can bring about legal action for battery or assault.
9. Describe the rights of students in relation to theory and practice grades and due process.

The growing strength of the consumer movement is having an increasing effect on the health care delivery system. Once health professionals, and especially physicians, were considered unquestionable experts, and patients put themselves in those "expert" hands, grateful if they got minimal information. People were admitted to the hospital after signing general releases and permits for treatment without even reading them because "the doctor knows best." They gave up even basic rights to human dignity and control over their bodies. They may have grumbled quietly but most often did not confront the staff, sometimes because of fear of reprisals. Perhaps their only way to fight back was to file malpractice suits when things went wrong.

However, as people learned more about health and illness, and consumer activists not only told them what their basic rights were but demanded more, the picture changed. *Malpractice*, a 1973 governmental commission report on medical malpractice, was among the first official reports to state bluntly that much of the malpractice crisis of the time was due to violation of patients' rights. In 1982, the President's Commission for the Study of Ethical Problems in Medicine and Biomedical and Behavioral Research (hereafter called the President's Commission) made equally strong statements and recommendations about respecting patients' rights.[1] Anyone following the appellate court decisions could also see the trend toward supporting patients' rights, although various individual decisions seem to flow against that tide.

Obviously, nurses are very much involved in situations concerning patients' rights. Nurses are at the bedside all the time or in the home. They are the ones who must deal with the patient and family in often emotional, always difficult, situations that may indeed be matters of life and death. Patients and families often look to nurses for advice and support. Nurses, besides being concerned about behaving ethically, must now also be aware of the legal implications of their actions. They must know what they can and can't do. Unfortunately, as in other legal situations, the answers are often far from clear. This chapter will highlight the major legal dilemmas with which nurses must deal in relation to people's rights in health care. The rights of students are also included, but the rights of RNs are discussed in Chapter 15 in the context of the workplace.

PATIENTS' RIGHTS

Most of the rights about which patients worry are their legal as well as moral rights and have been so established by common law. They are also stated in the codes of ethics of both physicians and nurses (although, to be honest, much is stated by implication and so is open to considerable interpretation). Moreover, they closely resemble the four basic consumer rights President John F. Kennedy listed in his message to Congress in 1962:

1. The right to safety.
2. The right to be informed.
3. The right to choose.
4. The right to be heard.

Since the well-publicized AHA's "Patient's Bill of Rights" was presented in 1972, many rights statements have followed for the disabled, the mentally ill, the retarded, the old, the young, the pregnant, the handicapped, and the dying. The AHA statement was revised in 1992 (Exhibit 9.1).

In some cases, these statements have been the basis for new statutory law. By the end of the 1970s, variations of the Patient's Bill of Rights had become law in many states. Some legislatures passed specific laws incorporating either the AHA statement or a similar version; state or municipal hospital codes were changed in somewhat the same manner, sometimes including mental institutions and nursing homes. In 1974, new Medicare regulations for skilled nursing facilities included a section on patients' rights. And, as with other laws, patients must be told what their rights are.

Since that time, the continuing scandals involving violation of patients' and residents' rights in so many LTC facilities have resulted in legislation in various guises, usually requirements under Medicare and Medicaid. For the LTC facilities not certified, there is still some control by state regulation. The regulations on rights are enacted and enforced erratically, sometimes depending on the political climate. However, nursing home residents now have the right to talk directly to state surveyors, who ensure that the facilities meet the standards set by the Health Care Financing Administration (HCFA), which include rights statements. Nursing homes also may have a volunteer ombudsman, and teaching nursing homes have students and faculty who observe what goes on. However, such facilities are not usually problem sites. Some states have also given legal attention to the rights of residents in continuing care communities, including such aspects as complete disclosure of costs and other financial data, posting of the last state examination report, freedom to form a residents' organization, and other mechanisms to avoid fraud and deception.

Many rights advocates have little enthusiasm for most of these declarations, as they tend to hedge about some rights, voluntary or legal. This is probably because few if any evolved out of some massive "goodness of heart" by the institutions or by government, but rather through consumer pressure. Nevertheless, the revised AHA statement shows progress.

Some statements are better than others, but Annas's Model Patient Bill of Rights, aimed at all facilities, is indeed a model, covering many of the loopholes in the various institutions' statements. Recognizing that most people are in health care facilities because they have a health problem and therefore are probably not as aggressive about ensuring their rights as they might otherwise be, the final statement in the model recognizes the right to all patients to have 24-hour-a-day access to a patients' rights advocate to assert or protect the rights set out in this document.[2]

It would seem that consumer action has had some ongoing effect on patients' rights. Annas says that the patients' rights movement is "as slow as a glacier, equally relentless in changing the landscape, but ultimately healthy.[3] In addition to the organizations built around specific populations and diseases (children, AIDS), there is a very visible national patient rights

EXHIBIT 9.1

A Patient's Bill of Rights

Introduction

Effective health care requires collaboration between patients and physicians and other health care professionals. Open and honest communication, respect for personal and professional values, and sensitivity to differences are integral to optimal patient care. As the setting for the provision of health services, hospitals must provide a foundation for understanding and respecting the rights and responsibilities of patients, their families, physicians, and other caregivers. Hospitals must ensure a health care ethic that respects the role of patients in decision making about treatment choices and other aspects of their care. Hospitals must be sensitive to cultural, racial, linguistic, religious, age, gender, and other differences as well as the needs of persons with disabilities.

The American Hospital Association presents *A Patient's Bill of Rights* with the expectation that it will contribute to more effective patient care and be supported by the hospital on behalf of the institution, its medical staff, employees, and patients. The American Hospital Association encourages health care institutions to tailor this bill of rights to their patient community by translating and/or simplifying the language of this bill of rights as may be necessary to ensure that patients and their families understand their rights and responsibilities.

Bill of Rights*

1. The patient has the right to considerate and respectful care.
2. The patient has the right to and is encouraged to obtain from physicians and other direct caregivers relevant, current, and understandable information concerning diagnosis, treatment, and prognosis.

   Except in emergencies when the patient lacks decision-making capacity and the need for treatment is urgent, the patient is entitled to the opportunity to discuss and request information related to the specific procedures and/or treatments, the risks involved, the possible length of recuperation, and the medically reasonable alternatives and their accompanying risks and benefits.

   Patients have the right to know the identity of physicians, nurses, and others involved in their care, as well as when those

* These rights can be exercised on the patient's behalf by a designated surrogate or proxy decision maker if the patient lacks decision-making capacity, is legally incompetent, or is a minor.

(continued)

involved are students, residents, or other trainees. The patient also has the right to know the immediate and long-term financial implications of treatment choices, insofar as they are known.

3. The patient has the right to make decisions about the plan of care prior to and during the course of treatment and to refuse a recommended treatment or plan of care to the extent permitted by law and hospital policy and to be informed of the medical consequences of this action. In case of such refusal, the patient is entitled to other appropriate care and services that the hospital provides or transfer to another hospital. The hospital should notify patients of any policy that might affect patient choice within the institution.

4. The patient has the right to have an advance directive (such as a living will, health care proxy, or durable power of attorney for health care) concerning treatment or designating a surrogate decision maker with the expectation that the hospital will honor the intent of that directive to the extent permitted by law and hospital policy.

   Health care institutions must advise patients of their rights under state law and hospital policy to make informed medical choices, ask if the patient has an advance directive, and include that information in patient records. The patient has the right to timely information about hospital policy that may limit its ability to implement fully a legally valid advance directive.

5. The patient has the right to every consideration of his privacy. Case discussion, consultation, examination, and treatment should be conducted so as to protect each patient's privacy.

6. The patient has the right to expect that all communications and records pertaining to his/her care should be treated as confidential by the hospital, except in cases such as suspected abuse and public health hazards when reporting is permitted or required by law. The patient has the right to expect that the hospital will emphasize the confidentiality of this information when it releases it to any other parties entitled to review information in these records.

7. The patient has the right to review the records pertaining to his/her medical care and to have the information explained or interpreted as necessary, except when restricted by law.

8. The patient has the right to expect that, within its capacity and policies, a hospital will make resonable response to the request of a patient for appropriate and medically indicated care and services. The hospital must provide evaluation, service, and/or referral as indicated by the urgency of the case. When medically appropriate and legally permissible, or when a patient has so requested, a patient may be transferred to another facility. The

institution to which the patient is to be transferred must first have accepted the patient for transfer. The patient must also have the benefit of complete information and explanation concerning the need for, risks, benefits, and alternatives to such a transfer.

9. The patient has the right to ask and be informed of the existence of business relationships among the hospital, educational institutions, other health care providers, or payers that may influence the patient's treatment and care.

10. The patient has the right to consent to or decline to participate in proposed research studies or human experimentation affecting his care and treatment or requiring direct patient involvement, and to have those studies fully explained prior to consent. A patient who declines to participate in research or experimentation is entitled to the most effective care that the hospital can otherwise provide.

11. The patient has the right to expect reasonable continuity of care when appropriate and to be informed by physicians and other caregivers of available and realistic patient care options when hospital care is no longer appropriate.

12. The patient has the right to be informed of hospital policies and practices that relate to patient care, treatment, and responsibilities. The patient has the right to be informed of available resources for resolving disputes, grievances, and conflicts, such as ethics committees, patient representatives, or other mechanisms available in the institution. The patient has the right to be informed of the hospital's charges for services and available payment methods.

The collaborative nature of health care requires that patients, or their families/surrogates, participate in their care. The effectiveness of care and patient satisfaction with the course of treatment depend, in part, on the patient fulfilling certain responsibilities. Patients are responsible for providing information about past illnesses, hospitalizations, medications, and other matters related to health status. To participate effectively in decision making, patients must be encouraged to take responsibility for requesting additional information or clarification about their health status or treatment when they do not fully understand information and instructions. Patients are also responsible for ensuring that the health care institution has a copy of their written advance directive if they have one. Patients are responsible for informing their physicians and other caregivers if they anticipate problems in following prescribed treatment.

Patients should also be aware of the hospital's obligation to be reasonably efficient and equitable in providing care to other patients and the community. The hospital's rules and regulations are designed to help

(continued)

the hospital meet this obligation. Patients and their families are responsible for making reasonable accommodations to the needs of the hospital, other patients, medical staff, and hospital employees. Patients are responsible for providing necessary information for insurance claims and for working with the hospital to make payment arrangements, when necessary.

A person's health depends on much more than health care services. Patients are responsible for recognizing the impact of their lifestyle on their personal health.

Conclusion

Hospitals have many functions to perform, including the enhancement of health status, health promotion, and the prevention and treatment of injury and disease; the immediate and ongoing care and rehabilitation of patients; the education of health professionals, patients, and the community; and research. All these activities must be conducted with an overriding concern for the values and dignity of patients.

A Patient's Bill of Rights was first adopted by the American Hospital Association in 1973. This revision was approved by the AHA Board of Trustees on October 21, 1992.
Source: © 1992 by the American Hospital Association, 840 North Lake Shore Drive, Chicago, IL 60611. Printed in the USA. All rights reserved. Catalog no. 157759. Reprinted with permission.

organization: The People's Medical Society. These groups generally provide excellent information. A list of addresses is found in Annas's *The Rights of Patients.*

INFORMED CONSENT

For years, when patients were admitted to hospitals, they signed a frequently unread, universal consent form that almost literally gave the physician, his or her associates, and the hospital a free hand in the patient's care. There was some rationale for this because civil suits for battery (unlawful touching) could theoretically be filed as a result of giving routine care such as baths. Patients undergoing surgery or a complex, dangerous treatment were asked to sign a separate form, usually stating something to the effect that permission was granted to the physician and/or his or her colleagues to perform the operation or treatment. Just how much the patient knew about the hows and whys of the surgery, the dangers, and the alternatives, depended on the patient's assertiveness in asking questions and demanding answers and the physician's willingness to provide information. Nurses were taught *never* to answer those questions, or few others, but to suggest, "Ask your doctor." Health professionals, especially physicians, took the attitude that "We know best and will decide for you."

Many patients probably still enter treatment and undergo a variety of tests and even surgery without a clear understanding of the nature of their condition and what can be done about it. Although they may be receiving care that is medically acceptable, they have no real part in deciding what that care should be. Most physicians have believed that anything more than a superficial explanation is unnecessary, for the patient should trust the doctor. Yet patients have always had the right to make decisions about their own bodies. A case was heard as early as 1905 on surgery without consent, and the classic legal decision is that of Judge Benjamin Cardozo (*Schloendorff v. The Society of New York Hospital*, 211 NY. 125, 129–130, 105 NE 92, 93–1914): "Every human being of adult years and sound mind has a right to determine what shall be done with his own body." This principle still stands, and treatment without consent is technically assault and battery.

Annas emphasizes this as he explains that in nonlegal terms, informed consent simply means that a doctor cannot "touch or treat a patient until the doctor has given the patient some basic information about what the doctor proposes to do, and the patient has agreed to the proposed treatment or procedure."[4] In what is still considered the most important study of informed consent, the President's Commission concluded that "ethically valid consent is a process of shared decision-making based upon mutual respect and participation, not a ritual to be equated with reciting the contents of a form that details the risks of particular treatments."[5] For this reason, some lawyers are advocating the use of the term *authorization for treatment*, implying patient control.

The patient's need for and right to this kind of knowledge is highlighted by the increasing number of malpractice suits that involve an element of informed consent. For many years, in such suits, courts have tended to rule that the physician must provide only as much information as is general practice among professional colleagues in the area, as determined by their expert testimony. However, courts are changing this attitude and emphasizing the need for *informed* consent. In 1995, for instance, the Court of Appeals of Washington ruled for the family of a patient who died during a biopsy done in a doctor's office. The physician knew that the patient had seizures, but did not tell her that she could have the procedure done at a hospital or clinic with backup resources, which would be safer in her situation. Therefore the signed consent form was not considered to be based on "informed" consent.[6]

Principles of Informed Consent

Consent is defined as a free, rational act that presupposes knowledge of the thing to which consent is given by a person who is legally capable of consent. *Informed consent* is not expected to include the tiniest details but to give the essential nature of the procedure and the consequences. The disclosure is to be "reasonable." The patient may, of course, waive the right to such explanation or any teaching. Consent is *not* needed for emergency care if there is an immediate threat to life and health, if experts agree that it is an emergency, if the patient is unable to consent and a legally authorized person can't be reached, and when the patient submits voluntarily.

Criteria for a valid consent are as follows: It must be written (unless oral consent can be proved in court); it must be signed by the patient or person legally responsible for him or her (a person cannot give consent for a spouse in a nonemergency situation); the procedure performed must be the one consented to; the essential elements of an informed consent must be present, including (a) an explanation of the condition; (b) a fair explanation of the procedures to be used and the consequences; (c) a description of alternative treatments or procedures; (d) a description of the benefits to be expected; (e) an offer to answer the patient's inquiries; and (f) freedom from coercion or unfair persuasions and inducements. The courts have ruled that explanations should be clear enough for the patient to make an "informed" decision, using language a lay person can understand. The relative importance of risks and facts to be disclosed should be judged on the basis of the understanding of a "reasonable man," not a reasonable medical practitioner. That the issue of informed consent crosses international borders was shown in the case of getting informed consent for chemotherapy, with criticism of Australian physicians because they did not give complete enough information about the pros and cons of this therapy. The patient should recognize that "It's OK to say no."[7]

Who Makes the Decision?

The competent patient (someone physically and mentally capable of making a choice) has the right to refuse consent, but a hospital can request, under certain circumstances, a court order to act if the refusal endangers the patient's life. If a patient is considered physically unable, legally incompetent, or a minor, a guardian has the right to give or withhold consent. The trend in court decisions seems to be that the patient, unless proven totally incompetent, has the right to refuse. For example, a Jehovah's Witness may be allowed to refuse a blood transfusion, even though it might mean his or her life, because taking such transfusions are against his or her religious beliefs.[8] In fact, the Witnesses and AMA in 1979 agreed upon a consent form requesting that no blood or blood derivative be administered and releasing medical personnel and the hospital for responsibility for untoward results because of that refusal. (This particular problem has been lessened to some extent as better blood substitutes have become available.) However, in 1990, a Jehovah's Witness sued a major medical center and five physicians because he was given blood after a serious automobile accident. Although he was unconscious and it was an emergency situation, he claimed that his rights were violated.

If a minor child of a Witness needs the blood and the parent refuses, a court order requested by the hospital usually permits the transfusion. This is based on a 1944 legal precedent when the Supreme Court ruled that parents had a right to be martyrs, if they wished, but had no right to make martyrs of their children.[9] On the other hand, if the child is deemed a "mature minor," able to make an intelligent decision, regardless of chronological age, the child is allowed to refuse the treatment. The rights of minors are discussed in some detail later.

In another type of case, a 79-year-old diabetic refused to consent to a leg amputation. Her daughter petitioned to be her legal guardian so that she (the daughter) could sign the consent. The judge ruled that the woman was old but not senile and had a right to make her own decision. In still another case, a young man on permanent kidney dialysis decided that he did not want to live that way and refused continued treatment. He was allowed to do so and died within a short time.

Other cases can also be cited. The right of a competent patient to refuse treatment seems more firmly established than ever, but when the patient is unconscious or in certain other situations, difficult legal questions arise. The question of assessing patient competence, particularly in the elderly, is being raised more frequently. Can a psychiatrist determine whether a patient is competent more accurately than the patient's primary case physician? Since senile dementia is estimated to affect from 25 to 47 percent of people above age 84, having proxy decision makers becomes more common, and whether their decision about a patient's treatment is what the patient would want may be in question, if the patient floats in and out of periods of intellectual functioning.[10]

Is Informed Consent Practical?

Some physicians do not believe that it is possible to obtain an informed consent because of such factors as lack of interest or education and high anxiety level, in which case a patient might refuse a "necessary" treatment or operation. On the other hand, the physician may invoke "therapeutic privilege," in which disclosure is not required because it might be detrimental to the patient.[11] Just what that means is not clear. Or information about certain alternatives may be withheld because the physician feels that they are too risky, unproven, or not appropriate. Although reasonable people would allow for *some* use of therapeutic privilege, this is seen as being rare enough to occur only once or twice in a career. There are physicians and

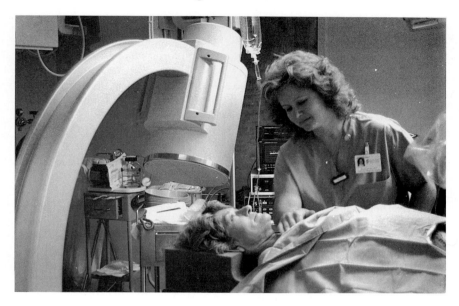

Ultimately it is the patient's right to choose whether or not to submit to diagnostic and therapeutic procedures. (*Courtesy of Somerset Medical Center, Somerville, New Jersey.*)

others who believe that despite the increasing number of rulings favoring patients' right to full knowledge, most patients are not given information in such a way that they really understand it (and the courts don't do enough about this problem). Surveys indicate that people *do* want full information even when they trust their doctor completely and will probably go along with his or her recommendations. They may not always remember the details later, but with a full explanation, given in lay terms, and with enough time for questions and answers, they can understand. However, many patients are still reluctant to ask for fear of appearing stupid or "bothering the doctor."

Ethicists have debated what alternatives for informed consent would be better. Presenting a list of plausible treatment options and letting the patients make a choice? Allowing a patient to choose a cadre of "well-being" experts with his/her "deep" values to make the decision? In all cases, the idea is to increase the patient's active, knowledgeable participation.[12]

The written consent form that is generally accepted as the legal affirmation that the patient has agreed to a particular test or treatment has undergone a number of changes in the last few years. The catchall admissions consent has already been ruled to be almost completely worthless for anything other than avoiding battery complaints, because it does not designate the nature of the treatment to be given. What has emerged are forms that contain all the required elements for the informed consent process, usually individualized by the physician of each patient and often in an appropriate foreign language. Although many people think of informed consent only in terms of hospitalization, there are already some court cases that indicate that the concept embraces the continuum of health care, such as a clinic or doctor's office. An interesting aspect of one of these cases was that the physician was held to have breached his duty by failing to inform the patient of the risk of *not* consenting to a diagnostic procedure, in this case a Pap smear. The patient died of advanced cervical cancer.[13]

The Nurse's Role in Informed Consent

What is the nurse's role in informed consent? To provide or add information before or after the doctor's explanation has been given? To refer the patient to the doctor? To avoid any participation? The advice given varies. Some suggest that getting involved in informed consent is simply not the nurse's business and is best left to the doctor; others consider it a professional responsibility.

It is generally agreed that nurses do not have the primary responsibility for getting informed consent. However, the President's Commission noted that "nurses as a practical matter typically have a central role in the process of providing patients with information,"[14] and that NPs, including nurse-midwives, have *full* responsibility for informing patients about their conditions, tests, and treatment, and obtaining consent. There was also at least one serious court case in which a patient sued because the physician *and* nurses withheld information about his condition. Both were held liable.[15] Nevertheless, the question asked by most nurses is how much can be told, especially if the physician chooses not to reveal further information. The Tuma case (Chapter 11) did not resolve the nurse's right to supply the missing information, and the nurse may be taking a personal risk. Greenlaw suggests that patients' questions may range over a variety of topics, including what you are doing to the patient and your qualifications (if so, answer honestly) to interpretation of what the doctor said (explain in lay terms) to "What's wrong with me?" (don't answer directly) or "Is my doctor any good?" (tell patients that they have a right to ask their doctor for his or her qualifications and experience or to get a second opinion).[16]

A variety of other opinions are offered, but a point that is always made is that the patient's lack of information should always be discussed with the doctor (tactfully) and, if there is no response, with administrative superiors. There is nothing wrong with questioning the patient to see what he or she really understands and clarifying points, providing that you know what you are talking about. If you decide to give further information, it should be totally accurate and carefully recorded, and the fact that it was given should be shared with the physician and others. Nurses have found ways to make the patient aware of knowledge gaps so that they ask the right questions, but it's unfortunate that many are still employed in situations in which it could be detrimental to them to be the patient's advocate.

Of course, if the patient is coaxed or coerced into signing without such an explanation, the consent is invalid. Moreover, if the patient withdraws consent, even verbally, the nurse is responsible for reporting this and ensuring that the patient is not treated. This is a legal responsibility not only to the patient but also to the hospital, which can be held liable. In one case, a competent patient refused intubation and, although persuaded by nurses to agree, the delay caused her to die of lack of oxygen. The family sued for wrongful death and won initially, but on appeal, a court held that if a competent patient had refused treatment, the physician could not be held responsible for her death.[17]

Hospitals are beginning to use a clerk to witness the consent form, after the physician provides an explanation, on the theory that only the signature is being witnessed, not the accuracy or depth of the explanation. Other hospitals ask the physician to bring another physician, presumably to validate the explanation. Where nurses still witness the form, it should be clear *what* they are witnessing—the signature or the explanation. Hospital policy can clarify this situation. Usually, nurses' chances of liability in such acts are considered to be minimal.[18]

It has been suggested that the nurse's role in informed consent is threefold: to perform a patient assessment, i.e. to evaluate the patient's readiness to understand and respond intelligently to the consent form; to determine the best approach to obtain informed consent (time, environment, presence of a supportive person); patient and staff follow-up (reaffirmation that the patient understood), supporting the patient's decision, reinforcement of information, apprising staff and physician of the patient's understanding.[19]

The nurse's specific responsibility is to explain nursing care, including the whys and hows. An interesting idea to think about is whether you should tell patients about the risks of the *nursing* procedures you do, even though this is not a legal requirement. (Nor does it prevent you from doing so.) The answer seems to be maybe, but carefully.[20] However, as also noted in the President's Commission report, nurses who *independently* perform treatments that might put the patient at risk (NPs, nurse-midwives, nurse anesthetists) *are* responsible for giving appropriate information to patients and getting consent.[21]

THE RIGHT TO DIE

Perhaps because improved technology has succeeded in artifically maintaining both respiratory and cardiac functions when a person can no longer do so, the definition of *clinical death* as the irrevocable cessation of heartbeat and breathing is no longer pertinent. In 1968, faculty of the Harvard Medical School identified certain characteristics of a permanently nonfunctioning brain. In the years since, all states have passed legislation using variations of those criteria to define *brain death*. Translated into statutory language, the concept is typically expressed as follows:

> An individual who has sustained either (1) irreversible cessation of circulatory and respiratory functions, or (2) irreversible cessation of all functions of the entire brain, including the brain stem, is dead. A determination of death must be made in accordance with accepted medical standards.[22]

Experts say that the use of the term "brain death" has been unfortunate. It has perpetuated the mistaken notion that there are two *kinds* of death, brain death and real death. The more accurate term and the one less likely to confuse both professionals and the general public is "death as determined by neurological criteria." Such semantic precision is important. Twenty-five years after the concept was developed, otherwise careful nurses and physicians still betray their confusion by such inappropriate behavior as labeling as "brain dead" patients who are comatose or by hesitating to remove life support from patients who are certifiably dead.

The determination of death by neurological criteria is a common diagnosis only in specialized units, particularly trauma centers. In such settings, staff members are clear that "dead is dead." They recognize that the diagnosis, though painstaking and time-consuming, is rarely difficult. They speak to family members in terms of "death" as they continue to test for signs of brainstem responsiveness. Finally, when they are convinced that death has occurred, they turn off the ventilator rather then asking family permission to do so. Thus "brain death" illustrates a general truth: There is nothing so practical as a clear concept and nothing so mischievous as a confused concept. For instance, in 1994, at the hospital's expense, the family of a brain-dead teenager took her home on life support, in the determined belief that she was alive. In a time of talk about rationing, stated some ethicists, it was appalling that a dead person continues to be treated, and doctors cannot discontinue life support. Whether the hospital feared prolonged litigation and thought that sending her home was less costly in the long run is unknown.

The popular label of "right to die" has been applied to a long series of famous court cases in which patients and, more often, their surrogates have fought to have life-sustaining treatment discontinued. The label is misleading because, strictly speaking, there is no "right to die." The rights to which these patients and their families have actually appealed are either (1) the right to freedom from undue state interference, often called the right to privacy, and (2) the right to self-determination. The first of these rights involves an appeal to constitutional guarantees. The second is based in our long tradition of common law.

Most of the "right to die" cases have been heard exclusively in state courts because they have not entailed legal questions appropriate to federal judicial review. Hence, it is not surprising that different states have evolved different standards. A review of selected "landmark" cases will illustrate the point.

In the Saikewicz case, the high court in Massachusetts upheld a decision not to give a severely retarded 67-year-old more chemotherapy that would be unpleasant for the sake of a short extended life span. (He died a month later of pneumonia.) That court ruled that such decisions on behalf of incompetent patients should be made only with explicit permission of the courts. A very different procedure was established by the New Jersey Supreme Court in the Quinlan case. In this case, a 22-year-old woman received severe and irreversible brain damage that reduced her to a persistent vegetative state (PVS). Her father petitioned the court to be made her guardian with the intention of having all extraordinary medical procedures sustaining her life removed. The court ruled that the father could be the guardian and have the life support systems discontinued with the concurrence of her family, the attending physicians, who might be chosen by the father, and the hospital ethics committee. (After disconnection of the respirator, Karen Quinlan continued to live another ten years, sustained by fluids and other maintenance measures, in a nursing home.) In a long series of subsequent cases the New Jersey Supreme Court has held to its initial stance that such decisions belong in the traditional control of family and primary caregivers. However, courts in some other jurisdictions have continued to insist on a role for judicial review.

One might suppose that nonemergency cases involving competent patients would be clearer. In such cases, there can be no question about whether the elements of informed consent have been satisfied. When someone wants to discontinue kidney dialysis today because the quality of life is unacceptable, there is relatively little objection. That may be because the patient is ambulatory and may simply choose not to come back for treatment. Yet when a competent 77-year-old California man with multiple serious ailments, but not at the point of dying, wanted the right to have his respirator turned off because *he* found the quality of life unbearable, neither the hospital, nor the doctors, nor the court would allow him to do so, and no other hospital or doctor would accept him. (He had signed a living will and other documents.) His arms were restrained to prevent any action on his part; the hospital said he continued to "live a useful life." His medical and hospital expenses were by then almost $500,000.[23] William Bartling died the day before the state appeals court heard his case. Six weeks later the court ruled that he did have the constitutional right to refuse medical treatment, including the respirator. The family sued the hospital.

Also in California, a 26-year-old woman almost totally paralyzed from cerebral palsy found the quality of her life intolerable and had herself admitted to a hospital and asked the staff to keep her comfortable and pain-free, but to let her starve herself to death. They refused, and a court supported that decision. She was described by psychiatrists as "mentally stable," not clinically depressed. She finally signed herself out to a nursing home in Mexico, but found that she would have been force-fed there also and consented to eat. Later that year Elizabeth Bouvia returned to California and again appeared in court because doctors in the facility in which she was now a patient cut down her medication for pain. The court supported her.[24] Ironically (or, perhaps, understandably from a psychosocial point of view), the patient ceased her efforts as soon as her right to do so had been affirmed by the court.

In New Jersey, a lower court agreed to removal of a nasogastric tube on an 84-year-old incompetent (but not brain-dead) woman, Ms. Conroy, at the request of her nephew. The case was appealed, but the patient died before a final appellate decision was reached. In the Conroy decision, the New Jersey Supreme Court ruled that termination of any medical treatment, including artificial feeding, on incompetent patients is lawful as long as certain procedures are followed. (Ms. Conroy had indicated, but not in writing, that she would not have wanted to live under those conditions.) The decision came too late for Ms. Conroy, who died with the feeding tube in place. This case was considered different because the person was in a nursing home, but Annas maintains that the distinction should not have been made. Another problem with the final decision was that, although the court articulated the right of competent adults to refuse treatment, it failed to provide any way to allow proxies to exercise the right on behalf of incompetent patients.[25]

This was demonstrated again in the similar Hilda Peters case in New Jersey, this time in part because the ombudsman mandated by the Quinlan decision forbade the removal of her feeding tubes even though the man with whom she lived had her medical power of attorney and there was verbal (not written) evidence that she, too, would not have wanted to survive in this condition. The ombudsman said that he didn't want to rule in this way because he believed Peters would not want to live, but that he had a legal obligation to do so because a 1985 ruling by the Supreme Court said that a feeding tube could be removed only if the patient were expected to die within a year. (Expected by whom?) However, in 1987, the New Jersey Supreme Court made three rulings, for Peters and two others, that was expected to influence other states. The court said, first of all, that these life-or-death decisions should be made not by a court, but personally or through a surrogate. The rulings also provided immunity from civil and criminal liability for those making such decisions "in good faith."

It is interesting to note that the New Jersey court decided that the care setting *did* matter. Because Ms. Conroy was in a nursing home, rather than in a hospital, the court modified its principle of leaving such decisions entirely in local hands. Citing a history of rights abuses in nursing homes and noting that nursing homes are less open to multidisciplinary scrutiny by highly trained professionals, the court insisted on review by the independent state office of the ombudsman before any withholding or withdrawing of life-sustaining treatment. This outside review applies only to elderly persons institutionalized in nursing homes and psychiatric hospitals and is justified wholly in terms of their preceived special vulnerability.

In the years since the Conroy decision, nursing homes have increasingly come under scrutiny. In most states, regulatory oversight has been extended and, in some ways, improved. The efforts of professional organizations and the further development of geriatric specialization in medicine, nursing, and social work are having a general, if unevenly distributed, effect. Even ethics committees are becoming more common in nursing homes.[26]

These cases are presented in some detail to show some of the legal and ethical factors that can affect decisions that would seem to be relatively clear-cut, although very painful to the family or other surrogate. Especially during the 1980s, many similar situations were reported, with court decisions varying in each state according to the way the judges interpreted the law or how they were influenced by their own moral or religious beliefs. Most often these cases arose when physicians or an institution refused to allow treatment to be discontinued.

Such legal processes can take a long time. The Paul Brophy case in Massachusetts is an example.[27] It took 2 years and the refusal of the US Supreme Court to review the case (which would have taken even longer) before, after many contrary rules, his wife, a nurse, could have him transferred to a hospital that was willing to do what he would have wished and removed his feeding tube. He died 8 days later, kept comfortable but not fed, and cared for by his wife.

People like Mrs. Brophy and the parents of Karen Ann Quinlan, though motivated by the plight of their own family member, have ended by doing a service to the entire community. These cases are called "landmark" because the decisions had implications far beyond the persons whose names they bear.

As noted in Chapter 8, the idea of having a loved one die of thirst or starvation, as the pro-life group describes it (although there is little evidence that a PVS patient has such sensations),[28] is naturally repugnant to families, and the pressures on them are great. Some advocates with a religious affiliation are strongly opposed to removal, although others are not.[29] Physicians and nurses are likewise divided in their feelings and, as noted in Chapter 8, are often confused as to whether their discipline and the public consider removal of food and hydration unethical. Nurses have occasionally criticized families contemplating removal of life support (especially artificial feeding) and in some cases have reported them to authorities or alerted right-to-life organizations. The nurse who had cared for Ms. Conroy testified in the case, in detail, as to Ms. Conroy's condition; she thought that the tube should not have been removed. Others have stated the opposite point of view. In all such cases, the nurses are the ones in intimate contact with the patient; if the decision is to let the patient die, it is their responsibility to keep the patient as comfortable as possible.

Because of the confusion, it may be helpful to cite, specifically, the AMA or ANA statements on the issue. In 1986, the AMA Council of Ethical and Judicial Affairs issued a statement on "Withholding or Withdrawing Life Prolonging Medical Treatment," declaring that "life-prolonging medical treatment and artificially or technologically supplied respiration, including nutrition and hydration, may be withheld from a patient in an irreversible coma even when death is not imminent."[30] In January 1988, the ANA Committee on Ethics issued guidelines on the subject, saying, in essence, that there are few instances under which it is morally permissible for nurses to withhold or withdraw food and/or fluid from persons in their care.[31] This position is now outdated. In 1992, the ANA Board of Directors adopted a new "Position Statement on Forgoing Artificial Nutrition and Hydration." This new stance is in essential agreement with that of the AMA and the Hastings Center's "Guidelines on the Termination of Life-Sustaining Treatment." Its central assertion is "Like all other intervention, artificially provided hydration and nutrition may or may not be justified."[32] Thus the ANA has distinguished tube feeding from assisting dependent people with feeding by mouth, an ancient and continuing form of care that is always obligatory.

It was inevitable that, given the controversy on these issues and the fact that there may be several hundred thousand PVS patients, a case would eventually reach the US Supreme Court, probably as a privacy (Fourth Amendment) issue. The first right-to-die case to go before the Court was that of Nancy Cruzan, a 32-year-old woman who was injured in an auto accident in 1983 and was eventually determined to be in a persistent vegetative state. In 1988, her case was the first in Missouri to raise the question of whether feeding tubes can be equated with other life-sustaining medical treatments and whether patients in Nancy's condition have any rights regarding their care. The parents, stating that this would have been Nancy's wish, wanted to have the implanted gastrointestinal tube removed. A probate judge ruled that they could, but was overruled by the Missouri Supreme Court, which relied on a Missouri statute requiring "clear and convincing" evidence of a patient's prior wish that life support be removed.

The United States Supreme Court's decision in *Cruzan* is complex. The court upheld the general concept, implied or asserted in so many cases from *Quinlan* onward, that there is a constitutional right to refuse life-sustaining treatment. Moreover, the court ruled that artificially delivered nutrition and hydration is not legally distinct from other kinds of medical intervention and thus may be withheld or withdrawn in the same way as other treatment.

Finally, the court upheld the right of the Missouri legislature to insist on "clear and convincing" evidence of prior wishes.[33] While clearly not requiring other states to adopt such a strict standard, the court ruled that Missouri's statute does not violate the United States Constitution. (Only New York and Missouri have laws insisting on "clear and convincing" evidence, a test difficult to meet by any means short of a "living will.")

Although this decision is considered, legally, as very narrow, since it relates only to Missouri, and is considered by some as embracing form over substance, it is perhaps also indicative of the new conservative bent of the Supreme Court. In his dissenting opinion, Justice William Brennan argued that the Missouri rules are out of touch with reality; that people do not write elaborate documents about how they might die and what interventions physicians might have to prolong life; and that, after all, friends and family are most likely to know what the patient would want, even without written instructions. He added that by ignoring such evidence, the Missouri procedure "transforms [incompetent] human beings into passive subjects of human technology."[34]

One positive aspect of this case is the agreement of almost all the justices that competent people *do* have a constitutional right to refuse life-sustaining treatment, and if there is clear and convincing evidence that the person would refuse further treatment, as demonstrated by a living will or a "duly appointed surrogate," the person's wishes should be upheld. Another important point made by Justice Sandra O'Connor was that "artificial feeding cannot readily be distinguished from other forms of medical treatment" and that, therefore, an individual's decision to reject such treatment is constitutionally protected. It seems that at least this decision will prevent some of the terrible things that can happen to patients.[35]

As for Nancy Cruzan, after a friend came forward to say that Nancy would not have wanted to be kept alive under the conditions present, the state withdrew its objections and Nancy was allowed to die, with her family at her bedside. An interesting point on this general issue is that a study of court decisions on withdrawing or withholding treatment found that they are affected by gender. Whereas men's treatment preferences, even without a living will, were considered by judges, those of women, even with a living will, were rejected or not considered.[36] This is particularly true of pregnant women; several states limit the applicability of their advance directives during a pregnancy.[37]

Advance Directives

"Advance Directives" is the generic name embracing both instruction directives (living wills) and proxy directives (appointment of someone to act when the directive maker is incapacitated). Living wills are written documents or statements by competent persons setting forth how they wish to be cared for at the end of their lives. The beginning statement of a living will generally say that the maker is "emotionally and mentally competent" and that he or she directs the physician and other health care providers, family, friends, and any surrogate appointed by him or her to carry out the stated wishes if the maker is unable to do so. The intent is to withhold life-sustaining treatment if there is no reasonable expectation of recovery from a seriously incapacitating or fatal condition. The directive also has space for specific directions about treatments the individual may refuse, such as "electrical or mechancial resuscitation of my heart when it has stopped beating"; "naso-gastric tube feedings when I am paralyzed or unable to take nourishment by mouth"; "mechanical respiration if I am no longer able to sustain my own breathing." If such a list is already present in the document, the person is directed to cross out all that do not reflect his or her wishes and/or to add others. Two witnesses sign the document; sometimes it must be notarized. Of course, the living will can be withdrawn at any time by the maker, but otherwise it stands as a clear indication of his or her wishes.

In 1977, California enacted a Natural Death Act, the first "legal" state living will. The next year, Arkansas, Idaho, Nevada, New Mexico, North Carolina, Oregon, and Texas followed with similar statutes. All states and the District of Columbia have now enacted such laws. All grant civil and criminal immunity for those carrying out living will requests.

In 1984 California enacted a law entitled the Durable Power of Attorney for Health Care, which was the first of its kind. This law allowed terminally ill patients to designate another individual to make life-or-death decisions in the event that the patient was unable to do so. The agreement conveys the authority to consent, refuse, or withdraw consent "to any care, treatment, service, or procedure to maintain, diagnose, or treat a mental or physical condition." Like living wills, durable power of attorney provisions are now recognized throughout the United States. They are also known as "proxy directives," and the person who has been designated may variously be known as the "proxy" or the "health care representative" or the "person with durable power of attorney for health care." Some forms include designation of an alternate surrogate, "should my surrogate be unwilling or unable to act in my behalf." This document must also be witnessed. Sometimes both components, will and proxy, are combined in one document. A sample generic form is shown in Exhibit 9.2.

Although probably a generic living will, that is, not the official state document, would be seen as a clear indication of a person's intent, legally the forms specific to the particular state in which the individual lives should be used. These can be obtained from the state or from the organization, Choice in Dying, 200 Varick Street, New York, NY 10014-4810; phone 1-800-989-WILL. (They also offer advice, a newsletter called *Choices*, and a number of informational publications for the public and professionals.)

EXHIBIT 9.2

Example of a Generic Combined Advance Directive for Health Care*

As a competent adult, I have the right to make decisions about my health care. If a time comes when I have been determined to be incapacitated due to a mental or physical condition, I, _____
_____, am now declaring my wishes regarding the health care to be given. If I am diagnosed as having an irreversible or incurable disease or condition, and this has been determined to be terminal, or if I am permanently unconscious, I direct that all life-sustaining measures be withheld or discontinued even if this would hasten my death. All appropriate care necessary to provide for my personal hygiene, dignity, and alleviation of pain should be given.

Specifically, I do not want the following life sustaining measures [Example—artificially-provided fluids and nutrition]:

_____

_____

I hereby designate the following individual as my health care representative [declares durable power of attorney]:

_____

(Name, address, telephone number).

If, at any time, that person is unwilling, unavailable, or unable to serve in this capacity, I designate the following person(s):

_____

(Name, address, telephone number of one or more persons).

_____

Signature of person making this directive

Witnesses (names, addresses)

_____

* This example is presented merely to show the *type* of information in an advance directive. Each state has its own, which should be used.

Federal law now requires all health care institutions receiving Medicare or Medicaid reimbursement to maintain policies and procedures regarding advance directives. The Patient Self-Determination Act of 1989 (PSDA) applies to hospitals, nursing homes, hospices, and home health agencies. It further requires that each newly enrolled patient be asked whether he or she has an advance directive. If the answer is "yes," a copy is to be placed in the patient record. If the answer is "no," the patient must be offered information about the right to execute such a document. The PSDA also requires institutions to provide education on advance directives both to staff and to the community.

Having an advance directive would seem to give a person a guarantee that his/her wishes would be carried out, but this is not necessarily so. There are a number of problems. To begin with, the vast majority of people do not have an advance directive of any kind, probably fewer than 25 percent. Health care professionals themselves don't have a much better track record and fewer than 10 percent of patients have advance directives. It is constantly recommended that physicians, nurses, and social workers educate patients about the need for advance directives. One study showed that even one simple educational intervention significantly increased the completion of forms for durable power of attorney health care.[38] Most health institutions provide educational materials of some kind on admission, and theoretically, there is follow-through by nurses and/or social workers. Nurses cite particular problems. One is that nurses often are unsure of their prerogative to discuss advance directives with patients and family members. Some are uncomfortable in either initiating such a discussion or responding to patient or family queries, often because they lack appropriate information themselves. Staff education and policies that fully inform nurses about the law and advance directives should help resolve this. Another concern is that whether or not the patient has a written directive, it is not always clear as to whether that is what he or she really wants, whether there was undue influence from someone to either consent to, or forgo treatment. And patients do change their minds about which treatments they may want under particular circumstances. Nurses may be aware of inaccuracies and inconsistencies because of their prolonged contact with patients. There are cases where patients have living wills but haven't told anyone, including their doctors. Facilitating self-determination in relation to end-of-life decisions is emphasized by the PSDA. The well-informed nurse can help patients think through just what they do want. Finally, a third concern, whether a patient has fully taken into account the consequences of a treatment decision before completing a written directive is another opportunity for nurses to use their knowledge and interpersonal skills to help a patient. Furthermore, "assuring nurse–physician collaboration in counseling patients would go a long way to assure that patients have a realistic understanding of the consequences of their treatment decisions," notes one group of nurse-authors.[39]

It is clear that simply legislating that patients know about advance directives is not enough. The advantages and disadvantages of various written documents have been analyzed in an attempt to improve the quantity and quality of advance directives. Gibson states that a belief that future medical conditions or treatments can be thought of in advance underlies the execution of an advance directive, and that this is a fallacy. Recommended is the use of a document from the center of Health Law and Ethics entitled "Values History Form." The form is not copyrighted and can be reproduced. It is seen as assisting patients in communicating their attitudes toward life, independence, control, illness, death and dying, which should give any advance directive more meaning and value.[40]

Because so few of the elderly have advance directives, and many decision-making dilemmas arise when their wishes and values are not documented, the barriers to such documentation was investigated in one nursing home. As is true of other patients, few physicians discuss advance directives with the elderly, in part not to provoke undue anxiety. Reasons cited by the patients for not having a living will included ignorance about what it is, a notion that God, family or doctors would decide what to do, and general fatalism. Those who did have documents often did not update them, and their verbal statements of what they wanted was sometimes different from that recorded. Interestingly, contrary to national statistics, in this particular nursing home, about half the patients had living wills.[41] (In reality, the numbers commonly cited may well be only educated guesses.) Nevertheless, the findings of this study regarding impediments are similar to what is often seen in the elderly population. In one study, it was found that an additional problem is that sometimes when the elderly person is admitted to an acute care facility, the advance directives are not available. (One of the things that people should know is to discuss and give copies to the health care provider, family, friends or spiritual advisors and store the original in a safe but available place.) When they are available, they appear to influence treatment in the vast majority of the cases.[42] Why not in *all* cases was not explained, but other studies indicate that physicians' attitudes are a major factor. Another study found that, with other factors controlled, physicians who were more willing to withdraw life support were young, were specialists, practiced in tertiary care settings and spent more time in clinical practice; those less willing were Catholic or Jewish. There was no difference in the physician's sex, in attitude, or practice of life support withdrawal. An unexpected finding was that almost half of those queried were either neutral or unwilling to withdraw life support, once started, regardless of supportive legal actions and statements by AMA and ethicists.[43] Physicians (or nurses) who will not or cannot in good conscience honor an advanced directive should withdraw from the case, first arranging that the care is taken over by someone whose values are the same as the patient's.

The ANA position paper on the nurses' role regarding the PSDA states that the nurse should assume a major role in facilitating informed decision making by patients, including, but not limited to, advance directives. The position paper recommends that the legally mandated questions about advance directives be made a part of the nursing admission assessment.[44] In fact, this recommendation has not been implemented in most hospitals. Where it has been, nurses are obliged to learn about advance directives and about the applicable state law regarding advance directives. On the whole, nurses who are thus aware and knowledgeable feel empowered in their role as patient advocates.[45]

Nurses have also realized that it would be helpful to know whether, when a surrogate has been selected by a person, both agree on what the future patient really wants done. In one study, it was found that they did indeed have general agreement on treatment issues, with the exception of use of chemotherapy. The surrogate was more likely to have chemotherapy used.[46] This reinforces the need for clear understanding between patient and surrogate.

Can a third party interfere with a surrogate's decision? They have certainly done so. Usually, these are people with strong "right to life" beliefs and affiliations, and they seek court orders to act as guardians or otherwise try to stop discontinuation of treatment. Two cases illustrate the problems. One is that of Sue Lawrence, who after brain surgery was in a permanent vegetative state. After several years, the family realized that her situation was hopeless; family physicians and clergy agreed. Nevertheless the nursing home wanted a court order authorizing removal of treatment and absolving the facility of any related liability. In March 1991, the parents petitioned the court to remove Sue's feeding tube. The court agreed, and she was transferred to a hospice where artificial nutrition and hydration was stopped. Nearly two weeks later a religiously oriented group petitioned in Superior Court to appoint an emergency guardian so that treatment could be restarted. This was done, but the guardian resigned shortly thereafter and was succeeded by an attorney affiliated with the group. Although the Indiana Supreme Court expedited consideration, the ruling supporting the family and stating that an emergency guardian should never have been appointed, did not come down until September 1991. Sue had died in July, still connected to the feeding tube. The family had suffered great pain and outrage, with the only consolation being that the court's ruling would make it much less likely that other families in Indiana would suffer third-party intrusion. The other situation concerned Christine Busalacchi who, in 1987 when she was 17, was involved in a serious auto accident and suffered severe brain damage. After a year of intensive therapy that could not help her, and after consultation with physicians, priests and ethicists who affirmed the principle that when medicine has nothing further to offer a person, it is appropriate to stop therapy, her father, Peter, decided that continued treatment was keeping Christine in a condition she never would have wanted. However, Christine was in the same facility as Nancy Cruzan, and he knew that with the media attention to Nancy's case, which had not yet reached the Supreme Court level, it would be impossible to get court permission to stop treatment. His attempt to move her to a facility outside of Missouri was blocked by the rehabilitation center and the Missouri Department of Health. Even with lower court victories for Peter Busalacchi, the attorney general and governor were determined to block the transfer. Fortunately, a new elected attorney general stopped the state's appeal; however, the judge accepted a petition for guardianship from a total stranger and granted a 10-day restraining order, which was dismissed after 10 days. Christine died shortly afterward. The father noted, "These people didn't care about Chris. They didn't want to know who she was, what she was like, or what she wanted. They cared only about what they wanted."[47]

Third-party intervention creates both emotional and financial problems. Even though the courts tend to support the family and/or surrogate eventually, the family is thrust into judicial and media spotlight during the process, which only adds to their pain in having to make difficult decisions in the first place. The best remedy to prevent interference is for people to have carefully thought-out advance directives and a designated surrogate. The other is to have legislation that clearly defines who has a legitimate interest in making treatment decisions.

When an individual has no living will and has not designated a specific surrogate, physicians have traditionally consulted the "next of kin" or close friends. With increased litigation, they are becoming more reluctant to use such an informal process, and with more third-party interference, cases often end in court. Now over 20 states and the District of Columbia have passed laws that establish a prioritized list of surrogate decision makers with the authority to make medical decisions for patients who cannot make such decisions themselves and did not or could not record their treatment preferences in advance. If the surrogate does not know what the patient would have wanted, he or she must base the decision on what he or she believes is in the patient's best interest.[48]

In what is probably the most comprehensive part of their 1983 report, *Deciding to Forgo Life-Sustaining Treatment*, the President's Commission supported the patient's right to refuse treatment and the right of the family of an incapacitated patient to make that decision with the physician. (The data presented are unusually detailed.) The next year, a group of experienced physicians from various disciplines and institutions came to the conclusion that in relation to these issues, "the patient's role in decision-making is paramount, and a decrease in aggressive treatment when such treatment would only prolong a difficult and uncomfortable process of dying" is acceptable.[49] In summary, several important points were made. In dealing with a competent patient, the treatment should "reflect an understanding between patient and physician and should be reassessed from time to time." Patients who are assessed as brain-dead require no treatment. With patients in a persistent vegetative state, "it is morally justifiable to withhold antibiotics and artificial nutrition and hydration, as well as other forms of life-sustaining treatment, allowing the patient to die. (This requires family agreement and an attempt to ascertain what would have been the patient's wishes.)" Severely demented and irreversibly demented patients need only care to make them comfortable. It is ethically appropriate not to treat intercurrent illness. Again, the patient's previous desires and the family's wishes must be considered. With elderly patients who have permanent mild impairment of competence—the "pleasantly senile"—emergency resuscitation and intensive care should be provided "sparingly." A later review of this stance reaffirmed the conclusions.[50]

RIGHTS OF THE HELPLESS

Children, the mentally ill, the mentally retarded, and certain patients in nursing homes are often seen as relatively helpless, because they have been termed legally incompetent to make decisions about their health care for many years. Often the rights overlap, as when a child or elderly person is mentally retarded. Some of the rights of the elderly are being protected by a legalized bill of rights.

The Mentally Disabled

For mental patients, state laws and some high court decisions have served the same purpose. Both have focused on mental patients' rights in the areas of voluntary and involuntary admissions; kind and length of restraints, including seclusion; informed consent to treatment, especially sterilization and psychosurgery; the rights of citizenship (voting); the right of privacy, especially in relation to records; rights in research; and, especially, the right to treatment. Although rulings have varied, the trend is toward the protection of these rights, even to the point of giving a voluntary mental patient the right to refuse psychiatric medication.[51] In some situations, a structured internal review system in which patients can appeal treatment decisions has seemed to work. On the other hand, follow-up on patients who refused treatment showed a deterioration in their functioning when they were released to the community.[52]

In large and small cities, the evening television news shows disquieting pictures of apparently undermedicated, mentally ill persons whose lives are endangered by harsh environments they are not equipped to negotiate safely. There is disagreement between the federal government and individual states as to whether an institution is or isn't a legitimate home for some mentally disabled. This is particularly true of the mentally retarded; parents often feel an institution is the safest long-term solution for care of their children. And while group homes may be seen as a more human alternative for the mentally ill, who cannot manage themselves, their presence in many neighborhoods is bitterly opposed by the residents of a large number of presumably suitable neighborhoods.

In issues of informed consent, other rulings have determined that if the mentally incompetent cannot understand the benefits or dangers of treatment, the family must be fully informed and allowed to make the decision. However, if there is no family to make these decisions, an ethical–legal debate still rages as to whether the patient should be treated.[53] According to a Supreme Court decision in 1990, prison officials are permitted to treat mentally ill prisoners with psychotropic drugs against their will without first getting permission in a judicial hearing. The prisoner who objects is entitled to a hearing and other protections first.

Some legal decisions relate to sterilization of the retarded, which came to a head when it was found that retarded adolescent black girls were being sterilized with neither the girls nor their mothers apparently having a clear notion of what that meant. Restraints were increasingly put on sterilization until, in 1979, DHEW tightened the regulations for federal participation in funding of sterilization procedures. Regulations included requirements of written and oral explanations of the operation, advice about alternative forms of birth control to be given in understandable language, and a waiting period. In addition, no federal funding was allowed for sterilization of those under 21, mentally incompetent, or institutionalized in correctional facilities or mental hospitals. However, this does not mean that a parent cannot have a mentally disabled child sterilized; it means that more precautions are being taken by the courts and the government to ensure that the child's rights are not violated. There is general concern for the rights of young people in the mental health system, but parents maintain considerable control. In 1979, the Supreme Court upheld the constitutionality of state laws that allow parents to commit their minor children to state mental institutions; several states have such laws.

Rights of Children and Adolescents

The rights of young people and children in health care relate primarily to consent for treatment or research and protection against abuse.[54] Other aspects of the law in relation to minors are given in some detail elsewhere.[55] It is a general rule that a parent or guardian must give consent for the medical or surgical treatment of a minor except in an emergency when it is imperative to give immediate care to save the minor's life. Legally, however, anyone who is capable of understanding what he or she is doing may give consent, because age is not an exact criterion of maturity or intelligence. Many minors are perfectly capable of deciding for themselves whether to accept or reject recommended therapy. In cases involving simple procedures, the courts have refused to invoke the rule requiring the consent of a parent or guardian for this *mature minor*.[56] If the minor is married, a member of the armed services, or has been otherwise *emancipated* from his or her parents, there is likely to be little question legally.

States cite different ages and situations in which parental permission is needed for medical treatment. The almost universal exception is allowing minors to consent to treatment for venereal disease, drug abuse, and pregnancy-related care. Although it has been understood that health professionals have no legal obligation to report to parents that the minor has sought such treatment, a few states are beginning to add statutes that say that the minor does not need parental permission, but that parents must be notified. In 1983, the Reagan Administration issued a rule that would require parents to be notified whenever children under 18 years of age received any contraceptives from federally funded family planning clinics. After a number of court challenges, this was overruled as infringing on a woman's right to privacy. However, some states continue to set up obstacles, and nurses who counsel teenagers should check the current law.

The entire question of permission for contraception, abortion, and sterilization is in flux. The key appears to be a designation of *mature minor*; emancipated minors are treated as adults. In general, there has been a national trend toward granting minors the right to contraceptive advice and devices, but the political power of conservative groups who oppose this trend is being felt.[57]

Since 1976, when the Supreme Court held that states may not constitutionally require the consent of a girl's parents for an abortion during the first 12 weeks of pregnancy, the reproductive rights of teenagers have been gradually eroded by state legislation and federal edicts influenced by conservatives and right-to-life groups. More than half the states have laws requiring teenagers to notify one or both parents, even if divorced, and/or to get permission from them before an abortion. Most of these laws had not been enforced on constitutional grounds. However, that picture changed when the Supreme Court heard two cases requiring parental notification. The justices ruled five to four, in June 1990, that states had a right to make such a requirement of unmarried women under 18 as long as there was an alternative of judicial bypass (speaking to a judge instead) if the law required notice to both parents. This judicial bypass alternative did not apply to the Ohio case, where only one parent had to be noticed. The Minnesota law is so restrictive that it applies even when a parent has never lived with the child or does not have legal custody. (Only one-half of the teenagers in Minnesota live with both natural parents.) The five conservative justices did not allow for the fact that one or both parents might be abusive, alcoholic, or drug-addicted or even that the pregnancy might be due to incest. While pro-choice forces continue to work to overturn these restrictive state laws, the more conservative Congress and Supreme Court, as well as the political power of conservative forces in the mid-1990s, make this an uphill battle. Ironically, should the young woman decide against an abortion and elect to bear the child, she can receive care related to her pregnancy without parental consent in almost every state. An unwed mature minor may also consent to treatment of her child.

The question of whether parents may make a decision for a child, if the child's well-being is their prime consideration, has not been decided with any consistency. The legal principles involved are *parental autonomy*, a constitutionally protected right; *parens patriae*, the state's right and duty to protect the child; the *best interest doctrine*, which requires the court to determine what is best for the child; and the *substituted judgment doctrine*, in which the court determines what choice an incompetent individual would make if he or she were competent.

In 1986, two-year-old Robyn Twitchell died of a bowel obstruction because his parents, who were Christian Scientists, did not seek medical help. They believed prayer would take care of the situation. In 1990, a jury found them guilty of manslaughter and they were sentenced to probation and community service; they also had to pledge to seek medical care for their other children. Yet, other Christian Scientists have interpreted their religion's precepts differently, considering surgery a purely "mechanical" intervention, which is permitted. Understanding some of the nuances of this religion as related to health care is helpful to the nurse and other health professionals who have difficulty with the concept that illness is caused by "mental" rather than physical factors and that seeking medical care "departs from the practice of Christian Science."[58]

Courts will override the parents' decision to withhold treatment if the treatment clearly would be beneficial. In another case, a New York court overruled a mother who refused surgery for a 15-year-old who had a massive tumor on his face, because the surgery held some danger. There are also similar cases.[59] The situation is more complex when it comes to refusal of treatment of badly deformed or damaged neonates. Court decisions are not consistent.

Several landmark cases occurred in the early 1980s. In Illinois, newborn Siamese twins joined below the waist and sharing an intestinal track and three legs were not expected to live. "Do not feed, in accordance with parents' wishes" was written on the chart. However, several nurses did feed the babies, and someone reported the situation to a government agency. A court order was obtained to gain temporary custody of the children, and a neglect petition was filed. The parents (a doctor and nurse) and the doctor were charged with attempted murder, a charge that was later dismissed. Four months later, they regained custody of the children, whose care had mounted to several hundred thousand dollars. They were also in danger of losing their licenses.[60]

In Indiana, about a year later, a Baby Doe was born with Down's syndrome and a correctable esophageal fistula. The parents refused surgery, and their decision was upheld by the courts. The child was deprived of artificial nutritional life support and died. Although similar action had been taken in other Baby Doe cases, this one came to the attention of President Reagan. It resulted in an HHS regulation that threatened hospitals that neglected such children with loss of funds under Section 504 of the Rehabilitation Act of 1973 (which protects the handicapped). Large signs had to be posted alerting people to a "hot line" number to call to report such incidents. After a series of legal challenges, this regulation was ruled unconstitutional—"arbitrary and capricious," among other things. Eventually, an alternative suggestion by the American Academy of Pediatrics was agreed on: establishment of infant bio-ethics committees (IBCs) with diverse membership whose responsibility, in part, would be to advise about decisions to withhold or withdraw life-sustaining measures.[61] This was encouraged in the "Baby Doe" law, the federal Child Abuse Amendments of 1984, which labeled withdrawal or withholding of medically indicated nutrition "child abuse." However, a regulation basically left the decision as to whether such nutrition might be "virtually futile" up to the physician.[62]

The courts have also supported refusal of treatment for infants. A child born HIV positive with cocaine withdrawal and numerous other problems was placed under the guardianship of the Illinois Department of Children and Family Services to make decisions on the child's medical treatment. A requested DNR order eventually went to an appeals court where the child's condition was evaluated and the DNR order supported.[63] In another case, the parents of Cody Glasner sued because Cody, one of twins delivered by cesarean section, was resuscitated, although the parents had been told he was dead *in utero*. The doctors never let the parents make any decisions about Cody's treatment. They took home a fragile baby requiring extensive medications and treatments, and they still had the other twin to care for. After 33 months, Cody died at home after the parents decided not to put him back on a ventilator.[64] In still another, the physician father of a very premature baby with probable brain damage, who took the baby off the respirator, was prosecuted but acquitted. He and his wife had asked doctors not to resuscitate the baby at birth, but they did so anyhow.

The pain—and cost—of futile medical care for babies is periodically reported in the media, as in the cases where the infant has only brainstem activity. Sometimes, as in the case of Baby K in Virginia, the court supported a mother with a firm Christian faith who insisted on further care, including tube feedings for an anencephalic baby, which the hospital considered futile and inappropriate care. This prompted a debate on costs and ethics, since the baby could never be a sentient human being and the public money spent could have provided many health care services for other children. On the other hand, physicians in one Washington state hospital considered the dialysis of another premature baby, Ryan Nguyen, futile, inappropriate and immoral. The parents sought and obtained an emergency order from the Spokane County Superior Court requiring the hospital to give any care necessary to stabilize and maintain the child's life. Because of the media reports, physicians from another hospital offered to accept Ryan for treatment. He had surgery and recovered well, requiring no dialysis and taking food by mouth. This case led to a discussion of how the "Baby Doe" regulations did or did not serve their purpose.[65]

At the other end of the age spectrum regarding children is whether teenagers should be permitted to forgo treatment. The trend is to letting them do so under the "mature minor role." In several cases, the young men had cancer and either chose not to have additional transplants and medication (after others had failed) or discontinue chemotherapy. Choice in Dying recommends that mature minors make their wishes known through family discussions and advance directives. This is considered particularly important for children with chronic or potentially life-threatening conditions. A few states allow emancipated minors to complete advance directives, but usually makers must be 18 or over. Four states allow parents to complete advance directives for children suffering from a terminal illness.[66]

An interesting right-to-die situation involving a minor came to the Maine courts in 1990. Chad Swan, in a PVS and being tube-fed after an accident, developed several medical complications. With the concurrence of his physician, his family filed for a court order permitting the termination of the feeding. The court ruled that there was clear evidences, based on Chad's statements reported by his family, that he would not want to be maintained in a PVS, but the state attorney general appealed because Chad was only 17 years old. The Maine Supreme Court then expanded a previous right-to-die decision to include minors capable of making a serious decision to forgo treatment.

A basic right that children have is not to be abused. Child abuse is reportable in every state, although defined differently. Hospitals, all health professionals (including nurses), and sometimes schoolteachers, are required to report reasonable suspicion of child abuse. Failure to do so may expose the individual to civil and, perhaps, criminal charges. In most states, those reporting in good faith are rendered free from civil liability (lawsuits) for having made the report.[67]

Nurses should ask three questions about a child's injury: Has the child suffered injury or harm? Does the injury appear nonaccidental or inconsistent with the history given? Did the parent or caretaker cause the injury or fail to prevent it? If yes, the nurse should report a case of suspected child abuse and carefully gather and report specific information.[68,69]

Sexual abuse is usually part of the statutory definitions of child abuse even if no physical injury has occurred. Among the specific forms of sexual assault identified are rape, incest, sodomy, lewd or lascivious acts upon a child under 14, oral copulation, penetration of a genital or anal opening by a foreign object, and child molestation.[70]

The entire issue of identification and reporting has become particularly sensitive since sexual abuse of children has become more visible, and children have died. The question has been raised as to whether it is always in the best interest of the child and family to report the situation, if changes are being made. On the other hand, health professionals, teachers, and social agencies have been sued for *not* reporting or following through on these cases. The minor's right of protection extends to her or his school where, in most states, the law stipulates what punishment a teacher can employ to maintain discipline in a classroom or school. Private schools are not always subject to the same legal restrictions as public schools in this respect.

Children also have a right to an education. A recent development concerns the rights of AIDS children in the classroom. Children linked with AIDS have been excluded, but courts have generally ruled that exclusion is not permitted under the Rehabilitation Act of 1973.[71]

RIGHTS OF PATIENTS IN RESEARCH

The use of new, experimental drugs and treatments in hospitals, nursing homes, and other institutions that have a captive population—for example, prisons or homes for the mentally retarded—has been extensive. Nurses are often involved in giving the treatment or drugs. DHHS regulations require specific informed consent for any human research carried out under DHHS auspices, with strong emphasis on the need for a clear explanation of the experiment, the possible dangers, and the subject's complete freedom to refuse or withdraw at any time. However, there has been some argument as to whether "deferred consent" is appropriate for persons incapable of communication, so that they can be immediately entered into research protocols.[72] Lack of consent is a delicate subject, since research without consent continues to be reported and involves some very prestigious organizations and universities.

An interesting trend is toward including very young children in making decisions about research in which they are asked to participate. In the past, as a rule, parents were asked whether they consented to their child's participation in research—medical, educational, psychological, or other. There has always been some concern as to whether the child should be subjected to such research if it was not at least potentially beneficial to him or her (such as the use of a new drug for a child with cancer). The child was seldom given the opportunity to decide whether or not to participate. New knowledge of the potential harm that could be done to the child, however innocuous the experiment, and appreciation of the child as a human being with individual rights, have now resulted in recommendations that even a very young child be given a simple explanation of the proposed research and allowed to participate or not, or even to withdraw later, without any form of coercion. Given that choice, some children have decided not to participate. Overall, though, the support for using healthy children in research or being volunteered for procedures not beneficial to themselves is eroding. In 1983, DHHS published rules requiring children's consent to participate in research.

Nurses were in the forefront of the move to protect research subjects, with a statement in the ANA Code of Ethics, "The nurse participates in research activities when assured that the rights of individual subjects are protected," as well as an extensive ANA document on research guidelines. (See Chapter 8.) When you are participating in research, at whatever level, ensuring that the rights of patients are honored in both an ethical and a legal responsibility. Know the patients' rights: self-determination to choose to participate; to have full information; to terminate participation without penalty; privacy and dignity; conservation of personal resources; and freedom from arbitrary hurt and intrinsic risk of injury; as well as the special rights of minor and incompetent persons previously discussed. For instance, nurses have been ordered to begin using an experimental drug knowing that the patient has not given an informed consent. The nurse is then obligated to see that that patient does have the appropriate explanation. This is one more case in which institutional policy that sets an administrative protocol for such a situation is helpful.

If you are the investigator, observe all the usual requirements, such as informed consent[73] and confidentiality. The quality of research in which human subjects are involved is particularly important. Peer review, such as that offered by a hospital institutional review board (IRB), can be helpful. Although sometimes there are no nurses on the board, when they are, they bring a useful perspective to the review.[74] An influential nurse executive is in a good position to propose nurse participation. Although there are some criticisms about how these boards function, an IRB is generally seen as a safeguard to patients.[75]

Finally, the increase in scientific misconduct defined as fabrication, falsification, plagiarism, or other practices that seriously deviate from those commonly accepted within the scientific community, although thus far primarily involving physicians, also has implications for nursing research.[76] There have been some incidents involving faculty and graduate students in nursing and even faculty–faculty accusations of plagiarism or other scientific misconduct. These are often handled quietly (or not so quietly) within the school or institution.

PATIENT RECORDS: CONFIDENTIALITY AND AVAILABILITY

There is some evidence that, in situations other than the legally required ones, confidentiality of patients' records is frequently violated. From birth certificates to death certificates, the health and medical records of most Americans are part of a system that allows access by insurance companies, student researchers, and governmental agencies, to name a few. The information is often shared illegally with others, such as employers.

One physician, after completing a survey of the number of health professionals and hospital personnel who had access to the chart of one of his patients, called the principle of confidentiality "old, worn-out and useless; it is a decrepit concept." An average of 75 people had a legitimate access to that medical record,[77] and this is confirmed by the American College of Hospital Administrators. Annas also says that it is not realistic for hospital patients to think that medical information about them will be kept confidential, even when staff follow all the basic rules about not discussing patients except in clinical situations. In part, of course, confidentiality is even less likely since the advent of computerized record-keeping, which has grown tremendously in the last decade. The American Medical Records Association (AMRA) stated their concerns in a position paper in the 1970s. By 1994, the organization's concern was even greater, and the AMRA suggested that reproductions of health records provided to authorized outside users should be accompanied by a statement prohibiting use for other than the stated purpose.[78]

Nevertheless, maintaining patient confidentiality is a part of both nursing and medical ethical codes, and practitioners have a responsibility to safeguard patients' privacy as much as possible. That includes the privacy of patient records. Nurses are advised to record only information pertinent to the patient's case on the patient's chart, to make sure that only those who *need* to see the patient's records are allowed to do so, and that requests for information are documented in writing with an accompanying written consent by the patient or an order of the court.[79]

Many states have enacted laws to protect medical records, and the federal Freedom of Information Act (FOIA) denies access to an individual's medical record without that person's consent. In addition, the Fair Health Information Act of 1994 addresses the need for federal law to protect confidential material. Still some feel that the law would not be able to protect the confidentiality of records because of computerization. There are also practical problems: if certain data are needed, as in following through on occupational health hazards, can exceptions be made for research that would be beneficial to the well-being of people? The problem does not lie in the aggregate figures but occurs when individual records must be scrutinized. The Supreme Court, recognizing the right of privacy, which protects certain personal information from public disclosure, has applied a test that balances the individual's constitutional right against the state's interest in maintaining open records. Most states have followed suit.[80]

While many health care institutions and individual practitioners have been hostile to the concept of sharing the patient's record with him or her, choice in the matter is ending. Whereas it is legally recognized that the patient's record is the property of the hospital or physician (in his office), the information that the record contains is not similarly protected. The Privacy Protection Study Commission, created by the 1974 Privacy Act, included recommendations on patient access, and now both states and the federal government have legislated access—either direct patient access, with or without a right to copy, or indirect access (physician, attorney, or provision of a summary only). The majority of states allow patients direct

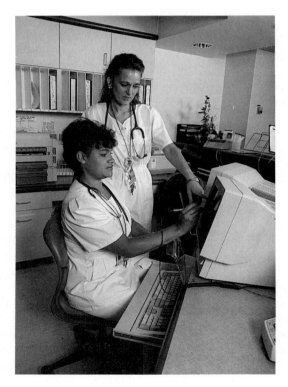

With the use of electronic patient records comes the responsibility to assure confidentiality. (*Courtesy of Robert Wood Johnson Hospital, New Brunswick, New Jersey.*)

access to their records. In the others, individuals have a probable legal right to access without going to court.[81] States may differentiate between doctors' and hospital records and have other idiosyncratic qualifications. Of course, one certain way in which the patient can get access is through a malpractice suit in which the record is subpoenaed, a costly process for both provider and consumer.

Do you have any legal responsibility to be an intermediary? The answer is more complex than just "yes" or "no." Certainly, you would not hand a patient the chart at request. Most states, as well as health care agencies, that permit access to records have a protocol to be followed. This usually involves providing both privacy and an opportunity for the physician and/or another person to explain the content. However, patients often don't want to see their charts if they feel that they are being given full information and are treated decently. Nurses certainly have a role in giving that open and humane care, but if the patient does ask, they should know the specific procedure in their agencies so that they can tell those patients.

OTHER ASPECTS OF PATIENTS' RIGHTS

Privacy

Nurses and others who work with patients must be especially careful to avoid invading the patient's right to privacy, which is identical to that of any other person. There are a number of special concerns. Consent to treatment does not cover the use of a picture without specific permission, nor does it mean that the patient can be subjected to repeated examinations not necessary to therapy without express consent; and undue exposure during examination must also be avoided. It has been recommended that the patient should be informed as to what confidentiality can be expected both ethically and legally. If the patient is the subject of a clinical conference, identifying aspects of the patient should be disguised to maintain anonymity.

Exceptions to respect for the patient's privacy are related to legal reporting obligations. All states have laws requiring hospitals, doctors, nurses, and sometimes other health workers to report on certain kinds of situations, because the patient may be unwilling or unable to do so. Nurses often have responsibility in these matters because, although it may be the physician's legal obligation, the nurses may be the only ones actually aware of the situation. Even if such reporting is not required by a law *per se*, regulations of various state agencies may require such a report. Common reporting requirements are for communicable diseases, diseases in newborn babies, gunshot wounds, and criminal acts, including rape. As noted earlier, child abuse is always reportable, and more recently, so is spouse and elder abuse.

Procedures vary greatly, but in elder abuse, in each state, the nurse is included as a reporter. In most states, the abuses covered are physical abuse, fiduciary abuse, neglect, and abandonment.[82] The nurse may be obligated to testify about otherwise confidential information in criminal and abuse cases.

As the AIDS epidemic grew, new reporting problems arose. By 1987 all states had added AIDS to the list of reportable diseases. Many, but by no means all, require reporting of AIDS carriers, that is, the reporting of positive test results for the human immunodeficiency virus (HIV). Physicians have been willing to make these reports because of the virulence of the disease and the need to maintain the best possible epidemiological records. However, the problem arises of whether to notify the family, especially a spouse or lover, of a person with AIDS. Many patients object to notification and therefore will not come for testing, creating a situation that may be even more serious. The laws are not clear on notification, although in cases related to other infectious diseases judges have ruled that the physician had a duty to inform the third party. Theoretically the third party could sue the physician if infected and not warned. As a rule, this kind of reporting is a public health department's responsibility, but it hasn't yet been determined whether, for instance, a home health nurse with information on AIDS-related conditions has a duty to tell the family.[83] What Northrop described as a breach of duty is the action of a nurse, formerly in an AIDS clinic, who passed on an AIDS-infected person's confidential record to the physician in charge of pre-employment physicals when the individual applied for a job in the hospital. Northrop said that the nurse could have been sued for breach of confidentiality and violation of privacy, although in this instance she was not named in the suit. The hospital paid.[84]

Confidential information obtained through professional relationships is not the same as *privileged communication*, which is a legal concept providing that a physician and patient, attorney and client, and priest and penitent have a special privilege. Should any court action arise in which the person (or persons) involved is called to testify, the law (in many states) will not require that such information be divulged. Not all states acknowledge that nurses can be recipients of privileged communication, but there are specific cases in which the nurse–patient privilege has been accepted, especially in the case of advanced practice nurses.[85] In one unusual case, when an office nurse revealed to a parent that her adult daughter was pregnant and considering abortion, the daughter sued. Because the nurse was calling at the direction of the physician, she herself was not sued (the doctor was), but her action was called violation of the *doctor–patient* privilege to the level of outrageous conduct.[86] Another issue is that psychiatric nurses, like other psychotherapists, have a responsibility to warn potential victims about their homicidal clients (the "Tarasoff principle," named after a case in which a psychiatrist did not do so). The same may be true of NPs in the case of warnings to the sexual partners of AIDS patients.[87]

Assault and Battery

Assault and battery, although often discussed with emphasis on the criminal interpretation, also has a patients' rights aspect that is related to everyday nursing practice, especially when dealing with certain types of patients. In many cases, where the action taken could come under this legal category, it is particularly important to chart fully and accurately. Grounds for civil action might include the following:

1. Forcing a patient to submit to a treatment for which he or she has not given consent either expressly in writing, orally, or by implication. Whether or not a consent was signed, a patient should not be forced, for resistance implies a withdrawal of consent.
2. Forcefully handling an unconscious patient.
3. Lifting a protesting patient from the bed to a wheelchair or stretcher.
4. Threatening to strike or actually striking an unruly child or adult, except in self-defense.
5. Forcing a patient out of bed to walk postoperatively.
6. In some states, performing alcohol, blood, urine, or health tests for presumed drunken driving without consent. There are some "implied consent" statutes in motor vehicle codes that provide that a person, for the privilege of being allowed to drive, gives an implied consent to furnishing a sample of blood, urine, or breath for chemical analysis when charged with driving while intoxicated. However, if the person objects and is forced, it still might be considered battery. Several states, acknowledging this, have enacted legislation to insulate hospital employees and health professionals from liability.

As a rule, intentional torts, such as assault and battery, are not covered by malpractice insurance. In a 1995 case, a couple's religious belief did not permit the woman to be seen unclothed by a male, and the physician and hospital were so informed. During her cesarean section, a male nurse allegedly observed and touched her naked body. In the legal suit, this was considered both battery and violation of the Right of Conscience Act by the Appellate Court. [88]

False Imprisonment

As the term implies, *false imprisonment* means "restraining a person's liberty without the sanction of the law, or imprisonment of a person who is later found to be innocent of the crime for which he was imprisoned." The term also applies to many procedures that actually or conceivably are performed in hospital and nursing situations *if they are performed without the consent of the patient or his or her legal representative.* In most instances, the nurse or other employee will not be held liable if it can be proved that what was done was necessary to protect others.

Among the most common nursing situations that might be considered false imprisonment are the following:

1. Restraining a patient by physical force or using appliances without written consent, especially in procedures where the use of restraints is not usually necessary. This is, or may be, a delicate situation because if you do not use a restraint, such as siderails, to protect a patient, you may be accused of negligence, and if you use them without consent, you may be accused of false imprisonment. This is a typical example of the need for prudent and reasonable action that a court of law would uphold.

2. Restraining a mentally ill patient who is dangerous neither to himself nor to others. For example, patients who wander about the hospital division making a nuisance of themselves usually cannot legally be locked in a room unless they show signs of violence. If they do, you must still be careful.

3. Using arm, leg, or body restraints to keep a patient quiet while administering an IV infusion may be considered false imprisonment. If this risk is involved—that is, if the patient objects to the treatment and refuses to consent to it—the physician should be called. Should the doctor order restraints for the patient, make sure that the order is given in writing before allowing anyone to proceed with the treatment. It is much better to assign someone to stay with the patient throughout a procedure than to use restraint without authorization.

4. Detaining an unwilling patient in the hospital. If a patient insists on going home, or a parent or guardian insists on taking a minor or other dependent person out of the hospital before his or her condition warrants it, hospital authorities cannot legally require him or her to remain. In such instances, the doctor should write an order permitting the hospital to allow the patient to go home "against advice," and the hospital's representative should see that the patient or guardian signs an official form absolving the hospital, medical staff, and nursing staff of all responsibility should the patient's early departure be detrimental to his or her health and welfare. If the patient refuses to sign, a record should be made on the chart of exactly what occurred, and an incident report probably should be filed. Take the patient to the hospital entrance in the usual manner, if possible.

5. Detaining for an unreasonable period of time a patient who is medically ready to be discharged. The delay may be due to the patient's inability to pay the bill or to an unnecessarily long wait, at his or her expense, for the delivery of an orthopedic appliance or

other service. In such instances, you may or may not be directly involved, but it is always wise to know the possibility of legal developments and to exercise sound judgment in order to be completely fair to the patient and avoid trouble.

LEGAL ISSUES RELATED TO REPRODUCTION

Laws permitting abortion have varied greatly from state to state over the years. In early 1973, the Supreme Court ruled that no state can interfere with a woman's right to obtain an abortion during the first trimester (12 weeks) of pregnancy. During the second trimester, the state may interfere only to the extent of imposing regulations to safeguard the health of women seeking abortions. During the last trimester of pregnancy, a state may prohibit abortions except when the mother's life is at stake (*Doe v. Bolton* and *Roe v. Wade*).

More than 20 years after the *Roe v. Wade* decision, opinions are still strong on abortion issues and now appears to be even more so; generally the same arguments are heard.[89] The major related court cases have concerned legislation attempting to outlaw or limit abortion. Immediately after *Roe v. Wade*, with a liberal Supreme Court, the rulings were almost consistently directed at freedom of choice, in opposition to restrictions on abortion being enacted by the states and later by the conservative Reagan Administration. The rulings changed dramatically with appointments of conservative judges by Presidents Reagan and Bush, until there was a five-to-four conservative majority, with the only woman Justice, Sandra O'Connor, considered the sometime swing vote. (However, she tended to be conservative on abortion issues.)

The case *Webster v. Reproductive Health Services*, in 1989, was considered a turning point.[90] The Court provided the states with new authority to limit a woman's right to abortion by upholding a Missouri law that banned abortions in tax-supported facilities except to save the mother's life, even if no public funds are spent; banned any public employee (doctors, nurses, others) from performing or assisting with abortions except to save a woman's life; and required testing of *any* fetus thought to be at least 20 weeks old for viability. Then in 1990, the Court ruled constitutional the Ohio and Minnesota laws requiring parental notification by unmarried teenagers. (Whether the girl was pregnant through incest or if there were other problems to make this difficult were ignored.)

Probably of even more concern to pro-choice advocates and even others who did not necessarily support *Roe v. Wade* was the 1991 decision on *Rust v. Sullivan*. The Court ruled that federal regulations that barred employees of clinics that receive federal funding "from discussing abortion with their patients, even if the women ask for the information or if the health care provider believes that an abortion is medically necessary" were constitutional. What shocked health care professionals was not just that poor women who had no other source of family planning would be denied full information, but that physicians, nurses, and other health care workers would be forced to withhold full information from patients, which is not only an ethical but a legal problem. Part of the majority opinion written by Chief Justice William Rehnquist stated that the women's right to have an abortion was not infringed because it was her indigence, not the regulations, that prevented it. Other statements by proponents indicated that, after all, physicians didn't *have* to work in such clinics if this "gag rule" bothered them. Because so many clinics depend on Title X money, some indicated that they would abide by the regulations, others that they would figure out a way around them. A number of Planned Parenthood clinics noted that they would simply have to do without federal funding. People turned to Congress for action, but late in the session, a bill invalidating the regulations was vetoed by President Bush and Congress did not override the veto. In addition, later, DHHS announced that only physicians were allowed to counsel women on abortion as a health care option. Of all the actions relating to family planning, this one probably affected nurses most, since it prevented nurses working in Title X clinics from giving their patients full and accurate information. However in 1993, one of President Clinton's first actions was to reverse this gag rule.[91] What the future holds is not clear, since the conservative Congress of 1994 planned more restrictions.

The aim of many of these cases, usually brought by a state, was to force the overturn of *Roe v. Wade*. That did not quite happen, but some state legislatures passed increasingly restrictive laws (even forbidding abortion in cases of incest and rape), in part to try to force the Supreme Court to hear the cases. Governors vetoed some of these laws, but the very fact that they had gotten through two Houses was appalling to many men and women alike. Both pro-choice and pro-life forces concentrated their efforts on legislators and candidates to bring about state laws that supported their particular point of view. The end is not in sight. After particularly restrictive laws were overturned by federal courts in Pennsylvania, Guam, Utah, and Louisiana, their advocates planned to take the cases to the Supreme Court. Because of the clear majority of conservative justices, particularly after the retirement of Justice Thurgood Marshall in 1991, an overturn of *Roe v. Wade* was predicted by some. As a matter of fact, in 1992 in *Planned Parenthood v. Casey*, the Court upheld most of the restrictions passed by the Pennsylvania legislature; and in doing so it established a new legal standard: restrictions are constitutional so long as they do not impose "undue burdens" on a woman's right to choose.[92] However, it is important to remember that the US Supreme Court rules only on issues related to the Constitution. In these cases, the Court rules that the state or another petitioner does or does not have a constitutional right to behave in a particular way. The trend now is to give states more freedom to act.

How does this affect nurses? Nurses support both sides of this issue, as was clear by the anger or joy expressed by nurses when ANA took a pro-choice stand. But regardless of their personal feelings, they will care for women and young girls who either made their choices or couldn't. Some girls have already sought back-alley abortionists, with the expected dire results. Theoretically, all hospitals are required to perform abortions within these guidelines, and it is legal to assist with such a procedure; actually, the right to an abortion cannot be withheld unless *Roe v. Wade* is overturned. However, for religious and moral reasons, some institutions are exempted from complying with the law, and individual doctors and nurses have refused to participate in abortions. Individual professionals or other health workers may make that choice, and there is legal support for them (the conscience clause). This does not preclude the right of the hospital to dismiss a nurse for refusing to carry out an assigned responsibility or to transfer her to another unit. There have been some suits by nurses objecting to transfer, but rulings have varied.

Ethically, nurses must give all patients good care, but who gets what care and why, as in the Webster case, may affect nurses professionally as well as personally. As citizens, nurses must stay abreast of such important issues. For instance, many pro-life groups also object to sex education and contraceptive use, yet an astounding number of teenagers get pregnant every year. What should the role of the nurse be in this situation? It is educational to see how other countries handle these issues.[93] It is also important to see how some of these issues interrelate. For instance, groups opposed to abortion are now becoming involved in right-to-die issues, taking a "life-is-sacred" stand.

In one case, a dying woman was forced to have a cesarean to "save" her fetus. Both died, and later the action was ruled illegal. In still another case, a woman in a coma was denied an abortion, but later, in a similar case, one was permitted—even though a right-to-life lawyer who didn't even know the woman tried to become her guardian to prevent it. And what of the Baby Doe-saved children? Who will be responsible for them? Will the family be forced to care for and pay for a severely deformed child? What of all the issues related to the fetus? Will new technology that has been successful in intrauterine surgery save some of these babies? Cure them? How will new techniques of birth control, including the abortion, pill, RU 486 and the use of other new drugs or changed use of drugs already approved for other conditions that are found to act as abortifacients, change the family planning scene? Laws on *family planning*, in general, also vary greatly. Some laws appear to be absolute prohibitions against giving information about contraceptive materials, but courts usually allow considerable freedom. Because there are still some state limitations and because, as noted earlier, the federal government is becoming more involved, it is important to keep up-to-date in this area. For instance, there are some legislative moves directed at "coerced contraception," requiring poor women on welfare and/or women who have abused their children to have Norplant implanted.[94] As in other cases of coerced contraception, it is expected that such judgments/ laws will be appealed on the constitutional basis of "right to privacy".

There are a number of other reproduction-related rights that are also important, such as sterilization, artificial insemination of various kinds, and surrogate parenthood. *Sterilization* means termination of the ability to produce offspring. Both laws and regulations have been in the process of change. Most refer to women. There seems to be little legal concern about male sterilization, *vasectomy*, which is being done with increasing frequency. The legal consequences of unsuccessful sterilization, both male and female, have resulted in suits. Called *wrongful birth*, these suits usually seek to recover the costs of raising an unplanned or unwanted child, normal or abnormal— but usually the latter. Judgments have varied but are more likely to favor the plantiff if the child is abnormal.

Artificial insemination, the injection of seminal fluid by instrument into a female to induce pregnancy, is evolving into an acceptable medical procedure used by childless couples, although there has been some abuse reported. (Consent by the husband and wife is generally required.) When a woman, for a fee, is artificially inseminated with a man's sperm and bears a child, who is then turned over to the man and his wife, this is termed *surrogate motherhood*. It has already created some legal problems when the woman decided not to give up the child and again when neither wanted a baby born with a birth defect. Even the legality of the process is in doubt.

Among the most controversial legal concerns related to reproduction are *in vitro sterilization* and *surrogate embryo transfer*, each of which is intended to enhance the fertility of infertile couples. One of the issues is related to patenting the process, which requires quality control and reproductive privacy. Other questions are being raised, such as: will the government put restrictions on such techniques as embryo freezing? (There has already been a case in which frozen embryos were awarded to a woman in a divorce settlement, somewhat like a child!) There are also cases of lesbian couples, one of whom has borne a child by artificial insemination, fighting for custody of the child in court when they separate. Still another issue seen as ethical, but possibly becoming legal, is whether lesbians or "geriatric" women have the right to have children.[95]

A relatively new legal aspect of human reproduction concerns the field of *genetics*, with which nurses, physicians, and lay genetic counselors must be concerned. Some of the issues have to do with human genetic disease, genetic screening, *in vitro* fertilization, and genetic databanks. In addition, legislation, such as the *National Sickle Cell Anemia, Cooley's Anemia, Tay–Sachs, and Genetic Diseases Act*, has encouraged or forced states to expand genetic screening to cover other disorders. Neonatal screening, for instance, will probably be expanded considerably and offers new opportunities and responsibilities for nurses. But with what is still a relatively new science, many legal questions will arise. Confidentiality is of major importance. If a genetic disease is discovered, the counselor should not contact other relatives, even if it would benefit those relatives, without the screenee's consent. One emerging problem is *wrongful life*, which occurs when a deformed baby is born, although abortion was an option, because the physician or other counselor neglected to tell parents of the risk. Informed consent that enables the patient to make such serious decisions as having an abortion, sterilization, or artificial insemination is also very important.

Finally, there are an increasing number of issues that affect the autonomy of women. For instance, over half of the state living-will statutes have a clause that suspends activation if the woman is pregnant. Also, some courts have ordered Cesarean sections against a woman's wish. One positive action is the 1991 Supreme Court decision that prohibits an employer from excluding a fertile female employee from certain jobs because of concern for the health of a fetus a woman *might* conceive.[96] There had been lower court rulings that barred women from jobs (usually higher-paying) that might endanger the fetus of a pregnant woman, even if the woman wasn't pregnant and didn't plan to have children.

TRANSPLANTS

Since Dr. Christian Barnard performed the first human heart transplant in 1967, the question of tissue and organ *transplants* has become a point of controversy. Tissue may be obtained from living persons or a dead body (at a certain point). With living persons, the major legal implications relate to negligence and informed consent.

The greatest legal problems arise from getting tissue and organs from a dead body. The big question is: when is an individual dead? When the definition of death as brain death has not been clarified, there have been suits against doctors and hospitals concerning removal of organs before "death," as seen by the family, even if it was a desire of the patient.

Common law once prevented the decedent from donating his own body or individual organs if the next of kin objected, and statutes prohibited mutilation of bodies. However, all 50 states have adopted, in one form or another, the *Uniform Anatomical Gift Act* (UAGA), approved in 1968 by the National Conference of Commissioners on Uniform State Laws. The basic purposes are to permit an individual to control the disposition of his own body after death, to encourage such donations, to eliminate unnecessary and complicated formalities regarding the donation of human tissues and organs, to provide the necessary safeguards to protect the varied interests involved, and to define clearly the rights of the next of kin, the physician, the health care institution, and the public (as represented by the medical examiner) in relation to the dead body. As a practical matter, however, organs are ordinarily not harvested without the explicit permission of the next of kin, regardless of the decedent's prior wishes. Of course, such permission is very likely if the newly dead family member had previously expressed a desire to donate. The UAGA does grant immunity to hospitals that harvest organs after making a "good faith" effort to locate family for permission.

Since 1987, hospitals have been required to ask the next of kin of all potential donors whether or not they wished to donate. (Among the barriers to organ donation are nonsupportive institutions and physicians, difficulty in explaining brain death to families, health professionals' lack of knowledge about organ and tissue procurement, and fear of intruding during grief.)[97] This "required request" law has resulted in widespread changes in hospital policies and stimulated some staff education. Most importantly, it resulted in designation of a person or set of persons who could be called when a prospective donor is identified. Such designated requesters are often both more knowledgeable about donation and more psychologically skilled than the primary physicians and nurses.

An ideal hospital procedure for securing organ donation might include such features as these:

1. The attending physician tells the family the patient has died (usually brain death).
2. The physician, nurse, chaplain, or organ-procurement coordinator makes the request for donation.
3. The donor's spouse (or other family in a specific legal order) may consent.
4. Find out what you can about the family before you make the request.
5. Explain to the family that they can donate as few or as many organs as they like.
6. If the family is opposed, support their decision, thank them, and leave them a number to call in case they change their minds.
7. If the family is uncertain, give them time alone to discuss it.
8. If the family agrees, have the appropriate donation card ready.
9. Answer the family's questions honestly; do not misrepresent what is to be done to the donor's body.[98]

For a quarter of a century, various attempts to get people to donate organs have been generally disappointing. The need for organs continues to far exceed the supply. While most people express positive attitudes toward organ donation, few take specific steps to make it more likely that their own organs will be harvested. Chief among those steps would be to have repeated, open conversations within families about organ donations and other aspects of end-of-life care. The scarcity of organs donated by African-Americans is considered a serious problem. Barriers include lack of transplant knowledge, religious fears, myths and superstitions, mistrust of the medical community, fear of premature death, and racism.[99] The problem for those who seek quick solutions to the persistent shortage of organs is that the discomfort of professionals and the public is not readily addressed by legislative initiatives and institutional rule-making.

RIGHTS AND RESPONSIBILITIES OF STUDENTS

When you began your nursing program, you also in effect, if not in writing, entered into a contract with the school that does not expire until you graduate (or leave). It is understood that both students and the school will assume certain responsibilities, many of which have legal implications. The first legal commitment the school has is to fulfill the minimum requirements for curriculum, faculty, and other resources set by the state board of nursing. Although you are responsible for your own acts in a clinical setting, you are expected to be under the supervision of a qualified teacher. Having your own professional liability insurance is important.

Perhaps you want to work as an aide to earn extra money. You will have to be especially careful because you can legally function only in those capacities not restricted to licensed nursing personnel. State laws governing the practice of nursing vary widely and are subject to misinterpretation by the employing agency. Most laws classify students working part time as employees. In this capacity, if you perform tasks requiring more judgment and skill than the position for which you are employed, you are subject not only to civil suits but also to criminal charges for practicing without a license.

Undesirable student conduct may result in some discipline, including suspension or expulsion, and there has been considerable disagreement on the school's power in such circumstances. Generally, it is expected that the school's rules of conduct are made public and that the student has the right to a public hearing and due process. Legal rulings may be different when applied to private or public universities. Private universities have greater power in many ways.

Constitutional rights are most frequently cited by students in complaints: the First Amendment (freedom of speech, religion, association, expression); the Fourth Amendment (freedom from illegal search and seizure); and the Fifth and Fourteenth Amendments (due process of law). The courts recognize the student first as a citizen, so that they will consider possible infringements of these rights. Most commonly, First Amendment rights involve dress codes and personal appearance. Although schools do not possess absolute authority over students in this sense, some lower court rulings have approved the establishment of dress codes necessary for cleanliness, safety, and health.

One case concerning a student's appearance found its way to the US Supreme Court. Sharon Russell was dismissed from her nursing program at Salve Regina College because she failed to lose weight, as she had agreed to do. Although her grades were good, her weight rose to 303 pounds and she was withdrawn from her senior year. She completed her degree elsewhere but sued for damages, partly because the faculty humiliated her about her obesity. She charged intentional infliction of emotional distress, handicap discrimination, invasion of privacy, and breach of contract. All charges were dismissed except the last. Throughout the various appeals, her award of damages was upheld. The Supreme Court heard the case on narrow procedural grounds, and the case was sent back to the First Circuit Court, and her award of damages was upheld. The question of whether obesity is a handicap (to fall under the Rehabilitation Act), whether the way she was treated was "atrocious" in a legal sense, and whether she or the college violated a contract were points of dissension. The court did comment negatively on how the faculty treated her in relation to her obesity.[100]

Random, unannounced searches that schools had carried out previously are no longer allowed without student permission or a search warrant; otherwise, evidence found is inadmissible in court. If material uncovered is proscribed by *written* institutional policy, it may be used in institutional proceedings.

Due process has been a major issue of legal contention. The rule or law must be examined for fairness and reasonableness. Are the student and faculty understanding of the rule the same? Did the student have the opportunity to know about the rule and its implications? What is the relationship between the rule and the objectives of the school? The National Student Nurses' Association (NSNA) developed grievance procedure guidelines as part of a bill of rights for students.[101] Besides suggesting the makeup of the committee and general procedures, such points as allowing sufficient time, access to information and appropriate records, presentation of evidence, and use of witnesses were included. The usual steps in any grievance process are also followed for academic grievances: an informal process first, consisting of a written complaint and a suggested remedy by the student grievant, a written reply, a hearing with presentation of evidence on both sides, a decision by the committee within a specific time, right of appeal, and sometimes arbitration. With students, the right to continue with classwork throughout the whole process is considered necessary, although in nursing, if the situation relates to a clinical problem and the safety of patients is considered a risk, further clinical experience may be put on hold until the matter is settled. At any rate a complete record of the hearing should be made.

Due process is considered crucial for students who are expelled or suspended for disciplinary reasons or who feel that they are discriminated against in their extracurricular activities because of race, religion, sex, or sexual preference. For instance, it became a major issue in the landmark case of *Dixon v. Alabama State Board of Education* (1961) where several black students were expelled during civil rights activities. The court held that they had a right to notice and disciplinary hearings.[102]

There seem to be an increasing number of grievances filed or legal complaints made because of academic concerns, especially grades. The courts have been reluctant to enter this area of academic freedom. There has yet to be a definitive ruling on curriculum and degree requirements. Most colleges now have grievance procedures for students who think that they have received unfair grades, and these procedures must be followed first before any lawsuit can be filed. In one case a nursing student was dismissed in her second year of a community college program for "unsafe clinical behavior." After a grievance procedure, in which her dismissal was upheld, she sued, alleging bad faith on the part of the faculty. The court refused to overturn the decision. A similar case in a diploma school resulted in the same decision by another court.[103] In still another case, a nurse who refused to take a predoctoral exam she had failed twice was terminated as a student of the university and not permitted to enter the doctoral program. She sued. The court could find no showing of bad motive or ill will on the part of the faculty, "which would warrant reviewing academic records based upon academic standards that are within the peculiar knowledge, experience, and expertise of the academicians."[104]

Before the student wages an all-out battle, the situation should be considered practically. It must be proved that the grade is arbitrary, capricious, and manifestly unjust, which is generally very difficult (especially when problems have been documented). Furthermore, unless that particular grade is extremely important to a student's career, the cost and time involved are greater than even a favorable result might warrant.

Cases in which the results have been more favorable to the student are related to inadequate program advisement[105] and the school catalog as a written contract.[106] A school has to deal with the nursing student according to the statements in the catalog the year she or he entered, not the later, more restrictive requirements. The Salve Regina case also had a school-catalog-as-contract component. A landmark case was heard by the Supreme Court, which ruled that an all-women's nursing school could not refuse to admit a male student.[107]

Because those schools receiving federal money directly are subject to federal laws, the Americans with Disabilities Act of 1990, the Civil Rights Restoration Act of 1987, and Section 504 of the Rehabilitation Act of 1973 have created rights for students with disabilities. In one case, a prospective student with a severe hearing problem sued because she was not admitted to a community college nursing program. The court upheld the school's decision because the applicant's hearing disability made it unsafe for her to practice as a nurse. At another school, an applicant with Crohn's disease was refused because her disease process would probably cause her to miss too many classes. Although the court required the school to admit the student, the decision was later overturned on a procedural issue. In other disciplines, students have been dismissed because of contracting tuberculosis, AIDS, and other diseases; this may yet occur in nursing.[108]

Another type of student right involves school records. The types of student records kept by schools vary. They may consist of only the academic transcript, or may include extracurricular activities and problem situations, which are kept in an informal file. The enactment of the Buckley Amendment has clarified the issue of student access to records. The individual loses the right to confidentiality by waiving the right or by disclosing the information to a third person. A student's academic transcript is the most common document released, particularly to other schools and employers.

As more student activists, most of whom are now voting citizens, request or demand certain rights as part of the academic community, more legal decisions are made such as the "truth in testing" laws. But school rules that were once ironclad have become flexible, even without legal intervention. The concept of rights need not be seen as an adversary proceeding. Both the student and the school have a new accountability. In the long run, it might be more meaningful to look at certain student rights as freedoms and responsibilities.

KEY POINTS

1. Patients are beginning to assert themselves in demanding their legal rights, and generally courts are supporting them.
2. In order to have a legal informed consent, the patient must be competent and not coerced; the process must include an explanation of the condition, the proposed treatment, alternatives, and dangers or benefits.
3. Nurses are not legally responsible for getting consents, but they should try to be sure that the patient knows what he or she consented to.
4. Court decisions, statutory law, and organizational actions seem to be favoring the patient's right to die.
5. The living will is designed to allow individuals to express to their families, health care personnel, and institutions in advance their desires about their care if they are later not able to do so.
6. Legal issues related to abortion, sterilization, family planning, and artificial insemination are becoming more complex as technology offers new options and as advocates for or against certain points of view become more aggressive.

7. The law is changing rapidly in relation to the rights of children and the mentally ill.
8. Even though an action is intended for the patients' own good, forcing them to do something can be considered assault or battery.
9. The grievance procedure is necessary in settling disputes in the educational setting.

REFERENCES

1. President's Commission for the Study of Ethical Problems in Medicine and Biomedical and Behavioral Research. *Making Health Care Decisions.* Washington, DC: US Government Printing Office, 1982.
2. Annas G. *The Rights of Patients: The Basic ACLU Guide to Patient Rights*, 2nd ed. Carbondale, IL: Southern Illinois University Press, 1992, pp 9–12.
3. Ibid, p 1.
4. Ibid, p 83.
5. President's Commission, op cit, pp 2–3.
6. "Office biopsy"—death results: Informed consent. *Regan Rep Nurs Law* 36:4, June, 1995.
7. McGrath P. It's OK to say no! *Cancer Nurs* 18:97–103, No 2, 1995.
8. Annas, op cit, p 204.
9. Ackerman T. The limits of beneficence: Jehovah's Witnesses and childhood cancer. *Hastings Center Rep* 4:13–18, August, 1980.
10. Dresser R, Whitehouse P. The incompetent patient on the slippery slope. *Hastings Center Rep* 24:6–10, July–August, 1994.
11. Somerville M. Therapeutic privilege: Variation on the theme of informed consent. *Law Med Health Care* 12:4–12, February, 1984.
12. Veatch R. Abandoning informed consent. *Hastings Center Rep* 25:5–12, March–April, 1995.
13. Creighton H. The right of informed refusal. *Nurs Mgmt* 13:48, September, 1982.
14. President's Commission, op cit, p 147.
15. Court case: What went wrong? *Nurs Life* 2:88, March–April, 1982.
16. Greenlaw J. When patients' questions put you on the spot. *RN* 46:79–80 March, 1983.
17. Nurses persist in persuading patient to be reintubated. *Regan Rep Nurs Law* 35:1, June, 1994.
18. Murphy E. Informed consent doctrine: Little danger of liability for nurses. *Nurs Outlook* 39:48, January–February, 1991.

19. Varricchio C, et al. Issues related to informed consent. *JET Nurs* 20:14–20, January–February, 1993.

20. Trimberger L, et al. Should you tell your patients about the risks of nursing procedures? *Nurs Life* 3:26–32, November–December, 1983.

21. Murphy, op cit.

22. Black P. Brain death. *New Engl J Med* 229:398, August 24, 1978.

23. Annas G. Prisoner in the ICU: The tragedy of William Bartling. *Hastings Cent Rep* 14:28–29, December, 1984.

24. Annas G. Transferring the ethical hot potato. *Hastings Cent Rep* 17:20–21, February, 1987.

25. Annas G. When procedures limit rights: From Quinlan to Conroy. *Hastings Cent Rep* 15:24–26, April, 1985.

26. Price D. The ombudsman experience: Administrative protection for vulnerable patients. *Trends Health Care Law Eth* 8:49–56, April, 1993.

27. Annas G. Do feeding tubes have more rights than patients? *Hastings Cent Rep* 16:26–27, February, 1986.

28. Crawford R. The persistent vegetative state: The medical reality (getting the facts straight). *Hastings Cent Rep* 18:27–32, February, 1988.

29. Meilaender G. On removing food and water: Against the stream. *Hastings Cent Rep* 14:11–13, December, 1984.

30. American Medical Association Council on Ethical and Judicial Affairs. Opinion: withdrawing or withholding life prolonging treatment, March 15, 1986.

31. Fry S. New ANA guidelines on withdrawing or withholding food and fluid from patients. *Nurs Outlook* 36:122–123, 148–150, May–June, 1988.

32. American Nurses Association. Position statement on forgoing artificial nutrition and hydration, April 2, 1992.

33. Aroskar M. The aftermath of the Cruzan decision: Dying in a twilight zone. *Nurs Outlook* 38:256–257, November–December, 1990.

34. Annas G. Nancy Cruzan and the right to die. *New Engl J Med* 323:670–672, September 6, 1990.

35. Death at a New York hospital. *Law Med Health Care* 13:261–282, December, 1985. This series of articles was written by the patient's friend and a hospital representative, with additional commentaries.

36. Miles S, August A. Courts, gender, and the "right to die." *Law Med Health Care* 18:85–95, Spring–Summer, 1990.

37. Fade A. Advance directives: Keeping up with changing legislation. *Today's OR Nurse* 16:23–26, July–August, 1994.

38. Rubin S, et al. Increasing the completion of the durable power of attorney for health care. *JAMA* 271:209–212, January 19, 1994.

39. Mezey M, et al. The Patient Self-determination Act: Sources of concern for nurses. *Nurs Outlook* 42:30–37 January–February, 1994.

40. Colvin E, et al. Moving beyond the Patient Self-determination Act: Educating patients to be autonomous. *ANNA J* 20:564–568, October, 1993.

41. Palker N, Nettles-Carlson B. The prevalence of advance directives: Lessons from a nursing home. *Nurse Pract.* 20:7–21, February, 1995.

42. Morrison R, Emanuel L. The accessibility of advance directives on transfer from ambulatory to acute care settings. *JAMA* 273:478–482, August 9, 1995.

43. Christakis N, Asch D. Physician characteristics associated with decisions to withdraw life support. *Am J Pub Health* 85:367–372, March, 1995.

44. American Nurses Association. Position statement on nursing and the Patient Self-determination Act, November 18, 1991.

45. Price D, Murphy P. PSDA: Practical help for conscientious nurses. *J Nurs Law* 1:51–56, January, 1993.

46. Libbus MK, Russell C. Congruence of decisions between patients and their potential surrogates about life-sustaining therapies. *Image* 27:135–140, Summer, 1995.

47. Third parties—can they take away your rights? *Choices* 4:1, 4–6, Spring, 1995.

48. Laws protect the family's role. *Choice in Dying News* 1:4, Winter, 1992.

49. Wanzer S, et al. The physician's responsibility toward hopelessly ill patients. *New Engl J Med* 310:955–959, April 12, 1984.

50. Wanzer S, et al. The physician's responsibility toward hopelessly ill patients: A second look. *New Engl J Med* 320:844–849, March 30, 1989.

51. Clayton E. From Rogers to Rivers: The rights of the mentally ill to refuse medication. *Am J Law Med* 13:7–52, 1, 1987.

52. Oriol M, Oriol R. Involuntary commitment and the right to refuse medication. *J Psychosoc Nurs* 24:15–20, November, 1986.

53. Backlar P. Will the "Age of Bureaucracy" silence the rights versus needs debate? *Comm Mental Health J* 31:201–205, June, 1995.

54. Holder A. Disclosure and consent problems in pediatrics. *Law Med Health Care* 16:219–228, Fall–Winter, 1988.

55. Kelly L, Joel L. *Dimensions of Professional Nursing*, 7th ed. New York: McGraw-Hill, 1995, pp 393–397.

56. Rhodes AM. A minor's refusal of treatment. *MCN* 15:261, July–August, 1990.

57. Isaacs S, Swartz A. *The Consumer's Legal Guide to Today's Health Care.* New York: Houghton Mifflin, 1992, pp 183–185, 244–247.

58. May L. Challenging medical authority: The refusal of treatment by Christian Scientists. *Hastings Center Rep* 25:15–21, January–February, 1995.
59. Isaacs, op cit, pp 246–247.
60. Cushing M. Do not feed. *Am J Nurs* 83:602–604, April, 1983.
61. Taub S. Withholding treatment from defective newborns. *Law Med Health Care* 10:4–10, February, 1982.
62. *The Rights of Patients*, op cit, pp 213–214.
63. Rhodes A. Guardianship and the refusal of treatment. *MCN* 20:109, April, 1995.
64. Minors and the right to die. *Choices* 3:1, 4–5, Winter, 1994.
65. Capron A. Baby Ryan and virtual futility. *Hastings Center Rep* 25:20–21, March–April, 1995.
66. Kavolius A. Refusal of treatment for minors and the law. *Choices* 3:4, Winter, 1994.
67. Fiesta J. Protecting children: A public duty to report. *Nurs Mgmt* 23:14–17, July, 1992.
68. Rhodes AM. Identifying and reporting child abuse. *MCN* 12:399, November–December, 1987.
69. Devlin B, Reynolds E. Child abuse: How to recognize it, how to intervene. *Am J Nurse* 94:26–31, March, 1994.
70. Switzer J. Reporting child abuse. *Am J Nurs* 86:663–664, June, 1986.
71. Equal opportunities: Protecting the rights of AIDS-linked children in the classroom. *Am J Law Med* 15:376–430, 4, 1989.
72. Levine R. Research in emergency situations: The role of deferred consent. *JAMA* 273:1300–1302, April 26, 1995.
73. Floyd J. Research and informed consent. *J Psychosoc Nurs* 26:13–17, March, 1988.
74. Robb S. Nurse involvement in institutional review boards: The service setting perspective. *Nurs Res* 39:27–29, January–February, 1981.
75. *The Rights of Patients*, op cit, pp 148–156.
76. Hansen B, Hansen K. Academic and scientific misconduct: Issues for nursing educators. *J Prof Nurs* 11:31–39, January–February, 1995.
77. *The Rights of Patients*, op cit, pp 178–179.
78. Computerized records' confidentiality a growing concern, attorney explains. BNA's *Health Reporter* 3:810–811, June 16, 1994.
79. Ibid.
80. Grad F. *The Public Health Law Manual*, 2nd ed. Washington, DC: American Public Health Association, 1990, pp 282–283.
81. Philipson N, McMullen P. Medical records: Promoting patient confidentiality. *Nurs Connect* 6:48–50, Winter, 1993.

82. Thobaben M, Anderson L. Reporting elder abuse: It's the law. *Am J Nurs* 85:371–374, April, 1985.

83. Brent N. Confidentiality and HIV status: A duty to inform third parties? *Home Healthcare Nurse* 8:27–29, April, 1990.

84. Northrop C. Rights versus regulation: Confidentiality in the age of AIDS. *Nurs Outlook* 36:208, July–August, 1988.

85. Silva A. Confidentiality crucial to nurse–patient relationship. *Am Nurse* 25:16, October, 1993.

86. Can nurse violate physician–patient privilege? *Regan Report Nurs Law* 35:1, April, 1995.

87. Henry P. Nurse practitioners and the duty to warn. *Nurse Pract Forum* 1:4–5, June, 1990.

88. Male nurse violates "Right of Conscience" Act. *Regan Report Nurs Law* 36:1, June, 1995.

89. McIntyre R. Abortions and the search for public policy. *Trends Health Care Law Eth* 8:7–16, 3, 1993.

90. Rhodes AM. Webster versus Reproductive Health Services. *MCN* 14:423, November–December, 1989.

91. Kelly L, Joel L. *Dimensions of Professional Nursing*, 7th ed., op cit, pp 447–449.

92. Benshoff J. *Planned Parenthood v. Casey. Trends Health Care Law Eth* 8:21–31, March, 1993.

93. Cohen S. Health care policy and abortion: A comparison. *Nurs Outlook* 38:20–25, January–February, 1990.

94. Mosely C, Beard M. Norplant: Nursing's responsibility in pro-creative rights. *Nurs Health Care* 15:294–297, June, 1994.

95. Curtin L. Lesbian, single and geriatric women: To breed or not to breed. *Nurs Mgmt* 25:11–16, March, 1994.

96. Murphy E. Are pregnant women autonomous decision makers? *Nurs Outlook* 39:144, May–June, 1991.

97. Lindsay K. Assisting professionals in approaching families for donations. *Crit Care Nurs Quart* 17:55–61, February, 1995.

98. When nurses obtain consent for organ donations. *Regan Report* 35:1, January, 1995.

99. Simmons D. Significance of increasing organ donations by African–Americans and implications for nursing practice. *ANNA* 22:313–317, June, 1995.

100. Weiler K, Helms L. Responsibilities of nursing education: The lessons of *Russell v. Salve Regina. J Prof Nurs* 9:131–138, May–June, 1993.

101. National Student Nurses' Association. *The Bill of Rights and Responsibilities for Students of Nursing.* New York: NSNA, 1991.

102. Lessner M. Avoiding student–faculty litigation. *Nurse Educ* 5:29–32, November–December, 1990.

103. Parrott T. Dismissed for clinical deficiencies. *Nurse Educ* 18:14–17, November–December, 1993.

104. Creighton H. Right of nursing student to pursue higher degree. *Nurs Mgmt* 14:16–17, December, 1983.

105. Jones J. University liability in program advisement. *Nurs Health Care* 4:83–84, February, 1983.

106. Creighton H. Nursing school catalog is written contract. *Nurs Mgmt* 15:68–69, February, 1984.

107. Greenlaw J. *Mississippi University for Women v. Hogan*: The Supreme Court rules on female-only nursing school. *Law Med Health Care* 10:267–296, December, 1982.

108. Helms L, Weiler K. Disability discrimination in nursing education: An evaluation of legislation and litigation. *J Prof Nurs* 9:358–366, November–December, 1993.

10

Politics and Public Policy

OBJECTIVES

After studying this chapter, you will be able to:

1. Define statutory law, regulatory law, judicial law, criminal law, and civil law.
2. Explain how judicial law derives its authority.
3. Explain how a bill becomes a law.
4. List ways in which you can get information about legislation.
5. Describe how nurses and others can influence the legislative process.
6. Name and explain briefly four federal laws that have a major effect on nurses.

Every nurse today needs to know something about law and legislation because there is so much in health care and nursing that is affected by law. Some federal laws influence how health care is given and how it is reimbursed. On a more personal level, other laws have to do with the rights and privileges of individuals, whether they are providers or consumers. State laws regulate our practice. Laws are implemented through the administrative process of rule-making. These rules and regulations carry the weight of law and specify provisions of the law. Court decisions also outline certain rights, and they pinpoint liability in cases of negligence or other malpractice. Few nurses set out to break or violate anyone's rights, but there are so many complex situations in health care today that there is a tendency to feel helpless about knowing what is *legal*. Yes, you can always consult with your employing institution's attorney, but that isn't very practical on a day-to-day basis. Worse yet, everyone dealing with the law knows that there is no final or absolute answer—something that is quite frustrating for those who want to know exactly what they can or cannot do. Yet, there are certain principles that may serve as guidelines to avoid problems and as a basis of understanding American law and influencing it. Providing this basic, practical know-how is the focus of this and the following chapters. [For more details, read any nursing law book, or Chapter 17 in Kelly and Joel, *Dimensions of Professional Nursing*, 7th ed. (New York: McGraw-Hill, 1995). Chapter 18 discusses legislation in considerable detail.]

INTRODUCTION TO LAW

As the American colonies were founded one by one, the way in which they would be governed was a primary consideration. Gradually, a system similar to that of the common law then in effect in England was adopted. However, the problems within the colonies varied so widely that each eventually developed its own procedures and laws, both common and statutory, based on its own needs.

From this evolved the concept of *states' rights*, which has played an important role in the history of the United States. Any infringement of these rights, either by the federal government or by other states, is usually strongly opposed. States do adopt the same or similar laws as others, such as voting age, seat belt use, and drinking age. However, a state can retain, revise, or repeal its own laws without interference from other states or the federal government. Variance in state laws creates a great deal of confusion, misunderstanding, and red tape. How much simpler it would be, for example, if the laws regulating the practice of nursing were uniform throughout the country.

Federal law is based on the US Constitution, ratified in 1789. Since then, the volume and complexity of problems facing the legislature have increased tremendously, but the Constitution always guides the action.

The Constitution has been amended 26 times. The first 10 Amendments, known as the Bill of Rights, were adopted within three years of the Constitution's ratification. These amendments guarantee certain freedoms, such as freedom of speech, press, religion, assembly, and due process. They are the basis of the civil rights we hear so much about. In recent years, the Bill of Rights has had relevance to health care issues, such as when the Fourteenth Amendment's protection of personal liberty is used in defense of a woman's right to choose to have an abortion or when the right to assemble allows nurses and others to rally as an expression of concern over labor issues. It is interesting to note that the Constitution does not specify access to health care as a guaranteed right. Nor do state constitutions.

THE UNITED STATES LEGAL SYSTEM

Under the US government, the law is carried out at a number of levels. The Constitution is the highest law of the land. Whatever the Constitution (federal law) does not spell out, the states retain for themselves (Tenth Amendment). Because they can create political subdivisions, units of local government—counties, cities, towns, townships, boroughs, and villages—all have certain legal powers within their geographic boundaries. On all levels, but most obviously on the federal and state levels, there is a separation of power: legislative, executive, and judicial. The first makes the laws, the second carries them out, and the third reviews them, a system that the founders of the United States believed would create a balance of power.

There are three basic sources of law: statutory law, executive or regulatory law, and judicial law.

Statutory law refers to enactments of legislative bodies declaring, commanding, or prohibiting something. Statutes are always written, are firmly established, and can be altered only by amendment or repeal. They are published in *codes*. The Nurse Education Act is one example of a federal law. The Social Security Act, which includes Medicare as Title XVIII and Medicaid as Title XIX, is another. Statutory laws also exist at the state level. Licensing laws for professional nurses, requiring them to be licensed before they can legally practice nursing, are examples of a state statute.

Executive, administrative, or *regulatory law* refers to the rules, regulations, and decisions of administrative bodies. In a sense, they spell out the specifics of a statutory law. For example, the DHSS Division of Nursing develops the regulations that determine the requirements for the various programs in the Nurse Education Act; the State Board of Nursing spells out the requirements for a nursing school; a city health code may adopt a patients' bill of rights as a requirement for all hospitals in the city. All have the effect of law but are more easily changed than statutory law.

Judicial law, also called *decisional, case,* or *common law*, is a body of legal principles and rules of action that derive their authority from usage and custom or from judgments and decrees of courts. Courts are agencies established by the government to decide disputes. (The term *court* is also sometimes used to refer to the person or persons hearing a case.) *Superior, supreme, common pleas, district,* and *circuit courts* are all courts of appeal (appellate). The kind of court in which a case is brought depends on the offense or complaint.

Federal courts established in all states hear cases related to the Constitution. With the introduction of written decisions, one of the most important principles known in the law was born, the principle of *stare decisis*, which means to stand as decided, or "let the decision stand." This means that if a case with similar facts has been decided finally in that particular jurisdiction, the court will probably make the same decision on a like case, citing the *precedent* of the previous case. If the precedent is out of date or not applicable, a new rule will be made.[1]

THE LEGISLATIVE PROCESS

It is not unusual for hundreds of health-related bills to be introduced during a legislative term. If nurses want to have some control over the laws that affect their practice, it is important that they learn how to influence the legislative process. The first step is to get the necessary information, as discussed in the next section.

The Legislative Setting

Even with the best intentions, no legislators can be experts on all the issues that come up. For instance, in one two-year session in Congress, 25,000 or so bills were introduced. Not all are acted on, but even reading them all is almost impossible. Therefore, all national and most state legislators have staffs of varying size, depending on seniority and other factors. Some staffs are in the capital; others are in home offices in the legislator's district in order to keep in touch with and help constituents. Some perform administrative duties, and others act as legislative aides, assistants, and/or researchers. These are individuals who summarize background material on key bills and brief the legislator on specific issues and on constituents' feedback. The legislator generally uses this information to decide how to vote. The administrative assistants share the power of the legislators, if not the glory. Committee staff do the preparatory work that comes before committees and subcommittees, drafting bills, writing amendments to bills, arranging and preparing for public hearings, consulting with people in the areas about which the committee is concerned, providing information, and frequently writing speeches for the chairman.

Because these assistants get information from numerous sources, it is a good idea to become acquainted with them, maintain good relations, and provide accurate, pertinent information about the issues in which you are interested. Do not ignore them; they are very influential.

A measure of the prestige a legislator has is the nature of committee appointments, where most of the preliminary action on bills occurs. Appointments are influenced or made by party leaders in the House of Representatives or the Senate. Chairmanships of committees, extremely powerful positions, are awarded to members of the majority party, usually senior members of the House or Senate. Some committee assignments are more prestigious than others and are eagerly sought. Although there are cases in which the chairpersons of some of these committees, particularly on the national level, have remained for years, the makeup of a committee may change with each new session. It is important to know on which committee your legislators sit, because the action of committees affects the future of a bill. The same process and relationships exist, for the most part, on the state level.

How a Bill Becomes a Law[2]

A lot of compromise goes into the legislative process, and often there is behind-the-scenes negotiating that is never seen in the open committee hearings or on the floor of the House or Senate. Nevertheless there is a formal process by which a bill becomes a law. This is charted in Exhibit 10.1. Here the bill starts in the House, but it could just as well be the Senate. Note particularly the steps at which you can influence the process by the various lobbying techniques described later. Some important details follow.

1. Anyone can initiate a bill. Common sources include the President and his administration; a group or organization, such as ANA; and private citizens who can convince a legislator about a need. The bill is put in the appropriate format by legal specialists.

2. One or more lawmakers sponsor the bill, with the major sponsor (the author) introducing the bill and guiding it through the legislative process. The more powerful that sponsor, the better. Bipartisan sponsorship is also desirable, because then it does not become a party issue.

3. The bill is introduced (commonly referred to as "put in the hopper") and given a number. Numbers are consecutive within each two-year session and begin with "HR" in the House or "S" in the Senate. If the bill does not become law, it can be reintroduced the following session and is given a new bill number.

4. After the bill is introduced and printed in the *Congressional Record* (*first reading*), it is assigned to one or more committees that have responsibility for that subject. You can obtain a copy of a federal bill from your representative or, preferably, from the House or Senate Documents Room. State legislatures also have document or bill rooms. Addresses for Document Rooms can be obtained from your representative. It is a good idea to call the Documents Room first to verify the proper procedure. Be sure to have the bill number whenever requesting information. A section-by-section analysis of the bill is usually easier to understand than the bill itself,

EXHIBIT 10.1

The Legislative Process
How a Bill Becomes a Law at the Federal Level

HOUSE

SENATE

Idea for bill
Any individual, or group,
any legislator,
legislative committee or
subcommittee or
executive branch

OR

Selection of Sponsors

Selection of Sponsors

Formal drafting of bill

Formal drafting of bill

Introduction and first reading
Bill given number

Introduction and first reading
Bill given number

* Referral to appropriate
committee / subcommittee

* Referral to appropriate
committee / subcommittee

May die in committee; if
reported out, with or
without amendments,
proceeds

* Hearings
(if requested or required)

* Hearings
(if requested or required)

Rules committee
"Rule" required
to reach floor

May be defeated,
amended, or sent
back to committee;
if passed, proceeds

* Second reading; debate;
floor action

* Second reading; debate;
floor action

* Third reading
Roll call vote on floor

Third reading
Roll call vote on floor

Same steps in other House

If passed,
proceeds to

Returned to first House
for another vote if
amendments have been
added by other House

If no
concurrence,
proceeds to

If passed,
proceeds to

* House-Senate
Conference Committee

If agreement
reached,
proceeds

* President for approval

If vetoed,
dies unless
both Houses
override the
veto

House vote

Senate vote

President's signature

Signature of Speaker

Signature of
President of Senate

Becomes a law

* Appropriate administrative
agency for formulation of
rules and regulations

* Points at which fate of bill is
usually influenced most

and can be obtained from your congressman or from the *Congressional Record*, which is available in many libraries.

5. Legislators spend a lot of time in committees. The committee chairperson is very powerful and can influence the fate of the bill by introducing it for discussion very quickly or by keeping it off the agenda for the entire session. Committees also conduct hearings, which are usually open to the public. Often nurses testify on health care issues by representing professional nursing organizations or appearing as individual witnesses. When a committee decides on a bill, it is either killed or passed with amendments or as a new bill. The process of deliberating and voting on a bill is called *mark-up*.

6. If the bill is passed, the Director of the Congressional Budget Office submits an estimate of the cost of the measure, and this is included in the Committee Report.

7. The bill then goes to the full House for action on the floor (*second reading*). Visitors can watch from the gallery but may not speak during floor deliberations. If you want to know when a particular bill will be brought to the floor, it is best to contact the leadership of the appropriate house. A bill is usually brought to the chamber of one house independent of events in the other.

8. At the end of floor action, the *third reading* is called for and the vote taken. Amendments added in committee or on the floor are a big factor in determining the fate of the bill. Adding amendments to a bill that seems sure to pass is a technique for putting through some action that might not succeed on its own and that may be only remotely or not at all connected to the content of the original bill. On the other hand, amendments that are totally unacceptable to the bill's sponsors may be added as a mechanism to force withdrawal or defeat of the bill. In general, amendments are introduced to strengthen, broaden, or curtail the intent of the original bill or law. If passed, they may change its character considerably. When debate is closed, the vote is taken by roll call and recorded. Passage usually requires a majority vote of the total House.

9. If the bill is passed, it goes to the Senate for a complete repetition of the process it went through in the House, and with the same opportunities to influence its passage. A bill introduced in the Senate follows the same general route, with certain procedural differences. Also, the President of the Senate is the Vice-President of the United States. Filibustering is a unique senatorial process whereby senators opposed to a motion to consider a bill may speak to it for extensive periods, thus preventing or defeating action by long delays.

10. At times, the same or a similar bill is introduced in both houses on certain important issues. If these bills are not the same when passed

by each house, or if another single bill has been amended by the second house after passing the first and the first does not agree on the amendments, the bill is sent to a conference committee consisting of an equal number of members of each house. The conference committee tries to work out a compromise that will be accepted by both houses. Usually an agreement is reached.

11. After passing both houses and being signed by each presider, the bill goes to the President, who may obtain opinions from various sources. If he signs it or fails to take action within 10 days, the bill becomes law. He may also veto the bill and return it to the house of origin with his objections. A two-thirds affirmative vote in both houses for repassage is necessary to override the veto. Because voting on a veto is often along party lines, overriding a veto in both houses is difficult. However, the National Center for Nursing Research was established in 1985 through a veto override of the NIH reauthorization bill, demonstrating the political strength of nurses and others who lobbied for the bill. If the Congress adjourns before the 10 days in which the President should sign the bill, it does not become law. This is known as a *pocket veto*.

12. Another type of legislation is a resolution. Joint resolutions originating in either house are, for all practical purposes, treated as a bill but have the whereas-resolved format. They are identified as *HJ Res.* or *SJ Res.*

13. All bills that become law are assigned numbers, beginning with "PL" (different from their original number), and then are printed and attached to the proper volume of statutes.

14. The last step is sending the new law to the appropriate administrative agency for rules on implementing the law. This is another juncture at which nurses can have input. Proposed and final rules are published in the *Federal Register*, which is available in many libraries.

15. It is important to keep in mind that the federal government's fiscal year is designated by the calendar year in which it ends. Thus, the period from October 1, 1995, to September 30, 1996, is fiscal year 1996 (FY96).

INFLUENCING THE LEGISLATIVE PROCESS

There are many factors to be considered before a legislative body or even individual legislators make a final decision on how to vote on a piece of legislation. Some are probably personal—how the legislator feels about an issue. Some are internally political—support of the party leadership or a favor owed to a colleague. But likely to be the most influential is the voice of the legislator's constituency, "the folks back home." Most legislators want to be reelected to the same or a higher office. If their constituents are not pleased with them, their voting record, or their attitude, they are replaced.

Just who are these powerful constituents? Actually, they range from the ordinary householder to the powerful conglomerate, and include individuals as well as interest groups. An *interest group* is an association of people who come together to promote or protect a common cause through the political process. They represent the issues of their constituents and use the power of the group to influence public decisions that affect them. In recent years, nurses have become increasingly influential with their legislators. Professional organizations at all three levels of government, as well as individual nurses with expertise in various aspects of health care, have knowledge of the health care system and patients' needs that make them valuable resources to legislators.

One method used to influence legislation is to support a candidate, either for election or for reelection. For many decades, making political contributions has been illegal for certain groups such as ANA, and more recently, tighter constraints have been placed on contributions and spending.

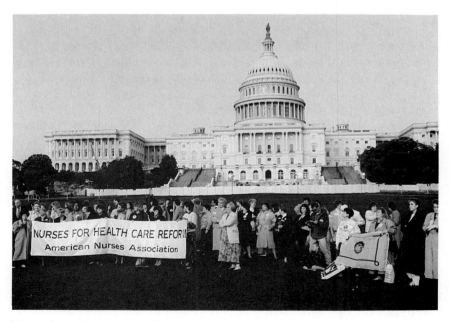

Nurses have become a significant force in shaping public policy. They are trusted by the public and are the largest group in the health care field. (*Courtesy of the American Nurses Association.*)

Because the law requires that, for some groups, campaign contributions be kept as a separate fund and that no organizational money may be used for this purpose, many groups have created separate organizations for political activity. These are known as *political action committees* (PACs).[3] They may be located in the same office as an organization, such as ANA–PAC in ANA's Washington office, but by law their funds and activities are carefully separated from the rest of the organization's work.

Many state nurses associations have formed state PACs based on the ANA model. They have endorsed candidates, contributed to campaigns, and encouraged fellow nurses to run for office. It is important to remember that the success of any nurse PAC depends on the input and support of individual nurses. You can always start by volunteering a small amount of time, and, in so doing, have a voice in advancing the political strength of nursing. State professional nursing organizations are a good source of information on PACs and political groups at the state level. (ANA–PAC is described in Chapter 13.)

In recent years, many political participants have criticized PACs, claiming that they make it easy for certain groups to "buy" legislators and their votes. Although it is hard to prove the exact relationship between campaign contributions and voting patterns, there is no doubt that substantial contributions help with access to public officials and create an atmosphere of familiarity. The first priority of any legislator is to get elected, and campaigning is becoming extraordinarily expensive. Recently, tighter constraints have been placed on contributions and spending. While limits are set by law on the amounts that can be given to candidates, there are ways of manipulating the system. For instance, AMA, often identified as one of the largest contributors in congressional races, has in some years contributed as much as $3 million to various campaigns.

In 1994, ANA–PAC could boast of a "war chest" of $1.2 million, significant growth from $300,000 in contributions during 1988. The PAC has also demonstrated an over 70 percent success rate in its endorsements for many years. ANA–PAC is the 30th largest federal PAC among the over 4000 PACs that exist in the United States. In 1995, it was identified as the second fastest growing federal health care PAC in the nation.[4]

Another important, if sometimes unofficial, component of lawmaking is lobbying. *Lobbying* is generally defined as an attempt to influence a decision of a legislator or other governmental body. Since it is a type of petition for redress of grievances, lobbying is constitutionally guaranteed. Lobbying exists at several levels, from a single individual who contacts a legislator about a particular issue of personal importance to the interest groups that carefully (and often expensively) organize systems for monitoring legislation, initiating action, or blocking action on matters that concern them.

Professional lobbyists must be registered with Congress, and there are regulations concerning the types of organizations that may employ lobbyists. They spend all or part of their time representing the interests of a particular group or groups. Lobbyists provide information to legislators and their staffs (not necessarily objectively) and introduce resource people to them. Lobbyists are knowledgeable in the ways of legislation and are often familiar with legislator's personalities and idiosyncracies. They keep their interest group informed about any pertinent legislation and the problems involved, and help them to take effective action.

This organized approach to lobbying, effective though it is, should not overshadow the efforts of the individual who, in effect, lobbies when contacting the appropriate legislator about an issue. Groups such as nurses have proved to be very effective in lobbying by coordinating the efforts of individuals for unified action.

NURSES AND POLITICAL ACTION

Organizations such as the ANA and various specialty groups have taken leadership roles in mobilizing nurses in grassroots lobbying. They have started educational programs and political consciousness-raising sessions, both to teach nurses techniques and strategies and to make them aware of the issues. Networks have been established which can be set in motion at a moment's notice on behalf of an issue, a candidate or a piece of legislation. The network is constituted of volunteer activists with an interest in politics, experts on particular topics, or they may be drawn from a social, ethnic or age group that is strategic.

The ANA's N-STAT program is described in Chapter 13. It is a network of trained volunteers from a variety of state and specialty organizations. Once activated, both a Leadership Team and a Rapid Response are triggered. The leadership are volunteers who have already established a relationship with specific legislators. The Rapid Response creates a high volume of calls, letters and faxes which are also focused on specific elected officials. All the activity is aimed at the grassroots, and conveys a message about support for reelection.

N-STAT is highly acclaimed for its ability to penetrate every state and district in the country. Many state nurses associations have created similar networks for state politics. Additional participants are always welcome. However, grassroots lobbying need not occur through an organization or special interest group, it can be your personal action plan to participate more fully in government through those who represent you.

Grassroots Lobbying

There are certain ways to lobby that give a better chance of success than if you approach it with good will but little organization. One of the first steps is making personal contact. It is sensible to become acquainted with your legislators before a legislative crisis occurs. This gives you the advantage of having made personal contact and shown general interest, and gives the legislator or staff member the advantage of a reference point. In small communities, legislators often know many of their constituents on a first-name basis through frequent contacts at town meetings or as other opportunities arise. This personal relationship may be more difficult to manage in large areas, but the effort to meet and talk with legislators is never wasted.

Having identified and located the legislator, call for an appointment or find out when the legislator is available in his local office (or in his capital office if this is convenient for both). Before the visit, it is helpful to know the following about the legislator:

1. Geography of the legislative district and district number.
2. Present or past leadership in civic, cultural, or other community affairs.
3. Voting record on major controversial issues recently under consideration.
4. Voting record in the past on major bills of interest to nurses.
5. Subject areas of special interest, such as health, consumer affairs, and so on.
6. Political party affiliation and committee assignments.
7. Previous occupation or profession, and whether there is still some involvement.
8. Bills of major importance which have been authored or co-authored.
9. Previous contacts with nursing organizations in the area.
10. Nursing organizations' endorsements or support to opponents in past elections.

This information may be available from the SNA, political action groups, or literature from the legislator's office.

No one can say how such a visit should be conducted—it is obviously a matter of personal style—but generally it is wise to be dressed appropriately, to be friendly, to keep the visit short, to identify yourself as a nurse and, depending on your level of expertise, to offer to be a resource. Comment on any of the legislator's bills or votes of which you approve. If the first visit coincides with pending health legislation, ask whether a stand has been taken and perhaps add a few pertinent comments. Probably not more than three major issues should be discussed. A *brief* written account of the key points and/or documentation of facts can be left, along with an offer to provide additional information when needed. Legislators respond best if what is discussed is within the context of what their other constituents might want. In other words, is it good for the public and not just for nursing?

It is important to be prompt for the visit, but be ready to accept the fact that the legislator may be late or not able to keep the appointment. The administrative assistant who substitutes will probably be knowledgeable and attentive, and the time will not be wasted. If distance and time make visiting difficult, a telephone call is a good approach. The same general guidelines can be followed, and here also, speaking to the legislator's administrative assistant serves as good a purpose as speaking to the legislator directly.

Although personal visits and calls are considered useful in trying to influence a legislator, letter writing is also effective, especially if an initial introductory visit has already been made. It is also the most frequent way to communicate. Legislators are particularly sensitive to communications from constituents. They give far less attention to correspondence from outside their state or district and are often annoyed by it. If you don't know the legislator's local address, address the letter to the state or federal house or senate. However, addresses should be on hand before the need arises, and some say that mail received in the local office is apt to get more attention, since the letters don't compete with other mail at the capital. Accepted ways of addressing public officials are found in Exhibit 10.2. Then, follow these guidelines:

Do:

1. Identify yourself as a nurse and a constituent.
2. State the specific reason for the letter.
3. Be brief and to the point.
4. Use local examples (legislators like to use these anecdotes in their speeches).
5. Give reasons for your objections or support.
6. Use correct spelling and grammar and a typed business letter format.
7. Include the bill number and title or at least its popular name, for instance, the Nurse Education Bill.

Don't:

1. Be trivial.
2. Be insulting, sarcastic, or threatening.
3. Use a form letter.

If speed is important, as when a vote is pending, use the telephone, a fax, or a telegram. Night letters are generous in the number of words allowed and inexpensive; a 20-word public interest telegram can be sent to any senator, congressman, or to the President or Vice-President, for a minimal cost.

If you support the legislator (or any candidate), then it is politically

EXHIBIT 10.2

How to Address Public Officials

Official	Address	Official	Address
President	The President of the United States The White House Washington, DC 20500 Dear Mr. President:	Assemblywoman	The Hon. Mary Doe The State House Trenton, NJ 08625 Dear Ms. Doe:
Governor	The Hon. John Doe Executive Chamber Albany, NY 12224 Dear Governor Doe:	Mayor	The Hon. John Doe City Hall New York, NY 10007 Dear Mayor Doe:
US Senator	Senator John Doe Senate Office Building Washington, DC 20510 Dear Senator Doe:	City Councilman	The Hon. John Doe City Council New York, NY 10007 Dear Mr. Doe:
Congressman	The Hon. John Doe House Office Building Washington, DC 20515 Dear Mr. Doe or Dear Congressman:	Judge	The Hon. Mary Doe (Address of Court) Dear Judge Doe:
State Senator	The Hon. John Doe Senate Chambers Albany, NY 12224 Dear Senator:	Other officials	(Not included above) The Hon. John Doe Dear Mr. Doe

Note: Addresses for state and local officials vary by locale.

smart to contribute to their election campaign and/or volunteer your services in the campaign. These might include house-to-house canvassing to check voter registration or to survey public support; supplying transportation to the polls; making telephone calls to stimulate registration and voting; acting as registration clerk and watcher, poll clerk and watcher, block leader, or precinct captain; raising funds; preparing mailing pieces; planning publicity; writing and distributing news releases; making speeches; answering telephones; staffing information booths; planning campaign events; or having "coffees" to meet the candidate.

Nurses who are knowledgeable about a particular issue are sometimes asked by ANA or another group to testify before a congressionl committee. This requires both know-how and assurance but it can be a very interesting and satisfying experience. However, it is important to be properly prepared and do it right. [For details on how to testify, see Kelly and Joel, *Dimenions of Professional Nursing*, 7th ed. New York: McGraw-Hill, 1995, pp 418–420.]

Nurses should never loose sight of the critical mass they represent, and the fact that public demonstrations, if done tastefully, can make a point that is impossible to ignore. On March 31 of 1995, 35,000 nurses marched on Washington DC to protest the dangerous conditions which exist in health care as cost-cutting becomes the driving force for change.

OVERVIEW OF FEDERAL AGENCIES

The federal agencies with responsibility for health care are primarily within the Department of Health and Human Services (DHHS), although certain health-related programs are administered by other departments. An example is the Food Stamps Program, which the Department of Agriculture administers. Within DHHS, there are several major agencies: the Public Health Service (PHS), Health Care Financing Administration (HCFA), and Administration for Children and Families (see Exhibit 10.3). Other divisions, such as the Administration on Aging and the Office for Civil Rights, also lie within DHHS. Most of the programs discussed in this chapter are under the auspices of the HCFA or the PHS. In 1994, Congress passed legislation that authorized a separate Social Security Administration, effective March 31, 1995. Until then, the Social Security Administration was an agency within DHHS, but legislators figured that making it a separate entity might help increase its visibility, accountability, and administrative efficiency.[5]

The HCFA administers the Medicare and Medicaid programs. The PHS includes the Agency for Health Care Policy and Research (AHCPR), Agency for Toxic Substances and Disease Registry, Centers for Disease Control and Prevention, Food and Drug Administration (FDA), Health

EXHIBIT 10.3

Department of Health and Human Services

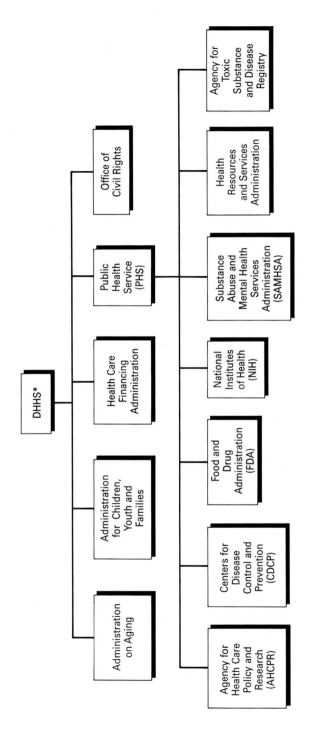

*The Social Security Administration was part of DHHS until 1995, when it became a separate agency.

Resources and Services Administration (HRSA), Indian Health Service, National Institutes of Health (NIH), and the Substance Abuse and Mental Health Services Administration (SAMHSA). The Division of Nursing within the HRSA and the National Institute of Nursing Research (NINR) at the NIH are focal points for nursing initiatives at the federal level and are discussed later in this chapter. However, nurses are involved in every agency listed, and the activities of each agency have an impact on nursing practice.

MAJOR LEGISLATION AFFECTING NURSING

Both federal and state laws have a major impact on nursing practice and education. At the state level, nurses need to know about their own nursing practice acts and should be acquainted with the licensure laws of other health practitioners. These are discussed in Chapter 11. Other state legislation affecting the health and welfare of nurses may be equally important, and you should keep abreast of both proposed and enacted legislation.

In this section, the focus is on federal legislation that affects the practice of nursing and the rights of nurses; occasionally, state laws that are almost univeral or closely related to federal laws are included. Obviously, all health legislation fits into that category, but those laws that seem to have particular significance are highlighted here.

Social Security

The Social Security Act, passed in 1935 and amended many times since, is the origin of most health and social welfare programs in this country. The act includes many titles or components, each covering a different program. The average person who talks of Social Security is most likely referring to the Old-Age, Survivors' and Disability Insurance (OASDI), which provides benefits after retirement age or in case of total disability. Contributions to OASDI are withheld from the employee's wage, and matched by the employer. Deductions appear on the employee's paycheck under "FICA" (Federal Insurance Contributions Act). Self-employed individuals are also required to contribute. In recent years, the aging of the US population has raised concerns about the solvency of the Social Security Trust Fund. In response, Congress has periodically enacted legislation to protect the program while ensuring that beneficiaries receive adequate payments.

Medicare

Medicare, authorized under Title XVIII of the Social Security Act, is a nationwide health insurance program for the aged and certain disabled persons. In both of the two parts (A and B) of Medicare, the benefits are limited to those who are 65 years of age or older and some disabled persons under 65.

Most Americans are automatically eligible for Part A, which consists of hospital insurance (HI), upon turning 65. Others, who are disabled or in need of kidney dialysis, qualify regardless of age. Under Part A, the patient pays a small deductible (which has been increasing) for hospital care, and the federal government pays the rest. Part A also covers skilled nursing facilities, home health care, and hospice care, with certain limits in each category.

Part B of Medicare is an optional supplemental medical insurance (SMI) program available to those over 65 upon payment of a monthly premium. SMI is financed through these premiums, along with general government funds. Most Part A beneficiaries are eligible to enroll in Part B. Part B pays 80 percent of the established fee for physicians' services in excess of an annual deductible. Services covered include the physician's care in the hospital, home, or office; laboratory and other diagnostic tests; outpatient services at a hospital; therapeutic equipment such as braces; home health services; mammograms; and respite care for caretakers of homebound Medicare beneficiaries. Certain services, such as long-term and preventive care that the elderly often need, are still unavailable under Medicare. Long-term care, in particular, is likely to be an area to which Congress will devote more attention in the near future as the demand for such services increases and the costs escalate.

The Medicare program is the responsibility of HCFA. HCFA enters into contracts with Blue Cross-Blue Shield, commercial carriers, and group practice prepayment plans to serve as administrative agents.

Medicare Legislation

Since 1966, Congress has enacted a number of Medicare amendments aimed primarily at controlling the soaring costs of the program. There are now rigid regulations regarding the length of the institutional stay that will be reimbursed and payment for specific services. Another major concern, quality of care, has also resulted in amendments.

The most far-reaching legislative changes were the provisions of the *Tax Equity and Fiscal Responsibility Act* (TEFRA) of 1982 (PL 97-248). This legislation required the Secretary of DHHS and certain congressional committees to develop Medicare prospective payment legislative proposals for hospitals, skilled nursing facilities (SNFs), and, to the extent feasible, other providers. Other cost-cutting mechanisms affecting health care facilities and providers were also included.

The work on the prospective payment mechanisms resulted in enactment of PL 98-21, variously called the *Social Security Amendments of 1983*, the *Social Security Rescue Plan*, or simply the *DRG law*. This legislation established a prospective payment system based on 467 Diagnostic Related Groups (DRGs) categories that establish pretreatment diagnosis billing amounts for almost all United States hospitals reimbursed by Medicare.

What DRGs mean to a hospital is that if a patient uses more resources (days and services) than designated by the patient's DRG category, the extra costs must be absorbed. If the patient uses less, the dollar amount designated is the hospital's clear profit.

Needless to say, the DRG system had a direct effect on nursing. (See the References for specific articles on how nurses work within the DRG system.) In some cases, hospitals desperate to cut costs chose to retain lower-paid nursing personnel, rather than RNs. Others chose to turn to all-RN staffs that could actually save money by teaching patients or by anticipating potential complications, so that the patient would be discharged before the DRG-set time. As noted in Chapter 6, the job market for nurses became tighter for a while. However, some nurses felt that this was a good time to cost-out nursing services so that they could be separated from general daily charges. Others identified ways of determining patient-specific variations in nursing resource use[7] so that these could be considered in the DRG system.[6] In general, the Medicare prospective payment system has encouraged all health care providers, including nurses, to be more aware of the cost components in health care. For nursing, this has been an advantage. Increasingly, nurse researchers have been able to document the cost effectiveness of nurse providers. This, in turn, contributed to the enactment of legislation providing for reimbursement of nurses under federal and state health programs. Prospective payment also resulted in hospitals discharging patients "quicker and sicker." This led hospital administrators to appreciate, more than they previously did, the indispensable role that nurses have in caring for patients with higher levels of acuity in all types of health care settings.

The 1983 Medicare legislation also mandated the formation of peer review organizations (PROs) to replace the then existing professional standards review organizations (PSROs). The intent of the legislation was to establish mechanisms for quality assurance by private entities in a competitive market. PROs review only Medicare services (appropriateness of admission, discharge and the use of resources during the episode in the delivery system). In general, each state has one PRO. However, some larger states have subcontracts with regional units. Nurses have been involved with PROs as staff and as members of PRO review boards. Consumers also play a significant role in PROs, because the 1983 law mandated that a certain proportion of the members of the PRO boards be composed of consumers. PROs are organized through the American Medical Peer Review Organization (AMPRO), based in Washington, DC.

Since the enactment of prospective payment in 1983, there have been a series of revisions in Medicare through legislation and regulation. Many of the new laws deal with prospective payment rates and Part B reimbursement based on recommendations of the Prospective Payment Assessment Commission (ProPAC) and the Physician Payment Review Commission (PPRC) respectively. Nursing has had an impact on these deliberations through the nurse representatives on the Commissions, through studies of the costing out of nursing services under DRGs and the practice of APNs, and through the lobbying of major nursing organizations. Congress has also approved changes in the scope of services provided under Medicare. In 1990, Pap smears, mammography, and expansion of hospice benefits were added.

In addition to increasing the scope of services provided, Medicare revisions have included reimbursement for a variety of providers once excluded from the program. In recent years, nurses have successfully lobbied for Medicare reimbursement. The year 1989 was a major one for legislation on nursing and physician reform under Medicare. First, certified registered nurse anesthetists (CRNAs) succeeded in obtaining legislation (PL 99-509) that authorized direct reimbursement under Medicare to CRNAs for anesthesia services that they are legally authorized to perform in the state.

Second, the 1989 reconciliation bill authorized nurse practitioners (NPs) and clinical nurse specialists (CNSs), working in collaboration with a physician, to certify and recertify the need for nursing home care under Medicare. A nursing home could be paid for the services of a gerontological nurse practitioner (GNP). As a result of other policy, APNs may be reimbursed when they practice in a Federally Qualified Health Center (FQHC), or in rural or medically underserved areas. The next step is legislation to allow direct reimbursement of all APNs regardless of practice site or geography.

Third, the reconciliation bill mandated a PPRC study of nonphysician providers, to be submitted to Congress by July 1, 1991. Nurses had input to the call for this study through their representatives on the PPRC and the lobbying of ANA and other nursing organizations.

The PPRC's work, in general, became the focus of attention when Congress began to reevaluate the system under which Medicare pays physicians' fees. Some of this concern was due to the dramatically rising costs of Medicare Part B, especially compared to the better controlled increases in Part A. The 1989 bill revamped the system of paying doctors on the basis of "customary, prevailing, and reasonable fees" and replaced it with a standard based on the total cost of the service provided, including the cost of maintaining a practice, liability insurance, and the relative value of the technical skills needed.

The new system is based on a resource-based relative-value schedule (RBRVS) that places emphasis on the service performed for a patient, instead of the traditional way of allocating fees according to the specialization of the provider. These changes in physician reimbursement under Medicare have provided incentives for review of nonphysician and noninstitutional reimbursement, including reimbursement for nurses.

In 1991, the PPRC recommended that nonphysician practitioners (including certain nurses) under Medicare should also be paid based on RBRVS, taking into account the differences in education and training between physicians and nonphysician providers.[7]

Medicaid

Medicaid was authorized in 1965 as Title XIX of the Social Security Act to pay for medical services on behalf of certain groups of low-income persons. It is a federal-state means-tested entitlement program, which HCFA also administers. Certain groups of persons (i.e., the aged, blind, disabled and members of families with dependent children, among others) qualify for coverage if their incomes and resources are sufficiently low. Each state designs and administers its own Medicaid program, setting eligibility and coverage standards within broad federal guidelines. As a result, substantial variation exists among the states in terms of persons covered, types and scope of benefits offered, and amount of payments for services. On the average, the federal government pays 56 percent of the benefit costs and states pay the rest. Until 1986, Medicaid eligibility was tied to welfare. In that year, Medicaid was extended to include certain women and children with low incomes who were not covered by the Aid to Families with Dependent Children (AFDC) program. This change was important because state poverty levels are considerably lower than the federal poverty level and were used as AFDC eligibility criteria, thus keeping many poor women and children from receiving necessary health care.

The expansion of Medicaid in recent years has occurred incrementally, with intense deliberations at state and federal levels of government. The discussions focused on what states were required and had the option to provide under Medicaid. The changes have had a significant impact on access to and financing of health care for America's women and children. However, the escalating costs have caused states to cut back services. Some, such as Oregon, have set up plans that will allow more primary care and preventive services and limit more expensive services that are seen as less necessary.

In 1989, nurses reached another milestone when Congress enacted legislation providing for coverage of family nurse practitioner and pediatric nurse practitioner services under Medicaid, as long as they are practicing within the scope of state law. Since July 1990, states have been required to cover the services of these two types of NPs, regardless of whether they are under the supervision of or associated with a physician.

Medicare and Medicaid in Later Days

The 104th Congress (1994–1996) created a new political landscape in the nation's capitol, as well as in many state legislatures. With the balance of power moving to the Republicans in both the House and the Senate in 1994, there was commitment to honor campaign promises which called for an eventually balanced budget, a reduction in the heavy hand of government, and a renewed emphasis on states' rights. Since very little of the federal budget is actually discretionary, reducing spending means inevitable cuts in public entitlement programs. The Medicare and Medicaid programs represent a major financial commitment and have always been shaped and reshaped as a political expedient. With increases in copayments and deductibles, older Americans are paying more out of pocket today (in dollars adjusted to a 1996 standard) than before Medicare. The prevailing technique to control Medicaid spending has been to offer a broad package of services but to pay so little to providers for delivering those services that Medicaid patients are rejected out-of-hand in many instances. The inappropriate use of hospital emergency rooms by the poor for primary care can be traced to the fact that other providers refuse to give care because of reimbursement which is inadequate to even sustain overhead in most cases. Hospitals cannot refuse and still qualify for federal and state monies in the form of either payment for services or programs. Financial games have allowed Medicare to survive because the poor elderly are eventually subsidized by the Medicaid program if their Medicare benefits terminate. But there are many elderly with personal resources, and they represent a large and powerful political constituency. Medicare reimbursement rates are within reason, and the requirement that providers accept the established rate as payment in-full for the poor elderly is the safety net. Medicare is fully federally funded, and so federal criteria can be imposed, resulting in equity for all recipients. In contrast, the poor are often voiceless, and states must only comply with broad standards to obtain federal matching dollars. The latitude in those standards can easily create inequity.

With the traditional games wearing thin and a new Congress mandated to cut federal spending, significant financial and structural changes are inevitable and those changes which do not require legislation are already well on the way. For Medicare and Medicaid, allowable growth will likely be capped at 5 percent and 4 percent respectively.[8] This holds serious implications for Medicare where growth has consistently been 10 percent per year. The shortfall will be the responsibility of the beneficiary, and from there to Medicaid. Medicaid faces bigger problems. In 1994, nursing home care accounted for 32 percent of Medicaid expenditures; and 53 percent of all nursing home residents are Medicaid beneficiaries.[9] Only 16 percent of the Medicaid dollars going to long-term care are used for home and community based services, but growth in this area is guaranteed.[10]

Medicare and Medicaid are on the fast track moving toward managed care. In some situations special federal waivers are necessary, but they have been easily forthcoming, with a Democratic administration anxious to support any strategy that might reduce the likelihood of deep program cuts or tax increases. For the most part, these managed care programs are marketed as Medicare or Medicaid Plans, thereby setting them apart and creating tiers. And they are different. For the poor, there are facilities and providers that need patients or need beds filled. They are willing to negotiate lower rates just to survive. These plans are offered by the same corporations that create networks (plans) for those insured through the workplace or by personal pay. Medicare recipients have been encouraged to select managed care through the "Medicare Select" Program which offers discounted "Medigap" coverage when you join a managed care program. The program was piloted in 15 states, but has not been properly evaluated. Despite this, the Congress has already expanded the program to all 50 states and extended its life, expecting eventual evaluation before it becomes permanent.[11] By the Fall of 1995, 10 percent of Medicare recipients were enrolled in managed care programs.

Block Grants

The block grant approach consolidates categorical programs into blocks and turns over control of money to the states, with little accounting to the federal government as to how the funds are spent. Block grants are funded through federal and state-matched funds. They shift much of the political and administrative accountability to the states, without subsequent increases in state funding, and they intensify inequities among states in terms of the populations covered by the programs. The major advantage of block grants is the streamlining they provide at the federal level by consolidating programs into clusters for legislative and programmatic purposes.

In 1981, three health block grants were formed: maternal and child health, preventive services, and mental health (including alcohol and drug abuse). Congress originally designated a primary care block grant that consisted of community and migrant health center programs, but it was never officially made a block grant, and today it remains a categorical program.

The Alcohol, Drug Abuse, and Mental Health Administration (ADAMHA) Block Grant is a high priority because it includes the drug abuse prevention programs that are part of the "war on drugs." The Maternal and Child Health Block Grant continues to gain support because of the country's unacceptably high infant mortality rate. The Prevention Block Grant is considered important because of the growing evidence that disease prevention and health promotion initiatives are cost effective and improve health status in many ways.

Sentiment remains strong for turning over the Medicaid programs to each state in the form of a "block grant." The debate will rage around what degree of oversight the federal government would retain, and what (if any) standard would be required.[12]

Health Services Legislation

Various other laws providing health care programs and services of interest to nurses include the following: *The Health Maintenance Organization Act* of 1973 authorized the spending of $375 million during the next five years to help set up and evaluate HMOs in communities throughout the country. The concept is an arrangement in which subscribers pay a predetermined flat fee monthly or yearly that entitles them to basic health care services as needed. Emphasis is on preventive care and self care and life-style changes through health teaching (see Chapter 3).

During the 1980s, federal funding for AIDS became a hot topic. The federal AIDS policies are extremely fragmented, lacking well-coordinated programs in health care or education. Nonetheless, the government supports a wide range of programs, which many AIDS advocates believe is still insufficient given the needs for research, community-based alternatives, and support for health professionals.

The *Ryan White Act*, named after an Indiana teenager who died of AIDS, provided $633 million in 1995 for economic assistance to cities with the highest incidence of AIDS to help absorb the cost of care. In the four years since its initial funding, Ryan White will have awarded more than $2 billion.[13] By the end of fiscal year 1996, Medicare will be spending about $690 million on AIDS treatment and care.[14] The rising cost to Medicare represents the increased lifespan of people with AIDS, who also need long-term care and support in their disability. Though the Ryan White dollars may sound positive, they are too little, given the extent of the problem. In 1994 alone, 80,691 new cases were identified and this only represents cases that were reported.[15]

One of the most controversial issues pertaining to AIDS is whether the federal government should be allowed to limit immigration to this country of people who are infected with HIV. AIDS activists are against such measures, arguing that it violates human rights. Other more conservative players and government officials, even within the Clinton administration, have taken a different stand. They claim that AIDS is a public health threat, that neither the federal government nor the American taxpayer can afford to care for these individuals, and that lenient immigration policies with regard to HIV/AIDS increase the public's risk of transmission. This policy was enacted into law under the 1993 NIH reauthorization bill (PL 103–43). However, the US attorney general has the right to grant waivers from the exclusion. Nurses, public health professionals, and other civil rights groups continue to challenge this exclusionary policy, because HIV is not spread by casual contact, and the policy restricts the freedom of many individuals, in particular refugees seeking political asylum here.

Also in the 1980s, one of Congress's attempts to combine concerns about the cost and quality of health care was the establishment of the *Agency for Health Care Policy and Research* (AHCPR) within the PHS. The agency was authorized under OBRA 1989 (PL 101-239), replacing what had been the National Center for Health Services Research and Health Care Technology Assessment. The mission of the AHCPR includes conducting research on the quality and effectiveness of health care services, developing practice guidelines, and assessing technology. The agency has the primary responsibility for implementing the Medical Treatment Effectiveness Program (MedTEP) within the DHHS. The purpose of MedTEP is to improve the effectiveness and appropriateness of health care services through better understanding of the effects of health care practices—including nursing—on patient outcomes. The effectiveness initiatives are of particular importance because many policymakers look to effectiveness research as a way of controlling health care costs, empowering the consumer, reducing malpractice claims and providing equity in treatment and care. The AHCPR, through a series of expert panels, each with nursing representation, has issued guidelines describing the professional consensus on the management of specific disease conditions. The conditions chosen for guideline development were: present in high volume; costly to the public; considerably variable in the manner of diagnosis and treatment; yet supported by a large body of knowledge which should have resulted in more agreement on the proper course of clinical management. Legal opinion cautions that these guidelines establish a standard for practice.[16] Guidelines are available in postoperative pain management, depression in ambulatory care, incontinence, prevention of decubiti, cataracts with lens implantation, to name a few.

Nursing Education and Research

In the 1960s, as the federal government urged the enactment of legislation to provide health care for the aged under Social Security, health facilities and personnel became matters of urgency to Washington. More and more funds were channeled into health and education projects. At the same time, nurses were becoming more vocal, and their organizations stronger, more self-assured, and more convincing when their representatives met with legislators and appeared before legislative committees. As a result of these and other factors, several new laws were enacted in the early 1960s that supported nursing and the individual nurse.

Most significant among these was the *Nurse Training Act* of 1964 (Title VIII of the Public Health Service Act). (For more details on federal funding of nursing education, see Chapter 19 in the fifth edition of *Dimensions of Professional Nursing*.) The purpose of this law was to increase the number of nurses through financial assistance to diploma, associate degree, and baccalaureate degree nursing schools, students, and graduates taking advanced courses, and thus to help ensure more and better schools of nursing, more carefully selected students, a high standard of teaching, and better health care for people.

Renewal of the law has had its ups and downs over two decades, especially during the era of retrenchment in the early 1980s. However, due to the successful lobbying of nursing organizations, and individuals across the country, the program remained on the books. In 1985, federal legislation for nursing education was renamed the *Nurse Education Act* (NEA). That year was also a landmark year for nurses because it marked the establishment of the National Center for Nursing Research (NCNR) at NIH. Nurses claimed victory on November 20, when the Senate voted 89 to 7 to override President Reagan's veto of the NIH bill. The House had already supported the bill in its 380 to 32 vote to override the veto the previous week. The bill culminated several years of negotiations among the various interest groups, legislative chambers, and branches of government. Within a short time, the center was up and running. Since its inception, the center has begun collaborative intramural research (within NIH) on topics such as the frail elderly, extramural grants to schools of nursing, a research program in bio-ethics and clinical practice, and research initiatives for low-birthweight babies and patients with HIV infections. In 1993, NCNR became the National Institute of Nursing Research (NINR).

The NEA and the NINR have maintained competitive funding levels and even grown in the toughest of economic times. NEA was appropriated $63.5 million in 1995, and NINR reached close to $53 million.[17] Of significant concern is the President's interest in consolidating funding for education of the health professions. Of further concern is the fact that most nursing education monies are concentrated in the NEA, as opposed to smaller amounts buried in a range of legislative initiatives. The need to diversify has been raised by a number of seasoned public policy experts. Since its inception in 1965, the Medicare program has contributed dollars to the training of health professionals. *Graduate Medical Education* (GME) expenditures for nursing have traditionally gone to hospital-based nursing education programs. The Tri-Council for Nursing is actively lobbying to shift funding from programs culminating in a diploma to the education of APNs and "RN to MSN" programs.

Support for other health professions education (medicine, osteopathy, dentistry, veterinary medicine, optometry, podiatry, and pharmacy), known by its acronym, MODVOPP, has been through such early laws as the *Health Professions Education Assistance Act* of 1963 and its successors. This law has a funding history similar to that of the NEA.

Employee Protections

Workmen's compensation is becoming ever more important to nurses as the hazards of their work and workplace increase. These include exposure to environmental hazards, some of which are described in Chapter 15, and potentially fatal diseases such as AIDS and hepatitis B. The first such insurance to be held constitutional was the *Workmen's Compensation Act*, enacted by the state of Washington in 1911. Today all states require employers in industry to carry workmen's compensation, but in some states, nonprofit organizations, including hospitals, are exempt. However, most nurses are covered by some version of this type of insurance. Federal employees are usually covered by the *Federal Employees' Compensation Act*, enacted in 1952.

Workmen's compensation insurance, the cost of which is carried entirely by the employer, pays to employees who are injured on the job a proportion of their regular salaries for the time they are unable to work because of their injuries. If they are permanently disabled, they are entitled to additional compensation. Workmen's compensation insurance laws do away with the requirement of proof that the employer was negligent or that the employee was free from contributory negligence. They also prevent court action for injuries and provide instead an administrative procedure for securing awards of compensation.

Many states have extended the coverage provided by workmen's compensation laws to include occupational diseases; other states have enacted separate occupational disease acts, some of which cover all types of occupational disease; others specify which ones are covered.

The major breakthrough on the federal level was the enactment of the *Occupational Safety and Health Act* of 1970 (also discussed in Chapter 3), which established administrative machinery for the development and enforcement of standards of occupational health and safety.

In recent years, health professionals and policy experts have placed growing attention on the importance of occupational health and safety, largely because of the increases in rates of many infectious diseases, such as tuberculosis, hepatitis, and HIV/AIDS. In December 1992, the *Occupational Safety and Health Administration* (OSHA) released standards on prevention of bloodborne diseases, requiring nurses and other health workers to receive protection. The standards require all employers to provide hepatitis B immunizations, as well as protective equipment and procedures, to prevent transmission of hepatitis B, HIV, and other infectious diseases.

More information on HIV/AIDS and the workplace is included in Chapter 15. In 1994, the CDCP issued guidelines for preventing the transmission of tuberculosis in health care facilities. OSHA has resisted requiring compliance with this standard.[18] In the summer of 1995, OSHA released a draft of voluntary guidelines on workplace violence.

Another occupational safety and health development occurred in May 1993, when a new *Office of Occupational Health Nursing* was established at OSHA "to underscore the major role such nurses play in striving for safe and healthful workplaces." The office will increase the visibility of nurses within OSHA and in related activities across the country.

Finally, nurses have joined with others involved with occupational safety and health to push for reform of the *Occupational Safety and Health Act*, which has not been revised since its original enactment in 1970. One of the most important proposals for reform is to extend coverage under the law to public employees. Approximately 323,000 nurses work in national, state, or local governmental hospital settings, and they, as well as other public employees, are often exposed to bloodborne pathogens (as well as other risk factors) and are entitled to the same protection as their colleagues in the private sector.[19]

Civil Rights, Employment, and Labor Relations

Beginning in the 1960s, a number of laws were passed to prohibit discrimination on sex as well as race, color, religion, and national origin. Many of these are particularly important to women and are referred to in Chapter 15. Some of the most important ones are discussed below. (Comparable worth issues and other rights are discussed in Chapter 9.)

Title VII of the *Civil Rights Act* of 1964 (Equal Employment Opportunity Law) has affected the job status of nurses because it includes a section forbidding discrimination against women in job hiring and job promotion among private employers of more than 25 persons. Executive Order No. 11246, as amended, extended the law to include federal contractors and subcontractors. Hospitals and colleges are subject to this order because of their acceptance of federal grants of various kinds.

Among other civil rights that have been given new protection are the rights of patients, children, the mentally ill, prisoners, the elderly, and the handicapped. Actions to protect these rights have come through a variety of legal means at state and national levels. Protection has increasingly been specified through regulations of various laws such as the amendments and subsequent regulations of the Social Security Act. Another is the *Rehabilitation Act* of 1973. Section 504 of that law reads, "no otherwise qualified handicapped individual in the United States shall, solely by reason of his handicap, be excluded from the participation in, be denied the benefit of, or be subjected to discrimination under any program or activity receiving federal financial assistance." The definition of *handicapped* includes drug addicts and alcoholics, as well as those having an overt physical impairment such as blindness, deafness, or paralysis of some kind. A major issue now is whether and under what circumstances AIDS patients and HIV-infected people come under this law. Some state and local jurisdictions have ruled that AIDS-related illness does come under their laws as a protected handicap. Those that do not consider communicable diseases as protected have ruled differently. In recent years, there have been two types of renewed civil rights activities. First, the *Americans with Disabilities Act* was enacted in 1990 with the intent of barring firms from denying jobs to individuals solely on the basis of disability, as long as reasonable accommodations can be made. The legislation is aimed at protecting the nearly 43 million disabled Americans, including people infected with HIV. Discrimination is prohibited in areas such as public accommodations, transportation, and private employment. This did not prevent an applicant to a nursing school who was hearing impaired from being refused. The Supreme Court upheld the decision.

In 1991, following a veto the previous year, President Bush signed the *Civil Rights Act* of 1991. The legislation was in response to 1989 Supreme Court rulings that shifted the burden of proof from employer to employee in cases where employees experience discrimination. The 1991 bill restored the previous standard by requiring employers to prove that the hiring practice is required for the job in question. The bill pertains mostly to women and minority members who claim to have experienced discrimination in job hiring situations. Its enactment was an important step in sustaining the civil rights of all Americans.

The right to privacy also affects nurses. One of the most important federal laws in this area is the *Freedom of Information Act* (FOIA) of 1966 and the *Privacy Act* of 1974. The purpose of the FOIA is to give the public access to files maintained by the executive branch of government. Recognizing that there are valid reasons for withholding certain records, the law exempts broad categories of records from compulsory public inspection, including medical records. It also gives access to their hospital records to patients in federal hospitals.

Another step in providing access to the individual's own records was enactment of the *Family Educational Rights and Privacy Act* of 1974, also known as the *Buckley Amendment*. The basic intent of this law was to provide students, their patients, and guardians with easier access to and control over the information contained in academic records. Educational records are defined broadly and include files, documents, and other materials containing information about the student and maintained by a school. Students must be allowed to inspect these records within 45 days of their request. They need not be allowed access to confidential letters of reference preceding January 1975, records about students made by teachers and administrators for their own use and not shown to others, certain campus police records, certain parental financial records, and certain psychiatric treatment records (if not available to anyone else). Students may challenge the content, secure the correction of inaccurate information, and insert a written explanation regarding the content of their records.

The law also specifies who has access to the records (teachers, educational administrators, organizations such as testing services, state and other officials to whom certain information must be reported according to the law). Otherwise, the records cannot be released without the student's consent. The law applies to nursing education programs as well as others.

The right of research subjects have also been incorporated in diverse federal laws, especially in the last decade. PL 93-348, the *National Research Act* of 1974, not only provided some funds for nursing research but also set controls on research, including the establishment of a committee to identify requirements for informed consent, and required an institutional committee to review a research project to protect the patient's rights. The 1974 *Privacy Act* required a clear, informed consent for those participating in research. The 1971 *Food and Drug Act* also gave some protection in regulating the use of experimental drugs, including notification to the patient that a drug is experimental. The *Drug Regulation Reform Act* of 1978 took further steps to protect the patient receiving research drugs. Other drug and narcotics laws also affect nursing.

The *Comprehensive Drug Abuse Prevention and Control Act* of 1970 (Controlled Substance Act) replaced virtually all other federal laws dealing with narcotics, depressants, stimulants, and hallucinogens. It controls the handling of drugs by providers, including hospitals. The *Drug Regulation Reform Act* of 1978 took further steps in protecting the patient; at the same time, the FDA set requirements about sharing product information on drugs with consumers.

Also within the broad categories of rights are those laws related to labor relations. The first was the *National Labor Relations Act* (NLRA), one of several laws enacted to pull the country out of the Great Depression. The thesis was that labor unions could prevent employers from lowering wages, resulting in higher incomes and more spending. To achieve the growth of unions, employers had to be limited; for instance, they could no longer legally fire employees who tried to unionize. The National Labor Relations Board (NLRB), created by law, was empowered to investigate and initiate administrative proceedings against those employers who violated the law. (If these administrative actions did not curtail the illegal acts, court action followed. Only employers' violations were listed.)

In 1947, the NLRA was substantially amended, and the amended law, entitled the *Labor Management Relations Act* (or *Taft–Hartley Act*), listed prohibitions for unions. Section 14(b), for instance, contained the so-called right-to-work clause, which authorizes states to enact more stringent union security provisions than those contained in the federal laws.

In 1959, a third major modification was made. One of the purposes of the law, the *Labor-Management Reporting and Disclosure Act* or *Landrum–Griffin Act,* was to curb documented union abuses such as corrupt financial and election procedures. For this reason, it is sometimes called the union members' Bill of Rights. The result is a series of rights and responsibilities of members of a union or a professional organization, such as ANA, that engages in collective bargaining. Required are reporting and disclosure of certain financial transactions and administrative practices and the use of democratic election procedures. That is, every member in good standing must be able to nominate candidates and run for election and must be allowed to vote and support candidates; there must be secret ballot elections; union funds must not be used to assist the candidacy of an individual seeking union office; candidates must have access to the membership list; records of the election must be preserved for one year; and elections must be conducted according to the procedures specified in the bylaws.

Highly significant for nurses is the 1974 law that again amended the Taft–Hartley Act, PL 93-360, the *Nonprofit Health Care Amendments.* This law made private nonprofit health care facilities that had, through considerable lobbying, been excluded in the 1947 law, subject to national labor laws. These employees were now free to join or not join a union without employer retribution, a right previously denied to them unless they worked in a state that had its own law allowing them to unionize. It also created special notification procedures that must precede any strike action. The definition of *health care facility* included a broad range of acute care and community health care facilities.

In 1991 and 1994, there were Supreme Court decisions of major significance to nursing and labor representation. The 1991 ruling upheld the NLRB's rule-making which sanctioned a separate collective bargaining unit for nurses. And further found LPNs appropriately included with technical employees in light of their skill level. In 1994, the court decided that a licensed practical nurse employed by a nursing home was a statutory supervisor because of her relationship with nurses aides. Therefore, she was ineligible for the legal protections offered to other employees. These issues are also discussed in Chapter 15.

The inadequacies of labor law observed in the 1994 decision have been a continuing frustration to the courts, management and the labor community. The Commission on the Future of Worker–Management Relations was created to review existing labor laws and speak on the need for corrective legislation. Observation tells us workers are different today. They want personal expression in their work, job security, and control over their day-to-day life in the workplace. In the existing economic environment, that is only possible when labor and management come together to save their industries. Commonly referred to as the *Dunlop Commission*, the panel reported in 1995 and recommended the creation of labor–management committees. (It will be this provision that is suspicious, given the existing strict definitions of company-created unions.) Otherwise, the important recommendation is to narrow the definition of supervisor with the intent of protecting professionals.[20] The report has gone to the Congress with drafting of legislation at the Congress' pleasure.

The strike is the ultimate weapon in collective bargaining, and used respectfully. The effect is weakened and retribution towards striking workers permitted when permanent striker replacements are hired. If the primary goal of collective bargaining is to level the playing field between labor and management, the strategy of permanent striker replacement frustrates that aim. In 1995, through issuance of an Executive Order, the President barred federal contractors from hiring permanent striker replacements.[21]

The nursing shortage of the late 1980s put us into a tailspin. Commissions were created to study the problem, our organizations came together in national recruitment efforts, and we looked to enhance our pool of registered nurses through foreign recruitment and immigration. *The Immigration Nursing Relief Act* of 1990 established a 5-year pilot project for use of a special work visa (H-1A) specific to foreign educated nurses who enter the United States. An INS crackdown in 1990 threatened deportation of a large number of nurses. Rather than chance a significant reduction in employed nurses during a time of shortage, those with expired visas were given an opportunity to convert to permanent status. Others were recruited on the new status, and employers were required to produce assurances that no US citizen was available to fill the position, and that steps were being taken to decrease dependence on foreign-educated nurses. In 1995, ANA and unions representing nurses opposed reauthorization in light of the downsizing in hospitals and current surplus of nurses.[22] The program sunsetted in August 1995.

Another piece of nursing legislation in the labor arena was the *Nurse Pay Act* of 1990. It was intended to enhance recruitment and retention of nurses in the Veteran's Administration (VA). Since the bill was implemented in April 1991, recruitment of VA nurses has improved. However, retention has been difficult due to the unintended salary compression of certain nurses, especially those earning a mid-range salary.

A different type of right that should be reported is the revision of the *Copyright Law*, amended in 1976 to supersede the 1909 law. The categories of work covered include writings, works of art, music, and pantomimes. The owner is given exclusive rights to reproduce the copyrighted work. The new law has some significance in this time of photocopying from journals and books; there are certain limits and need for permission to copy anything beyond certain minimums. Libraries can provide the appropriate information. Some books and journals specify their copying permission requirements.

A National Health Plan

Our patchwork system of health care delivery and insurance has resulted in approximately 37 million individuals lacking health insurance, one third of whom are children and an equal amount with inadequate coverage. Furthermore, contrary to popular belief, the majority of uninsured people are working or dependents of people who are working.

In the 1980s and 1990s, policymakers discussed various proposals to provide health coverage for the uninsured. The major obstacles to all of these proposals were that the burden of cost would fall on different groups, depending on the policy scheme, and that invariably the plans involved increased costs and spending. In addition, each plan targeted a different group and, unless Congress accepted some form of national health plan, there was no way to provide coverage for everyone.

Underlying all of these proposals are unanswered questions about health care as a right or a privilege. If one assumes that access to affordable health care is a right, then which level of government is responsible for it? The issue of equity needs to be addressed. Are all individuals entitled to the same level and quality of health care, regardless of their ability to pay for their care? Or can we accept a two-tiered system of care wherein those who can afford to pay more are entitled to the better quality and quantity of services their money can buy? Although the answers to these questions seem elusive, they raise important issues for nurses to consider as they become increasingly involved with the health care system.

In 1989, Congress took action to alleviate the burden of health insurance on the disabled by passing a law extending the period in which employers must let former workers who are disabled keep the group rate. The period was extended from 18 to 29 months, and the law is expected to protect the disabled, including individuals infected with HIV.

In 1990, the US Bipartisan Commission on Comprehensive Health Care (renamed the Pepper Commission after its chairman, the late Congressman Claude Pepper) issued one of the most noteworthy reports. It called for extensions of job-based insurance, a national health insurance plan for those not covered by an employer, and a proposal for long-term care including a nursing home plan that was a catalyst for discussion on these issues.

In the fall of 1990, for the first time in years, the Senate Committee on Labor and Health, chaired by Senator Edward M. Kennedy, approved health reform legislation. The following year, proponents of health care reform seemed to have more support, especially as they focused on the needs of the uninsured. Legislators talked seriously about "pay or play" options, whereby employers with a minimum number of employees would have to provide health insurance ("play") or "pay" a fee that would go to a national fund to cover the costs of insuring the uninsured. By the early 1990s, most health care organizations had designed or endorsed at least one plan for health care reform. In 1991, many nursing organizations supported *Nursing's Agenda for Health Care Reform*, calling for a "basic 'core' of essential health care services to be available to everyone."

These activities were accompanied, or perhaps inspired, by two important developments that altered the political landscape. First, the business community became increasingly vocal about the financial burden of health care costs. Second, organized medicine, traditionally opposed to major social reform in medicine, shed its inhibitions and called for changes in the current health care system. With congressional leadership also pushing for health care reform and with public opinion polls pointing to the growing concern about rising health care costs, there was no doubt that health care would be a visible and determining campaign issue in 1992.

The momentum around health care reform continued well into the second year of the Clinton presidency. The best minds were brought together at the White House and the final product was the *Health Security Act* of 1993. By September of 1994, Health Care Reform was dead for the 103rd Congress. The reasons for the turnabout are interesting and so predictable. Americans had become distracted from the health care agenda by more basic threats: safe streets and neighborhoods, the economy, jobs with a future, GATT and NAFTA, illegal immigrants. Most voters have access to health care, even if it's of limited and questionable value. Given that picture, there is fear of sweeping change that would in fact jeopardize one-sixth of the American economy. Incremental change—proceeding cautiously, building on successes and allowing one step to be assimilated before another is proposed—is the preferred process. But the content was flawed too:[23]

1. Americans value freedom of choice, and the plan seemed to limit their options.
2. There is a strong distaste for the heavy hand of government.
3. A bloated federalism is particularly unacceptable.
4. Proposals that are naturally offensive to states' rights are bound to bring dissension.

Meanwhile, the Clinton Administration aroused the passion and the conscience of the nation. In the absence of national policy and perhaps because of that absence, states have begun to move forward, launching programs on behalf of the health and welfare of their citizens. It seems a given that we will, over time, have universal coverage, but with a less robust benefit package than proposed by the administration. Financing will be through a combination of private and public sector resources. Managed care will dominate, but with the opportunity, for an additional cost, to select providers who are not members of the network. Indeed, the principle of reform may not be "the greatest good for the most people," but rather "a basic guaranteed standard for everyone, and the opportunity for those who are able to buy more." Prevention is guaranteed to be a driving force, as will direct access to a range of provider professionals. Care will be actively managed, primary providers will fulfill the role of gatekeeper (hopefully in a manner to help you make the best decisions on your own behalf, not to bar access to the system).

OTHER LEGISLATION

Even a cursory look at *The American Nurse* or *The Nation's Health* makes it clear that there is a tremendous amount of legislation that is of interest to nurses, in relation both to their own profession and to their role in health care or as individuals. While some of these laws have been reviewed in this chapter, Chapter 9, concerned with the rights of people, also points out how judicial rulings affect them. For instance, after the Supreme Court ruled (*Rust v. Sullivan*) that regulations preventing doctors and others from discussing abortion in clinics receiving Title X federal funds were constitutional, the House and Senate immediately went to work to write a bill (or section of a bill) that would invalidate the decision. They could do this since the regulation that forbade such discussions was an administrative interpretation of a law they had passed, which some legislators said was a misinterpretation of what they intended. (Although such a bill did pass, it was vetoed by President Bush, and Congress was not able to override the veto.) This issue is discussed further below.

The one area that Congress was able to reach consensus on was the right to obtain access to abortion clinics. The bill, enacted in 1994 with strong bipartisan support, makes it a federal offense to physically obstruct women's access to a clinic, or to use force, threats, or other tactics intended to intimidate women seeking abortion.[24] The legislation was introduced in response to the rise in violent incidents at abortion clinics, and killings of physicians who performed abortions. It also provides protection to abortion clinic employees, places of worship, and pregnancy counseling centers operated by groups that are against abortion.

The 1988 Supreme Court ruling, known as the "gag rule," banned health care practitioners from providing abortion counseling in federally funded (Title X) clinics. In the following years, many legislators introduced legislation to overturn the gag rule, but they always were defeated. In the meantime, the ruling was declared constitutional by the Supreme Court, in May 1991, but its implementation was delayed, owing to political protests and squabbles over its implications. In 1992, HHS announced that only physicians were allowed to counsel women regarding abortion as a health care option under Title X. Nurses were outraged, and argued that this infringed on their rights to practice their profession and to assist women make informed choices. The uproar over the gag rule continued until early 1993, when as one of President Clinton's first actions, he reversed it, relaxing the restrictions placed on all practitioners in Title X clinics.

The controversies over the gag rule, the Freedom of Choice Act, and even the clinic access bill reflect how abortion remains one of the most controversial issues on the domestic political agenda. The debate over abortion continues in 1995. The DHHS 1996 appropriations bill contained several provisions on abortion with the following outcomes:

1. Title X family planning monies were restored.
2. States may refuse to pay for abortions for Medicaid recipients where incest or rape are involved.
3. There is no requirement for training in abortion in accredited medical residency programs.[25]

In addition to abortion, there are several other family-related issues that Congress and interest groups such as nursing have been discussing. Two that received considerable attention during the late 1980s and early 1990s are family leave and child care. The first bill that President Clinton signed into law was the *Family and Medical Leave Act* of 1993.[26] It went into effect on August 5 of that year. In previous years, Congress came close to enacting legislation on family and medical leave that would require employers to give unpaid time off to parents of newborn or sick children or dependents. Women's rights groups and organized labor supported such legislation. However, business groups (and President Bush) opposed any type of family leave bill that made benefits mandatory.

The 1993 law allows employees to take up to 12 weeks a year of unpaid leave for the birth or care of a child born to an employee; placement of a child for adoption or foster care with the employee; care for an employee's immediate family member with a serious health condition; or a serious health condition that makes the employee unable to perform at work. Under the terms of the act, an employer must maintain health insurance benefits during the period of leave at the level and under the conditions coverage would have been provided if the employee had not taken leave. An employer can recover health insurance premiums paid during leave from an employee who does not return, unless due to serious illness. It applies to all private sector businesses with 50 or more employees within 75 miles of a given workplace. Employees may take leave intermittently or at one time.[27] Upon returning from leave, the employer must give the employee the same position, or an equivalent one in terms of benefits, responsibilities, and pay. This legislation was very important for signaling the federal government's support for the millions of families that shoulder responsibilities for caring for family members, while also maintaining full-time jobs.

As for child care, Congress enacted a landmark bill as part of the 1990 budget reconciliation act. It featured a new *Child Care and Development Block Grant* to assist states in improving the quality and availability of child care facilities, and it expanded the earned income tax credit. Both the block grant and the tax credit target low-income working families with children. President Clinton expanded the earned income tax credit under his 1993 reconciliation bill, and demonstrated his commitment to young children with large increases in Head Start funding, enacted in 1994.

Agencies and Regulations

Follow-up of federal legislation requires close attention. It is not just the law itself that affects the public, but the proliferating federal regulations. Legislators have charged that regulations have been used specifically to circumvent the intent of the law; at the least, regulations often shape the legislation they are intended to carry out.

Equally important are the agencies created by the various laws, such as the FDA and Federal Trade Commission (FTC). The FTC, for instance, goes back to 1914, when the Federal Trade Commission Act was passed. It has extensive power; it can represent itself in court, enforce its own orders, and conduct its own litigation in civil courts, and it seems to have relative freedom from the executive branch of government. Its forays into the health field, with rulings on professional advertising, licensure, and other aspects of health care delivery never thought of in 1914, may indicate a direction for other administrative agencies such as FDA. On the other hand, some subjects of the FTC rulings have banded together to lobby for limitation of FTC powers. This occurred, for instance, in 1982, when attached to the FTC reauthorization bill was an amendment exempting state-licensed professionals from its jurisdiction. AMA was a major supporter; ANA was an opponent.

WHAT NEXT?

Pressure to enact legislation for the uninsured and to hold down the spiraling health care costs of this country will dominate the political scene in the next few years. These problems will be compounded by complex bioethical issues raised by new technologies and the need to meet all of these demands in an era of continued budget deficits. Family concerns will also play an important role. Lawmakers will view health care policy within the context of broad social and environmental issues, both nationally and internationally. Without doubt, nurses will want to have a role in making these decisions.

KEY POINTS

1. The balance of power in the US legal system is due to the fact that statutory law, executive law, and judicial law all have separate functions.
2. The judicial system is made up of courts at national, state, and local levels, each handling different kinds of cases, with appeals courts providing further legal options.
3. Important aspects of the legislative process include committee hearings and decisions, debate, amendments, possible conference committee agreements, final vote, administrative signature, and assignment to an administrative agency.
4. Information needed to influence legislation can be acquired from many sources, including consumer organizations, nursing organizations, governmental offices at various levels, and many publications.
5. Nurses can influence legislation in many ways by keeping legislators informed of their opinions and by supporting PACs in which they are interested.
6. Federal laws influence both the education and the practice of nurses, and have a major impact on the quality of the workplace.

REFERENCES

1. Aiken T, Catalano J. *Legal, Ethical and Political Issues in Nursing.* Philadelphia: Davis, 1994.
2. The legislative process is described in full detail in many political action handbooks and pamphlets from organizations, as well as in the introduction to annual issues of the *Congressional Quarterly Almanac.*
3. Curtis BT, Lumpkin, B. Political action committees. In Mason DJ, et al. *Policy and Politics for Nurses,* 2nd ed. Philadelphia: W.B. Saunders, 1993, pp 562–576.
4. ANA–PAC ranks among top PACS in nation. *Capital Update* 13:7, May 19, 1995.
5. Katz, JL. Conference oks bill creating independent agency. *Congress Quart Wkly Rep* 2054, July 23, 1990.

6. Joel L. DRGs and RIMs: Implications for nursing. *Nurs Outlook* 32:42–49, January–February, 1984.

7. Middelstadt P. Medicare fee schedule recommended. *Am Nurse* 22:8, May, 1991.

8. *Changes in Medicare and Medicaid: A Report to the 1995 ANA House of Delegates.* Washington, DC: American Nurses Association, June, 1995.

9. Levit KR, et al. National health expenditures. *Health Care Finan Rev* 16:264, Fall, 1994.

10. Gallagher, RM. *Community-Based Long Term Care.* Washington, DC: American Nurses Publishing, 1995, pp 39–42.

11. Senate approves Medicare Select expansion. *Capital Update* 13:3, June 2, 1995.

12. American Nurses Association calls proposed Medicaid cuts devastating. *News Release*, April 13, 1995.

13. New AIDS data and Ryan White CARE Act update. *Capital Update* 13:7–8, March 10, 1995.

14. From the Health Care Financing Administration. *JAMA* 266:3404, December 25, 1991.

15. Different faces of AIDS are conjured up by politicians. *New York Times*, July 8, 1995.

16. Joel L. Seizing an exceptional moment: The effectiveness initiative. *Am Nurse* 22:6, April, 1990.

17. Early returns show generally favorable reactions to budget. *Legis Network Nurs* 12:19, February 8, 1995.

18. Flanagan L. *What You Need to Know about Today's Workplace.* Washington, DC: American Nurses Publishing, 1995, pp 30–35.

19. Occupational Safety and Health Act reform. *Capital Update* 13:6, January 27, 1995.

20. Dunlop Commission releases long-awaited report. *Am Nurse* 27:15, March, 1995.

21. Clinton issues Executive Order on replacement workers. *Capital Update* 13:1, March 24, 1995.

22. ANA dissents from INRAC recommendations. *Capital Update* 13:5–7, May 19, 1995.

23. Joel LA. Health care reform: Getting it right this time. *Am J Nurs* 95:7, January, 1995.

24. Clinic access bill clears House. *Congress Quart Wkly Rep*, May 14, 1994.

25. Labor–HHS–Education appropriations. *Capital Update* 13:2, August 18, 1995.

26. FMLA: a first step towards equitable leave policies. *Am Nurse* 93:21, September, 1993.

27. Flanagan, op cit, pp 27–28.

11

Health Care Credentialing and Nursing Licensure

OBJECTIVES

After studying this chapter, you will be able to:

1. Define licensure, certification, registration, and accreditation.
2. List three criticisms of licensure.
3. Describe the major controversies about institutional licensure.
4. Explain the difference between mandatory and permissive licensure.
5. Explain the meaning of a "grandfather clause."
6. List the key components of a nursing practice act.
7. List four reasons for which a license may be revoked or suspended.
8. Describe two current problems related to nursing certification.
9. Differentiate among the various ways of legalizing advanced practice.
10. Explain the meaning of "sunset legislation."
11. Identify the problems related to proving continuing competence.

For most nurses, licensure after graduation is a primary goal. For some this will be the only credential they will attain after the diploma or degree they earned from their entry-level educational program. To both the nurse and the public, being licensed is something special and important— and they're right. However, licensure is not the only credentialing mechanism in health care. (See Exhibit 11.1 for definitions.) Nor is it (or the others) without problems. Health manpower credentialing has been criticized by consumers and the government as being one of the factors responsible for

EXHIBIT 11.1

Definitions

Accreditation:[a] The process by which an agency or organization evaluates and recognizes an *institution or program* of study as meeting certain predetermined criteria or standards.

Licensure:[a] The process by which an agency of government grants permission to *persons* to engage in a given profession or occupation by certifying that those licensed have attained the minimal degree of competency necessary to ensure that the public health, safety, and welfare will be reasonably well protected.

Registration:[b] The process by which *individuals* are assessed and given status on a registry attesting to the individual's ability and current competency. Its purpose is to keep a continuous record of the past and current achievements of an individual.

Certification:[a] The process by which a nongovernmental agency or association grants recognition to an *individual* who has met certain predetermined qualifications specified by that agency or association. Such qualifications may include (1) graduation from an accredited or approved program; (2) acceptable performance on a qualifying examination or series of examinations; and/or (3) completion of a given amount of work experience.

---

[a] US Department of Health, Education, and Welfare, *Report on Licensure and Related Health Personnel Credentializing* [DHEW Publ. No. (HSM) 72–11], 1971.
[b] *The Study of Credentialing in Nursing: A New Approach*, Vol. 1. The Report of the Committee (Milwaukee, Wisc.: 1979).

---

some of the serious problems in health care: fragmentation of services, accelerating costs, and poor use and distribution of health manpower.

In the 1970s health manpower credentialing was the object of considerable attention, especially by the federal government. The strong recommendations of the various reports created an uproar among both health practitioners and employers, for there was the implied threat that if the credentialing problems were not resolved, the federal government would step in and take control away from the professions. What resulted was both internal and external scrutiny, with minor changes that improved the system to some extent. Action on the federal level has almost died out, since more conservative administrations have shifted responsibility to the states. Because the credentialing issues are not resolved, the states have responded with actions that affect every health care practitioner, including nurses. Therefore, knowing about the pros and cons of licensure and other credentialing options can help you think through some of these issues before they come to the inevitable crisis stage.

LICENSURE AND OTHER TYPES OF CREDENTIALING

Licensure is a police power of the state; that is, the state legislative process determines what group is licensed, and with what limits. It is the responsibility of a specific part of the state government to see that the law is carried out, including punishment for its violation. Although licensure laws differ somewhat in format from state to state, the elements of each are similar. For instance, in the health professions laws, there are sections on definition of the profession that describe broadly the scope of practice; requirements for licensure, such as education; exemptions from licensure; grounds for revocation of a license; creation of a licensing board, including members' qualifications and responsibilities; and penalties for practicing without a license.

Licensure laws are either mandatory (compulsory) or permissive (voluntary). If mandatory, the law forbids anyone to practice that profession or occupation without a license or face a fine or imprisonment. If permissive, the law allows anyone to practice as long as they do not claim to hold the credential (such as RN).

Licensing of the health occupations was advocated in the early nineteenth century, but it was not until the early 1900s that a significant number of licensing laws were enacted. They were generally initiated by the associations of practitioners that were interested in raising standards and establishing codes for ethical behavior. Because they could not count on voluntary compliance, the associations tried to get legislation. To some critics, this movement is also seen as a way of providing members of an occupation or profession as much status, control, and compensation as the community is willing to give. It is true that as the health occupations proliferate, each group begins to organize and seek licensure. Because many of these occupations are subgroups of the major health professions or are highly specialized, licensure creates problems of further fragmentation and increased cost in health care—according to the critics.

In all of the proposals for changes in health manpower credentialing, criticism of individual licensure is implicit or explicit. Particularly in the last 15 years, the evils were cited; changes (often slow in coming) were dismissed as too little and too late. Some of the key criticisms were (and are) as follows:

1. The minimal standards of safety, theoretically guaranteed by granting the initial license, are often no longer met by some (perhaps many) practitioners because there is no organized system of monitoring continued competence. There is even the question of whether any written exam can determine safe practice in the actual work setting.
2. There is too much rigidity in the rules and regulations in relation to curriculum, so that minimal standards may lag behind the times and educational innovations are stifled.
3. Definitions of practice are so general that, when challenged, allocation of specific tasks may be determined by legal opinions or interpretations by lay people who cannot make an accurate judgment about what is or should be done in practice.
4. Definitions may be so limiting that impractical or unrealistic boundaries are established between practitioners of different kinds.
5. Too many licensing boards are still composed of members of that particular profession (or, in some cases, the professional superior of that group), without representation by competent lay members or allied health professions. This is seen as allowing these professionals to control the kind and number of individuals who may enter their field, with the possibility of shutting out other health workers climbing the occupational ladder and limiting the number of practitioners for economic reasons.
6. There are always some licensed practitioners who are unsafe, and even if they lose their license in their own state, boards in other states are not notified, and the individual simply crosses a state line and continues to practice.

Despite the criticism of individual licensure, it is this model that assures the allegiance of the professional to the consumer rather than to any employer. This is essential to preserve as more and more professionals become salaried employees. This issue is further discussed in Chapter 4. The fact that employers cannot force the professional to compromise their practice as defined in their practice act is a fact of law.

Of the licensed occupations, only 14 are licensed in every state (but not every territory): chiropractors, dental hygienists, dentists, nursing home administrators, optometrists, pharmacists, physical therapists, physicians (MD and DO), podiatrists, professional and practical nurses, psychologists, and veterinarians. Other practitioners find their mobility restricted as they discover that they must be licensed in one state but not another. Even those licensed in all states may need to take licensing exams again when they relocate. Each state controls its own licensing exam. Nursing, with its state board examinations, now called the *National Council Licensure Examination* (NCLEX), is accepted in every state. This allows for licensure by endorsement.

That is, assuming that other criteria for licensure are met, a nurse need not take another examination when relocating to another state.

Despite these problems, it seems that almost all of the established or fledgling health occupations, more than 250 at last count, consider licensing as a primary means of credentialing. This preference is largely due to the fact that reimbursement for services has become associated with governmental recognition through licensure. The licensure problems of one health occupation obviously are not necessarily the same as those of all the others.

Institutional Licensure and Other Challenges to Individual Licensure

Because so many health workers function in institutional settings, one suggested alternative to individual licensure is institutional licensure. *Institutional licensure* is a process by which a state government regulates health institutions; it has existed for more than 35 years. Usually, requirements for establishing and operating a health facility have been concerned primarily with such matters as administration, accounting requirements, equipment specifications, structural integrity, sanitation, and fire safety. In some cases, there are also minimal standards of square footage per bed and minimal nursing staff requirements. The issue in the "new" institutional licensure dispute is whether personnel credentialing or licensing should be part of the institution's responsibility under general guidelines of the state licensing authority.

There are various interpretations of just what institutional licensing means and how it could or should be implemented. The general idea, according to Nathan Hershey, who originated the concept, is that since health care institutions are held accountable for the actions of their employees, they should be given the responsibility of regulating them. The state licensing agency would establish certain basic standards of education and experience, but the institution's administrators would decide just what kind of position that individual could hold. An example given was that of a nurse returning to work after 10 or more years. Her RN licensure would not count. Instead, she would be placed first in an aide position, then an LPN position, and gradually raised to a staff nurse level when she "regained her skills and became familiar with professional and technological advances through inservice programs"[1] In fact, this represents the ultimate in decentralization, allowing the organization to use personnel in varying ways, theoretically as long as safety is assured and some very broad guidelines are respected. Hershey was, then and later, rather evasive as to the place of the physician in this new credentialing picture, implying that the current practice of hospital staff review was a pioneer effort along the same lines and might as well continue to function. However, he did list as logical sites for institutional licensure organizations providing health services, such as hospitals, nursing homes, physicians' offices, clinics, and the all-inclusive "et cetera."

The advantages for the employer are obvious: potential financial savings and almost total control, including the ability to place employees where and when they would be most useful, without needing to consider individual licensing laws. For instance, an aide trained on the job might do procedures that now only RNs are permitted to do. This may or may not give the public cheaper care, but it certainly won't be better. The disadvantages for the licensed person are great. Particularly for nursing, it raises the specter of a return to the corrupted apprentice system of early hospital nursing in the United States. Probably a hospital's own personnel would be used as teacher-preceptors. Who then would do their job? How would they be compensated? How long would "students" be expected to function in their current positions with their current salaries while they "practice" the new role? And with what kind of supervision? What kind of testing programs would exist for each level? Testing by whom? With what kinds of standards? Such sliding positions might well cut personnel costs, but might they not also indenture workers instead of freeing them with new mobility?

Problems of criteria for standards are obvious. If 50 states cannot now agree on criteria for individual licensure, why would institutional licensure be any different? Instead of making interstate mobility easier, institutional licensure would more likely limit even interinstitutional mobility. A worker could qualify for position X in institution A, with absolutely no guarantee that this would be acceptable to institution B.

It is true that many of these practices already exist in hospitals, but it hardly seems progressive to make an unsatisfactory system legal. Expecting the state licensing agency to prevent abuse is overly optimistic. The number of inadequate and even dangerous caregiving facilities, supposedly inspected by the state but still in existence, is evidence of the problems in assuring even minimum quality. Checking who does what how well will be almost impossible, resulting in one more paper tiger—inspection by paperwork.

In the late 1970s the leadership of ANA pointed out these problems to other health professionals and the public. The resulting furor forced the federal government to stop encouraging the institutional licensure approach. Does this eliminate the threat of institutional licensure? Not really, for it seems now that the concept is reappearing, if it ever disappeared.

The 1990s have been particularly active in controversy over regulation as we know it. Lack of flexibility in defining the roles of this nation's health workers, the observation that the professions seem to drag their feet rather than responding creatively to change, and the absence of any comprehensive and rational public policy addressing supply, distribution, and competencies of the workforce are forcing a new look at licensure. The Pew Health Professions Commission has been particularly aggressive in criticizing the shortcomings of the current licensing systems (nursing is one field among many in health care that the Commission scrutinized) with claims that they constrain managerial flexibility, offer no guarantee of continuing competence, provide a weak link to quality, are costly, actually reduce access and create jurisdictions which deter changing models of care and development of new health occupations.[2] Pew has expanded the Commission's report into a grant program with one focus being to move the regulatory environment. Pew grants have been awarded to 8 states, and institutional licensure is being addressed in some form in 7 states.[3]

Similarly, other national professional and philanthropic organizations are advocating for the restructure of regulatory systems, but they are doing it through the back door. The American Hospital Association has developed a policy promoting the expanded use of unlicensed personnel. The Robert Wood Johnson Foundation is conducting demonstration projects on cross-training and shared governance throughout the country, which will invariably strengthen the voice of the workplace on issues of competency.[4]

An additional cautionary note comes from the *Ontario (Canada) model* of regulating nursing practice, which has drawn significant attention because of the North American Free Trade Agreement (NAFTA). In 1993, the *Regulated Health Profession Act* (RHPA) became effective in Ontario, and it is currently under study in other provinces. Simply put, RHPA defines what you may not do as a nurse, and the concept of an exclusive scope of practice is eliminated.[5] Advocates see this as an opportunity to expand into the territory of other disciplines. Adversaries believe that additional pronouncements on the scope of practice will be forthcoming from employers, they being responsible for the services rendered. (And so, in fact, we walk into institutional credentialing of some variety.) Maine and Washington have been looking seriously at RHPA as a basis for change in their own regulatory systems.

Different, but equally as challenging a possibility is the *"superboard"* or *"umbrella board"* which represent the merger and consolidation of the work of a variety of boards to presumably reduce cost and increase efficiency. Often staff do not adequately understand the discipline-specific issues, and some appointees may be disadvantaged because of their social status relative to other members of the board.[6]

In the same way that it is expedient to increase flexibility and to merge all health care interests into one board, it is equally expedient to rethink the possibility of a national license. Corporate acquisitions ignore the presence of state lines. A national license would facilitate geographic mobility and standardization which is a critical quality of the large health care chains.

Certification

Certification was and is attracting considerable attention as a substitute for, or an adjunct to, licensure; in the latter case, it is a means of identifying competence in specialty practice. For instance, many of the health occupations described in Chapter 3 are only certified, but physicians with general (plenary) licensure increasingly use certification to differentiate specialists. Nurses are also starting to do so.

Still, certification is not a clearly understood credentialing mechanism. Two points are essential for understanding: (1) certification is voluntary on the part of the individual, and (2) the organization or agency that certifies is nongovernmental and is usually made up of experts or peers in that particular field. This "private credentialing" differs fundamentally from "public credentialing" (licensure) in that the latter can legally prohibit unlicensed practice. Those who lack private credentials can still legally practice, although they may be disadvantaged in the marketplace because consumers, hospitals, insurers and managed care plans often look for certification as an assurance of quality. Private credentialing can be described as serving solely informational purposes, a sort of "seal of approval" from the professional association or nongovernmental board that grants it. It gives the consumer an opportunity to make more informed decisions, in that certification indicates that the certified person has voluntarily met certain standards that similar caregivers have not.

In general, criticisms of certification are remarkably like those of licensure. First, the validity of written examinations is challenged. Second, there is the question of grandfathering, also a licensure problem. Usually those who practiced a specialty before certification existed are "grandfathered in," that is, permitted to hold certification without fulfilling the usual requirements. Thus, the information given the public—that these persons fulfill certain criteria—is not accurate. Here the answer may lie in requirements to demonstrate ongoing competence for recertification—providing that measures are valid. More certifying groups now have a recertification mechanism.

Finally, there is concern when certification is done by the professional organization that also accredits the educational program the candidate must complete in order to qualify for certification, or when the certifier also establishes the practice standards. Clearly, either situation gives the occupation inappropriate control and can also shut out potential candidates. Professions gradually separated these functions into independent entities. Two examples are the nurse-midwives and nurse anesthetists, whose organizations are described in Appendix 5. They were also the first nursing specialties to have certification.

Despite these criticisms, certification is generally advocated as a way to help the consumer make choices. Certification rather than specialized licensure is the route preferred by ANA to identify nurses in advanced or specialty practice. ANCC certifications are described in Chapter 13, and other specialty certifications are noted in Appendix 6.

Because the public needs to know that the certifying group and its standards have some legitimacy, there is a second-tier credentialing organization (to certify the certifiers). A number of these organizations exist and they do set certification standards, to which most legitimate certifying groups adhere. Nursing set up a central organization to establish guidelines and approve existing and future nursing certification programs in 1990. As the result of a project funded by the Josiah M. Macy Foundation, the National Board of Nursing Specialties (NBNS) was established. It was the consensus of a group of nursing leaders meeting with the Foundation that both the quality of our service to the public and the profession would profit from standardization of specialty practice. Further, the most logical way to accomplish this would be through standardization in certification. Although there was initial interest among the certifiers of nurses, a considerable number refused to conform to the new standard which included upgraded educational credentials on the part of applicants.

Though there were many criticisms of the criteria proposed by the NBNS, the most controversy was generated by the BSN requirement for some certifications. For many groups, the majority of those certified did not have a BSN. Regardless of opposition from groups who represented half of certified nurses, the NBNS is a reality. A core group of 8 certifiers became the charter members and subjected their programs to the scrutiny of the review process.[7] In ensuing years more groups have joined. The future of ABNS is uncertain. Its growth has been slow but consistent.

Accreditation

Accreditation, another voluntary nongovernmental method of credentialing, occurs on an institutional, not an individual basis. Both educational programs and institutions and health care institutions often seek accreditation because it is presumably a mark of excellence, that is, it indicates that higher standards are met than those required by the government. Quite often, accreditation is necessary for hospitals, for instance, to have medical residency programs and for educational institutions to receive federal or state funds for scholarships or other purposes. (However, in 1991, the Secretary of Education recommended that the link between federal aid and accreditation be cut.) As with certification, there has been a great deal of criticism, with questions about the standards and procedures as well as the cost. In 1991, one regional accreditation group was under fire from the federal government because of a standard that required an educational institution to have a "sufficient" number of minority faculty. This was labeled governmental "interference" and drew an angry response from the American Council on Education, which represents many colleges and universities. The rigidity of accreditation standards was also seen to stifle creativity. Most of all, the lack of public representation on accrediting bodies (which has been rectified somewhat), and the lack of scientific development and validation of accreditation criteria, are still seen as serious problems.

In nursing, accreditation has also been a controversial issue. All nursing programs, including PN programs, are eligible for NLN accreditation, which is seen as an important asset. It is not a simple process. Certain fees are required, and the program must complete a self-study report. If the report indicates that NLN criteria have been met, there is a site visit by a team of nurse educators from the same level of program. After consideration by a board, recommendations are made to accredit for a certain period of time or not, a decision that may be appealed. (This is a very brief overview; changes in procedure are made periodically.) Besides the criticisms of accreditation in general, another in nursing is that a university or college already goes through a regional accreditation process and that NLN accreditation is duplicative and costly, a point that is being made by academic administrators about other kinds of specialty accreditation, too. A unique issue concerns which nursing organization should be accrediting. Both ANA and the American Association of Colleges of Nursing (AACN) have periodically expressed the thought that this is their role, although neither has made any progress in wresting accreditation from NLN.

As noted in Chapter 3, the JCAHO accredits a number of health care institutions and agencies. Whereas once it was involved only in hospital accreditation, its expanded activities now clash with nursing in at least one area. An independent subsidiary of the NLN, the Community Health Accreditation Program (CHAP), has been involved with accreditation of home health care agencies for some time. CHAP also provides management consultation to assist agencies in meeting its high standards for accreditation. Both groups require a self-study report and send a team for a site visit, but CHAP's visits are unannounced. CHAP, considered by many as the only consumer-oriented health care accreditation body, has an interdisciplinary board. Perhaps because of this, and its high standards, in 1992, CHAP was the first home care accrediting group to be awarded "deemed status" by DHHS. This means that HCFA grants CHAP authority to determine home care agencies' eligibility for Medicare reimbursement. The JCAHO has membership by organizations, with AMA and AHA having the majority of the 21 corporate seats, with fewer from the American College of Physicians, the American College of Surgeons, and the American Dental Association. There are five public members. In 1992, the nursing community was awarded a seat on the JCAHO board, and traditionally one of the AHA seats is filled by a nurse. By the end of 1992, the JACHO home health accreditation had also been awarded "deemed status" by DHHS. Like certification, accreditation is not likely to disappear, but issues will continue to be raised.

Sunset Laws and Other Public Actions

Besides considering alternatives, improving the licensure process has become a national mandate. Although the speed of the action taken has varied from state to state, steps taken almost universally at one level or another include adding consumers and sometimes other functionally related health professionals to each board, giving more attention to disciplinary procedures, and gradually developing proficiency and equivalency examinations. In a number of states, boards have been consolidated, sometimes under committees of lay people (or at least a majority of consumers), who make the decisions about licensing, with the individual boards acting in an advisory capacity. Although one reason given is improved efficiency, some nurses fear that this is an indirect approach to institutional licensure because these reorganizations tend to weaken nursing's control over its practice.

For some professions, improving the licensure laws to protect the public was a new experience. A motivating factor was the enactment of "sunset laws" that require the periodic reexamination of licensing agencies to determine whether particular boards or activities should be eliminated. Most of the states have now enacted such laws, a result of a lobbying campaign by Common Cause, a consumer group, to bring about legislative and executive branch oversight of regulating boards and agencies of all kinds. Common Cause identified 10 principles to be followed, including a time schedule. An important component was that an evaluation was to allow for public input, as well as that of the boards and occupations involved. Consolidation and "responsible pruning" were encouraged. Although the review would be done by appropriate legislative and executive committees, safeguards were to be built in to prevent arbitrary termination of boards and agencies. These principles are generally adhered to, but states do vary in their management of sunset reviews. If a sunset law is in effect, the data and justification for existence are a joint staff-board responsibility, although the professional organizations are also usually helpful.

By 1985, most nursing boards had undergone sunset reviews, and the new or amended laws usually reflected changes in practice and the environment. Most practice acts have broadened the scope of practice, added consumers to their boards, and sometimes required evidence of current competence through various means, including CE. State boards have given increased attention to removing and/or rehabilitating incompetent nurses. Meanwhile, educators are working seriously on equivalency and proficiency examinations and other methods of providing flexibility and upward mobility for nursing candidates. Nurses in the field have continued to improve techniques of peer evaluation, implement standards of practice, and encourage voluntary CE.

OVERVIEW OF NURSING LICENSURE

Mandatory and Permissive Laws

Enactment of nurse licensure laws was one of the primary purposes of ANA at its inception (as described in Chapter 2). The first state laws were permissive. The first mandatory nursing practice act was enacted in New York in 1938, but it was not put into effect until 1947. One of the dangers of permissive licensing is that schools with poor curricula and inadequate clinical experience produce workers who can legally nurse, although they are potentially dangerous practitioners.

As of 1991, all states had mandatory licensure laws for professional and practical nurses. However, some states are loose in their interpretation of *mandatory*. States that have global exemption clauses in licensure laws stating that almost anyone can be a nurse, providing that there is some kind of supervision, are sometimes seen as permissive states regardless of a mandatory clause.

The Grandfather Clause

One concern about mandatory laws is that those already practicing in the field will be abruptly removed and deprived of their livelihood. This is, however, untrue because mandatory laws are forced, for constitutional as well as political reasons, to include a grandfather clause. A *grandfather* or *waiver clause* is a standard feature when a licensure law is enacted or a current law is repealed and a new law enacted.

The grandfather clause allows persons to continue to practice the profession/occupation when new qualifications are made law. Although the concept goes back to post-Civil War days, it is also related to the Fifth and Fourteenth Amendments of the Constitution. The US Supreme Court has repeatedly ruled that the license to practice a profession/occupation is a property right and that the Fourteenth Amendment extends the due process requirement to state laws. Many nurses currently licensed were protected by the grandfather clause when a new law was passed or new requirements were made, although most probably never realized it. For instance, when various states began to require psychiatric nursing as a condition of licensure, those who had not had those courses in their educational programs did not forfeit licensure.[17]

When the grandfather clause is enacted in relation to mandatory licensure, those who can produce evidence that they practiced as, say, a PN, if applying for LPN status, must be granted a license. However, grandfathering does not guarantee employment. Thus, some employers chose not to employ "waivered" LPNs, just as they had not employed them as unlicensed practitioners.

ANA and NCSBN

Over the years, it was generally accepted that ANA, as the professional organization, developed models that SNAs used when introducing new practice acts (licensure laws). This was when a Council with representatives from state boards across the nation was more or less a part of ANA. When the group broke off to become an independent organization, the National Council of State Boards of Nursing (NCSBN), there was initially limited coordination between the two groups. In 1980 an ANA committee developed guidelines for state legislation to replace the 1976 Model Practice Act, and NCSBN chose to go its own way and published a Model Practice Act in 1982. Despite months of negotiating, the two organizations could not agree on a similar philosophy or even a common language. Some chose to explain that each group had its own constituents: NCSBN, with its representatives from all the state boards of nursing, who deal with state officials and legislatures on a day-to-day basis; and ANA, with its diverse group of nurses committed to setting standards for nursing.

In retrospect, there was wisdom in separating the Council of State Boards of Nursing from ANA, and the difference of opinion over suggested form and language for state legislation was inevitable. This point was already made in Chapter 4 during the discussion on definitions of nursing. Definitions and models presented by the state boards will reflect nursing as it is practiced today, while the professional association is committed to presenting nursing as it should be, in the hope of moving the profession to a more ideal future.[8] Further, the state boards have the responsibility to award credentials, and thus should be insulated from the peer group (the professional association) that sets the standard for practice. The same principles apply here as with separating certifying bodies from their standard-setting constituencies. Currently, after going through a sometimes painful adjustment period, the NCSBN and ANA enjoy a rich liaison relationship and aim for a very broad consensus on issues, realizing that they will disagree on detail. The more consistency between the policies and statements of these groups, the more the real and ideal mirror one another.

Over the years both ANA and NCSBN have provided suggested legislation/ model practice acts to serve as a guide to nurses, state nurses' associations, state boards of nursing, legislators, the public, and anyone else who is interested in considering revisions to their Nursing Practice Act.[9,10] Model Administrative rules usually accompany the legislative models, since the detail is worked through in regulations which operationalize the law (administrative rules). ANA's proposed "bill" is consistent with other association policies, especially reflecting the thinking of *Nursing's Social Policy Statement*, which is essentially the profession's contract with the public. Neither of these documents has authority, but they are a significant influence in shaping the public policy agenda at the state level. Realistically, these statements are taken as seriously as are the associations which created them. In recent years both ANA and NCSBN have proven their sophistication, integrity, and the desire to move closer to speaking with one voice.

The emphasis on states' rights in this country makes legislative conformity difficult. For instance, in 1986, the North Dakota Board of Nursing put into effect revised administrative rules for nursing education programs. Graduates entering programs after January 1, 1987, must have completed an approved nursing program that awards the appropriate academic degree in order to be eligible for licensure. For the RN, this is the baccalaureate; for the LPN, the associate degree. The North Dakota law does not allow equivalency preparation in determining eligibility for licensure, so licensing for out-of-state graduates not fulfilling those criteria has had to be worked out.

CONTENT OF NURSING PRACTICE ACTS

Because each state law differs to a degree in its content, it is important to have available a copy of the law of the state in which you practice and, if possible, the regulations that spell out how the law is carried out. You can get these from the state board or agency in the state government that has copies of laws for distribution. The language in all laws often seems stilted because the laws are written in legal terms, but the following sections can help you understand the key points.

Most nursing practice acts have basically the same major components, although not necessarily in the same order: definition of nursing, requirements for licensure, exemption from licensure, grounds for revocation of the license, provision for reciprocity (or endorsement) for persons licensed in other states, creation of a board of nursing, responsibilities of the board, and penalties for practicing without a license. Only the RN (not the LPN) licensure law or component of the nursing practice act is discussed in the following sections.

Definition and Scope of Practice

The definition of *nursing* in the licensure law determines both the legal responsibilities and the scope of practice of nurses. Inevitably, the definition of nursing in all nursing practice acts is stated in terms that are quite broad. This is generally frustrating to nurses who turn to the definition to find out if they are practicing legally, because it does not spell out specific procedures or activities. Often such activities are not even spelled out in the regulations of the laws, and require specific interpretation by the board. A broad definition is preferable because changes in health care and nursing practice often occur more rapidly than a law can be changed, and the amending process can be long and complex. If particular activities were named, the nurse would be limited to those listed. Not only would the list be overwhelmingly long, but it is possible that any new technique performed by a nurse would require an amendment to the law. An occasional state law does specify certain procedures but always includes the phrase "not limited to."

Until 1974 the nursing practice acts of most states had as their definition of nursing one similar to a model suggested by ANA in 1955. The definition distinguished between independent acts that the nurse might perform, but also identified certain dependent acts and prohibited diagnosis and treatment (not preceded by the word *medical*). In the 1970s, with expanded functions (advanced practice roles) being assumed by nursing, SNAs increasingly became concerned about the adequacy of this definition. Therefore, the first states to change their laws concentrated on broadening the definition to encompass these roles. The ANA counsel suggested that a new clause be added to the ANA model definition (commonly called an additional acts amendment):

A professional nurse may also perform such *additional acts*, under emergency or other special conditions, which may include special training, as are recognized by the medical and nursing professions as proper to be performed by a professional nurse under such conditions, even though such acts might otherwise be considered diagnosis and prescription.

Later revisions of the ANA Practice Act model called for one act and one scope of practice to address nurses in advanced practice, RNs and LPN/LVNs (advanced practice was not specified in the law). It further held the profession responsible for more specific delineation of the advanced practice role. Practically speaking, the absence of any mention of advanced practice in the law worked to the disadvantage of the profession. Some states even denied that such a person existed in their jurisdiction. This last ANA legislative strategy was an attempt to keep any discussion of advanced or specialty practice out of the domain of government, just as medicine had done successfully over the years. But advanced practice nurses, most specifically nurse practitioners, were adamant that they needed to be recognized in the law, and their militance resulted in a situation whereby in 1992, almost every state legally regulated advanced practice in some manner and those mechanisms were varied and inconsistent. In an effort to create some order, NCSBN issued a draft position paper which proposed a second license for advanced practice.[11] The current organizational positions on this matter are unclear. NCSBN seems to favor the second license approach, whereas ANA is promoting the development of administrative statements as opposed to legislation or rules and regulations, with sole right of the Board of Nursing to authorize and regulate nurses in advanced practice. This is considered the most professionally empowering approach. More detail on this issue can be found in the seventh edition of *Dimensions of Professional Nursing.*

The debate between ANA and NCSBN over the regulation of advanced practice is a good example of their complementary roles. A comparison of their evolving positions show movement through compromise and a continued allegiance to their individual constituencies and mission. Other points of comparison in ANA and NCSBN proposed statutory language and process are interesting and are presented in Exhibit 11.2.

While organizations search for the best language and the most representative definitions, there is reality. Definitions vary from state to state, and what most nurses are concerned about is whether the care expected in the employment situation is legal or in the domain of another health profession. Many of the activities in health care overlap. A common example is the administration of drugs, which may be done by the physician, RN, LPN, or various technicians in other hospital departments if related to a diagnostic procedure or treatment. Yet dispensing a drug from the hospital pharmacy, commonly done by some hospital nursing supervisors at night when no pharmacist is on duty, is in most states a violation of the pharmacy licensing law.

Obviously, one of the greatest concerns for nurses is the possible violation of the Medical Practice Act. Nurses have gradually come to perform more and more of the technical procedures that once belonged exclusively to medicine, but often these are delegated willingly by physicians. Whether nurses are always properly prepared to understand and perform them well is seldom questioned. However, as some nurses have assumed more comprehensive overall responsibilities in patient care, questions have been raised by both nurses and physicians. Some are resistant to such changes; others are supportive but worry about the legality of such acts. Therefore it is useful to know how states have legislated for advanced nursing practice, which is related to both statutes and regulations. This area of legislative and regulatory change is monitored carefully by both ANA and the NCSBN and an annual update published in the January issue of *Nurse Practitioner.*

Up to now, state governments have chosen three general means of dealing with expanded nursing practice in the legal definition of the licensure law. All have their advantages and disadvantages. The first trend was the use of administrative rules. These are statements that permit nurses expanded duties (additional acts) as authorized by the professional licensing boards: nursing alone, nursing and medicine, or medicine alone. Both regulations and legislation are important parts of this process, since the administrative rule may not exceed the intent or restrictions of the law or regulatory policies. However, no public

EXHIBIT 11.2

Comparison of ANA and NCSBN Suggested Legislation/Model Practice Act on Select Issues

Issue	ANA[a]	NCSBN[b]	Comments
Definition of nursing	"... the performance of any acts to care for the health of the patient that require substantial specialized knowledge, judgment and skill based upon principles of the biological, physical, behavioral, and social sciences as defined through rules promulgated by the Boards of Nursing."	"... assisting individuals or groups to maintain or attain optimal health, implementing a strategy of care to accomplish defined goals, and evaluating responses to care and treatment. This practice includes, but is not limited to, initiating and maintaining comfort measures, promoting and supporting human functions and responses, establishing an environment conducive to well-being, providing health counseling and teaching, and collaborating on certain aspects of the health regimen. This practice is based on understanding the human condition across the life-span and the relationship of the individual with the environment."	The definition should distinguish nursing from work of other providers, yet be broad enough to include all levels of practice: APRN, RN, LPN/LVN. The ANA relies on further definition in rules. This is probably a strategy to allow more flexibility and to avoid opening the practice act for periodic changes.

Scope of practice

"Skills which may be utilized in the performance of this profession include:

- observing, assessing and recording of physiological, behavioral and social signs and symptoms of health, disease, and injury, including the performance of examinations and testing and their evaluation;

- providing family assessment, discharge planning, therapeutic, preventive and restorative nursing care and services;

- counseling and educating patients about the promotion of health, prevention of disease, illness and injury and promotion of peaceful death;

- administering, supervising, delegating and evaluating of nursing services;

- teaching nursing;

- executing nursing and medical regimens consistent with the education and clinical expertise of the registered nurse;

"Practice as an **RN** means practice of the full scope of nursing which includes but is not limited to:

- assessing the health status of individuals and groups;

- establishing a nursing diagnosis;

- establishing goals to meet identified health care needs;

- planning a strategy of care;

- prescribing nursing interventions to implement the strategy of care;

- implementing the strategy of care;

- delegating nursing interventions to qualified others as provided in this act;

- providing for the maintenance of safe and effective nursing care rendered directly or indirectly;

- evaluating responses to interventions;

- teaching the theory and practice of nursing;

- managing and supervising the practice of nursing;

Again ANA seems to leave a lot to be worked through in rules. Additionally, the ANA statement on scope is written to accommodate APRNs and RNs; LPN/LVNs are not mentioned.

Both versions include delegatory language, and all steps of the nursing process. The ANA uses bolder words about medical diagnosis and treatment in this section, but there is no other section where APRNs are discussed.

(continued)

459

EXHIBIT 11.2 (*continued*)

Comparison of ANA and NCSBN Suggested Legislation/Model Practice Act on Select Issues

Issue	ANA[a]	NCSBN[b]	Comments
	• performing acts of nursing and medical diagnosis and prescribing nursing and medical therapeutic, corrective measures and devices; • performing other acts consistent with the education and training recognized by the nursing profession as properly performed by registered nurses; • conducting research relevant to nursing practice."	• collaborating with other health care professionals in the management of health care."	
Advanced practice	"Advanced Practice Registered Nurse means a registered professional nurse who has successfully completed a master's degree in nursing or a related area of specialized knowledge and skills to provide health care (as determined by the BON through administrative	"Advanced Practice Registered Nursing by NPs, CRNAs, CNMs, and CNSs is based on knowledge and skills acquired in basic nursing education; licensure as an RN; and a graduate degree with a major in nursing or a graduate degree with a concentration in the advanced	Again the ANA looks to administrative statements for the details, and to the BON to either deem or recognize professional certification. The NCSBN claims they cannot accept professional certification as a qualification for licensure as an

rule-making). Registered professional nurses with certification deemed appropriate by the BON include NPs, nurse anesthetists, nurse midwives, and CNSs as advanced practice registered nurses."	nursing practice category, which includes both didactic and clinical components, advanced knowledge in nursing theory, physical and psychosocial assessment, appropriate interventions, and management of health care." (A list of activities follows with recognition that the APRN diagnoses and treats medical problems. There is no mention of a need for supervision or collaboration, except in terms of referral, seeking consultation, and recognizing the limits of your own education.)	APRN unless they have first established the criteria themselves. The term *licensed* is used in the NCSBN model for APRNs. NCSBN sees specific criteria for licensure in each APRN category, as well as scopes which are distinguishable from one another. The details will be worked out in rules external to the legislation. The title of *advanced practice registered nurse* is protected in both renditions.
Prescriptive authority	An overall scope statement included recognition of prescription of medical therapeutics, but no specifics. May again rely on rule-making. In past ANA has recommended a separate Prescriptive Authority Act.	Clear statutory prescriptive and dispensing authority for the APRN. Suggests caution so RNs and LPN/LVN may implement orders given by APRN.	Again there is the clear difference between reliance on rule-making as opposed to legislation.
Impaired nurse	Though a separate Disciplinary Diversion Act was favored in the past, this revision includes language on voluntary surrender of license and limitations on practice.	Dealt with under the section on discipline.	Clearly appropriate to approach the issue differently based on the mission of each organization.

(continued)

461

EXHIBIT 11.2 (*continued*)

Comparison of ANA and NCSBN Suggested Legislation/Model Practice Act on Select Issues

Issue	*ANA*[a]	*NCSBN*[b]	*Comments*
Duties and powers of the board	Among other duties, the ANA includes: • ascertaining and enforcing reasonable and uniform standards for delegation … • enforcing reasonable and uniform standards for all levels of practice.	Among other duties, the NCSBN includes: • develop and enforce standards for nursing education and practice.	ANA sees the profession as the author of the standard that is applied by the BON. NCSBN claims the right to develop standards.
Education for entry into practice	Baccalaureate as educational requirement for entry into professional practice; no other distinctions made.	Graduate of an approved nursing education program.	

[a] A bill to regulate the practice of nursing. In *Report to the Board of Directors from the Congress of Nursing Practice*. Washington, DC: ANA. June. 1995.

[b] *Model Nursing Practice Act*. Chicago: NCSBN. August. 1994.

Note: The title *advanced practice registered nurse* (APRN) is used here, whereas *advanced practice nurse* (APN) appears in other places in this text. They are synonymous.

hearings or publication of the rule is necessary; but, statements may be challenged.

Whether or not the additional acts clause is part of the law, the majority of state boards have now been granted the right to develop administrative statements for the NP. The primary regulatory method of authorizing advanced practice is accepting certification by an organization approved by the state board. (In a sense, this makes voluntary certification a mandatory legal process.) Separate licensure, using a term such as *advanced nurse practitioner*, is also favored by some states. With the exception of nurse-midwives and nurse anesthetists, this identification and the specific require-ments are part of the general nursing practice act, with, of course, appropriate regulations. The second approach could be called the use of nonamended statutes. These states either have made no changes from the 1955 ANA model and allow a liberal interpretation of the definition by the state board or have made minor changes. In some, the word *medical* has been inserted to describe prohibited acts. Thus, where the terms diagnosis and treatment are used it would presumably be identified as nursing. Other states have retained portions of the traditional definition but have omitted or substituted certain other phrases. Although all these states maintain that their acts allow expanded practice, interpretation is the key, so a change in attitude or political/medical pressures could bring a rapid about-face.

The last category of nursing definitions is termed *authorization*, which also has problems of interpretation. These states have developed a new definition of nursing that is intended to cover expanded or advanced practice as well as what might be considered ordinary practice at this time. The first of these states was New York (1972), which pioneered the use of the phrase "diagnosing and treating human responses to actual or potential health problems." A number of other states copied this terminology almost verbatim. However, New York NPs had difficulty in practicing "legally," and in 1988, legislation was enacted to authorize NPs certified by the State Education Department, to "engage in the performance of primary health care services well beyond the scope of practice of nursing," using the NP title. In 1995, only five states authorized NP practice under a broad practice act, with no specific title protection. Twenty-three give NPs and/or CNSs legislative authority to practice, and seventeen use rules and regulations exclusively. In 20 states the Board of Nursing is the sole authority, and in 24 states the scope of practice is either jointly authorized with the Board of Medicine or physician collaboration/supervision is a requirement for practice.[12]

A breakthrough may have occurred when the Missouri Supreme Court ruled in 1983 that a particular general definition did indeed allow advanced nurse practice.[13] This landmark case, *Sermchief v. Gonzales*, was the out-come of a threat by the Missouri Board of Registration for the Healing

Arts, which licenses physicians and osteopaths, to initiate proceedings against nurses in a family planning clinic. (Physicians in the area had lodged a complaint.) The nurses, working under standing orders and protocols signed by the clinic physicians, performed a variety of diagnostic and treatment functions. The trial court judgment was that the nurses were practicing medicine without a license, but the Missouri Supreme Court ruled that the acts of the nurses were "precisely the types of acts the legislature had contemplated when it granted nurses the right to make assessments and nursing diagnoses." The 1975 Missouri law was similar to the earlier ANA guidelines and used the phrase "including, but not limited to." The nursing board had not developed any rules and regulations regarding advanced practice, so the case stood on the interpretation of the definition alone. Although the judgment is limited to Missouri, it is considered a victory for NP practice, with the focus on how clearly a general definition can legally determine whether a nurse is practicing nursing in performing what was once considered the exclusive function of medicine. On the other hand, there is a question as to whether the case was a good example, since Missouri had been open to NP practice for some time, which is not true of other states.

It is clear that advanced practice is still in legal flux. (Nurse-midwives and nurse anesthetists may be included within a nursing practice act, a medical practice act, separately, or totally ignored legislatively. If mentioned, certification is usually a prerequisite for legal practice.) Short of a state supreme court ruling, the legality of certain practices can change in any state with attorney general appointments, the attitude of a judge, or simply the political climate. Health care facility lawyers can only advise on how they interpret the practice act (and they may be influenced by physicians' attitudes or advice). A strong statement for or against advanced practice made by a voluntary professional association (medicine or nursing, for instance) is quite common but has no legal authority; it *can* help mold public opinion.

The doctrines of common practice or custom and usage may also be invoked. This means basically that the act is performed in that particular community or at that current time and is accepted as being within the responsibility of the nurse by the individuals' employer and/or physicians in the area. It usually assumes appropriate training for that function. Although this has been considered acceptable in some courts, it has been denied in others. Practically speaking, statutes cannot be changed informally by mass violation, although they may be changed through the legislative process eventually, because of evidence that a nurse has been taught to perform such a function and is capable of carrying it out safely.

Creation of a Board of Nursing

The name of the state administrative agency varies from state to state, as does the number of members. *Board of Nursing* is used by the NCSBN.

The majority of states now have consumers or other professionals, as well as nurses, as members. These are appointed by the governor, with or without nursing input. Board size ranges from 5 to 19 appointed members, who make policy. Staff employed by the board carry out the day-to-day activities.

Responsibilities of the Board of Nursing

The major responsibility of a board is to see that the nursing practice act is carried out. This involves establishing rules and regulations to implement the broad terms in the law itself and setting minimum standards of practice and education. Among specific responsibilities are issuing licenses to qualified applicants; disciplining those who violate the law or are found to be unfit to practice nursing; and collecting data.

Other responsibilities include developing standards for continuing competency of licensed practitioners and issuing a limited license (for someone who cannot practice the full scope of nursing, perhaps due to a handicap). Nursing boards may also offer educational programs, collect certain data, and cooperate in various ways with other nursing boards or the boards of other disciplines. If they operate under an overall board, certain administrative responsibilities will be carried out on a central level.

The power of the board should not be underestimated. For instance, it was simply by changing their administrative rules that the North Dakota Board changed its requirements for RN and LPN licensure.

Requirements for Licensure

Licensure is based on fulfilling certain requirements. The following points are usually included:

1. The applicant must have completed an educational program in a state-approved school of nursing and received a diploma or degree from that program; usually the school must send the student's transcript. Some states ask for evidence of high school education. There is some legislative pressure that the applicant not be required to have completed the program, particularly if the uncompleted courses are in a nonnursing area such as liberal arts. Neither ANA nor NCSBN approves of this.
2. The applicant must pass an examination given by the board. This examination is currently the NCLEX-RN, developed under the direction of the NCSBN and given in every state.
3. Some states require evidence of good physical and mental health, but this is not recommended by either ANA or NCSBN. Actual

practice varies a great deal from state to state. Handicapped students have been admitted, have graduated, and have taken state boards in some states; in others, this opportunity has been denied. Court cases can result.

4. Most states maintain a statement that the applicant must be of good moral character, as determined by the licensing board, but this, too, is impractical. The Model Act suggests terminology that refers to acts that are grounds for board disciplinary action if the nurse were licensed.

5. A fee must be paid for admission to the examination. This varies considerably among states.

6. A temporary license may be issued to a graduate of an approved program pending the results of the first licensure exam.

7. Demonstrating competence in English is the newest recommendation.

It has been declared unconstitutional to make requirements of age, citizenship, and residence.

Provisions for Endorsement

Nurses have more mobility than any other licensed health professionals because of the use of a national standardized examination. However, usually the nurse must still fulfill the other requirements in the state in which licensure is sought and must submit proof that the license has not been revoked.

If all requirements are satisfactorily fulfilled, the nurse is granted a license without retaking the state board examination. A fee is also required for this process of endorsement. Endorsement is not the same as *reciprocity*; the latter means acceptance of a licensee by one state only if the other state does likewise.

Renewal of the License

Until the early 1970s, nursing licenses were renewed simply by sending the renewal fee when notified, usually every two years. For nurses licensed in more than one state, as long as the license was not revoked in any state, the process was the same. Usually the form asked for information about employment and the highest degree (and still does), but no attempt was made to determine if the nurse was competent. At about that time there was increased concern about the current competency of practicing health professionals, and an estimate was made that perhaps 5 percent of all health professionals were not competent for some reason. One outcome was the enactment of a mandatory CE clause in a number of licensure laws; that is, a practitioner's license would not be renewed unless she or he showed evidence of CE. A number of health disciplines have such legislation, but not all requirements are well enforced.

Forms of CE accepted by states include various formal academic studies in institutions of higher learning; college extension courses and studies; grand rounds in the health care setting; home study programs; in-service education; institutes; lectures; seminars; workshops; audiovisual learning systems, including educational television, audiovisual cassettes, tapes, and records with self-study packets; challenge examinations for a course or program; self-learning systems such as community service, controlled independent study, delivery of a paper, or preparation and participation in a panel; preparation and publication of articles, monographs, books, and so on; and research. The required number of hours of CE or continuing education units (CEUs) varies considerably among states. *No law requires formal education directed toward advanced degrees.* In fact, although additional formal education is acceptable, the emphasis is on continuous, *updated competence in practice.*

Objections to mandatory CE focus on the difficulty of assessing true learning; the question of whether learning can be forced (attendance does not mean retention of knowledge, change in behavior or application of what was learned to practice); the danger of breeding mediocrity; the lack of research on the effectiveness of CE in relation to performance; limitation of resources, particularly in rural areas; the cost to nurses; the cost to government; the usual rigidity of governmental regulations; the problems in record-keeping; and the lack of accreditation or evaluation procedures for many CE programs.

The issue is far from resolved. The trend toward mandatory CE slowed considerably in the 1980s for all occupations, although the call for continued competence did not. It is possible that another trend, peer evaluation, and other kinds of performance evaluation may provide a more effective answer to continued competence.

Exemptions from Licensure

This may also be called an *exception clause.* Generally exempted from RN licensure are basic students in a nursing program; anyone furnishing nursing assistance in an emergency; anyone licensed in another state and caring for a patient temporarily in the state involved; anyone employed by the US government as a nurse (Veterans Administration, public health, or armed services); any legally qualified nurse recruited by the Red Cross during a disaster; anyone caring for the sick if care is performed in connection with the practice of religious tenets of any church; anyone giving incidental care in a family (home) situation; and any RN or LPN from another state engaged in consultation as long as no direct care is given.

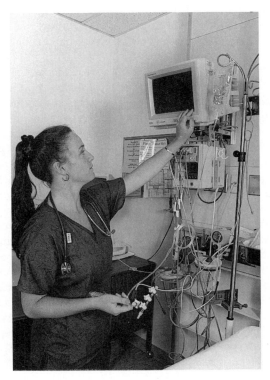

It is each nurse's responsibility to honestly assess their competence in clinical practice. This is what the individual license is all about (*Courtesy of Robert Wood Johnson Hospital, New Brunswick, New Jersey.*)

In all these cases, the person cannot claim to be an RN of the state concerned. Over strong nursing protests, some states have also incorporated in the exemptions nursing services of attendants in state institutions, if supervised by nurses or doctors, as well as other kinds of nursing assistants under various circumstances. This, of course, weakens the mandatory aspect of the law.

An interesting development is that the NCSBN model act suggests for this clause statements that permit the establishment of an independent practice.

Grounds for Revocation of Licensure

The board has the right to revoke or suspend any nurse's license or otherwise discipline the licensee, and reinstate a license if the conditions are corrected. The reasons most commonly found in practice acts for revoking a license are acts that might directly endanger the public, such as practicing while one's ability is impaired by alcohol, drugs, or physical or mental disability; being addicted to or dependent on alcohol or other habit-forming drugs or being a habitual user of certain drugs; and practicing with incompetence or negligence or beyond the scope of practice. Other reasons are obtaining a license fraudulently; being convicted of a felony or crime involving moral turpitude (or accepting a plea of *nolo contendere*); practicing while the license is suspended or revoked; aiding and abetting a nonlicensed person to perform activities requiring a license; and committing unprofessional conduct or immoral acts as defined by the board. The refusal to provide service to a person because of race, color, creed, or national origin has also been added in some states.

The most common reasons that nurses lose their licenses are the same as those that apply to physicians—drug use, abuse, or theft. Substance abuse has become a growing concern among professionals. The exact extent of the problem is unknown, but there are a growing number of disciplinary actions involving substance abuse.[14] Support programs have been developed by boards of nursing and state nurses associations. Despite what has been the establishment of a substantial number of peer assistance programs, little is known about the numbers entering or leaving treatment and the degree of recidivism. Almost every state provides services for impaired nurses, including referrals (42 states), education (46), intervention (21), reentry monitoring (19), hotline access (11), but only 13 states have enacted diversion legislation.[15] The diversion concept provides the impaired nurse with immunity from disciplinary action if there has been no harm to patients, and requires voluntary entry into treatment. The license may need to be voluntarily surrendered, but in some instances a limited license is issued after investigation of the case by the Board. (See also Chapter 8.)

As is true in obtaining or renewing licenses, a nurse can also lose his or her license because of physical or mental impairment. Legal blindness is the most common physical condition involved, but there are many exceptions, especially since the passage of the Americans with Disabilities Act (Chapter 10). It is possible that none of these conditions are specifically cited in the statutes, but if the nurse's practice is affected in any way, discipline is authorized by the ubiquitous "unprofessional conduct" clause.[16] Depending on the seriousness of the situation, nurses may also be given limited licenses in some jurisdictions, which restrict nursing practice to certain parameters.

Unprofessional conduct "as defined by the board" was at one time seldom defined in public rules and regulations. A turning point was the Tuma case. In Idaho in 1977, Jolene Tuma, an instructor in an AD program, went with a student to the bedside of a terminally ill woman to start chemotherapy after obtaining the patient's informed consent. When the patient asked Ms. Tuma about alternative treatments for cancer, she was told about several. Her son, upset because his mother stopped the chemotherapy, told the physician, who brought charges against Ms. Tuma. Subsequently, she was not only fired, but her license was suspended for six months by the Idaho Board of Nursing for unprofessional conduct, because her actions "disrupted the physician–patient relationship." The case aroused a national nursing furor. Ms. Tuma took her case through the courts, and on April 17, 1979, the Idaho Supreme Court handed down the decision that Ms. Tuma could not be found guilty of unprofessional conduct because the Idaho Nurse Practice Act neither defined unprofessional conduct nor set guidelines for providing warnings. The judge also questioned the ability of the hearing officer, who lacked "personal knowledge and experience" of nursing, to determine if Ms. Tuma's behavior was unprofessional.[17] Unfortunately, the court did not address itself to Ms. Tuma's actions, which leaves the nurse's right to inform the patient in some question—at least in Idaho.

While a number of states already had regulations defining unprofessional conduct, this court ruling spurred on those that did not. Depending on how licensure laws are structured, the regulations may apply to all licensed health professions (New York) or may be written into each separate law.

The courts have also played a major role in shaping interpretation. They have been opposed to trivializing the term and have held to the criteria of conduct that intellectually or morally creates jeopardy through practice. An example exists where the District Court in Nebraska reversed the Board of Nursing's denial of license finding that the plaintiff may be difficult to get along with and resistive to directions, but not unprofessional. Criteria originated by the state of Utah are especially clear and provide a good example:[18]

- Failing to utilize appropriate judgment in administering safe nursing practice based upon the level of nursing for which the individual is licensed.
- Failing to exercise technical competence in carrying out nursing care.
- Failing to follow policies or procedures defined in the practice situation to safeguard patient care.
- Failing to safeguard the patient's dignity and right to privacy.
- Violating the confidentiality of information or knowledge concerning the patient.
- Verbally or physically abusing patients.
- Performing any nursing techniques or procedures without proper education and preparation.
- Performing procedures beyond the authorized scope of the level of nursing and/or health care for which the individual is licensed.
- Intentional manipulation or misuse of drug supplies, narcotics, or patients' records.

- Falsifying patients' records or intentionally charting incorrectly.
- Appropriating medications, supplies or personal items of the patient or agency.
- Violating state or federal laws relative to drugs.
- Falsifying records submitted to a government agency.
- Intentionally committing any act that adversely affects the physical or psychosocial welfare of the patient.
- Delegating nursing care, functions, tasks and/or responsibilities to others contrary to the laws governing nursing and/or to the detriment of patient safety.
- Failing to exercise appropriate supervision over persons who are authorized to practice only under the supervision of the licensed professional.
- Leaving a nursing assignment without properly notifying appropriate personnel.
- Failing to report, through the proper channels, facts known to the individual regarding the incompetent, unethical, or illegal practice of any licensed health care professional.

The absence of very specific language in statutes and/or regulations is purposeful to avoid foreclosure on unanticipated types of behavior. This problem is sometimes resolved by using the phrase "not limited to," but if the legislature has a particular concern, this may be written into the law. Some states have also adopted the ANA standards of practice as criteria for incompetence. Another interesting point is the possibility of unprofessional kinds of nursing conduct once considered specific to medicine, such as fee splitting.

A particular problem in both statutory and regulating language relates to such terms as *moral*, *ethical*, and *moral turpitude*, since these can be interpreted in various ways. The model act uses phrases such as "has engaged in any act inconsistent with standards of nursing practice as defined by Board Rules and Regulations" and "a crime in any jurisdiction that relates adversely to the practice of nursing or to the ability to practice nursing."

Although the law seems to protect the public, data show that relatively few nurses have had their licenses revoked or suspended. In part, the reason is believed to be the reluctance of other nurses to report and consequently testify to these acts by their colleagues before either the nursing board or a court of law. Nursing associations and state boards are now emphasizing the responsibility of professional nurses to report incompetent practice. The Model Act makes nonreporting a disciplinary offense.

When a report is filed with the state board, charging a nurse with violation of any of the grounds of disciplinary action, he or she is entitled to certain procedural safeguards (due process). After investigation, the nurse must receive notice of the charges and be given time to prepare a defense. A hearing is set and subpoenas are issued (by the board, the attorney general, or a hearing officer). The accused has the right to appear personally or be represented by counsel, who may cross-examine witnesses. If the license is revoked or suspended, it may be reissued at the discretion of the board, and you have the right to appeal in the county court system in most states.[19] (Sometimes the individual is only censured or reprimanded.)

As pointed out earlier, one of the complaints about licensure is that incompetent practitioners so seldom lose their licenses, and if they do, they may simply go to another state, applying for a new license to practice. All too frequently, the license has been granted with inadequate checking to see whether the person had a record of incompetence. Another aspect of this problem in relation to physicians was that they could lose their hospital clinical privileges for incompetence, substance abuse, or similar reasons, and other hospitals at which they had or would seek privileges would be unaware of this situation. In all cases, patients were endangered, and the professions involved were accused of failing to police, rehabilitate, or remove their own. Therefore, as often happens, legislation follows. The Health Care Quality Improvement Act of 1986 (PL 99-660) mandated a National Practitioner Data Bank (NPDB), later enlarged by the Medicare and Medicaid Patient and Program Protection Act of 1987 (PL 100-93). Although it did not go into effect until September 1990, it will eventually influence all health care professionals.[20] The intent of the law is to "collect and release certain information" relating to the professional competence and conduct of physicians, dentists, and other health care practitioners. Reporting requirements vary among professional groups. The reporting of adverse licensure actions against nonphysician practitioners is not required at this time. Reporting of payments resulting from a claim or judgment on the part of malpractice insurers is mandatory for all health professionals. Copies are sent to state licensing boards. If a claim is settled on behalf of several named individuals, as often happens to nurses in hospital-related incidents, a separate report must be filed for each. APNs, nurse-midwives, and nurse anesthetists are particularly affected by another provision, although optional, that hospital-level professional disciplinary actions affecting clinical privileges or "action by professional societies" be reported. Institutions must check with the NPDB about new applicants and make an inquiry every two years about nurses with clinical privileges. Although there is limited access to the Data Bank—licensing boards, hospitals, professional societies, and health care entities involved in peer review—obviously any error in the information or leak in confidentiality can have a serious affect on a nurse's career. Therefore, nurses are advised to check their NPDB record, to which they also have access, to make sure that it is accurate.

Penalties for Practicing Without a License

Penalties for practicing without a license are included only in the mandatory laws. Penalties vary from a minimum fine to a large fine and/or imprisonment. Usually legal action is taken. Penalties are being strengthened to deter illegal practice.

PROCEDURE FOR OBTAINING A LICENSE

Almost all new graduates of a nursing program immediately apply for RN licensure, because it is otherwise impossible to practice. Although there is nothing to prohibit you from postponing licensure, it is generally more difficult, both psychologically and because of distancing from your educational experience, to take the state board examination (NCLEX) much later.

As a rule, your school makes available all the data and even the application forms necessary for beginning the licensure procedure. Should you wish to become licensed in another state because of planned relocation, request an application from that nursing board (see Appendix 4). The board advises you of the proper procedure, the cost, and the data needed. For this initial licensing, you must take the state board examination in the state where licensure is sought.

As of April 1994, NCLEX has changed its administration of the licensing examination from a paper-and-pencil, twice-a-year method to year-round using computerized adaptive testing (CAT). This change in testing methodology has resulted in a slightly altered candidate registration process. Applications for the examination are made to the board of nursing in the jurisdiction you want to be licensed. You will also need to register to take the NCLEX either with Educational Testing Service (ETS) or with the board of nursing, depending on the individual state procedures. Once the licensure application has been reviewed and eligibility approved by the board of nursing, you will receive an Authorization to Test (ATT) from the ETS Data Center. A bulletin, *Scheduling and Taking Your NCLEX*, will also be forwarded that describes the examination, procedures for making an appointment, a list of available test center locations and telephone numbers, and a toll-free number to call for information on any newly opened centers. The NCLEX is administered at more than 200 Sylvan Technology Centers, with at least one located in each state and territory. The individual candidate schedules his or her own date and time for the examination. For more information on specific candidate application procedures and requirements, contact your board of nursing.

The RN Field Tests found that candidates perform comparably on CAT and paper-and-pencil nursing examinations, and that demographic groups were neither advantaged nor disadvantaged.[21] The CAT has been determined to be psychometrically sound. The NCSBN has produced a video, *NCLEX using CAT: A Candidate's Viewpoint*, that walks the candidate through the test experience. It is designed to answer basic questions commonly asked by candidates, and shows the test site. The video is available for $50 from the National Council, Dept. 77-3953, Chicago, IL 60678-3953.

The CAT provides for each candidate to have a unique examination because it is assembled interactively as the individual is tested. A competence estimate based on all earlier answers is calculated by the computer as the candidate answers each question. A large question bank stores all the examination questions and classifies them by test plan area and level of difficulty. The questions are then searched and the one determined to measure the candidate most precisely in the appropriate test plan area is shown on the computer screen. This process is then repeated for each question, thus forming an examination unique to the candidate's knowledge and skills.

The result of testing is reported as a simple pass–fail score. Both NCLEX (RN) and NCLEX (LPN) are based on periodic job analyses. The exam consists of multiple-choice questions which test your judgment and decision-making, not just knowledge. The exam questions are based on client needs and the nursing process, with a predetermined percent of the total questions from each category.[22] Questions also represent differing degrees of difficulty, and so using CAT, the higher achiever will probably answer fewer questions and complete the testing process in a shorter period of time. (See Exhibit 11.3.)

The tests are the same for all nurses seeking an RN, whether graduating from a diploma, associate degree, or baccalaureate program. This has been the subject of considerable criticism, because the stated goals of all three programs are different. However, proponents of a single licensing exam state that the purpose is to determine safe and effective practice at a minimal level, and that this criterion applies to all levels of nurses.

Nurses who pass the licensing examination receive a certificate bearing a registration number that remains the same as long as they are registered in that state. The certificate (or registration card) will also carry the expiration date—usually one, two, or three years hence. Failure to renew promptly may mean that you must pay a special fee to be reinstated.

It is advisable to keep your registration in effect, whether actively engaged in nursing or not. The expense is nominal, and more and more nurses who "retire" temporarily return to nursing. These nurses do have the responsibility (and sometimes the legal requirement) to keep their nursing knowledge updated through CE.

To become licensed or registered by endorsement, you must already

EXHIBIT 11.3

Framework of the NCLEX Test Plan

	RN	PN
Nursing process:		
1. Assessment	15–25%	N/A
2. Analysis	15–25%	N/A
3. Collecting data	N/A	25–35%
4. Planning	15–25%	15–25%
5. Implementation	15–25%	25–35%
6. Evaluation	15–25%	15–25%
Client needs:		
1. Safe and effective care environment	25–31%	24–30%
2. Physiological integrity	42–48%	42–48%
3. Psychosocial integrity	9–15%	7–13%
4. Health promotion/maintenance	12–18%	15–21%

Note: Percentages listed are from the current NCLEX-RN test plan.

Source: NCSBN—Taking the NCLEX: Information every candidate should know. *Imprint* 42:9–19, January, 1995.

be registered in one state, territory, or foreign country. You then apply to the state board of nursing in the new state and present credentials, as requested, to prove that you have completed preparation equal to that required. A temporary permit is usually issued to allow you to work until the new license is issued.

Should you wish to be reregistered after allowing your license(s) to lapse, it's best to contact the state board for directions. If you wish to practice nursing in another country, investigate its legal requirements for practice. Members of the armed forces or the Peace Corps, or those under the auspices of an organization such as the World Health Organization or a religious denomination, will be advised by the sponsoring group. Licensure in one state is usually sufficient.

Nurses educated in other countries are expected to meet the same qualifications for licensure as graduates of schools of nursing in the United States. The procedure for obtaining a license is the same as for graduates of schools here. However, generally nurses from other countries are now expected to take the Commission on Graduates of Foreign Nursing Schools (CGFNS) Qualifying Examination, which screens and examines foreign nursing school graduates while they are still in their own countries to determine their eligibility for professional practice in the United States. The one-day examination covers proficiency in both nursing practice and English comprehension; both exams are given in English. If the applicant passes, she or he is given a CGFNS certificate, which is presented to the US embassy or consulate when applying for a visa (necessary to obtain a work visa) and to the state board in the state where the nurse wishes to practice. The nurse still must take the state board examination and otherwise fulfill the licensing requirements for that state. The vast majority of foreign nurses who have not passed CGFNS fail NCLEX, even after several repetitions. Specific information about requirements for licensure must be obtained directly from the board of nursing in the state in which the foreign nurse wishes to be licensed.

ISSUES, DEVELOPMENTS, AND PREDICTIONS

It seems that almost every month brings information about changes in nurse practice acts or challenges as to what they permit. The scope-of-practice issue will not be resolved for quite a while. Many changes relating to APNs are already occurring in nurse practice acts and other legislature and regulatory routes. For instance, in 1983, 18 states had formally given prescription-writing authority to certain categories of nurses. By 1995, the number had reached 47 and the District of Columbia. Two of the remaining states (Alabama and Oklahoma) introduced prescriptive authority legislation in 1995. Direct reimbursement to APNs for their services is another policy issue closely related to individual licensure and definition and scope of practice. All states with the exception of the District of Columbia and Ohio reimburse APNs directly for Medicaid clients. APNs are generally paid 80 to 100 percent of the amount a physician would bill for the same service. Thirty-five states have statutes which allow third-party reimbursement to APNs. Medicare limits direct reimbursement to rural and underserved areas.[23] The issues here are many and complex. You are referred to *Dimensions* for more detail.

Because of the hodgepodge of regulations and other legal means of giving nurses prescriptive authority, ANA has proposed separate legislation.

Certification for specialties will certainly grow, probably with an overview organization certifying the certifying groups. As noted earlier in this chapter, the ABNS has already been established to assume this function. The growth of the many certifying groups, sometimes overlapping in functions, is quite astounding.

At the other end of the educational scale is the growing concern about the competence of nurses' aides. New positions are growing for aides in hospitals, LTC facilities, and home care; 433,000 *new* jobs are predicted for the year 2000. As the least expensive and least prepared nursing person, the aide is still expected to detect behavioral changes that may signal a serious health problem—and isn't trained to do so. Although the need for national training standards has been recognized, just who will implement them is still undecided. Some states, such as New Jersey, now regulate home health aides. How can nurses who are ultimately responsible for nurses' aides ascertain that they are safe and competent? Will the state boards have a role? The NCSBN has developed standards for the regulation of nurses' aides and a testing program for certification of long-term care aides as required by the government.

Equal concern can be directed at the growing responsibilities of LPNs. Many state boards are put under pressure by employers to approve procedures for LPNs that are not in their curricula, such as venipuncture. Some boards approve and demand that PN programs include these procedures in their course of study. Schools say that there is already enough to cover in one year. The impact of this problem is uncertain. Will patients be endangered? What of the responsibility of nurses who supervise LPNs? Might these new demands escalate the move toward AD education for LPNs?

On a less happy note, nurse disciplinary problems are likely to increase. The stress of institutional staff cutbacks, caring for sicker patients with fewer people, and an uncertain job future can all be triggers for substance abuse. Programs sponsored by the state boards and state nurses association were mentioned earlier. They will probably increase in number and diversity, but be evaluated as to their efficacy.

Regardless of the outcome of health care reform efforts, it is clear that there will be an increasing push for more uniform licensing standards, and removal of statutory barriers to practice. The licensure examinations are expected to continue to change. Next on the agenda is computerized simulation testing (CST), augmented by interactive video, which will allow candidates to demonstrate competence in clinical judgment and decision making.[24] (The National Board of Medical Examiners has already developed such a computer-based test.) Another activity for NCSBN is a study to determine potential item bias. NCLEX has been criticized as not taking into consideration cultural, gender, and other factors. With the large immigrant population, some of whom may go into nursing, such aspects must be considered. Other issues about licensure will include concerns about developing a mechanism to ensure competence, including that of returning nurses; the great diversity of definitions of nursing and scope of practice; and developing better means of verifying licensure across state lines.

Finally, the credentialing issues in health care in general are not expected to improve greatly because they are so disorganized now. More health occupations will continue to seek licensure or other legal status. All these groups will have problems similar to nursing with definition, scope, discipline, and testing methods. And what of the uncredentialed health worker? How best can we guarantee at least safe care for the public?

Resolution of the problems posed here could help to resolve some of the other problems of health care delivery. And if someone must take the lead in initiating cooperative action, it may well be nursing.

KEY POINTS

1. There are a variety of mechanisms for credentialing nurses and other health care workers, all of which have some problems.
2. Mandatory licensure means that an individual cannot practice without a license and safeguards the public more than permissive licensure.
3. Among the criticisms of licensure are too much control by the profession or occupation, a tendency for practice requirements to be rigid and out of date, and primarily that the public has no guarantee of competence.
4. Institutional licensure, although favored by administrators for economic and other reasons, would not guaranteee improved care but would limit the autonomy and mobility of nurses who now have individual licenses.
5. Nursing practice acts may vary from state to state, but they generally have the same components that define and control practice.
6. Nursing practice acts must change with the times, but the current practitioner is protected by a grandfather clause.
7. The most common reasons for revocation of a license are drug abuse or misuse, or other failure to meet the standards of the profession.
8. One purpose of nursing certification is to recognize advanced practice, but because there is not yet coordination among certifying groups, the public may be confused.
9. The approaches to authorizing advanced nursing practice are interpreting current statutes to include advanced practice, developing rules and regulations, or legislation with new definitions of practice.
10. Sunset legislation, which requires a review of existing agencies to determine if they are fulfilling their purpose, has resulted in some good revisions of nursing practice acts.
11. A major problem with CE as a requirement for relicensure is that there is little evidence that it results in improved competence.
12. Many changes are occurring in the testing of individuals for nurse licensure.

REFERENCES

1. Hershey N. Alternative to mandatory licensure of health professionals. *Hosp Prog* 50:73, March, 1969.
2. Pew Health Professions Commission. *Commission Policy Papers.* San Francisco: University of California, 1994.
3. American Nurses Association. *Licensure and Registration of Registered Nurses: A Report to the 1995 House of Delegates.* Washington, DC: ANA, 1995.
4. Moore J, et al. Administrators and nursing directors expectation of primary care tasks to be done by extenders. *Nurs Home Med* 2:203, November–December, 1994.
5. Hadley E. *Description of the Ontario Approach to Professional Licensure.* Unpublished paper, October, 1994.
6. American Nurses Association. *Licensure and Registration of Registered Nurses,* loc cit.
7. Hartshorn J. A National board for nursing certification. *Nurs Outlook* 39:226–229, September–October, 1991.
8. Joel LA. Laying circles end-to-end. *Am J Nurs* 95:7, September, 1995.
9. American Nurses Association. A bill to regulate the practice of nursing. In *Report to the Board of Directors from the Congress of Nursing Practice.* Washington, DC: ANA, June, 1995.
10. National Council of State Boards of Nursing. *Model Nursing Practice Act.* Chicago: NCSBN, August, 1994.
11. National Council of State Boards of Nursing. *Position Paper on the Regulation of Advanced Nursing Practice.* Chicago: NCSBN, 1993.
12. Pearson LJ. Annual update of how each state stands on legislative issues affecting advanced practice. *Nurs Pract* 20:13–56, January, 1995.
13. Wolff M. Court upholds expanded practice roles for nurses. *Law Med Health Care* 12:26–29, February, 1984.
14. Megel MA. Nursing laws and regulations as they reflect societal issues. In Bullough B, Bullough V (eds): *Nursing Issues.* New York: Springer, 1994, pp 32–43.
15. American Nurses Association. *Addictions and Psychological Dysfunction in Nursing: The Profession's Response to the Problem.* Kansas City, MO: ANA, 1991.
16. Fiesta J. Why nurses lose their licenses, part I. *Nurs Mgmt* 24:12, 14, October, 1993.
17. Jolene Tuma wins: Court rules practice act did not define unprofessional conduct. *Nurs Outlook* 27:376, June, 1979.
18. Heinecke *v.* Department of Commerce, Division of Occupational and Professional Licensing, 810 P.2d 459 (Utah App 1991).

19. Calfee B. Going before the Board. *Nursing 95* 56–58, March, 1995.
20. Montague J. Should the public have access to the National Practitioners Data Bank? *Hosp Health Netw* 68:52–56, June 5, 1994.
21. What candidates can expect with NCLEX administered by computerized adaptive testing (CAT). *Issues* 14, 1993.
22. National Council of State Boards of Nursing. Taking the NCLEX: Information every candidate should know. *Imprint* 42:9–12, January, 1995.
23. Pearson, loc cit.
24. Computerized clinical simulation testing project (CST): Project overview and update. *Issues* 11:4–5, January, 1990.

12

Legal Aspects of Nursing Practice

OBJECTIVES

After studying this chapter, you will be able to:

1. Define basic legal terms.
2. Explain the elements of the standard of care as it might be applied in a court of law.
3. Give examples of legal problems nurses may encounter in caring for patients.
4. Present specific ways in which nurses may avoid malpractice suits.
5. Name three charting errors that may cause problems for the nurse in a malpractice suit.
6. Identify key points in selecting liability insurance.
7. Give examples of criminal activities for which nurses can be held responsible in their practice.
8. Explain how best to handle a situation calling for a critical incident report.
9. Explain the usual steps in a trial.
10. List the main points a nurse should know about testifying.

There are numerous ways in which nurses become involved with the law in their practice. The impact of statutory law has been previously discussed. In this chapter, other legal aspects will be considered, primarily within the common law of torts, that is, an intentional or unintentional civil wrong. This is the kind of law that relates to the daily practice of most nurses. When cases are used to illustrate a legal principle, it is important to remember that even a landmark decision may be overturned. The law is dynamic, not rigidly fixed, and changes with changing times.

LITIGATION TRENDS IN HEALTH CARE

Part of the doctrine of common law is that anyone can sue anyone if she or he can get a lawyer to take the case or is able to handle it personally (as is common in a small claims court). This does not necessarily mean that there is just cause or that the person suing (plaintiff) has a good chance of winning; in fact, the defendant might be protected by law from being found liable, as when someone, in good faith, reports child abuse.

Most people are reasonably decent in their dealings with others, and unless a person sustains a serious injury, they will not institute legal proceedings. Sometimes this is because legal services are expensive, perhaps more so than paying the medical bills, and the offended person is realistic enough to know this. Often the person inflicting the injury is also realistic and prefers to settle the matter out of court, knowing that it will be less costly in the long run; or insurance may pay for the damage inflicted. One or both parties may settle their difficulties out of court because one or the other or both wants to avoid publicity and does not want to have a court record of any kind.

Once people seemed particularly reluctant to "make trouble" for nurses, doctors, or health agencies such as certain nonprofit or voluntary hospitals, either out of respect for the services offered and/or because they presumably had so little money that it seemed unfair or pointless. The latter was probably always an inaccurate generality, but today patients and families who feel aggrieved are considerably more likely to sue any or all concerned, sometimes for enormous sums. Health care is big business. The number of claims and the monetary escalation of awards began to increase in the 1930s, declined during World War II, and then rose again, with the 1980s and 1990s seeing multi-million-dollar awards. Malpractice suits against hospitals, especially, have increased, and the doctrine of *charitable immunity*, which granted them freedom from liability, and *sovereign immunity* that does the same for government, is gradually being wiped out in the courts.

A variety of reasons have been cited: the "litigant spirit" of the general public, what seems to be a "sue if possible; I'm entitled" attitude; changing medical technology that has brought new risks, with a potential for exceptional severity of injury; sometimes high, unrealistic public expectations; the increase in specialization that has resulted in a deterioration of the physician–patient relationship; and patient resentment of depersonalized care and sometimes rude treatment in hospitals.

At the height of the malpractice crisis, a specially appointed inter-disciplinary committee reported that the *prime factor in malpractice was malpractice*. However, because there are so many more medical injuries than medical claims, another major factor might be interpersonal problems between the provider and patient and frustration with the way specific complaints were handled or not handled. This was reaffirmed in 1994, when "poor relationships with the provider before the injury" was cited as the second major reason for pursuing litigation, interrelated with the litigant's impression that the patient and/or family were not being kept informed or properly referred. However, there is also some evidence that people are being socialized into thinking that if something goes wrong, they should sue.

The main reason for suing was reported to be the influence of the ubiquitous advertisements of attorneys on radio and television, promising legal help for a multitude of injuries and accidents. Another was explicit recommendations by other health care providers to seek legal counsel.[1] Contrary to the belief of some physicians who decline to serve poor people because of their likelihood of suing, it was found that they actually tended to sue less, nor did they file inappropriate claims (not injured).[2]

Most suits are settled out of court. Moreover, the plaintiff generally does not win the suit. The dramatic multi-million-dollar suits seldom result in awards anywhere near the original figures, although they still may be large. Sometimes they are not won at all. The largest elements of compensation in the million-dollar awards are for pain and suffering, almost exclusively occurring after some negligently caused catastrophic injury, such as severe brain damage or paralysis, which obviously has an enormous effect on the victim's life. (In 1995, the AMA tried to persuade Congress to limit compensation for pain and suffering, but were unsuccessful in the Senate. Limits on punitive damages were considered.) The frequent suits and large awards were part of the reason for the mid-1970s' and 1980s' malpractice crisis, when many physicians could not get malpractice insurance, and neither hospitals nor physicians felt that they could afford it if they could get it. In 1990, malpractice fees were being reduced; state laws limiting awards and increased caution by physicians were cited as reasons. By 1992, a study of medical malpractice cases indicated that unjustified payments were rare. Nevertheless, the issue of tort reform was of major interest to Congress in 1995.

The vast majority of malpractice cases are against physicians or hospitals. Don't nurses get sued? Absolutely. As noted later, a good percentage of hospital and physician suits include nurses and may be based on the nurse's negligence. Because of the various legal doctrines, also explained later, the aggrieved patient has the option of suing multiple defendants. The *deep pocket* theory of naming those who can pay most has become traditional tort law strategy, as has the *fishnet theory* of suing every defendant available.

Thus the likelihood of recovery from one or more defendants is greater, and a favorite defense of admitting negligence but blaming an absent party, the so-called *empty chair defense*, is defeated. Because presumably either or both the physician or the hospital has more money than the nurse, either may have to pay the award or at least more of the award, even if it is the nurse who is clearly at fault. Particularly in the case of the hospital whose liability and responsibility may be only secondary (*vicarious liability*), it may recover damages from the employee primarily responsible for the loss through the process of *subrogation*, meaning that the employer can sue the employee for the amount of damages paid because of the employee's negligence.

In the last fifteen years, the number of legal suits involving nurses has increased significantly. It is difficult to say whether this is because there is actually more negligence, whether the public's litigious spirit now extends to nurses, or whether people simply are more aware of nurses' increased responsibilities and nurses are now seen as professionals responsible for their own actions. It may be that all of these factors are involved.

In late 1988, the ANA reported that each year an estimated 1900 nurses are named in liability and malpractice lawsuits. Half of those claims against nurses resulted in payment. The ANA followed this study by establishing a National Nurses Claims Data Base in order to have some reliable data about nurses in malpractice suits, in part because questions were being raised by insurance carriers about the cost of defending nurses. Preliminary information made available in 1990 came primarily from two major insurance carriers involved with nursing liability insurance. The results showed some similarity to a study of litigation against nurses between 1967 and 1977.[3] Sites of the alleged negligence were again, hospitals first, by a large margin, and then clinics (13.5 percent). The areas most involved were obstetrics, patient room, emergency room, and operating room. The chief reasons for the claims were improper treatment, birth related; improper treatment, miscellaneous; and patient falls.

In 1994,[4] the current statistics on a national level taken from data reported in the National Practitioner Data Bank (NPDB) from 1990 to 1993 indicated that as of 1990, about five nurses in 10,000 are sued in a given year. The malpractice claims ranged from patient falls (the greatest number of claims) to failure to impart vital information about a patient's changing condition. More cases are involving physical procedures, and courts are using policy and procedure documents increasingly.[5] Insurance reports for one state, which are rather typical of others, listed patient falls, burns, medication errors, failure to assess adequately, failure to remove foreign objects, mistaken identity of patients, failure to clarify the physician's instructions, "bad baby" cases, and failure to restrain, as some of the most recurring cases.[6] Again, many of these are the same as those reported in the Campazzi study cited earlier.

Some insurance companies have expressed concern about potential malpractice claims of advanced practice nurses, and APNs do have higher premiums than other nurses. In a 1994 readership survey by *Nurse Practitioner* that had 1610 responses, 25 NPs reported allegations, only one of which was entered into the NPDB, described in Chapter 11. (There is evidence that NPDB does not reflect current NP practice because the reported cases are 5 to 8 years old.) Most of the cases were dropped or the NP was dropped from the claim.[7]

An earlier survey of state boards, which included all kinds of advanced practice nurses, had a rather small sample of 45 complaints. It was found that nurse practitioners had the largest percent of complaints related to practice, such as failure to assess or intervene, misdiagnosis, and documentation errors. Almost 40 percent of all complaints about APNs were dismissed; 24 percent resulted in some kind of state board discipline. Clinical nurse specialists had the fewest complaints of any kind. It is important to note here that not all complaints to state boards are related to malpractice suits and it is possible to win a suit or have it dismissed without the information necessarily getting to the state board; this applies to all nurses. Also, some of the state board cases related to drug abuse (of which the highest percentage were nurse anesthetists).[8]

Given these circumstances, it makes sense to know (1) the kinds of situations that lead to litigation, (2) steps to take to avoid being sued, and (3) what to do if a patient is hurt. This chapter gives an overview of the legal problems in which nurses can be involved in their practice within the common law of *torts*, that is, an intentional or unintentional civil wrong. Criminal problems that are common are reviewed more briefly.

Some of the cases presented later are classic cases that are repeatedly cited in nursing law; others are more recent. At times, when two similar cases are judged in quite different ways, both are mentioned. Remember that the findings may change with the changing role of the nurse and a court's concept of what a nurse is and does.

APPLICATION OF LEGAL PRINCIPLES

The majority of incidents leading to legal action in which nurses are involved occur in an employment situation, generally the hospital. That is to be expected because that is where most nurses work and where patients are usually sickest and most helpless. When a person is injured, chances are that the hospital will be sued, even when an employee or a doctor has done the actual damage. In the case of the employee, the hospital is sued under the legal principle of *respondeat superior*: "let the master answer" or be responsible for the actions of the employees.

This does not prevent the employee from being sued, since the rule or doctrine of *personal liability* says that everyone is legally responsible for his or her acts, even though someone else may also be held legally liable, usually the institution. The latter is called *vicarious* liability, imposed without personal fault or without a causal relationship between the actions of the one held liable and the injury.

At one time, physicians were held directly responsible for any error of personnel who worked with them in a patient care situation (*borrowed servant*) on the basis of the *"captain of the ship"* doctrine; this has been overturned by most courts, but not all as shown in a case described later. The institution, however, can be held accountable for physicians' acts, even if they are not employees, under the principle of *corporate negligence*. A classic example is the 1965 landmark decision of *Darling v. Charleston Community Memorial Hospital*, which has set several precedents. Although other cases will be presented to exemplify some of these points, it also illustrates the elements that must be present in order to have cause for action based on malpractice or negligence:

1. A duty was owed to the plaintiff by the defendant to use *due care* (reasonable care under the circumstances).
2. *The duty was breached* (the defendant did not behave in a reasonable manner).
3. The plaintiff was injured or damaged in some way.
4. The plaintiff's injury was caused directly by the defendant's negligence (*proximate cause*).

CASE

Darling v. Charleston Community Memorial Hospital (1965)

A minor broke his leg playing football and was taken to Charleston Community Memorial Hospital, a JCAH-accredited hospital. There a cast was put on the leg in the emergency room, and he was sent to a regular nursing unit. The nurses noted and charted that the toes became cold and blue. They called the physician, who did not come. Over a period of days, they continued to note and chart deterioration of the condition of the exposed toes and continually notified the physician, who came once but did not remedy the situation. The mother then took the boy to another hospital, where an orthopedist was forced to amputate the leg because of advanced gangrene. The family sued the first doctor, the hospital, and the nurses involved.

The physician settled out of court; he admitted that he had set few legs and had not looked at a book on orthopedics in 40 years. The hospital's defense was that the care provided was in accordance with the standard practice of like hospitals, that it had no control over the physician, and that it was not liable for the nurses' conduct because they were acting under the orders of the physician.

The appellate court, upholding the decision of the lower court, said that the hospital could be found liable either for breach of its own duty or for breach of duty of its nurses. The new hospital standards of care set by that ruling were in reference to the hospital by-laws, regulations based on state statutes governing hospital licensure and criteria for JCAH accreditation. The court reasoned that these constituted a commitment that the hospital did not fulfill. In addition, the court held that the hospital had failed in its duties to review the work of the physician or to require consultation when the patient's condition clearly indicated the necessity for such action.

Nursing Implications
You must be persistent in reporting inadequate care. It is not enough to observe and record. For nurses, the crucial point in the court decision was the newly defined duty to inform the hospital administration of any deviation from proper medical care that poses a threat to the well-being of the patients. Specifically, the court said:

> Skilled nurses would have promptly recognized the conditions that signalled a dangerous impairment of circulation in the plaintiff's leg, and would have known that the condition would become irreversible in a matter of hours. At that point, it became the nurses' duty to inform the attending physician, and if he failed to act, to advise the hospital authorities so that appropriate action might be taken.

(The hospital was also expected to have a sufficient number of trained nurses capable of recognizing unattended problems in a patient's condition and reporting them.)

Two terms used here and almost inevitably in most suits are *malpractice* and *negligence*. Malpractice technically means "professional misconduct," and in the eyes of some courts this does not apply to nurses. *Negligence* means failing to conduct oneself in a prescribed manner, with due care, thereby doing harm to another or doing something that a reasonably prudent person would not do in like circumstances. The following case not only illustrates another incident of negligence, but presents one court's concept of the captain-of-the-ship doctrine that cost a hospital $5 million.

CASE

Nelson v. Trinity Medical Center (1988)

The physician of a woman in active labor ordered assessment of fetal heart tones, an IV, and analgesia. Standing orders in that labor unit called for continuous fetal heart monitoring, but the nurse, without checking, assumed that the monitors were all in use and did not place one on the patient until an hour later. It indicated fetal distress, and despite an immediate Cesarean, the infant was born with severe brain damage. According to the expert who testified, the damage was caused by placental separation, which could have been diagnosed by earlier fetal monitoring. The defendant hospital tried to invoke the captain-of-the-ship doctrine to cover the nurse's negligence. The court ruled that even though the doctor was in charge of the case, he had no direct control over what the nurse did (as opposed to an operating room situation) and that the nurse was performing a routine act.[9]

Nursing Implications
The entire area of obstetrics is high on the list of malpractice suits. As seen here, the problem is not always that of a nurse not knowing how to handle equipment (although this also is the basis of nurse negligence), but carelessness and false assumptions. Check whether equipment is available and working; don't guess. If it is not, notify your manager and the doctor so that other arrangements can be made. Check to see if equipment is in working order *before* it is needed. You are not at fault if equipment doesn't work, but it is your responsibility to report it and follow through. Again, use your nursing judgment! In this case, the nurse's neglect was considered the *proximate cause* of the child's injury. However, in another case, where the nurse was considered negligent in ignoring the fact that the patient was allergic to latex and catheterizing her with a rubber catheter, which caused her some problems, the court did not find that negligence was the direct *proximate* cause for the baby's being born with cerebral palsy. She was not held liable for the child's injuries.[10]

The following judgment again illustrates negligence but also demonstrates that courts vary in their interpretation of "borrowed servant" or "captain of the ship" in relation to a hospital's liability.

CASE

Parker v. Hosp. Auth. of City of Bainbridge (1994)

In 1990, a child was taken to a hospital emergency room after suffering a seizure in school. Shortly after a physician treated the boy with Dilantin, he went into cardiac arrest and subsequently died. The Medical Examiner listed the cause of dealth as "Dilantin overdose." The mother sued the hospital, two doctors and two nurses employed by the hospital, alleging negligent treatment. Because the nurse who gave the Dilantin and assisted with the care of the child was doing so under the express direction of the doctor, this court considered her participation a case of "borrowed servant," and because the physician was not an employee of the hospital, the hospital was not held liable for his or her actions. Nor did the jury hold the physician liable, although he admitted the overdose.[11]

Nursing Implications
This Georgia case has a number of peculiarities, but does demonstrate that judges and juries in various jurisdictions have vastly different notions of liability in a civil case. For instance, in other situations the nurse has been held individually responsible for giving a drug overdose, when she should have known it was an overdose. And a physician admitting to negligence has his insurance carrier rushing to settle out of court. You should be aware that the dosage of drugs is different for a child, and should not hesitate to question the doctor. (Remember tact is always appropriate.)

Criminal negligence and *gross negligence* are sometimes used interchangeably and refer to the commission or omission of an act, lawfully or unlawfully, in which such a degree of negligence exists as may cause a serious wrong to another. Almost any act of negligence resulting in the death of a patient would be considered gross negligence. In such a situation the plaintiff may be awarded *punitive damages*, over and above the ordinary damages.

CASE

Texarkana Memorial Hospital Inc. v. Firth (1988)

In Texas, a 33-year-old woman was brought to a hospital emergency room, where she was diagnosed as being depressed, possibly suicidal, unable to sleep and hallucinating. She was given medication and was supposed to be sent to a closed unit, but was not. On two occasions, the patient threatened to jump out of the hospital window and was ordered additional medication. At 6 P.M., because of the situation, the nurse on duty called for additional help. The supervisor "floated" an RN to the unit and she was advised that the patient needed someone with her constantly. At 11 P.M. the RN float called the hospital administrator, noting that the patient was asleep. She was given permission to go home, and no replacement was assigned. The patient jumped from the window to her death. The jury awarded almost one million dollars in damages to the decedents' estate.[12]

Nursing Implications
Unfortunately this is not an unusual situation, and the plaintiffs are almost always awarded damages. The courts rule that a reasonably prudent person (the nurse) would have realized the potential danger. In other cases, even the excuse of short-staffing was not acceptable.[13]

You are expected to use nursing judgment whether or not there are doctor's orders to stay with the patient. Not to do so violates the doctrine of *foreseeability*. What of restraints? Unless the patient is violent, and even then persuasion should be tried, restraints cannot be used without a doctor's orders.[14] Remember, too, that there is a long history of patient's getting out of restraints.

Contributory negligence is the rather misleading expression used when the plaintiff has contributed to his or her own injury through personal negligence. This may have been done accidentally or deliberately. Some authorities assert that a plaintiff who is guilty of contributory negligence cannot collect damages; others state that he or she may collect under certain conditions. As in most legal matters, decisions vary widely. Because contributory negligence must be proven by the defendant, as much written evidence as possible is needed. The following cases illustrate the concept.

CASE

Huckathorn v. Lester E. Cox Medical Center (1992)

A competent patient was ordered a heating pad to his back "as tolerated" in the evening. The next morning when the nurse asked the patient several times to turn so that she could check his back, he refused, saying that he couldn't. The heating pad was removed at 1 P.M. revealing burns to the back; he sued. The hospital contended that he was partially responsible since he wouldn't allow the nurse to check his back. An appeals court refused this defense, saying there was no evidence as to when the burns developed or whether he could turn himself, so the jury's award stood.[15] (Interestingly, an earlier, very similar heating pad situation, where the patient was mobile and alert resulted in a different verdict.)

CASE

Oxford v. Upson County Hospital (1993)

When a patient asked to go to the bathroom, because there was nothing in the woman's chart to indicate that she had dizzy spells nor did she say she did, the nurse helped her to the bathroom. She fainted while sitting on the commode and hit her head. She sued the hospital and nurse for negligence. Both the Superior Court and the appeals court ruled in favor of the defendants, noting that the patient had a responsibility to inform caregivers of her symptoms. (The doctor did know of her tendency to dizziness, but hadn't recorded it.)[16]

Nursing Implications
You must always do a careful nursing assessment, make sure that there is accurate and complete communication with the physician, and chart accurately what occurred between you and the patient. If the nurses in the first case had checked to see whether the patient's back was all right, and if either nurse had checked with the doctor as to whether the patient *could* be turned, the entire problem might not have occurred. Whether or not any of this was recorded is not clear in the information given, but charting that substantiates what happened at the time it was happening is almost always accepted by the court.

In the second case, questioning the patient before taking her to the bathroom might have avoided injury, as would have the doctor's accurate recording. (It is interesting that the patient did not sue him.) Even if a case is decided in favor of the nurse, an injury to the patient is, of course, always bad, and can cause other problems. This court ruled that the nurse was not responsible because she didn't know of the patient's tendency to become dizzy. Another court could well have said that she should have found out, and under the doctrine of *comparative negligence*, she would have had a partial responsibility.

An important legal concept is *res ipsa loquitor* ("the thing speaks for itself"), a legal doctrine that gets around the need for expert testimony or the need for the plaintiff to prove the defendant's liability because the situation (harm) is self-evident even to a lay person. The defendant must prove, instead, that he or she is not responsible for the harm done. Before the rule of *res ipsa loquitor* can be applied, three conditions must be present: the injury would not ordinarily have occurred unless there was negligence; whatever caused the injury at the time was under the exclusive control of the defendant; the injured person had not contributed to the negligence or voluntarily assumed the risk. Often such a situation occurs in the operating room.

In 1995, newspapers reported that a Superior Court jury in New Jersey ordered a doctor and two nurses to pay a woman $500,000 for leaving a pad inside her body during a Cesarean section, in 1990. She was forced to undergo several surgeries, first to remove the pad, and then, in 1993, to correct problems from that surgery. The nurses were blamed for miscounting the pads; they said the doctor was also responsible. Here the nurses did not exercise the *due care* that they owed the plaintiff. Another point to note is the length of time between the negligent action and the suit. The *statute of limitations* varies with states, but usually the length of time during which a person can sue is longer for nurses. The time involved begins when the injury is noted (*discovery*), which may be several years. In the case of infants, or children, it doesn't begin until age 18, the *long tail* concept.

Another case of *res ipsa loquitor*, reported in 1987, resulted in an award of over $2 million. A 4-day-old infant suffered trauma to her head as a result of being dropped or mishandled by the nursing staff. The hospital and staff denied responsibility, although the baby had been under the exclusive control of the hospital staff throughout her stay. Even when the parents visited, staff were present. It appears that whoever caused the injury chose to cover up the incident. The hospital paid under the *respondeat superior* doctrine, since all the staff members were employees.[17]

Assuming that you are at little risk because you don't work in the ICU, the emergency room, or some other high-pressure unit is a mistake. In reviewing cases in which nurses were found liable, the sad news is that most of the incidents are everyday situations in which nurses not only did not use nursing judgment but sometimes didn't even use common sense. Quite often they neglected basic principles that they learned in their first year of nursing, such as how to give medications, or were careless about communication. Not only are RNs found liable, but also students. The following hypothetical situation (although based on fact) provides a useful illustration as well as applying several other legal principles.

A first-year student nurse was assigned by the instructor to care for a thin, very ill patient who required an intramuscular injection. The student had only practiced the procedure in the school laboratory. She injected the medication in the patient's sciatic nerve and caused severe damage. The patient sued the doctor, hospital, head nurse, student, faculty members, and school of nursing, an example of the *fishnet* principle. This was a case of *res ipsa loquitor*. The student was clearly negligent because she should have known the correct procedure and should have taken special precautions with an emaciated patient. The student is held to the standards of care (*standards of reasonableness*) of an RN if she is performing RN functions. If the student is not capable of functioning safely unsupervised, she should not be carrying out those functions. The doctor may or may not be held liable, depending on the court's notion about the *captain-of-the-ship doctrine*. However, this would have nothing to do with the drug and injection itself, assuming that it was an appropriate order. The hospital would probably be held liable under *respondeat superior*, because students, even if not employed, are usually treated legally as employees. Also applicable is the doctrine of *corporate liability*, which relates to the legal duty of a health care institution to provide appropriate facilities (staff and equipment) to carry out the purpose of the institution and to follow established standards of conduct.[18] In addition, because the head nurse is responsible for all patients on the unit and presumably should have been involved in the student's assignment, or should have assigned an RN to such an ill patient, she too would be liable, because she did not make an appropriate assignment ("appropriate delegation of duties").

The instructor might be found liable, not on the basis of *respondeat superior*—just as the head nurse or supervisor would not be liable if the student had been an RN, because these nurses are not the employers in the legal sense, but on the basis of inadequate supervision. If a supervisor or other nurse assigns a task to someone not competent to perform that task and a patient is injured because of that individual's incompetent performance, the supervising nurse can be held personally liable because it is part of her or his responsibility to know the competence and scope of practice of those being supervised.[19] (Although theoretically, in dealing with other than students, this nurse could rely on the subordinate's licensure, certification, or registration, if any, as an indication of competence, if there is reason to believe that that individual would nevertheless perform carelessly or incompetently and the nurse still assigns that person to the task, the nurse is held accountable, as is the employer under the doctrine of *respondeat superior*.) The school might be found liable in the case of the student, if the court believed the director had not used good judgment in employing or assigning the faculty member carrying out those teaching responsibilities. Nevertheless, the bottom line is that the student *is* responsible for her own actions, a basic principle of law.

Another case involving a student reinforces the principle of individual and teacher responsibility. In *Central Anesthesia Associates v. Worthy* (1985), Bonnie Castro, a senior student nurse anesthetist, was accused of administering anesthesia improperly, causing the patient to have a cardiac arrest and brain damage; the patient was still in a coma at the time of the case. Castro was under the supervision of a PA employed by the professional corporation that had the nurse anesthetist program. The Supreme Court of Georgia held Castro, the PA, and the three anesthesiologist teachers liable.

It rejected her argument that she should be held to the student standard; she was held to the standards of a certified nurse anesthetist (CNA). The teachers were not on the scene and had not delegated supervision properly. The PA either did not supervise adequately or was himself not capable. This case has implications for nursing students and their staff nurse preceptors when faculty are absent.

MAJOR CAUSES OF LITIGATION

Certain practices are more likely than others to result in nurses being sued or included in a malpractice case. Sometimes legal problems are caused by lack of knowledge, as when a nurse simply does not know the most current use or dangers of a drug or treatment or how to respond to a complication. For instance, in a 1987 case, $7.3 million was awarded to a husband in Illinois when his wife died because nurses did not recognize or handle an emergency correctly. A central venous pressure line, which had been inserted through the patient's internal jugular vein during surgery, perforated the wall of her heart, allowing fluid to accumulate in the pericardial sac. Even though in the first five postoperative hours the blood pressure became undetectable and her heart rate rose, the nurses failed to call the physician. The suit alleged inadequate postoperative care because of the nurses' failure to act.[20]

Often problems result from poor nursing judgment, as when a nurse in the emergency room sends away a patient without consulting with or calling a physician, or does not question a doctor's order or behavior, despite having doubts that the action is correct.[21] The amount of responsibility now put on nurses to judge the actions of the physician and (within their scope of practice or knowledge) to stop and/or report a questionable action is increasing. For instance in one case, both nurse and physician knew that a baby was in footling breech position and the nurse observed symptoms of fetal distress, but the physician decided to perform a vaginal delivery anyhow. The nurse expressed her concerns to the physician (who ignored them), but she did not contact her supervisor or anyone else. The baby suffered brain damage. In the suit that followed, the courts ruled that the physician made an error, but that the nurse should have notified a supervisor immediately. The hospital was held responsible and the family was awarded damages.[22] A large number of cases are the result of poor physician–nurse communication.

Communication Problems

Do you have a responsibility to take action when a doctor writes an order that you think is incorrect or unclear? When he or she does not respond to a patient's worsening condition? When he or she does not come to see a patient even if you think it's urgent? When he or she does not follow accepted precautions in giving a treatment? What if the physician becomes angry and abusive? What if he or she was right? According to court decisions in the last few years, the answer to all these questions is that it *is* the nurse's responsibility to take action. The case noted above is a good example.

However there are also problems of communication when the nurse does not keep the physician properly informed and the situation is disastrous for the patient.

CASE

Glassman v. St. Joseph Hospital (1994)

A patient underwent coronary artery bypass surgery and the doctors ordered vital signs to be taken every 15 minutes in the ICU. The patient's temperature rose to over 105 degrees at 2 P.M., the nurse notified the doctor, and he ordered treatment, which was carried out. When the patient had seizures, medication was ordered and given; but by 11 P.M., when the patient continued to have seizures, the nurse neither medicated the patient further as directed nor did she notify the doctor. Neither did the nurse on the next shift. The patient suffered severe permanent diffuse brain damage. The family sued the hospital and the doctors. An expert witness testified that the nurses had not followed the applicable *standard of care* in not administering sufficient medication (that had been ordered) and that their failure to notify the doctors of the multiple seizures beginning at 10:40 P.M. had contributed to the patient's brain damage.[23]

Nursing Implications

Just why the nurses did not give the medications or notify the physician is not clear. Busy? Afraid to "bother the doctor" at night? Uncomfortable about giving the kind and amount of medication ordered? Whatever the reason, their decision or carelessness hurt the patient irrevocably. Whatever the reason, you *must* communicate with the doctor in any case. If he is given to temper tantrums at being questioned or awakened, your resource is your supervisor, who can act as a buffer, intermediary, and support, perhaps checking with the doctor herself. If he or she is no help, you simply have to talk with the doctor, get clear what the situation is, and record fully what transpired. You should also go up the administrative ladder for help if necessary. The patient's well-being comes first.

You have a right to question the physician when in doubt about any aspect of an order, and the nursing service administration should support you. In fact, there should be a written policy on the nurse's rights and responsibility in such matters, so that there is no confusion on anyone's part and no danger of retribution for justifiable questioning when faced with an irate physician. What if the physician refuses to change the order? You should not simply refuse to carry out an order, for you may not have the most recent medical information and could injure the patient by *not* following the order. You should report your concern promptly to your administrative supervisor and record your action on the chart. Remember, a nurse who follows a physician's orders is just as liable as the physician if the patient is injured because, for instance, a medication was the wrong dose, given by the wrong route, or was actually the wrong drug. If the order is illegible or incomplete, it is necessary to clarify that order with the physician who wrote it. If you doubt its appropriateness, check with a reference source or the pharmacist, and always with the physician who wrote the order.[24] A good collegial relationship and mutual courtesy can prevent or ease a doctor–nurse confrontation.

Verbal or telephone orders are another part of the problem.[25] Although they are considered legal, the dangers are evident. In case of patient injury, either the doctor, or the nurse, or both will be held responsible. There frequently are or should be hospital, sometimes legal, policies to serve as guides. If telephone orders are forbidden and a patient is injured through confused orders, the situation could be considered negligence. If telephone orders are acceptable, precautions should be taken to ensure that they are clearly understood (and questioned if necessary), with the doctor required to confirm the orders in writing as soon as possible. Some hospital policies require a repetition of the order; it is not unheard of to have two nurses listen together to a telephone order, with the second nurse cosigning the order. In states where PAs' orders have been declared legal (as an extension of the physician), the same precautions must be taken, with the physician again confirming the order as quickly as possible.

An incident that repeatedly shows up in litigation is the failure of a physician to see a patient either on the unit or in the emergency room. Often the nurse is held liable for not following through. More and more often, it is suggested that a system (or a policy) be set up specifying who the nurse then contacts. If you neglect to call a doctor when the patient needs help or simply because you are not aware of the seriousness of the patient's condition, simply charting is not enough. This was clearly demonstrated in the *Darling* case. But charting is important. Even if a nurse swears in court that she did call a doctor and he denies it, the lack of charting has been noted by courts as raising questions about the nurse's credibility.[26]

There are a number of actions you can take to resolve these problems of communication. Don't hesitate to call a physician; be persistent in tracking down the attending or substitute physician; stay on the phone until you get the information you need (use nursing judgment). Be especially careful about telephone orders. Make sure you're both talking about the same patient. Make certain you understand what the doctor is saying even if it requires repetition. Repeat the order. Document the order, noting physician's name, time, date, and name of the third party if there was a witness.

Still other judgments against the nurse have been given when a doctor has not followed through on appropriate technical procedures, such as the timely removal of an endotracheal tube. As noted earlier, if you know that a particular procedure is being done incorrectly or a wrong medication is ordered (because it's within the scope of your knowledge) and do nothing about it, you can be held liable as well as the physician. A nurse may also refuse to administer a drug or treatment because it is against hospital policy.[27] However, it is important to have support from nursing management, if discussion with the physician ends with an impasse. It cannot be repeated too often: if the supervisor refuses to help, it will be necessary to go up the chain of command.[28]

Medication Errors

Medication errors are a particularly serious problem. Studies have shown that drugs are the major cause of illness and injury to patients in hospitals, from treatment given by physicians and others. Twenty percent have caused a serious disability. The major errors, in order, are: wrong dose, wrong drug, omission of a dose, wrong rate of administration, wrong route, and wrong time.[29] In one group of claims studied, 75 percent of the errors were made by physicians, about 13 percent by nurses, 8 percent by pharmacists, and about 4 percent by others.[30] Nurses who take unsafe shortcuts or otherwise fail to follow what they know is competent nursing practice are being negligent. If harm to a patient or co-worker can be traced to a nurse, and it often can, she or he may be held liable. Negligence tends to involve carelessness as much as lack of knowledge.

Preventing medication errors is, in part, getting back to basics with the "5 rights":[31]

1. *Right drug.* Check the order, question any drug that seems inappropriate, and consult about any drug with which you are unfamiliar (drug references, drug inserts, or pharmacist). Listen to the patient who notes that the medication "looks different."
2. *Right patient.* Check the patient's identification band.
3. *Right dose.* Be sure that you understand all abbreviations and measurements used in your facility. Have a colleague recheck your calculations. Question any dose that you feel is incorrect.

4. *Right route.* Follow all procedures for each route of administration. If you question the route specified, clarify it *with the physician.*
5. *Right time.* Omit or delay a dose only when indicated by a specific time or condition. Record this.

If an order is illegible, guesswork is dangerous. Physicians are responsible for writing legible orders, with standard abbreviations.[32] Computers are solving some of these problems, but it is still important to make sure the order is complete, including dose and route of administration. Preprinted standardized forms should be carefully done, according to standard practices, so that the medication orders are not misunderstood.[33]

What if you make an error? The patient should be observed for untoward

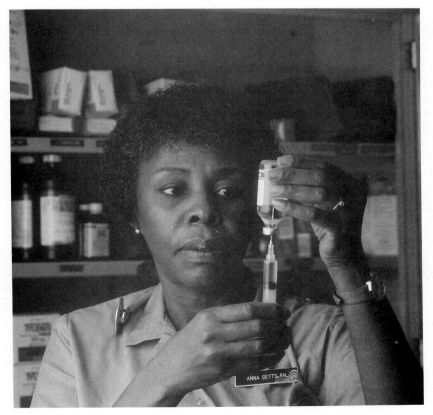

Because medication errors are a major cause of injury to patients, nurses must follow the appropriate procedure carefully. (*Courtesy of the American Nurses Association.*)

results, the error should be reported, and documented on the chart, and an incident report filed. If necessary, the patient is treated. Then review what happened to prevent another error.[34,35] The American Society of Hospital Pharmacists calls nurses "the final point of the checks and balances triad" that starts with the physician and pharmacist.[36]

Giving medication by injection is a common procedure, but again carelessness and haste can cause serious damage, and there is little question that the nurse is responsible.

CASE

Breid v. St. Luke's Memorial Hospital (1987)

A patient had had a laminectomy; by the next day he had full use of his extremities and could walk. When the patient complained of pain, the nurse took an unwise shortcut: she gave him a morphine injection when he was in an upright position. Soon he lost all sensory and motor function and became an invalid. Two expert nurse witnesses testified that the morphine should not have been given in that way, because it could cause hypotension, and the pooling of blood in the legs could precipitate a stroke. The nurse admitted that she knew this. She was found liable.[37]

Nursing Implications

Several points can be made here. It could be said that the nurse followed all five rules for giving medications safely, but she didn't use her nursing judgment. Just knowing the correct thing to do and then not doing it because you're in a hurry, and carelessness, almost always create later problems and, sometimes, as in this case, serious injury to the patient. One of the major reasons for negligence is failing to use adequate precautions to protect the patient against injury. When you have basic knowledge like the need to maintain the sterility of equipment such as needles, dressings or various catheters, but are careless about it, this can lead to court cases. This is clearly not a matter of the need for esoteric knowledge or management of complex equipment, but simply carelessness.

Other Common Acts of Negligence

Among the acts of negligence a nurse is most likely to commit in the practice of nursing are the following (not in order of importance):

1. *Abandoning a patient.* Abandonment simply means leaving a patient when your duty is to be with him. One example would be leaving a child or incompetent adult without the protection you would have offered. This may include leaving a patient in the bathroom or on a chair or stretcher while attending to something else. Falls often bring on suits. The results of abandonment can be more serious than a broken bone.

2. *Improper delegation and supervision.* Unless you work in a place that has all-RN staffing, you probably will be delegating certain patient assignments to an LPN or aide. Theoretically you can look to the LPN's licensure as evidence that this person is qualified to perform certain tasks. However, it is your responsibility to know an individual's competence before assigning an LPN or aide to patient care. The person, if not licensed, must be properly trained. In other words you can't simply say "You take the patients on that side of the hall" if any one of those patients requires the care of an RN. Should a patient be injured, you can be held responsible.

3. *Failure to use adequate precautions to protect the patient against injury.* As a nurse, you are expected to know that drugs, or hot liquids, or potentially harmful implements, such as scissors, must be kept out of the reach of a young child or a delirious or confused patient. You know the danger of falls or slips when weak, elderly, or disabled patients are walking or left alone. Patients often fall when trying to get out of bed or using the bathroom.

The following case is an example of these three acts of negligence.

CASE

Halby v. Humana Hospital–West Hills (1994)

A postpartum patient felt faint in the bathroom. An aide told the patient to hold on to the rail and grabbed the patient's arm. She fell back unconscious and hit her head. The patient sued, claiming that had the aide lowered her to the floor and called for help she wouldn't have been hurt.[38]

Nursing Implications
Whether or not the aide was properly trained was at issue here. Presumably, she should have known what to do. Did she forget? Misjudge? Should an LPN or RN have tended to that patient? You must use your nursing judgment to determine whether a patient can be cared for by a less-prepared person.

4. *Failure to respond, or to ask someone else to respond, promptly to a patient's call light or signal* if, because of such failure, a patient is injured.

CASE

Ard v. East Jefferson General Hospital (1994)

A 64-year-old patient with a history of myocardial infarction, stroke, and unstable angina was admitted to the hospital and subsequently underwent a coronary bypass. After a respiratory problem, he was transferred to a critical care unit. His wife maintained that nurses did not respond to her calls for assistance from 5:30 to 6:45 P.M. At that time he stopped breathing, and a code was called. He never regained consciousness and died two days later. His wife brought a suit for wrongful death. That no one had responded to her calls for assistance for one hour and 15 minutes was consistent with the medical record. An expert witness determined six breaches of the *standard of care* in relation to the patient's condition that the nurses should have recognized as a potential danger, and therefore should have checked the patient frequently themselves. Poor nursing assessment and incomplete nurses notes were also pointed out.[39]

Nursing Implications
The basic problem here, of course, was poor nursing assessment, but ignoring the patient's light resulted in what was called "*loss of chance*," that is, that the patient might have survived if someone had come right away and noted the seriousness of his respiratory problems. Ignoring call signals or waiting too long to respond is, unfortunately, not unusual in hospitals, especially with short-staffing. True, often the request is minor or trivial and could have waited, but you never know. A common mishap occurs when a patient gets tired of waiting, tries to get out of bed alone, and falls. At least a quick stop to see what is needed, even by an aide, who, if properly trained, knows when to get RN help, may forestall a disaster.

---

5. *Inadequate or dated nursing knowledge.* Since having current knowledge is a professional responsibility, there seems to be little excuse for this kind of negligence. However, on occasion, even the most competent nurse has a problem. If an entirely new type of treatment or piece of equipment is introduced on your unit, it is your responsibility, as well as that of the head nurse or supervisor, to get the appropriate information. (See also the *St. Paul Medical Center v. Cecil* case, cited later.)

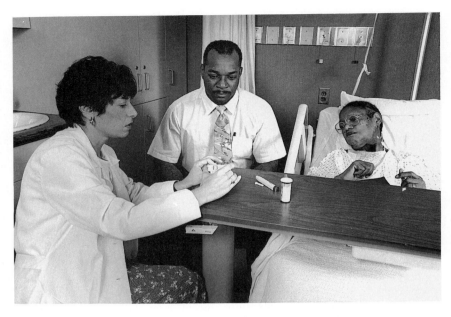

Teaching patients thoroughly can avoid malpractice claims. (*Courtesy of Robert Wood Johnson Hospital, New Brunswick, New Jersey.*)

6. *Failure to teach a patient.* Nurses sometimes neglect to teach a patient in preparation for discharge, either because of the time it takes or because the physician objects. An increasing number of suits are being filed because such teaching was not done or not done thoroughly or understandably. Written instructions are often considered necessary to help the patient and family remember the information.

7. *Failure to make sure that faulty equipment is removed* from use, that crowded corridors or hallways adjacent to the nursing unit are cleared, that slippery or unclean floors are taken care of, and that fire hazards are eliminated. This is an area of negligence that, in most instances, would implicate others just as much as, or more than, the professional nurse. For example, the hospital administration would certainly share responsibility for fire hazards and dangerously crowded corridors, and the housekeeping and maintenance departments would not be blameless either. This does not lessen your responsibility for reporting unsafe conditions and following up on them or for checking equipment you use. Report persistent hazards in writing and keep a copy for personal protection.

LEGAL PROBLEMS IN
RECORD-KEEPING

It is almost impossible to overemphasize the importance of records in legal action, especially nurses' notes. They are the only evidence that orders were carried out and what the results were; they are the only notes written with both the time and date in chronological order; they offer the most detailed information on the patient. Nurses' notes, like the rest of the chart, can be subpoenaed. No matter how skillfully you practice, if your actions and observations are not documented accurately and completely, the jury can judge only by what is recorded. If you are subpoenaed, comprehensive notes will not only give weight to your testimony, but will help you remember what happened. A case may not come up for years, and unless there was a severe problem at the time, it is difficult to remember exact details about one patient. General, broad phrases such as "resting comfortably," "good night," and "feeling better" are totally inadequate. How could a jury interpret them? How could even another professional who did not know that patient interpret them?

Some of the most serious problems arising from poor charting concern lack of data, which have resulted in liability judgments against nurses and hospitals, although in each case it was contended that the right thing had been done. One judge noted that insufficient notes indicated substandard care.[40] Moreover, there are instances when a patient might be legally harmed by inaccurate reporting, as in child or adult abuse or rape.[41]

The correct way to chart, with legal aspects in mind, is probably to chart as you were taught and to follow good nursing practice.

Do:

1. Be objective: write what you see, hear, smell, and feel.
2. Be complete: for medications, record what, where, and how.
3. Be accurate: if a mistake is made, recopy or cross out, with the original copy attached; never use white-out.
4. Be specific.
5. Record the patient's progress and any change in condition.
6. Record abnormal patient behavior.
7. Document any patient teaching.
8. Write legibly.
9. Use only standard abbreviations.
10. Be careful about how statements read. ("Bathed in wheelchair in lounge" can cause a legal problem.)
11. Record the time and date of entries; chart the *correct time* when events occurred.
12. Sign every entry.

Don't:

1. Use a pencil.
2. Make flip, derogatory, critical, or extraneous remarks about anyone or use labels to describe your patient's behavior, such as "non-compliant." (Describe what actually happened.)
3. Omit data such as amounts and kind of fluids, oxygen, or the physician's visits.
4. Guess at such things as output and vital signs.
5. *Ever* lie or cover up for anyone. *Never* alter a record other than as described above; this has been shown to influence a jury negatively. Every good malpractice attorney calls on experts to examine charts for alterations, erasures, and additions. This can also lead to criminal charges.
6. Let anyone chart for you or change what you have charted.
7. Chart for anyone else. When you must chart what an aide or student says he or she did or what occurred when you have not personally seen it, add a statement that clarifies the fact to protect yourself.
8. Fail to record verbal orders and have them signed.
9. Chart your actions in advance to save time.
10. Refer to staffing problems.
11. Mention that an incident report has been filed.
12. Use terms like "accidentally" or "somehow" to explain a mistake. Just record what happened.
13. Air "dirty laundry"—disputes with colleagues or criticisms of nurses or doctors.
14. Refer to another patient by name; use "roommate," initials, or bed number.
15. Withhold important information, such as conversations with family or health professionals.[42,43]

Computer records have changed correction procedures, since corrections can be made immediately. (Such "charting" does allow for more accurate, timely and legible charting, but the issue of confidentiality discussed in Chapter 9 may present a problem.)[44] Charting incorrect data in any form obviously does not give an accurate picture of your patient's condition, which could lead to life-threatening errors. It may also raise a question of fraud, so that your actions appear not just negligent, but criminal. It has been suggested that for proper patient care, you should:

1. Collect and analyze data from other parts of the medical record, for example, the physician's notes, lab and other diagnostic reports.
2. Use your data to identify patients at increased risk for complications.
3. Not focus so much on the diagnosis that you do not analyze the data accurately.

4. Periodically review and revise policy manuals to see if they conform to national standards. (This is also important should a legal situation occur, as shown later.)[45]

Some of the most serious problems arising from poor charting concern lack of data, such as omission of a temperature reading or other vital signs, lack of observations about a patient's condition, or no record of oxygen liter flow in a newborn infant; these and others have resulted in liability judgments against nurses and hospitals. Although it is often inaccurate, the statement "if it wasn't charted, it wasn't done" has evolved into a legal standard.[46]

Court cases in which nursing documentation is inadequate are many and often result in a judgment for the plaintiff.[47] While the current trend toward "charting by exception"—that is, charting only when something unusual or out of the ordinary happens—may save time, it frequently leaves gaps that raise questions about patient care.[48] A well-designed flowchart can be useful, but it should be consistent with the nurse's notes. You cannot simply check off what the nurses on the previous shift checked off. If you were sued, such discrepancies would damage your credibility. Moreover, you should not depend too heavily on flowcharts; it is still important to record the patient's *response* to care in your notes. Overall, any significant indicator of a change in the patient's condition, corresponding interventions, and the patient's response should be recorded. The chart must accurately reflect the patient's condition and progress. Cases such as the classic *Darling* one continue to occur.[49] The case described below is a particularly good example of what can happen if charting by exception is taken too literally.

CASE

Lama v. Borras (1994)

A patient underwent back surgery for a herniated disk, twice. For several days, nurses noted that the bandage was "soiled," "bloody," and "soiled again." They did not record the patient's complaint of pain, changing characteristics of the surgical wound, any nursing or medical interventions, or evidence that the doctor was alerted. Objective aspects of the patient's care such as vital signs and medication administration *were* recorded. The day after a night that had the patient screaming with pain, the doctor diagnosed the problem as diskitis, an infection between the disks, and treated it. The patient needed several months of hospitalization. He sued the hospital and doctor, claiming in part that because the nurses did not chart his changing condition in detail, his infection was not caught in time. The jury ruled in his favor; the appeals court concurred.[50]

Nursing Implications

Although the hospital tried to defend charting by exception, noting among other things that the patient didn't have a fever, a common sign of infection, which would have been charted, the appeals court concluded that "intermittent charting" and the failure of nurses to document early signs of impending infection delayed the diagnosis. You should be very clear about what needs to be charted to accurately document the patient's condition, regardless of a hospital policy on charting. Saving time is not worthwhile if a patient suffers. As in so many other cases, taking short-cuts, even approved short-cuts, can be calamitous. First of all, however, your nursing assessment is the key to what to chart, and reporting as well as recording is essential. Should a situation arise when you do notify a physician about a problem and he denies it, in court, your written documentation *at the time* of doing so generally carries weight over the doctor's testimony.[51]

THE PROBLEM OF SHORT-STAFFING

Can an injury to a patient be excused on the basis of short-staffing? Not really. Even if there is a staff shortage, nurses have a responsibility to use good judgment.

In *Harrell v. Louis Smith Hospital* (1992), the plaintiff alleged negligence on the part of the hospital because of short-staffing, and the president of the hospital did make several statements that created some question as to whether certain units, such as the emergency room, were well staffed. The court ruled that the hospital *must* provide staff "adequately trained to exercise a reasonable degree of care and skill when delivering healthcare."[52] There is some feeling that with all the unlicensed assistive personnel being hired and a cutback of RNs today, this point will come up again.

Further problems can come from "floating." In these cases, you may be placed in a specialty area with which you are not familiar, with or without a more experienced nurse. There is no clear answer to this dilemma, since some courts have ruled that shifting staff is the employer's privilege and refusal can be considered insubordination. Express your reservations and explore alternatives, for instance, to delay such an assignment until you're received in-service, or indicate a willingness to provide the care you are comfortable with.[53] This is equally important if you are an inexperienced new graduate. The supervisor, of course, is also responsible for any damage done because he or she is supposed to delegate safely. The float nurse must be especially careful and report any change in a patient's condition. Perhaps the best defense if injury occurs is to be able to document that you recognized your knowledge gap, but did not know that specialty and had asked for help. Meanwhile, some union contracts and some individual agreements in hospitals specify that a nurse is not to be floated to an unfamiliar unit without some training in that specialty. (See also Chapter 15.) Regardless, as shown in the next case, you are responsible for your own actions.

CASE

St. Paul Medical Center v. Cecil (1992)

A pregnant woman arrived in the hospital telling the nurse her water had broken. The nurse did a pelvic exam, assessed the patient's vital signs, contractions, and other conditions and checked the fetal heart rate. Over a number of hours, both the resident and the nurse checked a fetal monitor the nurse had attached, but there were a number of delays and the nurse left the patient for long periods of time. Then a wait for an anesthesiologist caused a further delay before the patient's physician performed what was supposed to be an emergency Cesarean. The baby was born with severe brain damage due to prolonged hypoxia. The attending physician settled before the trial, but the nurse and the hospital were each found 50 percent negligent, with an award of over $1 million. The patient alleged that the hospital should have known that the nurse was not qualified to perform the necessary tasks required by the position, that she sometimes fell asleep at her station, and that she was not adequately supervised. They cited an employee evaluation of 3 months before this incident that indicated that she did fall asleep, that she had trouble using electronic fetal monitors and that she was reluctant to seek guidance.[54]

Nursing Implications
One point that this case demonstrates is that you are responsible for your own actions. If you have difficulty with a procedure or a certain kind of nursing care, make it your business to learn. If a situation arises about which you are insecure, get help. The fact that this nurse was assigned to a unit in which she was not completely capable did not excuse her.

SPECIALTY NURSING

As nurses assume more responsibility in nursing, particularly in specialty areas, they often seek help in determining their legal status. Frequently their concern has to do with the scope of practice: are they performing within legal bounds? Negligence, whether in a highly specialized unit, an emergency, or a self-care unit, is still a question of what the reasonably prudent nurse would do. Therefore, although a nurse might look for a specific answer to a specific question, the legal dangers lie in the same set of instances described earlier, simply transposed to another setting. The Bibliography citations give some examples, such as office nursing and community health nursing.

STANDARD OF CARE

The standard of care basically determines nurses' liability for negligent acts. (Note its importance in the cases cited previously.) This standard requires an individual to perform a task as any "reasonably prudent man of ordinary prudence, with comparable education, skills, and training under similar circumstances" would perform that same function. It is often described as requiring a person of ordinary sense to use ordinary care and skill. Who makes that judgment on what the "reasonably prudent" nurse would do?

In litigation, it is the judge or jury, based on testimony that could include the following:

1. *Expert witnesses.* Did the nurse do what was necessary? A nurse with special or appropriate knowledge testifies on what would be expected of a nurse in the defendant's position in like circumstances. The expert witness would have the credentials to validate his or her expertise, but because the opposing side would produce an equally prestigious expert witness to say what was useful to them, the credibility of that witness on testifying is critical. A nurse would generally be judged by an expert in his or her particular kind of nursing.[55]

2. *Professional literature.* Was the nurse's practice current? The *most current* nursing literature would be examined and perhaps quoted to validate (or invalidate) whether the nurse's practice in the situation was totally up-to-date.

3. *Hospital or agency policies and protocols.* Were hospital policies, especially nursing policies (in-house law), followed?[56] For example, if restraints were or were not used, was the nurse's action according to hospital policy? On the other hand, if a nurse followed an outdated policy or followed policy without using nursing judgment (according to the expert witness), it could be held against her or him.

4. *Manuals or procedure books.* Did the nurse follow the usual procedure accurately? Example: If the nurse gave an injection that was alleged to have injured the patient, was it given correctly according to the

procedure manual? If the procedure book is not up-to-date and the nurse followed it, she or he might still be liable on the basis of needing to be aware of current practice.

5. *Drug enclosures or drug reference books.* Did the nurse check for the latest information? For example, if the patient suffered from a drug reaction that the nurse did not perceive, was the information about the potential reaction in a drug reference book, such as the *Physicians' Desk Reference* (PDR) or a drug insert?

6. *The profession's standards.* Did the nurse behave according to the published ANA standards, both general and in the specialty, if any?[57]

7. *Licensure.* Did the nurse fulfill her responsibilities according to the legal definition of nursing in the licensure law or the law's rules and regulations? For example, did she teach a diabetic patient about foot care?

If the judge or jury is satisfied that the standards were met satisfactorily, even if the patient has been injured, the injury that occurred would not be considered the result of the nurse's negligence. (If there is *no* injury, even if the health care provider was negligent, there is no tort.) Different judgments in different jurisdictions must be expected. Nevertheless, a nurse who knows the profession's standards and practices accordingly is in a much firmer position legally than one who does not.[58]

OTHER TORTS AND CRIMES

The average nurse probably will not get involved in criminal offenses, although in the last few years, a number of nurses have been accused of murder or other deliberate injury to patients.[59] Nurses, like anyone else, may steal, murder, or break other laws. But they can also be falsely accused. In a recent case, good documentation of patient care and the doctor's support helped clear one nurse.[60] Crimes most often committed are criminal assault and battery (striking or otherwise physically mistreating or threatening a patient); murder (sometimes in relation to right-to-die principles); and drug offenses. If found guilty of a felony, the nurse will probably also lose her or his license.

Whether the nurse is a perpetrator or victim, or simply has to deal with people who are, it is useful to know the definition and scope of the most common criminal offenses. These can be found in most nursing law texts. Several are discussed here. Not discussed but worth mentioning are some torts and crimes in which nurses occasionally are involved in their professional lives: *forgery*—fraudulently making or altering a written document or item, such as a will, chart, or check; *kidnapping*—stealing and carrying off a human being; *rape*—illegal or forcible sexual intercourse; and *bribery*—an offer of a reward for doing wrong or for influencing conduct. Other causes for action against nurses beyond negligence are false imprisonment (also discussed in Chapter 9), intentional infliction of emotional distress, and invasion of privacy.[61]

Assault and Battery

Any attempt to use force and violence with an intent to injure, or put one in fear of injury, constitutes an *assault*, such as striking at a person with or without a weapon; holding up a fist in a threatening way near enough to be able to strike; or advancing with a hand uplifted in a threatening way with intent to strike or put someone in fear of being struck, even if the person is stopped before he or she gets near enough to carry out the intended action.

Battery, as distinguished from assault, is the actual striking or touching of a person's body in a violent, angry, rude, or insolent manner. Every laying on of hands is not a battery: the person's intention must be considered. To constitute a battery, intent to injure or put one in fear of injury must be accompanied by "unlawful violence." However, the slightest degree of force may constitute violence in the eyes of the law. Legal action can result from any of these acts unless they can be justified or excused.

Defamation, Slander, and Libel

As is true of so many legal terms, there is some overlapping of meaning and interpretation of the terms *defamation, slander,* and *libel*. In general, however, it is correct to consider *defamation* as the most inclusive term because it covers any communication that is seriously detrimental to another person's reputation. If the communication is oral, it is technically called *slander*; if written or shown in pictures, effigies, or signs (without just cause or excuse), it is called *libel*. All three are considered wrongful acts (torts) under the law, and a person convicted in court is ordered to make amends, usually by paying the defamed person a compensatory fee.

In both slander and libel, a third person must be involved. For example, one person can make all kinds of derogatory statements directly to another without getting in trouble with the law *unless* overheard and understood by a third person. Then the remarks become slanderous. Likewise a person can write anything she or he wishes to another, and the communication will not be considered libelous unless it is read and understood by a third person. A malicious and false statement made by one person to another about a third person also comprises slander.[62]

Uncomplimentary statements are not necessarily slanderous or libelous.

They must be false, damaging to the offended person's reputation, and tending to subject him or her to public contempt and ridicule. The best and often the only defense allowed under the law is proof that she or he told the truth in whatever type of communication used.

Given the many "ifs," "ands," and "buts" associated with defamation, slander, and libel, it's better to avoid becoming embroiled in such litigations. Be careful in what you say or write about anyone. Also, proceed with caution when you are the victim of slander or libel. Litigation is expensive and time-consuming and, in many instances, hardly worth the trouble. On the other hand, don't be overly meek in accepting unfair and untrue statements about yourself that are likely to adversely affect your reputation. There have been documented cases in which nurses were slandered by a physician, for instance, and collected damages.

Homicide and Suicide

Homicide means killing a person by any means whatsoever. It is not necessarily a crime. If it is unquestionably an accident, it is called *excusable homicide*. If it is done in self-defense or in discharging a legal duty, it is termed *justifiable homicide*. The accused must be able to prove justification, however. *Criminal homicide* is either murder or manslaughter; murder is usually with intent.

Suicide is considered criminal if the person is sane and of an age of discretion at the time of his or her action. A person who encourages another to commit suicide is guilty of murder if the suicide is successful. Statutes vary from state to state.

As a professional person, it is not unusual for a nurse to become involved in cases of murder and suicide, usually associated with patients. Following are a few suggestions for keeping as free of legal involvement as possible:

1. Take seriously any indication on the part of any patient or employee that she or he has suicidal tendencies. Report this to the appropriate person.
2. Generally, don't leave a patient with known suicidal inclinations alone unless completely protected from self-harm by restraints or confinement.
3. Keep items that a depressed person might use for suicidal purposes out of reach.
4. Make and report observations accurately on the patient's chart.
5. Try to get help for individuals or their families immediately upon becoming aware of suicidal tendencies.
6. Cooperate with the police and hospital authorities guarding a patient who is accused of homicide.

7. Avoid unethical discussions of a homicide case involving a patient or employee.
8. Keep complete and accurate records of all facts that might have a bearing on the legal aspects of a case.

DRUG CONTROL

In 1914, the United States adopted an antinarcotic law, the *Harrison Narcotic Act*, to be administered by a bureau of narcotics within the Department of the Treasury. It was amended frequently to meet the demands of changing times. The *Comprehensive Drug Abuse and Control Act* of 1970 (*Controlled Substance Act*) replaced virtually all earlier federal laws dealing with narcotics, stimulants, depressants, and hallucinogens. Sections of this law prohibit nurses from prescribing controlled substances, but they may administer drugs at the direction of legalized practitioners (who are registered). All registrants must follow strict controls and procedures against theft and diversion of controlled substances. New state laws are based on the federal law, although there are variations. Controlled substances are identified as such in health care delivery sites. New drugs are also being given closer scrutiny because of misuse and consequent dangerous effects.

Knowledge of the laws controlling the use of drugs will help you to understand the reasons for the policies and procedures established by an institution or agency for the mutual welfare of the employer, employee, and patient. It will also help you to keep free of legal involvements and to direct and advise intelligently others whom you may supervise or who may look to you for guidance in such matters. Be alert to changes in drug laws at either the state or the national level.

GOOD SAMARITAN LAWS

The enactment of Good Samaritan laws in many states exempts doctors and nurses (and sometimes others) from civil liability when they give emergency care in "good faith" with "due care" or without "gross negligence." All states and the District of Columbia have Good Samaritan laws, but not all include nurses in their coverage. The law is intended to encourage assistance without fear of legal liability. As far as the law is concerned, there is no obligation or duty to render aid or assistance in an emergency. Only by statutory law can the rendering of such assistance be required. Emergency treatment in a health care setting such as hospitals, clinics and occupational health departments, is not covered under the Good Samaritan laws.

Because of the lack of clarity of terms and the many differences in the law from state to state, many health professionals are still reluctant to give emergency assistance.[63] One lawyer gives this advice:

1. Don't give aid unless you know what you're doing.
2. Stick to the basics of first aid.
3. Offer to help, but make it clear that you won't interfere if the victim or family prefers to wait for other help.
4. Don't draw any medical or diagnostic conclusions.
5. Don't leave a victim you've begun to assist until you can turn his or her care over to an equally competent person.
6. Whether you do or do not volunteer your services, be absolutely certain to call or have someone else call for a physician or emergency medical service immediately.[64]

PROFESSIONAL LIABILITY (MALPRACTICE) INSURANCE

Almost all lawyers in the health field now agree that nurses should carry their own malpractice or, as it is increasingly called, *professional liability* insurance, whether or not their employer's insurance includes them. The employer's insurance is intended primarily to protect the employer; the nurse is protected only to the extent needed for that primary purpose. It is quite possible that the employer might settle out of court, without consulting the nurse, to the nurse's disadvantage. The nurse then has no control and no choice of lawyer.[65]

There are a number of other limitations. The nurse is not covered for anything beyond the job in the place of employment during the hours of employment. If the nurse alone is sued and the hospital is not, the hospital has no obligation to provide legal protection (and may choose not to). Moreover, as noted earlier, if the nurse has been negligent, and carries no personal liability insurance, there is the possibility of subrogation.[66] Should there be criminal charges, the employer or insurance carrier may choose to deny legal assistance, or the kind offered could be inadequate. However, some professional liability policies held by the nurse personally, may also state that criminal action is not covered. Remember that no matter how trivial or how unfounded a charge might be, a legal defense is necessary and often costly, aside from the possibility of being found liable and having to pay damages.

Professional liability insurance should be bought with some care so that adequate coverage is provided. Certain features are optional. Decide which coverage meets your needs, but don't necessarily choose the least expensive. For instance, the most important distinction to be made in selecting insurance is whether it has an *occurrence-based coverage* or a *claims-made coverage.* If the insurance policy is allowed to lapse, an incident that occurred at the time of coverage will be covered in an occurrence-based policy but not in a claims-made policy. The latter may be less expensive but will require almost continuous coverage, which might be a problem for a nurse planning to interrupt practice for any reason or for one close to retirement.

Before deciding on a policy, check:[67]

1. What kinds of acts are covered on the job.
2. What kinds of acts are covered off the job.
3. Whether personal liability is covered.
4. Under what circumstances a lawyer will be provided.
5. Whether you have any choice of lawyer.
6. Whether a settlement can be made without your approval.
7. The term of the policy.
8. What affects renewability.
9. The cost.

Benefits usually include paying any sum awarded as damages, including medical costs, paying the cost of attorneys, and paying the bond required if appealing an adverse decision. Some policies also pay damages for injury arising out of acts of the insured as a member of an accreditation board or committee of a hospital or professional society, personal liability (such as slander, assault, or libel), and personal injury and medical payments (not related to the individual's professional practice).

Generally speaking, an ANA or SNA policy is the best buy. Premiums depend on the position of the nurse. Only nurse anesthetists and nurse-midwives are not covered, but NPs and nurses in private practice are, at a higher premium. In 1990, ANA also expanded its coverage to include students. Nurses who have retired are often advised to keep their professional liability insurance. Most nurses tend to help and advise neighbors, friends, and family about their health care. If the person advised feels that the advice was the cause of an emotional or physical problem later, he or she has been known to sue the nurse.

As noted earlier, most malpractice cases are settled out of court (although this still requires a lawyer) and multimillion-dollar awards are not as common as the newspapers may imply. However, for the careful nurse, professional liability insurance is a good investment, as well as being tax-deductible.

IN COURT: THE DUE PROCESS OF LAW

Yes, you can be sued. What happens if you become involved in litigation? What steps should you take to try to make sure that the case will be handled to your best advantage throughout? The answers to these questions will depend on: whether you are accused of committing the tort or crime; whether you are an accessory, through actual participation or observance; whether you are the person against whom the act was committed; or whether you appear as an expert witness.

Assuming that this is a civil case, five distinct steps are taken:

1. The filing of a document called a *complaint* by a person called the *plaintiff* who contends that his legal rights have been infringed by the conduct of one or more other persons called *defendants.*
2. The written response of the defendants accused of having violated the legal rights of the plaintiff, termed an *answer.*
3. Pretrial activities of both parties designed to elicit all the facts of the situation, termed *discovery.*[68]
4. The *trial* of the case, in which all the relevant facts are presented to the judge or jury for decision.
5. *Appeal* from a decision by a party who contends that the decision was wrongly made.

The majority of persons who are asked to appear as witnesses during a hearing accept voluntarily. Others refuse and must be subpoenaed. A *subpoena* is a writ or order in the name of the court, referee, or another person authorized by law to issue the same, which requires the attendance of a witness at a trial or hearing under a penalty for failure. Cases involving the care of patients often necessitate producing hospital records, x-rays, and photographs as evidence. A subpoena requiring a witness to bring this type of evidence to court contains a clause to that effect and is termed a *subpoena duces tecum.*

The plaintiff, defendant, and witnesses may be asked to make a *deposition,* an oral interrogation answering various questions about the issue concerned.[69] It is given under oath and taken in writing before a judicial officer or attorney. Tips given by experts on how to handle yourself at a deposition are basically the same as for testifying. You may be cross-examined by the opposing lawyer; the only limitation on the scope of questioning is that the inquiry must be relevant to the subject under suit. Since the primary purpose is *discovery,* the procedure is sometimes referred to as a "fishing expedition."

The trial itself follows a certain format: choosing the jury; opening statements by both sides, with the plaintiff going first; testimony and cross-examination; possible request for dismissal; and closing arguments. An appeal to a higher court may be filed.[70]

A witness has certain rights, including the right to refuse to testify as to privileged communication (extended to the nurse in only a few states) and the protection against self-incrimination afforded by the Fifth Amendment to the Constitution. The judge and jury usually do not expect a person on trial or serving as witness to remember all the details of a situation. Witnesses in malpractice suits are permitted to refer to the patient's record, which, of course, they should have reviewed with the attorney before the trial. Only under serious circumstances is someone accused (and convicted) of *perjury*, which means making a false statement under oath or one that the person neither knows nor believes to be true.

There are certain guidelines on testifying that are the same whether serving as an expert or other witness or if the nurse is the defendant:

1. Be prepared; review the deposition, the chart, technical and clinical knowledge of the disease or condition; discuss with the lawyer potential questions; educate the lawyer as to what points should be made. Trials are adversary procedures that are intended to probe, question, and explore all aspects of the issue.
2. Dress appropriately; appearance is important.
3. Behave appropriately: keep calm, be courteous, even if insulted; don't be sarcastic or angry; take your time (a cross-examiner attorney may try to put you in a poor light). Never argue with the attorney questioning you.
4. Give adequate and appropriate information: if you can't remember, notes or the data source, such as the chart, can be checked. Answer fully, but don't volunteer additional information not asked for. Don't answer until you understand the question. Wait for the question to be completed before you respond. Think about your answer before responding.
5. Don't use technical terminology, or, if use is necessary, translate it into lay terms. Enunciate clearly.
6. Don't feel incompetent; don't get on the defensive; be decisive.
7. Don't be obviously partisan (unless you're the defendant).
8. Keep all materials; the decision may be appealed.

In the expert witness role,[71] the same suggestions hold, but in addition the nurse should present her or his credentials, degrees, research, honors, and whatever else is pertinent, without modesty; the opposing expert witness will certainly do so. Expert witnesses are paid for preparation time, pretrial conferences, consultations, and testifying. Nurses are just beginning to act officially in this capacity, and several SNAs accept applications for those interested in placement on an expert witness panel, screen applicants in a given field for a specific case, submit a choice of names to attorneys requesting such information, and have developed guidelines and CE for nurse expert witnesses.

Should you be sued, here are some tips for defending yourself:

- Cut off all communication with the claimant; simply tell whoever contacts you that your insurer will be in touch. (Then find out why they haven't already done so.)
- Educate the insurer; claims adjusters may know little about nursing.
- Keep tabs on the claim. Don't be afraid to ask questions.
- Be sure that your claim is supervised adequately. You have a right to ask that it be handled by an experienced and attentive professional.
- Seek input on settlement decisions. You may not have the right, but you can ask your insurer to check with you before making an offer.
- Remember that the defense attorney is *your* attorney. If you really think his or her qualifications are inadequate, ask for a change.
- Dictate all memories of the patient to the attorney. Do it as soon as possible, but not until an attorney has been assigned to your case, or your information may not be considered "privileged."
- Retrieve medical records. You have access if you still work at the same place and can get access before the attorney does.
- Review the records.
- Compile a list of experts; the case may hinge on getting the best. (Although in some courts physicians have been allowed as expert witnesses on a nursing case, ordinarily it should be the nurse(s) who are most knowledgeable about the type of situation involved.)
- Have a reference list available.
- Speak up in court; you must project self-confidence.[72]

Other attorneys also point out that you shouldn't talk to anyone about the case at your hospital except the risk manager, or with anyone involved in any way with the plaintiff, or to reporters. Certainly don't hide any information from your attorney, and *never* alter the patient's record.

RISK MANAGEMENT

No matter how strong the defense, everyone agrees that prevention is better than any suit. Therefore, hospitals have now adopted risk-management programs in which nurses are very much involved, as part of the team and also sometimes in one of the risk-management positions, including patient representative or advocate. Risk management must be a team effort involving everyone.

Risk management initiatives are now required by JCAHO and more and more by state legislation. The purpose is not only to protect the interest of the hospital and its personnel but also to improve the quality of patient care. Risk management means taking steps to control the possibility that a patient will complain and minimizing any risks *before* complaints are filed. Nurses are often involved in risk management which includes focusing on the review and improvement of employee guidelines, personnel policies, incident reports, physician–nurse relationships, safety policies, patient records, research guidelines, and anything else that might be a factor in legal suits.[73]

Nevertheless, patient injuries do occur. In case of patient injury, most hospitals and health agencies require completion of an "incident report." The purpose is to document the incident accurately for remedial and correctional use by the hospital or agency, for insurance information, and sometimes for legal reasons. The wording should be chosen to avoid the implication of blame and should be totally objective and complete: what happened to the patient; what was done; what his condition is. The incident report may or may not be discoverable, depending on the state's law. It is considered a business record, not part of the patient's chart, but some courts rule that it is not privileged information. The incident *must* be just as accurately recorded in the patient's chart. This kind of omission casts doubt on the nurse's honesty if litigation occurs. However, the fact that an incident report was filed should not be charted.

Appropriate behavior by nurses and other personnel is often a key factor as to whether or not the patient or family sues after an incident, regardless of injury. Maintaining a good rapport and giving honest explanations as needed is very important.

AVOIDING LEGAL PROBLEMS

Malpractice continues to be an issue in health care from the point of view of both patient endangerment and cost. Physicians are said to practice "defensive medicine," that is, ordering every possible test to make sure that nothing was neglected that may eventually result in litigation. That and the rising cost of malpractice insurance adds to the overall cost of health care. Nurses are also concerned about their liability as they care for more patients, who are more sick, with less help. While it may be possible to get some information from your employing agency's legal counsel or state licensing board in relation to specific aspects of your practice, observing some basic principles will also help to avert problems:

1. Know your licensure law.
2. Don't do what you don't know how to do. (Learn how, if necessary.)
3. Keep your practice updated; CE is essential.
4. Use self-assessment, peer evaluation, audits, and the supervisor's evaluations as guidelines for improving practice, and follow up on criticisms and knowledge/skill gaps.
5. Don't be careless.

6. Be considerate of patients and their significant others.
7. Practice interdependently; communicate with others.
8. Record accurately, objectively, and completely; don't erase.
9. Delegate safely and legally; know the preparation and abilities of those you supervise.
10. Help develop appropriate policies and procedures (inhouse law).
11. Carry professional liability insurance.

There are those nurses who defend their patients from harm and others whose substandard practices make them a target for litigation. Never forget that licensure is a privilege and a responsibility mandating accountability to the consumer it is intended to protect; therefore, you have a legal and moral obligation to practice safely.

KEY POINTS

1. Malpractice suits of any kind are often stimulated by how the patient and family were treated, as well as by the possible injury.
2. The standard of care by which a nurse is judged in a malpractice case is based on what the "reasonably prudent nurse" of the same background and in the same situation would do.
3. The most common reason for legal suits against nurses is negligence.
4. Negligence frequently occurs in giving medication and treatments because the nurse has inadequate knowledge or is careless.
5. *Darling v. Charleston Community Memorial Hospital* is a landmark case pinpointing the corporate liability of hospitals for the actions of their employees and physicians. For nurses, it underlines the legal responsibility to follow through and ensure that patients get competent care.
6. Poor communication between doctors and nurses, and among nurses themselves, can endanger patients and result in litigation.
7. To avoid problems in law, be accurate, complete, and objective in charting. Never falsify a record for any reason.
8. When selecting professional liability (malpractice) insurance, among the points to consider is whether it is occurrence based or claims made.
9. When testifying in a court of law, be prepared and calm; give appropriate information without jargon, and be accurate and honest.
10. To avoid malpractice, it is especially important to know your licensure law, stay up-to-date in your practice, communicate with others adequately, be careful, and practice humanistic nursing.

REFERENCES

1. Huycke L, Huycke M. Characteristics of potential plaintiffs in malpractice litigation. *Ann Int Med* 120:792–798, May 1, 1994.
2. Burstin H, et al. Do the poor sue more? A case-control study of malpractice claims and socioeconomic status. *JAMA* 270:1697–1701, October 13, 1993.
3. Campazzi B. Nurses, nursing and malpractice litigation, 1967–1977. *Nurse Adm Quart* 5:1–18, Fall, 1980.
4. Lupia I. Who gets sued and why: Malpractice trends and issues update. *NJ Nurse* 24:14–15, July–August, 1994.
5. Moniz D. The legal danger of written protocols and standards of practice. *Nurse Pract* 17:58–60, September, 1992.
6. Lupia, op cit, p 14.
7. Pearson L, Birkholz G. Report on the 1994 readers' survey on NP experiences with malpractice issues. *Nurse Pract* 20:18–27, March, 1995.
8. Advanced practice discipline survey results. *Issues* 14:1, 4–5, 10, (2) 1993.
9. Cushing M. Law and orders. *Am J Nurs* 90:29–32, May, 1990.
10. Nursing negligence is not "proximate cause" of injury. *Regan Rep* 35:2, February, 1995.
11. Vicarious liability for nurses: a "borrowed servant" doctrine. *Regan Rep* 35:2, October, 1994.
12. Fiesta J. Malpractice damages—compensation or punishment? *Nurs Mgmt* 25:16–20, November, 1994.
13. Cushing M. Short staffing on trial. *Am J Nurs* 88:161–162, February, 1988.
14. George J, Quattrone M. Law and the emergency nurse. Restraining patients: Can you be sued? Part I. *J Emerg Nurs* 18:536–537, December, 1992.
15. When a patient refuses to cooperate. *Nurs 95* 25:27, February, 1995.
16. Failure to inform. *Nurse 94* 26:70, October, 1994.
17. Northrop C. Current case law involving nurses: Lessons for practitioners, managers and educators. *Nurs Outlook* 37:296, November–December, 1989.
18. Fiesta J. The evolving doctrine of corporate liabililty. *Nurs Mgmt* 27:17–18, March, 1994.
19. Feutz-Harter S. *Nursing and the Law*, 4th ed. Eau Claire, WI: Professional Education Systems, 1991, pp 18–19.
20. Cushing M. Hazards of the infiltrated IV. *Am J Nurs* 90:31–32, September, 1990.
21. Rhodes AM. Carrying out physicians' orders. *MCN* 15:193, May–June, 1990.

22. Calfee B. *Nurses in the Courtroom.* Cleveland: ARC Publishing, 1993, pp 40–41.
23. Nurses fail to keep physicians informed of multiple seizures. *Regan Rep* 35:4, June, 1994.
24. Legal questions: Dose dilemma. *Nurs 94* 24:23, June, 1994.
25. Carson W. What you should know about physician verbal orders. *Am Nurse* 26:30–31, March, 1994.
26. Nurse fails to chart call to doctor. *Regan Rep* 35:2, January, 1995.
27. Following hospital policy: A legal risk? *Nurs 94* 24:26, May, 1994.
28. Doctor's IV order: Edging toward liability. *Nurs 94*, 24:30, April, 1994.
29. Smith L. Those medication error dilemmas! *Adv Clin Care* 5:50–51, September–October 1990.
30. News item, *Am J Nurs* 95:72, January, 1995.
31. Lilley L. Getting back to basics. *Am J Nurs* 94:15–16, September, 1994.
32. Davis N. Confusion over illegible orders. *Am J Nurs* 94:9, January, 1994.
33. Davis N. Using standardized forms. *Am J Nurs* 95:16, February, 1995.
34. Parisi S. What to do after a med error. *Nurs 94* 24:59, June, 1994.
35. Lilley L, Guanci R. Now what? After an error. *Am J Nurs* 94:18, November, 1994.
36. Lippman H. Rx: Error-free meds. *RN* 56:65–66, June, 1993.
37. Cushing C. Two caveats: Listen and use your knowledge of science. *Am J Nurs* 89:1434, November, 1989.
38. Fiesta J. Legal update, 1994: Part II. *Nurs Mgmt* 26:10, March, 1995.
39. Nurses fail to respond: "Loss of chance" death. *Regan Rep* 35:2, August, 1994.
40. Calfee, op cit, pp 83–84.
41. Aiken MM. Documenting sexual abuse in prepubertal girls. *MCN* 15:176–177, May–June, 1990.
42. Calfee B. Seven things you should never chart. *Nurs 94* 24:43, March, 1994.
43. Mandell M. Not documented. *Nurs 94* 24:62–63, August, 1994.
44. Frawley K. Confidentiality in the computer age. *RN* 57:59–60, July, 1994.
45. Martin F. Documentation tips. *Nurs 94* 24:63–64, June, 1994.
46. Fiesta J. Charting—one national standard, one form. *Nurs Mgmt* 24:22–24, June, 1993.
47. Martin, op cit, p 64.
48. Tammelleo AD. Charting by exception: There *are* perils. *RN* 57:71, October, 1994.
49. Failure to chart circulation—amputation: proximate cause. *Regan Rep* 36:2, June, 1995.

50. On trial: Charting by exception. *Nurs 95* 25:29, April, 1995.
51. Tammelleo, op cit, p 72.
52. Fiesta J. Staffing implications: A legal update. *Nurs Mgmt* 25:34–35, June, 1994.
53. Sullivan G. When assignments don't match skills. *RN* 58:57–60, April, 1995.
54. Fiesta, Staffing Implications, op cit.
55. Rhodes AM. The expert witness. *MCN* 14:49, January–February, 1989.
56. Failure to follow protocols: Hospital vulnerability. *Regan Rep* 35:2, May, 1995.
57. Fiesta J. Legal aspects: Standards of care, Part II. *Nurs Mgmt* 24:16–17, August, 1993.
58. Falling short of the standard of care. *Nurs 94* 24:27, December, 1994.
59. Fiesta J. Legal update, 1994—Part III. *Nurs Mgmt* 26:21, April, 1995.
60. RN is cleared in murder probe: "It was a nightmare". *Am J Nurs* 94:85, 89, January, 1994.
61. Bhouin A, Brent N. Selected causes of action beyond professional negligence. *JONA* 25:11–12, 55, March, 1995.
62. Klein C. Defamation: libel and slander. *Nurse Pract* 11:59–60, January, 1986.
63. Northrop C. How Good Samaritan laws do and don't protect you. *Nurse 90* 20:50–51, February, 1990.
64. Horsley, J. You can't escape the Good Samaritan role—or its risks. *RN* 44:87–92, May, 1981.
65. Think twice about relying on employer liability coverage. *Am Nurse* 25:35, 40, March, 1993.
66. Brooke P. Shopping for liability insurance. *Am J Nurs* 89:171–172, February, 1989.
67. Northrop C. Six questions about malpractice insurance. *Nurs 87* 17:97–98, August, 1987.
68. Rhodes AM. Nursing and the discovery process. *MCN* 13:53, January–February, 1988.
69. Rosen L. Deposition procedure and preparation. *Today's OR Nurse* 16:49–50, July–August, 1994.
70. Rosen L. The legal process: A guide through the maze. *Today's OR Nurse* 16:47, 49, September–October, 1994.
71. Guido G. Be an expert witness for critical care nursing. *AACN Crit Issues* 5:66–70, February, 1994.
72. Quinley K. Twelve tips for defending yourself in a malpractice suit. *Am J Nurs* 90:37–38, 40, January, 1990.
73. Harrison B, Cole D. Managing risk to minimize liability. *Caring* 12:26–30, May, 1994.

Transition into Practice

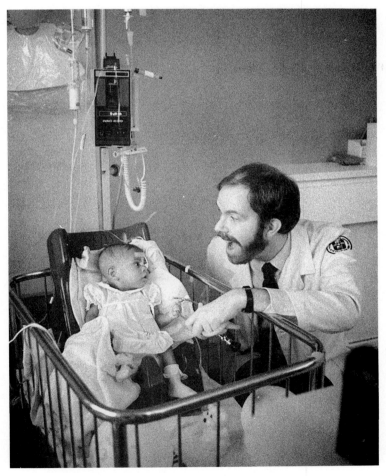

Your first job can set the tone of your nursing career.
(*Courtesy of Columbia University School of Nursing*)

13

Nursing Organizations
and Publications

OBJECTIVES

After studying this chapter, you will be able to:

1. Identify key issues related to nursing organizations.
2. Identify the major activities and programs of ANA.
3. Identify the major activities and programs of NLN.
4. Discuss the key differences between ANA and NLN.
5. Discuss ways in which nursing organizations have sought unity in working together.
6. Identify some of the types of nursing organizations that currently exist.
7. Identify aspects of the nursing literature with which nurses should be familiar.

DIVERSITY AND DIFFERENCES

In 1952, when the six major nursing organizations decided to restructure, the ANA and NLN absorbed the activities of all but the American Association of Industrial Nurses (later renamed the American Association of Occupational Health Nurses), which stayed separate. Students became part of the newly formed National Student Nurses' Association, NSNA. In general, ANA was (and is) considered *the* professional organization, one that every RN can join and find an interest group in which to participate.

There are several major differences between ANA and NLN. ANA membership is limited to RNs, but NLN includes anyone interested in the purposes of the organization, as well as agency members (health care facilities and educational programs in nursing). ANA is registered as a labor organization with the federal government, although it does not directly provide any workplace representation; rather those services are provided by the state nurses associations (SNAs). ANA, in its credentialing center, certifies certain clinical practitioners and nurse managers; it also has an accreditation program for CE programs. NLN is recognized for its accreditation of all kinds of nursing education programs and some health care agencies, primarily home health. Both make policy statements about health and nursing; they also overlap in their public statements about nursing education. Until the last few years, they seemed to cooperate in only a limited way, although often the nursing leaders belonged to both.

The first specialty organization, the American Association of Nurse Anesthetists, began in 1931. In the 1940s and 1950s several others were founded, but beginning in 1968, literally dozens of others were organized. They were usually splinter groups that broke off from ANA and formed their own association as the profession became more specialized. Later, still other organizations formed, as subspecialty groups or groups that felt they had certain needs that could be best met by uniting with the like-minded. These included ethnic nurses, male nurses, nurses with a certain philosophy of care or social concerns, and gay nurses. Some grew rapidly and acquired staff and headquarters. Others almost literally functioned out of a member's home or office. Special-interest groups seem to serve the same purposes: leadership development, certification, continuing education, peer support, and standard-setting.

COOPERATIVE EFFORTS

The proliferation of nursing organizations, although meeting the special needs of some nurses, has also caused some confusion among nurses, other health workers, and the public. Do these organizations speak for nursing in addition to ANA? In place of ANA? Members of the nursing organizations are also concerned. A perceived or real lack of unity in common health care interests can hamper the achievement of goals. Therefore, in November 1972, ANA hosted a meeting of 10 specialty groups and NSNA to explore how the organizations could work toward more coordination in areas of common interest. It was found that concerns were similar and that such a meeting was generally considered long overdue.

In its second meeting, hosted by the American Association of Critical-Care Nurses (AACN), the participants accepted the importance of the specialty groups, at the same time recognizing the unique role of ANA. They agreed "in principle" to certain statements. In 1973, the group adopted a name: the Federation of Specialty Nursing Organizations and the American Nurses Association. There were 13 charter members.

Meetings were held on a semiannual basis in the following years, with the member organizations alternating as hosts, responsible for arranging and conducting the meeting and writing the minutes. The nursing press and auditors were permitted to attend meetings. The focus of the meetings was usually on current issues but was often related to CE accreditation procedures and certification, about which ANA and the other organizations seldom agreed. However, the Federation did support ANA on some issues.

In 1981, the title of the organization was changed to *National Federation for Specialty Nursing Organizations* (NFSNO), which more clearly defined the membership, not all of whom represented clinical specialties. By 1985, NFSNO had changed its requirements for membership, so that membership was exclusive to specialty nursing organizations. ANA, which had been a charter member, moved from member to auditor status. ANA clinical practice councils were given the option to join. The purpose of NFSNO is now to foster excellence in specialty nursing practice by providing a forum for communication and collaboration and to assume a leadership position in activities that contribute to specialty nursing practice. The NFSNO mailing address is Box 56, East Holly Avenue, Pitman, NJ 08071. (See Appendix 5 for an overview of major nursing organizations.)

Another cooperative effort aimed at nurse specialists is the *National Alliance of Nurse Practitioners* (NANP), a coalition of nurse practitioner (NP) organizations formed in 1986. The purpose is to address the health care of the nation by promoting the visibility, viability, and unity of NPs. Among its major concerns is gaining reimbursement for NP services. Currently, NANP represents some 30,000 NPs through its organizational members. The address is 325 Pennsylvania Avenue SE, Washington, DC 20003.

ANA also made a direct effort to bring together the various nursing organizations. A change in the 1982 bylaws provided for the formation of a *Nursing Organization Liaison Forum* (NOLF) to promote unified action of allied nursing organizations under the auspices of ANA. In December 1983, ANA invited 45 nursing organizations to Kansas City to explore the possibilities. The meeting was cordial, but the results were somewhat noncommittal. There was a question of whether NOLF and NFSNO would be duplicative efforts, although ANA indicated that NOLF would focus on broad issues as opposed to specialty concerns. Over time, NOLF has grown and flourished, uniting 73 nursing organizations. Its members are regularly updated on the work of ANA, their opinions sought, and they frequently speak for both ANA and their specialty organization to the media, the Congress, and in a variety of instances. NOLF organizations have voluntarily shared their resources with ANA to help fund a variety of programs.

The *Tri-Council for Nursing* represents another successful cooperative effort. The Tri-Council traces its roots to the ANA–NLN Coordinating Council, established with the ANA reorganization in the 1950s. In time, the American Association of Colleges of Nursing (AACN) and the American Organization of Nurse Executives (AONE) were added to this coalition. The Tri-Council agenda addresses broad-based issues such as public image, nursing shortages, recruitment to the field, and legislative and regulatory concerns. Despite the addition of AONE as a fourth member in 1986, the name of Tri-Council was retained. The presidents and executive directors of the Tri-Council organizations meet regularly and frequently engage in joint lobbying on the federal level.

Such collaborative activities among nursing organizations show a new maturity in nursing that recognizes the importance of joining together on major health issues. Cooperative action will enable nurses to be a stronger force in the planning and delivery of health care services.

AMERICAN NURSES ASSOCIATION

The ANA was established in 1897 by a group of nurses who, even then, recognized the need for a membership association within which nurses could work together in concerted action. Its original name was the Nurses' Associated Alumnae of the United States and Canada, but in order to incorporate under the laws of the state of New York, it was necessary to drop the reference to another country in the organization's title. This was done in 1901; however, the name remained Nurses' Associated Alumnae of the United States until 1911, when it became the American Nurses Association. The Canadian nurses formed their own membership association.

History shows that ANA's primary concern has always been individual nurses and the public they serve. In its early years ANA worked hard for improved and uniform standards of nursing education, for registration and licensure of all nurses educated according to these standards, and for improvement of the welfare of nurses.[1] Similar efforts continue today. ANA headquarters is 600 Maryland Avenue SW, Washington, DC 20005.

Membership

ANA is made up of 53 state and territorial member associations (SNAs). Although the bylaws say constituent members, the "vernacular" is still the SNA. SNAs are made up of district nurses' associations (DNAs). At one time the individual nurse was a member of ANA, but with the adoption of a federation model at the 1982 House of Delegates, the constituent SNA is the member, and individuals join the SNA.

Only 10–15 percent of all RNs belong to ANA. Some belong to

specialty or special interest organizations, others to none. Why? Cost may be a factor; dues are more than $200 in most states, considerably more than for other organizations. Some nurses are simply not interested in nursing issues and don't know why it is important to be represented in legislation or other policy making. And, of course, others disagree with ANA positions, such as entry into practice and collective bargaining.

General Organization

The House of Delegates, which meets yearly, with full conventions in even years, is the policymaking body of ANA. Delegates are elected by each state. Between conventions, decisions based on House policies are made by the board of directors, which has been elected by the House. The board consists of 15 members, including the officers (president, first and second vice president, secretary, and treasurer). Terms are staggered to prevent a complete turnover at any one time and to provide continuity of programs and action.

The ANA has a largely RN professional staff, with supporting clerical and secretarial staff. They carry out the day-to-day activities based on policies adopted by the House and ANA's general functions. The executive director, a nurse, is the chief administrative officer and works closely with the board and SNAs.

Like other large organizations, ANA has its *standing committees*, those that are written into the bylaws and that continue from year to year to assist with specific continuing programs and functions of the association. *Special committees* and *task forces* of the House or board are appointed on an ad hoc basis to accomplish special purposes.

Other structural units include congresses which are organized, deliberative bodies that focus on long-range policy development essential to the mission of the association. There is a *Congress on Nursing Economics* and a *Congress of Nursing Practice.* Congresses are accountable to the board of directors and report to the ANA House of Delegates.

According to the bylaws, the major reponsibilities of the Congresses are to:

1. Develop long-range policy essential to the mission of the association.
2. Establish a plan of operation for carrying out its responsibilities.
3. Develop and adopt standards.
4. Develop and evaluate programs.
5. Address and respond to concerns related to equal opportunity and human rights, ethics, and to nursing education, research, and services.
6. Recommend policies and positions to the board of directors and the ANA House of Delegates.
7. Evaluate trends, developments, and issues.

In 1990, the House of Delegates established an *Institute of Constituent Members on Nursing Practice*, which reports directly to the Congress of Nursing Practice. It consists of one representative from each SNA.

The *Institute of Constituent Member Collective Bargaining Programs* was put into place in 1990. It consists of one elected representative from each SNA with a collective bargaining program and is autonomous in respect to the development of operational standards, positions, policies, practices, and all other matters related to SNA collective bargaining programs. More details about the institutes can be found in the ANA bylaws.[2]

The *Commission on Economic and Professional Security* is an organized, deliberative body which evaluates trends, developments, and issues related to the economic and professional security of individual nurses and groups of nurses on behalf of the Congress of Nursing Economics.

Councils have a clinical or functional focus and are established by the board. They provide the one mechanism through which the individual SNA member can participate or join directly in ANA activities. Their primary purpose relates to providing a forum for discussion; continuing education; consultation; and proposing standards and certification offerings. SNA members may choose from councils on Acute Care Nursing Practice, Advanced Practice Nursing, Community-Primary and Long Term Care Nursing Practice, Nursing Research, Professional Nursing Education and Development, and Nursing Services and Informatics.

The *Constituent Assembly* is made up of the president and chief administrative officer of each SNA or their designees. The purpose is to discuss nursing affairs of concern to ANA, SNAs, and the profession. *The Nursing Organization Liaison Forum* (NOLF), mentioned earlier, is made up of duly authorized representatives of ANA and other nursing organizations, who meet for the purpose of discussing issues of concern to the profession and promoting concerted action on them.

Major Programs and Services of ANA

The programs and services of ANA represent the efforts of members and staff, elected officers, committees, forums, cabinets, and councils. These include meeting with members of other groups and disciplines; planning or convening institutes, workshops, conventions, or committee meetings; developing and writing brochures, manuals, position papers, standards, or testimony to be presented to Congress; and implementing ongoing programs, planning new ones, or trying to solve the problem of how to serve the members best within the limitations of the budget. Every issue of the *American Journal of Nursing* and *The American Nurse* carries reports of these many and varied activities. Presented here are brief descriptions of some (but not all) of the major ANA programs and services.

Programs are implemented both through the internal administrative structure of ANA and in some cases by independent or affiliated organizational entities related to ANA. These allied structures are presented following this discussion of ANA activities.

Nursing Education

The important ANA function of setting standards and policies for nursing education has been demonstrated in many ways. The 1965 Position Paper was the beginning of a series of specific actions toward implementing the position that education for entry into professional nursing practice should be at the baccalaureate level. (See Chapters 2 and 5.) ANA has made a number of other important educational statements in the last few years; these are available from ANA.

ANA endorses the concept of continuing education for all nurses as a vehicle to maintain competence, but believes that the responsibility for maintaining competence is personal and not an area for government intrusion. ANA puts emphasis on the role of the SNAs in providing and approving the quality of continuing education offerings. To facilitate this work, in 1975 the Association established an accreditation program which currently operates through the American Nurses Credentialing Center (ANCC).

Nursing Practice

Nursing is practice, and so many would say that ANA's work in this area drives all of the other association activities. ANA is responsible for developing and disseminating the *Standards of Clinical Nursing Practice* (see Chapter 4). ANA has collaborated with countless specialty associations to assure that their standards are framed in the same model, and subsequently can be endorsed by ANA. Many excellent publications are part of the overall plan to assist SNAs and individuals in the utilization of the standards of practice. Workshops, seminars, and other programs are held to provide nurses with new knowledge to facilitate implementation and thereby improve nursing care. Major papers and/or proceedings of these conferences are made available. ANA's concern for quality nursing care is also manifested through its Center for Ethics and Human Rights and *Code for Nurses*. One of the center's purposes is to develop and disseminate information on ethical and human rights issues facing the profession of nursing. The center provides consultation and resources on addressing practice dilemmas and controversies. For example, the center helps nurses and SNAs with application of the *Code for Nurses* and prepares documents such as the position statement on the nurse's role in end-of-life decisions. This is only one example of a variety of position papers which ANA has authored and approved to provide guidance for the practice of nursing. A list of current position statements is presented in Exhibit 13.1.

EXHIBIT 13.1

Select ANA Position Statements, and Date of Approval

Ethics and human rights
- Promotion of Comfort and Relief of Pain in Dying Patients (September 1991)
- Nursing and the Patient Self-Determination Act (November 1991)
- Foregoing Artificial Nutrition and Hydration (April 1992)
- Nursing Care and Do Not Resuscitate Decisions (April 1992)
- Nurses' Participation in Capital Punishment (1983, revised 1988 and December 1994)
- Assisted Suicide (December 1994)
- Active Euthanasia (December 1994)

Bloodborne and airborne diseases
- Guidelines for Disclosure to a Known Third Party About Possible HIV Infection (April 1991)
- Support for Confidential Notification Services (April 1991)
- Post-Exposure Programs in the Event of Occupational Exposure to HIV/HBV (September 1991)
- Education and Barrier Use for Sexually Transmitted Diseases (STDs) and HIV Infection (September 1991)
- Availability of Equipment and Safety Procedures to Prevent Transmission of Bloodborne Diseases (September 1991)
- Travel Restrictions for Persons with HIV/AIDS (September 1991)
- Personnel Policies and HIV in the Workplace (September 1991)
- HIV Testing (September 1991)
- HIV Infection and Nursing Students (April 1992)
- HIV Infected Nurse, Ethical Obligations and Disclosure (December 1992)
- Needle Exchange and HIV (April 1993)
- HIV Exposure from Rape and Sexual Assault (April 1993)
- Tuberculosis and HIV (April 1993)
- Tuberculosis and Public Health Nursing (April 1993)

Social causes and health care
- Physical Violence Against Women (September 1991)
- Lead Poisoning and Screening (April 1994)
- Childhood Immunizations (March 1995)
- Informal Caregiving (March 1995)
- Longterm Care (July 1995)
- Cessation of Tobacco Use (July 1995).
- Health Promotion and Disease Prevention (July 1995)

Drug and Alcohol Abuse
- Polypharmacy and the Older Adult (December 1990)
- Opposition to Criminal Prosecution of Women for Use of Drugs While Pregnant and Support for Treatment Services for Alcohol and Drug Dependent Women of Childbearing Age (April 1991)
- Abuse of Prescription Drugs (April 1991)
- Drug Testing for Health Care Workers (December 1994)

Nursing Practice
- Psychiatric Mental Health Nursing and Managed Care (April 1993)
- A National Nursing Database to Support Clinical Nursing Practice (December 1994)

Nursing Research
- Education for Participation in Nursing Research (April 1993)

Workplace Advocacy
- Maintaining Professional and Legal Standards During a Shortage of Nursing Personnel (August 1992)
- Sexual Harassment (April 1993)
- Polygraph Testing of Health Care Workers (December 1994)
- Restructuring, Work Redesign, and the Job and Career Security of Registered Nurses (March 1995)

Unlicensed Assistive Personnel
- Registered Nurse Utilization of Unlicensed Assistive Personnel (December 1992)
- Registered Nurse Education Relating to the Utilization of Unlicensed Assistive Personnel (April 1992)

All of the programs of the ANA hold serious implications for practice. Some examples are the legislative and regulatory work to assure nurses staff privileges in health care facilities, prescriptive authority and direct reimbursement for services rendered to the public. Much effort has also been expended in having the National Library of Medicine (NLM) recognize the classification systems which are unique to nursing practice: the North Atlantic Nursing Diagnosis Association classification of nursing diagnoses, the McCloskey and Buelechek Classification of Nursing Interventions, and the Omaha and Saba systems for classifying home care encounters. This is part of a broader goal to have the government incorporate data necessary to distinguish nursing in its mandatory reporting systems. All of these pieces come together in activities related to the minimum data set (MDS) for nursing. Not only does this work promise to have us recognized for our practice, but it allows retrieval of information related to our practice both from government reporting systems and library databases.

Legislation and Legal Activities

ANA's legislative program is an important one that often affects, directly and indirectly, the welfare of both nurses and the public (see Chapter 10). ANA's legislative program has three main purposes: (1) to help SNAs promote effective nursing practice acts in their states in order to protect the public and the nursing profession from unqualified practitioners; (2) to offer consultation on other legislative and regulatory measures that affect nurses; and (3) to speak for nursing in relation to federal legislation for health, education, labor, and welfare, and for social programs such as civil rights.

The major responsibility for coordinating legislative information and action lies with the ANA's governmental affairs arm. The Washington staff's responsibilities include lobbying (through its registered lobbyists); development of relationships with congressional members and their staffs and committee staffs; contacts with key figures in the administrative branch of government; maintaining relations with other national organizations; preparing most of the statements and information presented to congressional committees; drafting letters to government officials; presenting testimony; acting as backup for members presenting testimony; and representing ANA in many capacities. Major newspapers and journals have commented on nursing's presence and influence.

Over the years, ANA has represented nursing in the capital on numerous major issues: funds for nursing education, Social Security amendments to cover nurses, national health insurance, quality of care in nursing homes, collective bargaining rights, health hazards, civil rights, Federal Trade Commission authority and regulations, problems of nurses in the federal service, tax revision, higher education, problems of health manpower, prescriptive authority and reimbursement for nurses, and general support for improvement of health care.

ANA has often cooperated and coordinated with other health disciplines, but has also faced areas of disagreement (such as early opposition of AMA and other groups to funding for nurse education). Such philosophical differences still occur, but there has been increasing cooperation with both health and other groups to achieve mutual legislative goals.

Communication about legislative matters is particularly important to help members keep abreast of key legislative issues. Prepared monthly by the legislative staff as a regular part of *The American Nurse*, are various articles that highlight major legislative and related developments. A monthly newsletter, *Capital Update*, is available by subscription.

Legislative information is also provided in the *American Journal of Nursing*, and special communications are sent out from the Washington office when membership support is needed for legislative programs. SNAs have a vital role in providing information and assistance to members on pertinent legislative issues, and when funds allow, there is often a legislative staff, a lobbyist, and perhaps a separate legislative newsletter at the state level.

In addition to specific legislative action, ANA becomes involved in various legal matters that affect the welfare of nurses. In some cases, ANA acts as a friend of the court, providing information about the issues involved. In other cases, ANA joins with an SNA if its issue has broader implications. One such situation was the class action litigation in the state of Illinois claiming salary inequity for women employed by the state, a large number of whom were nurses.

Economic and General Welfare

The ANA economic security program is often misunderstood by members, nonmembers, and others. Seeing that the economic security of its members is maintained is one of the classic roles of a professional association, and, especially in recent years, economic security has been seen as extending beyond purely monetary matters and conditions of employment to involvement of nurses in the decision-making aspects of nursing care. An example might be that, through an agreed-upon process, perhaps including a formal committee structure, nurses' objections to inadequate staffing or illegal or inappropriate job assignments would be instrumental in bringing about changes that would provide improved care.

ANA promotes the economic and general welfare of nurses through a host of publications and services, including supporting the work of 26 SNAs who provide formal workplace representation programs for nurses through collective bargaining. ANA does not serve as a bargaining agent for nurses itself; however, it does hold official consultation rights to the Office of Veterans Affairs on behalf of VA nurses. ANA supports collective bargaining states by developing principles and techniques for workplace representation, training SNA staff, maintaining a database on contract language and other useful information, providing on-sight consultation, and generally advising and assisting SNAs with their activities as much as possible. Other approaches to workplace advocacy are also critical. These include legislative, legal and regulatory concerns about confidentiality, at-will employment, discrimination, and a range of other issues which are discussed more extensively in Chapter 15. Additionally, ANA publications and programs educate nurses to their rights and develop skills for personal protection.[3]

Overall, ANA is concerned not only with improving salaries, fringe benefits, and working conditions but has also expanded its activities to improve the quality of nursing care, to assure the public of the individual and collective accountability of qualified professional nurses, and to increase accessibility of health care services for the public. This is accomplished by nurses achieving the right to make decisions affecting themselves, their practice, and the quality of care. Although this approach to collective bargaining might be considered new to individuals who think of economic security only in terms of salaries, fringe benefits, and working conditions, job action by nurses is more often in protest of inadequate patient care.

Human Rights Activities

ANA works toward integrating qualified members of all racial and ethnic groups into the nursing profession and tries to achieve sound human rights practices. From the time of its founding, ANA as a national organization has never had any discriminatory policies for membership in the association. Until 1964, however, a few of its constituent associations denied membership to black nurses. In these instances, ANA made provision for black nurses to bypass district and state associations and become members of ANA directly. At that point (1950), the National Association for Colored Graduate Nurses (NACGN) voluntarily went out of existence, on the basis that there was no longer a need for such a specialized membership association.

ANA's human rights activities are housed in the Center for Ethics and Human Rights. A major program with over 20 years of success is the Racial/Ethnic Minority Fellowship Program. The Program provides financial and personal support to minority candidates for doctoral study to prepare for research or clinical practice in psychiatric and mental health nursing.

Communication and Information Services

ANA is a veritable goldmine of information. The association publishes *The American Nurse* monthly which reports recent activities and happenings important to the nursing community. Many of the staff units, as already described, have specific newsletters that are published on a regular basis; such as *Capital Update, Center for Ethics and Human Rights Communique, Legal Developments*, and *E&GW Update*, to name a few. ANA is also a clearinghouse for information on the state-specific statutory requirements for nursing, language in collective bargaining contracts, the prevailing demographics of practicing nurses, as some examples.

American Nurses Publishing (an arm of ANA and ANF) publishes Standards of Practice, the Code for Nurses, major reports, monographs, papers presented at meetings; and certain publications of the AAN and ANCC. The association also publishes position statements, guidelines for practice, bulletins, manuals, and brochures for specialized groups within the organization and sends out news releases and announcements concerning activities of interest to the public. Available from American Nurses Publishing upon request is its periodically revised *Catalogue*. ANA also monitors news and public opinion trends affecting the profession. ANA has created "ANA Net," which enables the electronic exchange of information between ANA and the SNAs.

Other Activities and Services

Among other ANA benefits for nurses is insurance of various kinds, available at favorable group rates at national and state levels. Many educational programs, seminars, workshops, clinical conferences, scientific sessions, and so on are available at all levels at reduced rates for members. They are geared to current issues and new developments in health and nursing.

Nurses are also increasingly interested in international nursing. ANA was one of the three charter members of the ICN and is an active participant in the work of this international nursing organization. Essentially, ICN is a federation of national associations of professional nurses (one from each country), and ANA is the member association for the United States.

ANA established an International Nursing Center in 1992 through the ANF. The center sponsors an international talent bank comprised of nurses with expertise in international work and foreign language capability. The center was awarded a grant by the World AIDS Foundation in 1993 to train nurses in Sri Lanka and India in HIV/AIDS prevention and care.

Amercian Academy of Nursing

A significant action taken by the 1966 House of Delegates was the creation of the American Academy of Nursing (AAN) to provide for recognition of professional achievement and excellence. It was established in 1973. The members, designated as Fellows of the American Academy of Nursing, are entitled to use the initials FAAN following their names. They are selected on the basis of their outstanding contributions to nursing and their potential for continued contributions. The Academy holds a yearly Scientific Session combined with business meetings.

The Academy was constituted as a self-governing affiliate of ANA to insulate its work from the inevitable politics of membership associations. The Academy has its own dues structure, bylaws, and elected officials. Using AAN as the vehicle, the leadership corps for the profession provides thinking on the critical issues confronting nursing. Their ability to create, speak, and disseminate intellectual products must be unencumbered by political pressure. The AAN has responded well to the challenge of shaping the future. The Magnet Hospital Study of 1983 (see Appendix 1) set the stage for the current Magnet Hospital Recognition Program instituted by ANCC to pay tribute to departments of nursing service that are exemplary. The Teaching Nursing Home Program contributed significantly to the nursing home reforms of 1987.[4] The AAN Clinical Scholars Program accorded advanced practice nursing intellectual respect, and moved practice toward the level of distinction it currently enjoys. The faculty practice initiative of the 1980s gave credibility to service–education unification efforts that have since become the standard to bring the best of nursing to both students and patients. The AAN has accomplished its work through demonstration projects, annual meetings, smaller interest groups that are a mechanism for continuing problem solving and discussion around issues, dissemination of ideas through *Nursing Outlook* (the Academy's official journal), and the wide reach of its influential members.

The American Nurses Foundation

The American Nurses Foundation (ANF) was created by ANA in 1955 to meet the need for an independent, permanent, nonprofit organization devoted to nursing research. This tax-exempt foundation was organized exclusively for charitable, scientific, literary, and educational purposes.

ANF has a Competitive Extramural Grants Program, funded through the contributions of both corporations and individuals, that provides small grants to nurse researchers. In 1983, in collaboration with ANA and AAN, the ANF Distinguished Scholar Program was established. The purpose of the program is to permit nurse health policy scholars to analyze selected issues related to economics, delivery of nursing services, nursing practice, and nursing education.

The American Nurses Foundation solicits, receives, and/or administers funds for a variety of projects such as the W.K. Kellogg Foundation award of $1.3 million for the community-based Health Care Project. ANF also receives and administers funds for ANA and AAN. Grants have been received from various sources for work on HIV prevention, managed care, immunization, managing genetic information, and nursing informatics.

ANF is governed by its bylaws and directed by a nine-member board of trustees. All trustees are RNs. The executive director of ANA is also the executive director of ANF. There is a professional ANF headquarters staff involved in fundraising and grant management which also services ANA.

The American Nurses Credentialing Center

The ANA established a *certification* program in 1973 to recognize professional achievement in practice. More than 5000 applications were received for the first examination given in May of 1973. This program provides a *credential* which is rewarded by salary increases, prestige and promotion in many work settings, and recognized by many state governments as indicating competence in advanced practice. By 1995, 26 areas of certification were offered with certification for the clinical specialist in home health nursing in development for 1996 (see Exhibit 13.2). In 1995, over 100,000 nurses were certified by ANCC.

Two levels of certification are offered: competence in specialized areas of practice (generalist), and acknowledged achievement as a specialist. The former requires a bachelor's, and the latter calls for the master's degree. Each is based on the assessment of knowledge through examination, demonstration of current practice ability, and endorsement of colleagues. Once certified the certification is valid for five years and may be renewed by fulfilling stipulated requirements for practice and continuing education or by retaking the examination. Specific information on eligibility criteria

EXHIBIT 13.2

ANCC Current Certifications and Year First Offered

Clinical Specialist in Adult Psychiatric and Mental Health Nursing (1977)
Clinical Specialist in Child and Adolescent Psychiatric and Mental Health
    Nursing (1977)
Psychiatric and Mental Health Nursing (1974)
Medical–Surgical Nurse (1976)
Clinical Specialist in Medical–Surgical Nursing (1976)
Pediatric Nurse Practitioner (1974)
Pediatric Nurse* (1979)
School Nurse Practitioner (1979)
Gerontological Nurse (1974)
Nursing Administration (1979)
Nursing Administration, Advanced (1979)
Community Health Nurse (1975)
Maternal–Gynecological–Neonatal Nursing (1976, last admin 1978)
High-Risk Perinatal Nurse (1982, last admin 1988)
Maternal–Child Nurse (1982, last admin 1988)
General Nursing Practice (1988)
School Nurse (1988)
Perinatal Nurse (1989)
Clinical Specialist in Gerontological Nursing (1989)
Clinical Specialist in Community Health Nursing
    (cosponsored with American Public Health Association) (1990)
College Health Nurse
    (cosponsored with American College Health Association (1991)
Adult Nurse Practitioner (1976)
Family Nurse Practitioner (1976)
Gerontological Nurse Practitioner (1979)
Nursing Continuing Education and Staff Development
    (cosponsored with National Nursing Staff Development Organization
    and the ANA Council on Professional Nursing Education and Develop-
    ment) (1992)
Home Health Nurse (1993)
Cardiac Rehabilitation Nurse (1994)
Informatics Nurse (1995)
Acute Care Nurse Practitioner
    (offered in collaboration with the American Association of Critical-Care
    Nurses) (1995)
Clinical Specialist in Home Health Nursing (1996)

---

* Originally called Nursing of the Child/Adolescent with Acute or Chronic Illness or
Disabling Condition; name changed to Child and Adolescent Nurse in 1982; name changed
to present in 1988.

for each specialty area and the cost of the exam may be obtained by contacting ANCC.

An *accreditation* program was established in 1974 by ANA as a voluntary system for accreditation of continuing education in nursing. The essential purpose of this system is to provide professional nursing judgment on the quality of continuing education offerings. An organization may be accredited as either an approver or a provider of continuing education in nursing.

The Magnet *Recognition Program* was introduced in 1994, and is built on the 1983 Magnet Hospital Study conducted by AAN. The goal of this program is to identify excellence in nursing services and to recognize hospitals that act as a "magnet" by creating a work environment that values and rewards professional nursing. The first recipients of this status were the University of Washington Medical Center in Seattle and Hackensack Medical Center in New Jersey (awarded in 1995). A Magnet Nursing Home Program is in development.

Early certification and accreditation activities were conducted by ANA. In 1991, as a result of the action of the ANA House of Delegates, these credentialing programs were placed in a separately incorporated center (ANCC). The ANCC philosophy of credentialing is consistent with and based on the ANA ethical code, standards of practice, and positions on practice, education and service. The separation of ANA and ANCC removes the threat of conflict of interest which can result when the entity establishing the standard intrudes in the work of evaluating the practitioner according to that standard.

ANCC is governed by a Board of Directors whose members are appointed by the ANA Board of Directors. Six ANCC board members are also sitting members of the ANA board.

American Nurses Association Political Action Committee

Most professional organizations have a political action group which is independent of the organization but related to it. This is because a tax-exempt professional organization such as ANA is under definite legal constraints as far as partisan political action is concerned. In 1974, with a $50,000 ANA grant, a voluntary, unincorporated, nonpartisan political action group was formed. Initially called Nurses' Coalition for Action in Politics (N-CAP), the name was changed to the American Nurses Association Political Action Committee (ANA–PAC) in more recent years. ANA provides some dollars for administrative support, but none for the campaigns of candidates for election. ANA–PAC has a single purpose: to promote the improvement of health care through political action. Its two major activities are education and endorsement of candidates for public office on the national level who support ANA's public policy positions. This requires major fund-raising efforts. Many SNAs have their own political action committees that support candidates for state office.

The ANA–PAC has enjoyed significant growth in recent years. In 1995, contributions totaled more than $1.2 million, and ANA–PAC was awarded the distinction of being the second fastest growing health care PAC in the United States. Its candidate success rate has never been less than 70 percent and in some election cycles has been 98 percent. SNA members are more politically active than other citizen groups, giving many hours as well as dollars to political campaigns. About 58 percent donate to political campaigns and 91 percent are registered to vote.

ANA–PAC is noted for its grassroots network, Nurses Strategic Action Team (N-Stat). N-Stat educates members of the Congress to nursing issues and provides an immediate response in areas where "time is of the essence." N-Stat consists of a *Leadership Team* and a *Rapid Response* system. Members of the Leadership Team are individually assigned to a Congressperson or Senator. Their forte is the relationship. It becomes their task to monitor the record of this legislator, educate to nursing's issues, and seeing support for nursing's work to keep them in office. In contrast, the Rapid Response strength is speed and volume. Rapid Response is constituted of as many volunteers as show interest and are willing to write, call or fax their opinions to a specific legislator on specific issues as the need arises.

ANA–PAC is governed by its own Board of Directors, including some currently sitting ANA board members. ANA–PAC is headquartered at ANA's offices in Washington, DC.

The Individual Nurse and ANA

A classic article by sociologist Robert Merton lists the functions of any professional organization as including social and moral support for individual practitioners to help them perform their role as professionals, to set rigorous standards for the profession and help enforce them, to advance and disseminate research and professional knowledge, to help furnish the social bonds through which society coheres, and to speak for the profession. In carrying out some of these functions, the association is seen as a "kind of organizational gadfly, stinging the profession into new and more demanding formulations of purpose."[5]

Not all members agree with their organization's goals. However, the key to the success of any organization is the participation of its actual and potential members. Even though ANA has only a small percentage of working nurses, it is still the largest nursing organization (Sigma Theta Tau is second in membership). ANA speaks for nurses; nonmembers have no part in that organization and have no right to complain if it does not represent them. The strength in the organization and in nursing lies in thinking, communicating nurses committed to the goal of improving nursing care for the public and working together in an organized fashion to achieve this goal.

INTERNATIONAL COUNCIL OF NURSES

Nursing claims the distinction of having the oldest international association of professional women, the International Council of Nurses (ICN). Antedating by many years the international hospital and medical associations, ICN is the largest international organization primarily made up of professional women in the world. (There are, of course, men in ICN member organizations.) The originator and prime mover of ICN was a distinguished and energetic English nurse, Ethel Gordon Fenwick (Mrs. Bedford Fenwick) who first proposed the idea of an international nursing organization in July 1899.

ICN today is still a federation of national nurses' associations worldwide. The requirements for membership have been, essentially, that the national association be an autonomous, self-directing, and self-governing body, nonsectarian, with no form of racial discrimination, whose voting membership is composed exclusively of nurses and is broadly representative of the nurses in that country. Its objectives must be in harmony with ICN's stated objective: to provide a medium through which national nurses' associations may share their common interests, working together to develop the contribution of nursing to the promotion of the health of people and the care of the sick. A majority vote by the ICN's governing body determines the admission of national associations into membership.

Organization

The governing body of ICN is the Council of National Representatives (CNR), consisting of the presidents of the member associations (114 in 1995). This group, including ICN's board of directors, meets at least every two years to establish ICN policies. Carrying out ICN's day-to-day activities is its headquarters staff—a group of professional nurses, including ICN's executive director, currently an American nurse. These nurses represent ICN's executive staff, and in their relationships with and services to the member associations, they serve in an advisory and consultative capacity. Staff members are selected from various member countries.

ICN Congresses

Once every four years, the ICN holds its Quadrennial Congress: a meeting of the members of the national nurses' associations in membership with ICN.

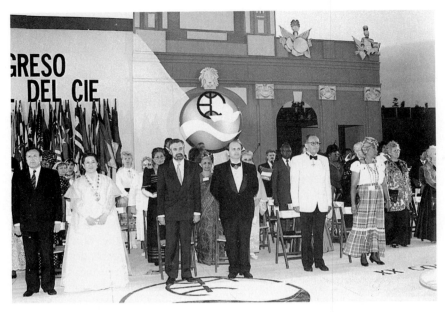

The ICN quadrennial Congress brings together nurses from around the world. (*Courtesy of the International Council of Nurses, Geneva.*)

Nursing students are usually eligible to attend ICN congresses, too, if they are sponsored, and their applications are processed, by their national nurses' association. Students have been meeting as a Student Assembly during the congresses.

During the last several congresses, discussions and resolutions ranged from those focusing specifically on nursing issues to general social concerns. Included, for instance, were career ladders, socio-economic welfare, educational and practice standards, research, autonomy, the nurse's role in safeguarding human rights, the nurse's role in the care of detainees and prisoners, and nurse participation in national health policy planning and decision making. Related to general health care were such topics as primary care, excision and circumcision of females, increased violence against patients and health personnel, the uncontrolled proliferation of ancillary nursing personnel, environment quality, care for the elderly, and affirmation of the World Health Organization's (WHO's) "Health for all by the year 2000" theme. On an even broader scale were the concerns about refugees and displaced persons, nuclear war, poverty, and the status of women.

The activities at ICN congresses are reported in the *American Journal of Nursing* (*AJN*) and other nursing journals, including *International Nursing Review* (the ICN journal).

Functions and Activities

From the very beginning, ICN has been concerned with three main areas: nursing education, nursing service, and nurses' social and economic welfare. Whenever possible, ICN has sought common denominators in education and practice throughout the world. One such common denominator, for instance, is the international Code of Ethics adopted by ICN and equally applicable to nurses in every country. At the same time, ICN has always recognized the autonomy of its member associations and the principle that each country will develop the systems of education and practice best suited to its individual culture and needs.

Providing liaison for nurses with other international groups is one of ICN's most significant contributions to world nursing. Among the organizations, government and nongovernmental, with which ICN is associated in some way are the World Health Organization, the World Federation of Mental Health, the International Labor Organization, the World Medical Association, the International Hospital Federation, the International Federation of Red Cross and Red Crescent Societies, the International Committee of the Red Cross, United Nations Educational, Scientific and Cultural Organization (UNESCO), Council of International Organizations of Medical Sciences (CIOMS), and the Union of International Associations.

ICN has sponsored a variety of projects to study issues critical for the development of nursing. Most recent ventures have been the International Classification of Nursing Project,[6] the Regulation Project,[7] costing nursing services,[8] nursing and AIDS, nursing research, the use of assistive personnel,[9] mental health services, to name a few. Most of these initiatives produce publications that are available through headquarters, some free and others for a fee.

ICN headquarters is located at 3 Place Jean Marteau, 1201, Geneva, Switzerland (mailing address: PO Box 42, CH-1201 Geneva 20, Switzerland).

NATIONAL LEAGUE FOR NURSING

The National League for Nursing (usually referred to as NLN or the League) was the first nursing organization in the United States. Established in 1893 under the title of the American Society of Superintendents of Training Schools for Nurses of the United States and Canada, it became the National League of Nursing Education in 1912. Its purpose was to standardize and improve the education of nurses. Originally for nurses only, it broadened its membership policies in 1943 to admit lay members.

In 1995, NLN revised its mission statement as follows:[10]

The mission of the NLN is to improve education and health outcomes by linking communities and information. It achieves its mission through: collaborating, connecting, creating, serving and learning.

As in the past, there remain two major classes of membership within NLN, individual and agency. Individual membership is open to anyone interested in fostering the development and improvement of nursing service, education, and health care. Agency membership is for organizations or groups providing various nursing services and for the various schools conducting educational programs in nursing. Agency membership includes two subdivisions, category 1 and category 2. Category 1 membership entitles an agency to 10 votes; category 2, 5 votes. Membership dues and available services vary within each category. There is another category of agency membership (allied) for agencies interested in the work of the NLN but not qualifying within the preceding categories. These agencies do not have voting power.

Individual members join NLN and one of the 48 constituent leagues in the area in which they live or work. If there is no league in that area, they may join NLN directly at the national level. Annual dues for each individual combine the national and constituent league dues. Agency members join NLN directly. Individual membership includes three avenues for influence and activity: at the national level, within a more local constituent league, and within a council focused on a more particular concern. Individual members may belong to any number of these membership councils.

General Plan of Organization

Both individual and agency members are concerned with the "further development and improvement of nursing services, education, and the achievement of comprehensive health care." The groups approach the task through membership opportunities in various NLN councils. At NLN business sessions held at the biennial conventions, decisions are made by the individual and agency members present, provided that there are enough to meet the League's quorum requirements.

Membership Councils

Through 11 councils, agency and individual members may influence the policies of the NLN, receive information, attend programs, participate on committees, present ideas, and vote. The four *educational* councils are:

- Council of Associate Degree Programs (CADP)
- Council of Baccalaureate and Higher Degree Programs (CBHDP).
- Council of Diploma Programs (CDP).
- Council of Practical Nursing Programs (CPNP).

The *practice and multidisciplinary* councils provide opportunities for participants to play key roles in shaping nursing practice and its relationship to nursing education. These are:

- Council of Community Health Services (CCHS).
- Council for Nurse Executives (CNE).
- Council for Nursing Informatics (CNI).
- Council for Nursing Centers (CNC).
- Council for Nursing Practice (CNP).
- Council for the Society for Research in Nursing Education (CSRNE).
- Council of Constituent Leagues for Nursing (CCLN).

Each council works within its own readily identifiable field of interest, but there are certain activities in which all engage. All are expected to facilitate collaboration among councils and non-NLN groups, ensure consumer involvement in council activities, and develop goals that are not only relevant to individual council activity but are also congruent with those of the NLN. Workshops and programs are held regionally and nationally. The four education councils also have accreditation of nursing education as part of their work. Council committees vary according to each council's needs.

Board of Governors, Officers, Committees

An 18-member NLN Board of Governors consists of three elected officers (president, president elect, and treasurer), the membership council chairs, three governors at large, and the chief executive officer of NLN, who is a voting member.

Balloting for national offices is done by mail, with both individuals and agency members entitled to vote. All of these offices and elected positions are open to both nurse and nonnurse NLN members.

Business sessions of the individual councils are held at annual meetings, and the full organization membership meets at a biennial convention. Decisions are made by the individual and agency members present. Each individual membership means one vote, and each member agency has 5 or 10 votes, depending on its membership category.

The NLN has two types of committees, standing and special, which may be elected or appointed. The composition and methods of election or appointment and the term of office of committee members are spelled out in the bylaws. The Committee on Nominations is currently the only elected committee of the overall organization. In the appointed category are three standing committees: the Committee on Constitutions and Bylaws, the Committee on Finance, and the Committee on Accreditation. From time to time the League appoints other special committees to deal with matters of general, and often continuing, concern to the organization as a whole.

Services and Programs

More or less permanent components within the League are a variety of services and programs carried out through its organized staff divisions. Among these are CE programs related to issues in education and service, accreditation, and research.

Division of Education and Accreditation

The NLN accrediting service has been a stimulant to the improvement of nursing education since it began in 1949 under the name of the National Nursing Accrediting Service. It is a service that reviews and evaluates nursing education programs of various types such as those preparing PNs, diploma, AD, and baccalaureate degree programs for RNs, and programs leading to a graduate degree in nursing. Those meeting NLN criteria within each category are granted NLN accreditation.

The published criteria for evaluation of each type of program, set by the appropriate council, are basic guides, as is the booklet on policies and procedures of accreditation. It is expected that a school will conduct a thorough evaluation of all aspects of their program through committees of faculty and students, use of studies, and review of other data. The results of the evaluation are incorporated in a self-evaluation report, which is sent to NLN (previously notified as to the program's intent to seek evaluation) in anticipation of a site visit to clarify, verify, and amplify the written document. NLN accreditation is a peer evaluation, and site visitors are faculty and/or faculty-administrators of like programs, who have been selected for and specially trained by NLN to review programs. Both reports (self-study and site visit) are then studied by a peer member board of review. There is a process of appeal if the Board's decision is not acceptable to the school, and, of course, the opportunity to correct the deficiencies and reapply for accreditation. In recent years, there has been greater flexibility in the acceptance of ways to meet accreditation standards, so that programs of greatly varying educational approaches are being accredited. The common denominator is quality. Increasingly, NLN accreditation is sought and worked toward, because of the significance of this accreditation to the prospective student, the faculty member, and the community. In addition, only NLN-accredited schools are eligible for the nursing education funds made available through the Nursing Education Act. NLN is officially recognized by the Council on Post-Secondary Accreditation and the US Department of Education as the accrediting agency for master's, baccalaureate, AD, diploma, and PN programs.

Each year, a list of NLN-accredited programs of nursing is published in the NLN journal. There are also pamphlets issued listing all state-approved and accredited nursing programs. By 1995, more than 1550 educational programs held NLN accreditation; over 75 percent of the total of basic RN programs were accredited by the League.

Community Health Accreditation Program (CHAP)

The Community Health Accreditation Program (CHAP) is an evaluating body for home care and community health care organizations driven by considerations of management, quality, and client outcomes. CHAP is a subsidiary of the National League for Nursing. CHAP's purpose is to employ accreditation to elevate the quality of home care in this country and to counter public fears about a quality crisis in this increasingly crucial health care arena. Its goal is to see home care organizations not only prosper but also gain strength in the overall health care industry. CHAP is committed to ensuring that this nation's home care and community health providers adhere to the highest standards of excellence and that those standards are maintained through specific guidance for self-improvement.

Agencies seeking CHAP accreditation perform an extensive self-study, which is submitted to CHAP offices for preliminary analysis of specific areas. A site visit is then performed by visitors selected to assure a range of expertise, including both management and service delivery areas, and come from an agency similar to that of the applicant organization. Site-visit findings along with the agency's self-report are then studied by a peer-member board of review. There is a process of appeal if the board's decision is not acceptable to the agency. Organizations are accredited for a three-year cycle, during which additional site visits occur, focusing on specific standards. CHAP holds deemed status with the Health Care Financing Administration. In other words, home care or community health care organizations accredited by CHAP are approved by Medicare for reimbursement without any additional surveys.

NLN Consultation Network

NLN's newly expanded consultation network offers a wide range of consultation services through a cadre of experts in the fields of nursing education, practice, research, testing and evaluation, and communication/ video. Traditionally, nursing schools have utilized NLN consultation services for help with their educational programs. Recent developments in the health care arena, such as spiraling costs and personnel shortages, have increased the demand for assistance from individuals, hospitals, and community health services.

Division of Testing and Evaluation

NLN conducts one of the largest professional testing services in the country. Test batteries have been developed by NLN using experts in tests and educational measurements and in nursing. The tests available through NLN fall into several categories: guidance and placement of students for schools of professional and practical nursing; achievement of professional and practical nursing students while in nursing school; the preimmigration screening examination and nursing tests prepared for the Commission of Graduates of Foreign Nursing Schools; tests designed for nurse practice settings; and certification tests for nursing specialties. The League's testing services are offered on a voluntary basis; no school or state is required to use them. The tests undergo continual evaluation and revision to maintain their validity and ensure appropriateness of content.

Division of Communications

The NLN distributes a wide variety of informative materials. Some of this information is promotional, explaining the nature and purpose of the League, at the same time providing the public with a glimpse of the League's newest products. Other publications are statistical or highly factual, such as school directories and lists of accredited schools of nursing. The bulk of NLN publications are references and texts, written by leading nursing and health care authorities on topics such as administration and management, career guidance, community health care, curriculum, ethics, public policy, research, theory, and long-term care. In addition, videotapes are available on a wide range of subject matters pertinent to the health care arena, with a growing segment developed for the general public.

Each year NLN issues a publications catalog that is available on request from its headquarters office and is also sent to all members. The official journal, *N&HC: Perspectives on Community*, is published bimonthly. A subscription to this journal is included with NLN membership. Periodic bulletins help members keep informed of current federal and state legislation, important health care issues, and League positions on major issues.

Division of Research

Activities of the Division of Research include data collection (as well as development of the data-gathering instruments), research studies, and special projects. Annually, for instance, NLN collects information on admissions, graduations, and enrollments in programs of practical and professional nursing education. Aspects of these data are reported in various NLN publications. The *NLN Nursing Data Review* is a compilation of statistical information on nursing education and newly licensed nurses. Also published are booklets and directions on state-approved programs preparing students for licensure as RNs or LPNs. The directories indicate types of programs, accreditation status, administrative control, financial support, and data on admissions, enrollments, and graduation. The biennial Nurse-Faculty Census and the biennial Newly Licensed Nurse Study are also published.

NLN, as need and resources permit, surveys or studies other selected aspects of nursing education or nursing service programs. In addition, it carries on both short-term and long-term research projects. Some of these projects are financed by the League itself; some are financed through grants from other agencies. (NLN, unlike ANA, enjoys tax-exempt status, and funds granted to it are not considered taxable income.)

Other Services and Activities

Because of its tax-exempt status as an educational and charitable organization, the League (and its constituent leagues) is prohibited from participating in any political campaign on behalf of or in opposition to any particular candidate, and no substantial part of its activities may consist of influencing legislation. However, this prohibition does not extend to dealing with administrative agencies or the executive branch of the government. The League is also permitted to inform members fully of proposed legislation, engage in nonpartisan analysis or study and disseminate results, and give factual testimony and information. Preferably these presentations are made on request of the legislators. Within this framework, NLN has been involved in legislation affecting nursing and has been helpful in its implementation. NLN works closely with ANA, AACN, and AONE (especially as part of the Tri-Council) on these and other issues. However, throughout its entire program, NLN also maintains active liaison with many other national agencies, both governmental and voluntary.

In 1973, the NLN chose the National Library of Medicine in Bethesda, Maryland, home of the world's largest collection of health sciences literature, as the official repository of NLN's historical documents and records. These include the history of NLN, old photographs of American nurses, correspondence by Florence Nightingale and other nursing leaders, and the history of the National Organization for Public Health Nursing (NOPHN).

The impact of NLN on nursing does not lie only in the services and activities of the organization and its component groups. It is equally important to look at some of the major pronouncements made by NLN in taking stands on nursing issues. Many are on education and practice. These were discussed earlier. Other position papers are on a national health plan and on nursing's responsibility to minorities and disadvantaged groups.

The NLN headquarters is located at 350 Hudson Street, New York, New York 10014.

NATIONAL STUDENT NURSES' ASSOCIATION

The National Student Nurses' Association, Inc. (NSNA), established in 1953, is the national organization for nursing students in the United States and its territories, possessions, and dependencies. According to its bylaws, NSNA's purpose is:

to assume responsibility for contributing to nursing education in order to provide for the highest quality health care; to provide programs representative of fundamental and current professional interests and concerns; and to aid in the development of the whole person, his/her professional role, and his/her responsibility for the health care of people in all walks of life.

The NSNA is autonomous, student financed, and student run. It is the voice of all nursing students speaking out on issues of concern to nursing students and nursing.

In its first few years, NSNA had little money, a small membership, no real headquarters of its own, and no headquarters staff. It did have financial and moral support from ANA and NLN. Today the association pays for headquarters offices, a staff, and all the other expenses incidental to running the business of a large association. It holds and finances its own annual convention. And, at the same time, it has initiated and financed several important projects in the interest not only of its members but of the nursing profession as a whole.

Membership

Students are eligible for active membership in NSNA if they are enrolled in state-approved programs leading to licensure as an RN or are RNs enrolled in programs leading to a baccalaureate degree in nursing. Students are eligible for associate membership if they are prenursing students enrolled in college or university programs designed to prepare them for programs leading to a degree in nursing. Associate members have all of the privileges of membership except the right to hold office as president and vice president at state and national levels. Application for membership is made directly to NSNA. Dues paid to NSNA are a combination of national and state association dues.

Organization

The policies and programs of NSNA are determined by its House of Delegates, whose membership consists of elected representatives from school and state associations. The delegates at each annual convention elect NSNA's three officers; six directors, one of whom will become editor of *Imprint*, the official journal of NSNA; and a four-member nominating committee. Officers serve for one year or until their respective successors are elected. The board of directors manages the affairs of the association between the annual meetings of the membership. There is only one standing committee (nominating), but the board has the authority to establish other committees as needed. Two consultants are appointed, one each by the ANA and NLN,

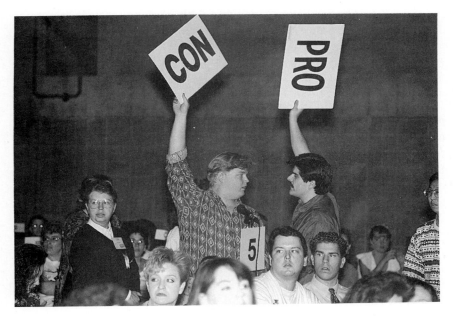

Student nurses at an NSNA convention are serious about the issues they vote on. (*Courtesy of the National Students Nurses' Association.*)

in consultation with the NSNA board of directors. Their role is to act as resource people and to provide an interchange of information between NSNA and their respective organizations. Constituent organizations may or may not function in a similar manner; their bylaws must be submitted to NSNA for review.

Projects, Activities, Services

NSNA has a wide variety of activities, services, and projects to carry out its purpose and functions. Even in its early years, the association sought participation in ANA and NLN committees and sent representatives to the ICN. Today, NSNA representatives sit on committees of ANA and other health organizations. It is a leading participant in the student assembly of the ICN. NSNA members are involved in community health activities such as hypertension screening, health fairs, child abuse, teenage pregnancy, and education on death and dying. Some of these activities are carried out in cooperation with other student health groups.

In addition to health- and nursing-related issues, social, women's, and human rights issues are supported by NSNA. Breakthrough to Nursing is a major project aimed at recruiting minority group members into nursing and helping them financially, morally, and educationally to undertake such a career. Their participation in legislative activities at the state and national level has also been impressive.

NSNA has shown a forward-looking interest in the health and social problems of society, often combined with like interest in interdisciplinary cooperation. With the American Medical Student Association (AMSA), Student American Pharmaceutical Association (SAPhA), and American Student Dental Association (ASDA), nursing students have participated in a variety of activities.

Scholarship Funds

The Foundation of the National Student Nurses' Association administers its own scholarship program. The fund is incorporated and has obtained federal tax exemption. Scholarship monies are obtained from various organizations, and contributions have included both commercial enterprises and professional organizations as well as individuals.

Publications

Imprint, the official NSNA magazine, came into existence in 1968, and a subscription is given to members. Subscriptions are also available to other interest groups, schools, and individuals. *Imprint*, published five times during the academic year, is the only publication of its kind specifically for students. It is the only nursing magazine written by and for nursing students, and students are encouraged to contribute articles and letters.

Other Professional Activities

At the tenth anniversary of its founding, NSNA had accomplished a great deal. Before its thirtieth, it had become an involved group whose activities demonstrated committed professionalism. Gone are the stunt nights and uniform nights of the early days. Now students are involved in many of the same issues as ANA and NLN and often seem to show more foresight. Resolutions have addressed such issues as nuclear war, abortion, licensure, patients' rights, environmental hazards, collective bargaining, quality of care, nursing education and practice.

As in other fields, nursing students have also fought for their own rights, and NSNA has maintained a commitment to students' rights. In 1970, a guideline for a student bill of rights was distributed to all constituents, a mandate of the 1969 delegates. In 1975, a comprehensive bill of rights, responsibilities, and grievance procedures was accepted and published. The statement was adopted in schools throughout the country. (See Chapter 9 for more on students' rights.)

NSNA offers the opportunity for nursing students to be heard, becomes a forum for debates on health and social issues as well as nursing issues, provides opportunities for interdisciplinary contacts, and is a testing ground for leadership skills. Participation and involvement can be a meaningful and valuable part of the nursing student's education.

NSNA headquarters is at 555 West 57th Street, New York, NY 10019.

HEALTH-RELATED ORGANIZATIONS

Many health-related organizations, both governmental and nongovernmental, frequently provide opportunities for participation by nurses through some form of membership, consultation, or inclusion on committees or programs. A number provide services specifically for nurses, such as workshops, conferences, publications, and audiovisual materials. Nurses may be invited to attend other program sessions, present papers, or serve on panels. Some examples include the American Cancer Society, the American Heart Association, the American Medical Association, and the Catholic Hospital Association.

There are also organizations in which there are large, active nursing components, such as the American Hospital Association and, particularly, the American Public Health Association (see Appendix 5). The American Red Cross, particularly, has many activities in which nurses are involved, including their disaster health services and educational programs. Nurses may give volunteer service and apply for enrollment as a Red Cross Nurse.

THE NURSING LITERATURE

Not long ago, text or reference books in nursing were generally limited to the major clinical fields. Now there is scarcely any area relating to nursing that does not have books on the subject. New titles show the extremely diverse nature of the subjects that nurses must read and write about today. Many of these books (this one, for instance) must be frequently revised and published in new, updated editions to keep up with new knowledge and expanding concepts.

Reading the book advertisements in the nursing magazines is almost an education in itself; by doing this, you are reminded of the "hot" topics of the day—or of tomorrow. Even more important is reading the reviews of these books, also published in the nursing journals. That way, you get a better knowledge of their content and the reviewer's estimate (and he or she is usually an expert in the field) of their value. Then it is easier to decide whether to buy it, borrow it from the library, glance through it there, or forget about it. It is impossible to read all the books published in the nursing field today, so you will want to select those that are most worthwhile for you.

It is the nursing journals, however, that will keep you up-to-date and well informed. Usually at least six months pass between the writing of a book and its appearance in print, and a few more months may pass before it is reviewed. But the nursing journals, especially those that are published monthly, make available news, reviews, and information promptly. Within the past 15 years alone, there has been a remarkable increase in the numbers and kinds of nursing magazines. Some you will want to subscribe to and keep for reference, others to look at each month in the library. It is helpful to have at least an idea of the content, purpose, and approach of all of them, whether for reading purposes or sometime to publish yourself. Writing for publication is becoming more important as changes in nursing and health care occur; therefore, learning how to write and publish is worth considering.

It is not feasible to review the content of all these periodicals; some are listed in Appendix 5, if they are associated with a professional organization. There are also other general and clinical journals, published by the nonprofit American Journal of Nursing Company, owned by ANA, journals owned by commercial publishers, journals of the SNAs, and national journals of other countries. It is worthwhile to review these journals sometimes if possible (they are not subscribed to by many libraries), as well as the other health-related journals, because they contain useful information. All nursing journals and serials are listed in *INI*, the *International Nursing Index*. A listing of nursing and allied health periodicals, with addresses, is given in the *Cumulative Index to Nursing and Allied Health Literature* (*CINAHL*). Other health-related journals are found in *Index Medicus*.

Other Reference Sources

Most schools of nursing today do not have a collection adequate to meet the needs of a serious scholar or even of someone who wants to go beyond the major nursing journals and books. Nevertheless, nurses who learn how to use the library, the interlibrary loan service, and the various computer information retrieval services will find a new world of reference sources. For instance, CINAHL indexing from 1983 to the present is available electronically as an online database and on CD-ROM. In these formats, abstracts from many of the journal articles are also available. The online database is updated monthly; the CD-ROM, every two months.

As noted elsewhere, the *International Nursing Index* (INI) is published by the American Journal of Nursing Company in cooperation with the National Library of Medicine (NLM), a federal agency. All of the citations

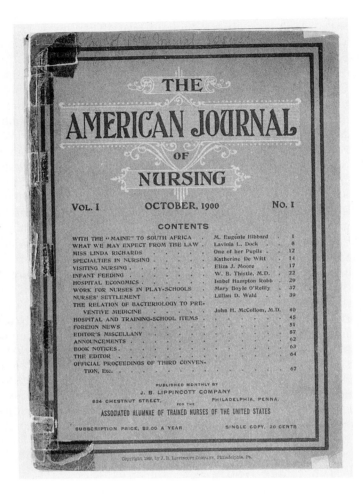

The *American Journal of Nursing* has been owned by nurses since its inception in 1900. (*Courtesy of the American Journal of Nursing Company.*)

appearing in INI are part of MEDLINE, the massive, world-renowned biomedical database produced by NLM and updated twice a month. Some 360,000 citations from 3500 journals are added each year to MEDLINE. A selected number of nursing journals appear in *Index Medicus*, its print counterpart.

Although an excellent source for general biomedical information, MEDLINE is not as efficient as CINAHL for retrieving nursing literature. However, because it is federally supported, MEDLINE is extremely inexpensive and is widely available in online, locally mounted, and CD-ROM formats. An advantage for the researcher is that it contains data as far back as 1966.

NLM provides access to a number of related databases of interest to nurses. Among some 30 NLM databases are AIDSLINE, which consists of citations on acquired immunodeficiency syndrome; BIOETHICSLINE, a database containing citations covering ethics and public policy in health care and biomedical research; several cancer databases; DIRLINE, a directory of organizations; and HEALTH, a database developed in cooperation with the AHA, on nonclinical aspects of health care delivery.

Located in Sigma Theta Tau's Center for Nursing Scholarship in Indianapolis, Indiana, the International Nursing Library serves as a comprehensive focal point for information relating to nursing research. This electronic library is designed to assist nurses with the development, utilization, and dissemination of nursing information and to provide the public with information about breakthroughs in nursing research.

Other reference sources of interest to nurses, such as directories, handbooks, review texts, and manuals, are too numerous to list in these pages. A number of guides regularly provide libraries and nurses with lists of recommended journals, books, and other materials. For specific needs, it is advisable to consult a professional librarian.

You will not want to confine youself to the limits of nursing's literature. The publications of medical and hospital groups, allied professions, education, administration, the social services, and other related fields frequently contain useful and interesting material. Understanding social, economic, educational, and other issues is as important to understanding current and future changes in nursing as knowledge of medical and scientific progress.

Of course, all the reference sources in the world are of little value if you can't use them properly. What follows are some of the ways students and professionals can maximize the benefit they receive from the library's services:

1. Establish personal contact with a professional librarian in the institution's library. Information management is the librarian's expertise, and he or she can provide valuable support in meeting educational and clinical goals. Librarians want to meet information needs, but they also can do so only if they know their patrons and their specific needs.
2. Take advantage of library orientations and tours, and keep up with regular library newsletters. Internal library operations are fast becoming totally computerized, and knowing how to retrieve needed data quickly from online catalogs and other systems will prove advantageous. Some training is also needed to use the library's electronic systems for searching the databases mentioned previously. It's also valuable to know how to request copies of articles or books from other libraries.

KEY POINTS

1. The rapid increase in various specialty nursing organizations resulted in some lack of coordination in advancing nursing goals.
2. NFSNO, NOLF, and the Tri-Council are examples of the way in which nursing organizations have established relationships that allow them to communicate and, at times, collaborate in areas of mutual interest.
3. Key differences between ANA and NLN are in the areas of size, membership, collective bargaining, credentialing, and legislative activity.
4. ANA focuses considerable attention on nurses' economic and general welfare, lobbying, standard setting, certification, accreditation of CE programs, and relationships with other groups. ANA sees itself as speaking for nurses.
5. NLN's major activities are in accreditation of educational and home care programs, consulting, and testing.
6. Specialty organizations include those that are clinical, have special interests in ethnic or other minority concerns, or maintain a scholarly, educational, or socially oriented focus.
7. Health-related organizations, such as AHA, APHA, and the Red Cross often have activities in which nurses participate.
8. There are a number of aids for nurses that will help them find the kinds of references they need; nurses should seek them out and become familiar with the use of computers for this purpose.

REFERENCES

1. Flanagan L. *One Strong Voice: The Story of the American Nurses Association.* Kansas City, MO: ANA, 1976.
2. American Nurses Association. *Bylaws.* Washington, DC: American Nurses Publishing, 1995.
3. Flanagan L. *What You Need to Know About Today's Workplace.* Washington, DC: American Nurses Publishing, 1995.
4. Mezey M, et al. The teaching nursing home program. *Nurs Outlook* 32:146–150, May–June, 1984.
5. Merton R. The functions of the professional association. *Am J Nurs* 58:50–54, January, 1958.
6. International Council of Nurses. *Nursing's Next Advance: An International Classification for Nursing Practice (ICNP).* Geneva: ICN, 1993.
7. Affara F, Styles MM. *Nursing Regulation Guidebook: From Principles to Power.* Geneva: ICN, 1993.

8. International Council of Nurses. *Costing Nursing Services.* Geneva: ICN, 1993.

9. International Council of Nurses. *Nursing Support Workers.* Geneva: ICN, 1993.

10. National League for Nursing. *Strategic Plan 1995–2000.* New York: NLN, 1995.

14

Job Selection

OBJECTIVES

After studying this chapter, you will be able to:

1. Assess your talents and interests in planning for your career.
2. Prepare for a job interview.
3. Put together a professional résumé.
4. Write an application letter.
5. Identify sources of information about jobs.
6. Terminate employment in an appropriate manner.
7. Deal with being fired or laid off.

Graduation at last! And now what? For most nurses, "what" means it's now time to get a job. For some, the job is predetermined—commitment to the armed services, the Veterans Administration, or another agency that funded their education. Others may have decided early on exactly the kind of nursing they prefer and the place they want to do it. If all goes well and there are no problems, such as an oversupply of nurses for that specialty or geographic area, at least one major decision is made. But for all graduates, choosing that crucial first job and preparing for it are big considerations.

There are many employment opportunities for nurses today, although the place of employment preferred may not offer the exact hours, specialty, opportunities, or assistance a new graduate may want. Pockets of unemployment most often result from budgeting factors and a tightening of the economy. Nurses may be *needed*, sometimes seriously, but some employers still tend to retain less qualified workers on lower salaries and to eliminate patient care services. Another problem is maldistribution, with not enough nurses opting to work in ghettos or poor rural areas, although the need there is serious. On the other hand, small communities may be flooded by nursing graduates of a community college who wish to stay in that area.

Even with these social and economic factors, new nursing opportunities are constantly emerging (these are described in some detail in Chapter 6). How, then, can you decide what is the best job for you? How do you maximize the chances of getting it?

BASIC CONSIDERATIONS

Personal and Occupational Assessment

It's a good idea to start thinking about career choices while you are still in your educational program. Since most schools have rotations through the various clinical specialty areas, this gives you a chance to compare as you learn. Generally, there is also access to someone who can advise you about the pros and cons of certain types of nursing—or at least there's a more experienced nurse, often a faculty member, to talk to.

More important than anything else, though, is to take a considered look at yourself—your own qualities and what you want out of life. There are a variety of approaches to this sort of self-assessment that are interesting to explore in depth,[1] but there are generally certain commonalities. Some questions you might ask are:

- *What are my personality characteristics?* Do I like to do things with people or by myself? Am I patient? Do I like to do things quickly? Am I good at details, or do I like to take the broad view? Do I like a structured and quiet environment or one that is constantly changing? Am I relatively confident in what I undertake or do I look for support? Am I easily bored? Do I like to tackle problem situations or avoid them? Do I have a sense of humor? Am I emotional? Am I a risk taker? Do I care about the way I look? Do I care what others think of me?
- *What are my values?* Do I believe in the right to life or the right to die? Do I think everyone should have access to health care? Do I have some religious orientation? Do I think that too many people today are too rigid or too loose in their beliefs and behavior? Can I accept and work with those who have very different values? How do I feel about my responsibility to myself, my employer, my patient, the doctors, my profession, and society? Do I believe strongly that my way is the right way? Am I intolerant of others' beliefs?

- *What are my interests?* In the broad field of nursing? In certain specialties? In the health field? In my private and social life? In the community? Do I like to travel? Do I long for adventure?
- *What are my needs?* Am I ambitious? Do I like to boss? Is money important to me? Status? Do I need intellectual stimulation? Is academic success important? What about academic credentials? Am I comfortable working where the majority of nurses have different educational credentials? Do I prefer working with a supervisor of the same or other sex? Am I willing to relocate? Does a city, suburb, or rural area fit my desired lifestyle? Is success in my field important? Am I willing to sacrifice personal and family time for success? Do I think that my first responsibility is to my family at this point? Do my spouse and I plan to have dual careers? Is part-time work an option? Do I want plenty of time for family, friends, and leisure activities? Do I see nursing as a career or a way to earn a living as long as that is necessary? Do I really like nursing? If not, why not, and what can I do about it?
- *What kinds of abilities do I have?* In manual skills? In communication? In intellectual/cognitive skills? In analyzing? In coordinating? In organizing? In supervising? In dealing with people? Do I have a great deal of energy and stamina? Are there certain times, situations, or climate conditions in which I have less? Am I good at comforting people? Am I able to give some of myself to others? Am I more comfortable with or enjoy more caring for children, the elderly, the chronically ill or some other group?

It's good to prioritize some of these lists, since life and a job are usually a compromise. What's most important? What would make you miserable? It might also be very helpful to share this list with others. Is this the way you are seen by them? Have you missed something? If some of your friends and peers are involved in their own decision making, get together with them and/or a trusted teacher or mentor to brainstorm about the possibilities in the field now or later in order to match your own profile most accurately with nursing opportunities. When compromises are necessary, you can decide ahead of time which ones are tenable or even perfectly acceptable at that point.

Since there will probably be economic constraints in the health care system for a long time, one way to look at the job market is in terms of future growth. For instance, you may choose a community hospital for a first job in order to hone your new skills, but have you considered an investor-owned hospital or, later, a long-term care facility, home care, a one-day surgical center, a wound-care center, or an ambulatory-care outreach center? Should you start thinking about further education? All are part of the trends in health care.[2] You should examine those job prospects as carefully as any other. They may have components that do not fit in with your own self-assessment. But don't close doors because of preconceived notions.

Licensure

Regardless of the results of your self-study, a basic and essential step in your professional nursing career is becoming licensed, since you cannot practice in any state without an RN. Information about how to apply to take the state board examination leading to licensure is found in Chapter 11. The procedure for becoming licensed is now very quick since the use of computer adaptive testing and the ability to take the test any time of the year at more than 200 testing centers.[3] Some state boards of nursing permit nurses to practice temporarily while their application for licensure is being processed, although this is changing. Check with the board or your school. You may be employed as a *graduate nurse* until you pass the licensure exam. However, in reality, many, perhaps most, hospitals will interview you but not employ you until you become licensed. The administration feels that the cost of orientation is too great to take a chance that the nurse will fail. If a nurse fails the test after employment, he or she may be dismissed or must work as some type of nursing assistant.

What if you decide not to work right away—for example, to stay home with your family or to take a long vacation? It's probably wise to study for and take the exam anyway. Unused knowledge has a way of disappearing from the mind, and it might be much more difficult to pass the exam later, without some ongoing learning and practice. Moreover, in most states, you are expected to take the exam within a certain time after graduation. Should you take a nursing board review course? It depends on the confidence you have in your nursing knowledge and test-taking ability. The *good* courses can be very helpful, and may provide backup materials as well as lectures. However, be careful to select a reputable company. Remember that these are profit-making operations, expensive to you, and always attracting some borderline operators. Another way of preparing is to study with a group of peers, perhaps using board review workbooks or texts designed for that purpose.[4]

PROFESSIONAL BIOGRAPHIES AND RÉSUMÉS

New nursing graduates today have a wider variety of personal and educational backgrounds than they did a few years ago. Many have held responsible positions in other fields, and even more have worked part- or full-time before or during their educational programs.

Therefore, the suggested procedures for application and resignation presented are just that. They review generally accepted ways to handle certain inevitable professional matters in a sophisticated and businesslike way, and may serve as a refresher for those already familiar with these or other equally acceptable ways of relating and communicating in professional business relationships. For the younger, less experienced nurse, this material provides a convenient reference and guide.

After self-assessment and thought about career alternatives, it's time to write a résumé. No matter how you obtain a position in nursing, you will probably be asked to submit a résumé or summary of your qualifications for the job before any interview is possible. In addition, a prospective employer may request a transcript of your educational record and names and addresses of references, but this may not occur until after the interview. Some universities and other educational programs still maintain a file with updated information about your career provided by you, as well as references that you have solicited. This has the advantage of eliminating the need to ask for repeated references from teachers who may scarcely remember you or to write again and again to a variety of places for records. However, this service is gradually fading away and that may not be bad. As you and your career develop, a reference from your first teacher or your first staff position says little other than how you were evaluated at that time. Newer references may be far more useful. Your academic record or simply evidence of your graduation may still be requested, and your school always provides that information. But today a well-prepared résumé is considered a must for a job applicant.

A résumé is a relatively short professional or business biography. In academia, a curriculum vitae (CV), which is somewhat lengthier and contains different and more detailed information, is the appropriate form of professional biography.[5] Résumés are usually shorter than CVs.

The résumé should be businesslike, typed neatly on one side of good-quality plain white or off-white paper measuring $8\frac{1}{2}$ by 11 inches, with a $\frac{3}{4}$ to 1 inch margin all around. No more than two pages are usually recommended, preferably one. A word processor is useful in writing résumés because it allows you to tailor the résumé to a particular job opportunity without making a total revision. However, make sure that the word processor prepares a good-looking product. Some experts suggest that you have a professional printer duplicate your résumé on a newer photocopier that produces a sharp copy, absolutely free of dark areas or smudges. It can be reproduced on paper with texture and a subtle tint. Quick-copy shops may specialize in making a résumé look good, doing layouts, typing, printing, and copying. The point is to have a neat, clean résumé with no misspellings, poor grammar, or typographical errors.

There are various ways to write a résumé.[6] Nursing articles on job search often include examples, as well as books in a general library. Remember that it is a marketing tool and should show you to advantage. Therefore, while you must never be dishonest, the way you present your talents and credentials, especially after you have had additional work experience, may make the difference between whether you are even interviewed or ignored, especially in a competitive situation. While format is a matter of taste, a sample résumé is shown in Exhibit 14.1.

EXHIBIT 14.1

Sample Résumé

LESLIE B. SMITH

120 Pine Street   Home Phone (415) 456-7890
North Ridge, CA 01302   Message Phone (415) 482-6132

PROFESSIONAL
OBJECTIVE: Staff nursing in a community hospital.

EXPERIENCE:
September 1994   Central Hospital, Alton, California
to August 1995   Unit clerk on medical–surgical units, evening shift.
                         Assisted charge nurse in (list activities); trained new clerks;
                         developed end-of-shift report between clerks.

Summer 1994   Central Hospital, Alton, California
                         Nurse's aide on medical–surgical units. Responsible for
                         care of thirty patients under direction of RNs, including
                         (list *major* activities).

EDUCATION:
1995–1997   Blank Community College
                         Associate in Science, May 1997

HONORS:
1995–1997   Dean's List
1996–1997   Member, Wings, college honor society
1995–1997   Honor Scholarship
1997   Outstanding Student Leader Award, Blank Community
                         College

PROFESSIONAL ACTIVITIES:
1996–1997   Member, National Student Nurses' Association
1997   Chair, Program Committee, NSNA
May 1997   Presented paper "When Students Teach Patients."
                         Blank Hospital, Nurses' Day
June 1996   Attended ANA Convention
April 1996   Debate: "Be It Resolved: Everyone Has a Right to Health
                         Care." Student Leadership Forum, Blank Community
                         College

COMMUNITY ACTIVITIES
1991–1997   Volunteer for public television telethon
1991–1997   Volunteer for March of Dimes
1990–1994   Candy-striper at Central Hospital, Alton, California

Some suggestions may be helpful. There is some disagreement as to whether a professional objective stated in the beginning is helpful, especially if you are not sure exactly what you want to do. Some experts say that it shows that you have a clear goal; others, that you may close the door to another opportunity that is available, but will not be offered because your stated goal is different. When you write a résumé, it should match the job for which you are applying, and thus may need to be changed accordingly. For instance, someone with a master's degree in perinatal nursing may be interested in either a teaching or a clinical specialist position. Both the objective and the emphasis in the résumé must focus on the position for which the person is applying. Needless to say, if you are applying for your first or second staff nurse position in a hospital, the decision on what to write is less complex. However, it is often recommended that you review and revise your résumé every year, not only to update, but to reassess what you've accomplished and, perhaps, to think again about your career goals.

All relevant work experiences should be included, with the most recent listed first. The usual format is to list the agency and date, followed by a *brief* description of the duties performed, using "action" verbs—*developed, initiated, supervised.* If you've done something exceptional in the line of your duties, certainly mention it. Some people suggest that if you have not had impressive positions, you should attempt to bury this fact in statements that focus on you personal qualities, such as "Leadership—Demonstrated my ability to lead others as night nurse on a pediatric unit at X hospital, such and such address." On the other hand, there are interviewers who see this as a deliberate attempt to hide lack of experience. No one really knows what is more effective, but again, style is a matter of personal choice.

The education section should also begin with the most recent academic credential, and should include the major and such additions as research projects, special awards, academic honors, extracurricular activities, and offices held. There is no need to go as far back as high school. Information on other honors, professional memberships and activities, and community activities might also be given in separate sections. If you have certification in a specialty area, include this. (You may also put the appropriate initials after your name.) Don't put down a heading such as "honors" and then write "none." Just omit such categories.

Under federal law, you cannot be required to include personal data such as your age, marital status, place of birth, religion, sex, race, color, national origin, or handicap. In fact, there is some feeling that including irrelevant personal data such as this and including height, weight, hobbies, and interests, unless they contribute to your ability to do the job you've applied for, is a negative. If you choose to do so, decide whether this makes you a more desirable candidate. For instance, a second language or extensive travel might be a plus in certain situations. When you are licensed as an RN, or if you later become certified in a specialty, that can be listed as well.

It is not necessary to say "References on request"; you would hardly refuse to give them. If your school does maintain a file, you can state this later, giving the correct address. When you do give the references, include the full names, titles, and business addresses of three persons who are qualified to evaluate your professional ability, scholarship, character, and personality. Most suitable are teachers and former employers. Ask permission to use their names as references in advance. Choose carefully. If the individual, no matter how prestigious, really doesn't know you, your talents, and your abilities, and the reference is noncommittal, it can do more harm than good. When you contact a reference, however, it is acceptable, even good sense, to offer to send a résumé to refresh that person's memory. For instance, almost everyone forgets the dates they knew you, as you are not likely to be the only student or employee they know. If the individual is reluctant, don't push; the result can be a reference that says nothing much, and the potential employer may read it as negative—and it may be. You should also keep in mind that prospective employers frequently telephone the reference, either because they want a quick answer or because they want to ask questions that are not on a reference form or to explore some aspect of the written reference (particularly if it was noncommittal). Therefore, if the individual you've chosen as a reference is inclined to be abrupt, unpleasant, or irritated on the phone, choose another. As a rule, don't ask for a "To whom it may concern" letter and have it recopied. Most sophisticated employers see that as an uninterested response. If you carry a reference with you to an interview, it may be regarded with some suspicion.

Suppose that you didn't get along with your last employer and, even though you left with appropriate notice, you fear a poor reference. Sometimes someone else who was your positional superior, or another person such as a clinical specialist who knows your work, can be substituted. (A peer's opinion may be discounted.) However, administrators often know each other, and your potential employer may know that you did not name the person who would be the usual reference and may check with him or her by phone. That could result in a really negative reference. Therefore, as lists of references are often not requested until after the interview, you could simply say then that you did not have a positive relationship. Be careful not to speak negatively of the former employer; try to be objective or neutral. Though references can be important, the impression you make in an interview can be much more important in the long run.

LOOKING OVER THE JOB MARKET

It's sensible to assess the potential for a particular job both before and after applying for and/or being offered a nursing position. Chapter 6 should be helpful as an overview of the opportunities available in terms of both specialties and professional development (career ladder, internships); but reading the literature, talking to practitioners in the field, and, if possible, getting exposure to the actual practice during your educational program will help answer some specific questions. Start thinking about that first job early, while you're a student. Start getting preliminary information and talking to people in your network.

Today, even if an employer is actively recruiting for nurses, an application, a formal letter of interest, and often a résumé are necessary before a position is actually offered. Although there are those who feel that going through the entire process is worthwhile for the experience alone, unless you have at least some interest, it is unfair to take an employer's time to review an application and go through an interview for nothing. Therefore, after self-assessment, do at least a potential job assessment in advance. The first logical consideration is a place with which you have already had experience.

Hospitals or other agencies affiliated with schools of nursing may offer new graduates staff positions. That has several advantages for the employer and usually for the student as well. Nurses who are familiar with the personnel, procedures, and physical facilities may require a shorter orientation period, which saves time and money. And, of course, to an extent, the former student is already known. There are also benefits for new graduates. During these first months after graduation, you can gain valuable experience in familiar surroundings. There are opportunities to develop leadership and teaching skills and to practice clinical skills under less pressure because the people, places, and routines will not be totally unknown. The potential trauma of relocating and readjusting your personal life is not combined with the tension of being both a new, untried graduate and a new employee. And it may be a wonderful place to work. Besides, if the job market is tight, making a good impression as a student (or even as a volunteer or employee in another capacity) may bring you a job offer or, at least, give you an advantage over another applicant.[7]

However, if the experiences offered do not help you to develop, if the environment is one that eventually makes you resistant, resentful, indifferent, unhappy, or disinterested, you may be set for a lifetime of nursing jobs, not a professional career. Of course, that can also happen in other places, but if you're alert, you can often get a pretty good notion of how it would be to work at the agencies in which you have had student or work experience. Be observant; look at how care is being given, the interaction between staff and management, with physicians, with other departments, and generally, the work environment.[8] This evaluation can be a little more difficult if you don't know a place at all, but the opinion of someone you respect, word-of-mouth information, the institution's newsletter and brochures, and even the way someone replies to your inquiry provides indirect as well as direct information.

On a more concrete level, you can give some thought to what you are willing to accept in terms of salary, shifts, benefits, and travel time. (Don't underestimate the value of the fringe benefits, which may not be taxable.) Balancing these with other advantages and disadvantages as determined by your self-assessment is important. And realistically, if the job market is tight in the geographic area of your choice, your opportunities may be fewer than they would be in times of nursing shortage. Whether or not this is so, spend the time, effort, and sometimes money to research institutions in which you are interested. Call for their information pamphlet/brochure, and perhaps the annual report. All this is public information, available from the public/ community relations office. The public library also has materials giving information about health care agencies.[9] If you're considering relocation and aren't familiar with the area, again check the library, write to that town's Chamber of Commerce, or get some copies of the local newspaper. However, some of your best information may come from your network, discussed later.

All of these factors must be considered seriously. You'll never have another first job in nursing, a job that could set the tone of your professional future. At best, you'll have wasted time. It's much better to act carefully and make sure that your choice is the best possible one for moving you toward your goal, whatever it may be.[10]

SOURCES OF INFORMATION ABOUT POSITIONS

Two principal sources of information are available to nurses who are looking for a position: (1) personal contacts and inquiries; and (2) advertisements and recruiters. Commercial placement agencies can be of some help at a later stage of your search, although they may be more interested in nurses with advanced experience, education or specialization.

Personal Contacts and Inquiries

The nursing service director or someone on the nursing staff of a student-affiliated agency, instructors, other nurses, friends, neighbors, and family members may suggest available positions in health agencies or make other job suggestions. Hospitals not affiliated with schools of nursing sometimes ask the heads of nursing schools to refer graduates to them for possible placement on their staff. Often, letters or announcements of such positions are posted on the school bulletin board or are available in a file. Your own inquiries are likely to be equally productive in turning up the right position.

Never underestimate the value of personal contacts—your network. People seldom suggest a position unless they know something about it. That gives you the opportunity to ask questions early on, and the information can help you decide as well as prepare you better for the interview. Moreover, if your contact knows the employer and is willing (better yet, pleased) to recommend you, your chances of getting the position are immediately improved. (This kind of networking, discussed more fully in Chapter 7, will be useful throughout your career.) One business executive has said, "Eighty percent of all jobs are filled through a grapevine ... a system of referrals that never sees the light of day." When equally qualified people compete for the same position, the network recommendation could make the crucial difference. Asking for job-seeking help is neither pushy nor presumptuous, but you should be prepared to discuss your interests intelligently. A résumé will help, too. Most people like to be asked for advice and want to be helpful, but they have to be asked. On the other hand, you need to use some common sense in deciding how much and how often you ask for help from whom.

Some aspects of networking are much less formal, but equally helpful. For instance, contacts you've made as a member of a national nursing organization, beginning with NSNA, can give you inside information on what it's like to work in a certain place and/or in a particular geographic region. They may help with anything from housing to introduction to professional, social, or community groups.

Advertisements and Recruiters

Local newspapers and official organs of district and state nurses' associations often carry advertisements of positions for professional nurses. National and regional nursing magazines and papers list positions in all categories of employment, usually classified into the various geographic areas of the country. National medical, public health, and hospital magazines also carry advertisements for nurses, but they usually are for head nurse positions or higher, or for special personnel such as nurse anesthetists or nurse consultants.

All publications carry classified advertisements for information only, and, of course, as a source of revenue. Rarely, if ever, does the publisher assume responsibility for the information in the advertisement beyond its conformity to such legal requirements as may apply. If you accept an advertised position that does not turn out to be what was expected, you cannot hold the publication responsible. Read the advertisement very carefully. Is the hospital or health agency well known and of good reputation? Is the information clear and inclusive? Does it sound effusive and overstress the advantages and delights of joining the staff? What can be read between the lines? How much more information is needed before deciding whether the job is suitable? Some of these questions can be resolved through correspondence or telephone contact or your network. Naturally, advertisers are putting "best foot forward." Unless you've been watching the advertisements for some time or know someone from that institution, you might not know, for example, that the turnover is high, generally a sign of some problems. Nevertheless, want-ads are one reasonable start to a job search.

At some time, you may want to place an advertisement in the "Positions Wanted" column of a professional publication. In that case, obtain a copy of the magazine and read the directions for submitting a classified advertisement. The editor will arrange the information to conform to the publication's style but will not change the material sent unless asked to. Therefore, all the information needed to attract a prospective employer within the limits of professional ethics should be included clearly and concisely.

Career directories published periodically by some nursing journals or other commercial sources are free to job seekers. They have relatively extensive advertisements with much more detailed information than appears in the usual ad. The other advantage is instant comparison and geographic separation, with preprinted, prepaid postcards that can be sent to the health agency of interest. (Most are geared to hospital recruitment.) Directories are frequently available in the exhibit section of student and other nursing conventions. Some carry reprints of articles on careers, licensure, job seeking, and other pertinent information. Some journals also do periodic surveys on job salaries and fringe benefits that can be useful when considering various geographic areas and may have special sections describing job opportunities in certain regions of the country.

Recruiters for hospitals and other agencies are usually present at representative booths in the exhibit areas of conventions; some have hotel suites where they have an open house. Recruiters, who may or may not be nurses, also visit nursing schools or arrange for space in a hotel for preliminary interviews. Notices are placed in newspapers or sent to schools. There are advantages to the personalized recruiter approach because your questions can be answered directly, and you can get "a feel" for the employer's attitude, especially if nurses accompany the recruiter. However, remember the recruiters are selected for their recruiting ability.

Commercial Placement Agencies

There are commercial placement agencies in some places that maintain a list of nurses who are looking for part-time work or who are job hunting. As might be expected, some are reliable and some are not. They can be checked out with the Better Business Bureau and your network. Almost always a fee must be paid to the registry, sometimes based on a percentage of the nurse's earnings. At another level of job seeking—executive positions —well-known agencies of good reputation (headhunters) are used by both employers and potential employees to match the best possible person to a suitable position.

Under ordinary circumstances, however, the so-called temporary nurse service is another option (see Chapter 6). These services function quite differently from agencies or registries, since they themselves employ the nurses and then, according to requests and a nurse's choices, send her or him to an institution—or other agency for a specific period of time. Nurses are usually placed in short-term situations in hospitals, but some services advertise home care. The single most important factor that seems to attract nurses to temporary nurse services is control over working conditions, including the time, place, type of assignment, and so on. New graduates may find this type of employment attractive as a temporary measure, since the nonavailability of fringe benefits may not be important to them. There is also an opportunity to try out different types of nursing, but for the new nurse, the lack of individual support and supervision is a disadvantage.

PROFESSIONAL CORRESPONDENCE

The first formal contact with a prospective employer is usually made by letter, probably accompanied by a résumé. Telephone conversations or informal contacts with a recruiter at a convention or job fair may precede this step. Telegrams, mailgrams, or, perhaps, a fax are also often part of the job search process at one point or another. Every business letter makes an impression on its reader, an impression that may be favorable, unfavorable, or indifferent. To achieve the best effect, the stationery on which it is written should be in good taste; the message accurate and complete, yet concise; the tone appropriate; and the form, grammar, and spelling correct.

Stationery and Format

Business letters should be neatly and legibly typed or, if necessary, hand-written in black ink on unlined white stationery. Single sheets no smaller than 7 by 9 inches or larger than $8\frac{1}{2}$ by 11 inches are more suitable than folded sheets. Personal stationery is acceptable if it is of the right size and color (white or off-white) and used with unlined envelopes. Notebook paper should never be used for business correspondence; neither should someone else's personal stationery or the stationery of a hospital, hotel, or place of business. Good-quality typing paper is always in good taste if a suitable envelope is used with it.

If at all possible, you should type the letter or use a word processor. This is considered most desirable; in fact, some employers react very negatively to a handwritten letter, even if neatly printed. They feel that it is always possible to get a letter typed and not to do so shows lack of interest or professionalism. In addition, the letter, like the résumé, should be error-free. Always keep a copy for future reference.

Books on English composition and secretary's handbooks include correct forms for writing business letters. Two or more variations may be given; the choice is yours. One example is shown in Exhibit 14.2. If personal stationery on which the name and address are engraved or printed is used, this information should be omitted from the heading of the letter and only the date is given. Another acceptable format is shown later in Exhibit 14.3.

In doing business correspondence, it is always advisable to address a person exactly as the name appears on her or his own letters. The full title and position should be used, no matter how long they may be. It is better to place the lengthy name of a position on the line below the addressee's name, and break up a long address, in the interest of a neat appearance, remembering to indent continuation lines.

It is always best to address your correspondent by name. This may be more difficult at a distance. If you are within reasonable telephoning distance, call and get the correct name and title from the person's secretary, telephone operator, or other staff. However, if the name of the person to whom you are writing to inquire about a position is not known, the letter may be addressed to the recruiter, the director or supervisor of the appropriate division, for example, "Director of the Department of Nursing." The salutation could then be "Dear Director." Using "Dear Sir" or "Dear Madam" may be incorrect, since you don't know whether the recipient is male or female. The inside address and the envelope address should be identical. People are sensitive about their names and titles; be accurate. Again, a little extra effort is worthwhile and may pay off in the favorable impression you make: get the correct name and title. If you've done the necessary research about the institution in which you're interested, this kind of information is available.

There is no agreement as to whether it is only correct to give a title before the name in an address in the heading and on the envelope—not in the form of initials after the name—for example, "Dr. Constance E. Wright" rather than "Constance E. Wright, EdD." Both forms seem to be used. In a signature, however, it is preferable to place the degree initials after the name of the signer of the letter. Never use both the title and the initials in an address; "Dr. Constance E. Wright, EdD" or Ms. Mary Jones RN are incorrect.

It is quite suitable, and even desirable, for a (licensed) nurse to use "RN" after his or her name, particularly in professional correspondence. Many nurses with doctorates place after their names RN PhD, or EdD RN to clarify that they are nurses as well as holders of a doctorate. They should be addressed as "Dear Dr. Whatever:"

EXHIBIT 14.2

Sample Application Letter

Date of letter
Applicant's address
Applicant's phone number

Employer's name and title (Use complete title and address)
Employer's address

Salutation:

Opening paragraph: State why you are writing. Name the position or type of work for which you are applying. Mention how you learned of the opening.

Middle paragraph: Explain your interest in working for this employer and the specific reason for desiring this type of work. Describe relevant work experience, pointing out any other job skills or abilities that relate to the position for which you are applying. If appropriate, state your academic preparation and how it relates to the job description. Be brief but specific; your résumé contains details. Refer the reader to your enclosed résumé.

Closing paragraph: Have an appropriate closing to pave the way for an interview and indicate dates and times of availability. A telephone number is useful. If you cannot be reached during the day, give a number for messages. Or you might also indicate a time and date in which *you* will call to check about making an appointment.

Sincerely,

Signature
Name typed

Enc. (probably your résumé)

A professional or businesswoman usually does not use her husband's name at all in connection with her work. However, she may use the title "Mrs." to identify herself as a person who is, or has been, married if she desires. "Mrs." goes in parentheses before her typed name. Many women prefer "Ms.," but this is not included in the signature.

Content and Tone

The information included in a business letter should be presented with great care, giving all pertinent data but avoiding unnecessary details. It is often helpful to outline, draft, and edit a business letter, just as you would a term paper. This requires you to think it through from beginning to end in order to ensure completeness and accuracy. It is also helpful to tailor it to fit a well-spaced single page, if possible, or two at the most.

Your writing style is your own, and how you word your message may be part of what you are judged on. The tone of a business letter has considerable influence on the impression it makes and the attention it receives. It is probably better to lean toward formality rather than informality. Friendliness without undue familiarity, cordiality without overenthusiasm, sincerity, frankness, and obvious respect for the person to whom the letter is addressed set the most appropriate tone for correspondence about a position in nursing. Although there are those who suggest very unusual dramatic, or "different" formats, the reality is that they may backfire.

If you feel that you need more information before seriously considering a position (for instance, whether tuition reimbursement is a benefit or a particular specialty area has an opening), you can indicate your interest in a letter beforehand, simply asking for the information, or ask directly within the same application letter. A courteous telephone call to the recruiter might take care of such questions more simply and avoid wasting time. The kind of response you get in terms of courtesy, promptness, and general tone will tell you a lot about the prospective employer.

If you decide not to apply for the position after all, or not to follow through with an interview, it is courteous to inform the person with whom you have corresponded. Specific reasons need be given (briefly) only if such a decision is made after first accepting the position. This is not only courteous but advisable, because you may wish to join that staff at another time or may have other contacts with the nurse executive.

Applications

Applications are not just routine red tape. Whether or not a résumé is requested or submitted, the formal application, which is developed to give the employing agency the information it wants, can be critical in determining who is finally hired. Even if the information repeats information offered in the résumé, it should be entered. It is usually acceptable to attach the résumé or a separate sheet if there is not adequate space to give complete information. It's a good idea to read the application first so that the information is put in the correct place. Neatness is essential. Erasures, misspellings, and wrinkled forms leave a poor impression. Abbreviations, except for state names and dates, or other standard abbreviations, should not be used as a rule.

If the form must be completed away from home, think ahead and bring anticipated data—Social Security and registration numbers, places, dates, and names. Although occupational counselors say that it is not necessary to give all the information requested (such as arrests, health, or race, some of which are illegal to request), it is probably not wise to leave big gaps in your work history without explanation. (See Chapters 9 and 15 regarding federal legislation on employment rights.)

PERSONAL INTERVIEW

An interview may be the deciding factor in getting a job. Anyone who has an appointment for a personal interview should be prepared for it physically, mentally, emotionally, and psychologically. The degree of preparation will depend on the purpose of the interview and what has preceded it. Assuming that you have written to a prospective employer about a position and an interview has been arranged, preparation might include the following:

- *Physical preparation.* Be rested, alert, and in good health. Dress suitably for the job, but wear something in which you feel at ease. It is important to be well-groomed. First appearances are important, and given a choice, no one selects a sloppy or overdressed person in preference to someone who is neat and appropriately dressed. Have enough money with you to meet all anticipated expenses. If you are to be reimbursed by the employing agency, keep an itemized record of expenses for submission later. Get accurate directions to the interview site. Arrive at your destination well ahead of time, but do not go to your prospective employer's office earlier than five minutes before the designated time.
- *Mental preparation.* Read some articles about interviews and think about how you would answer potential questions. Review all information and previous communications about the position. Showing that you know about the hospital or agency is desirable and impressive.

Make certain that you know the exact name or names of the persons you expect to meet and can pronounce them properly. (You can always ask the secretary.) Decide what additional information you want to obtain during the interview. Consider how you will phrase your leading questions, making notes if necessary. Think ahead about what you might need. Have your list of references with correct addresses typed on a separate sheet. You might also bring a copy of your transcript, although the interviewer may choose to send for it. Carry a small notebook or card on which you have listed data that you may need during the interview. If you bring an application form with you, place it in a fresh envelope, which you leave unsealed. Have it ready to hand to the interviewer when she or he asks for it; otherwise, offer it at an appropriate time. Some interviewers suggest that you bring another copy of your résumé; it *can* get lost.

- *Emotional and psychological preparation.* If you have any worries or fears in connection with the interview, try to overcome them by thinking calmly and objectively about what is likely to take place. (Role-playing an interview with a colleague who may have been through the experience can be helpful.) Be ready to adjust to whatever situation may develop during the interview. For example, you may expect to have an extended conversation with at least a nurse manager and find when you arrive that a personnel officer who is not a nurse will interview you. She or he may interview you in a very few minutes and in what seems to be an impersonal way. Or you may have visualized the job setting as quite different.

Accept things as you find them, reserving the privilege of making a decision after consideration of the total job situation. If a stimulating challenge is inherent in the position, you will sense it during the interview, or you may have reason to believe that it will develop. However, you can't demand a challenge, and if one is "created" for you spontaneously by the interviewer, regard the promise with some reservations; an employment situation rarely adjusts to the new employee.

During the Interview

Usually the interviewer will take the initiative in starting the conference and closing it.[11] You should follow that lead courteously and attentively. Shake hands firmly. Be prepared to give a brief overview of your experiences and interests, if asked. At some point, you will be asked if you have any questions, and you should be prepared to ask for additional information if you would like to have it. Should the interviewer appear to be about to close the conference without giving you this opportunity, say, "May I ask a question, please?" It is perfectly acceptable to ask, before the interview is over, about salary, fringe benefits, and other conditions of employment if a contract or explanatory paper has not been given to you. In fact, it would be foolish to appear indifferent. A contract is desirable, but if that is not the accepted procedure, it is important to understand what is involved in the job. The job description should be accessible in writing, and it is best that you have a copy. You should know if the staff is unionized, which often affects the job description.

Most interviewers agree that an outgoing candidate who volunteers appropriate information is likeable. On the other hand, many use the technique of selective silence, which is anxiety provoking to most people, to see what the interviewee will say or do. A good interviewer will try to make you comfortable, in part to relax you into self-revelation; most do not favor aggressive methods. Good eye-contact is fine, but don't stare. Be sensitive to the interviewer's being disinterested in a certain response; maybe it's too lengthy. Don't interrupt. Don't smoke. Don't mumble. Watch your body language (and the interviewer's). It can denote indifference, irritation or even nervousness. Be enthusiastic but don't gush.

Some questions that are likely to be asked in an average one-hour interview are:

1. What position interests you most? (Be specific.)
2. Why do you want to work here? (Know something positive.)
3. What are your strengths and weaknesses? (Play up your strengths, and, although you should be honest, play down your weaknesses. Give examples, perhaps of what people say about you.)
4. What would you do if ...? (Show your decision-making and judgmental skills.)
5. What can you do for us? (Tell about your special qualities and experience.)
6. Tell me about yourself. (Keep it short; don't give more information than necessary to reassure the interviewer that you are suitable for the job physically, mentally, and in terms of preparation. Stress your reliability.)
7. What did you like most and least in school or on your last job? (Be honest, but don't list a series of gripes.)
8. How would you describe your ideal job? (Take the opportunity to do so, but let the interviewer know that you know that nothing's perfect.)
9. Where do you think you'll be five years from now? (Emphasize goals that show your interest in growing professionally.)
10. Do you have any questions? (Be prepared.)

In a survey of directors of nursing service in various settings, the characteristics valued most highly in rating a nursing job applicant were punctuality, completion of the application prior to the interview, neatness and completeness of the application, well-groomed personal appearance, and questions asked. As other qualities that might be more important were bypassed, this list may show how important the external aspects of an interview can be.

When the interview is over, thank the interviewer, shake hands, and leave promptly. A tour of the facility may be offered before or after the interview. This gives you a chance to observe working conditions, ask questions, and, sometimes, note interpersonal relationships.[12] You may or may not have been offered the position. If it was offered to you, it's usually well to delay your decision for at least a day or two until you have had time to think the matter over carefully from every practical point of view. Perhaps you'll want more information, in which case you may write a letter, send a fax, a telegram or mailgram, or make a phone call to your prospective employer. It's always courteous and sometimes acts as a reminder to send a thank-you letter.

Follow-up Communications

Sometimes during the procedure of acquiring a position, you may have occasion to discuss some aspect of it over the telephone with the prospective employer. If you make the call, be brief, courteous, and to the point, with notes handy, if needed. It may be helpful to make notations on the conversation. It's sensible to listen carefully and not interrupt. If you receive a call and are unprepared for it, be courteous but cautious and, perhaps, ask for time to think over the proposal—or whatever may have been the purpose of the call.

Agreements about a position made over the phone should be confirmed promptly in writing. If it's your place to do so, you might say, while speaking with the person, "I'll send you a confirming letter tomorrow." If it's the responsibility of the other person to confirm an agreement but she or he doesn't mention it, ask, "May I have a letter of confirmation, please?"

After any interview or conversation, make notes about what happened for future use and reference. If any business arrangements are made by fax, e-mail or letter, file this information with other related correspondence.

For positions sought through a registry or employment agency, the same courteous, thorough, and businesslike procedures used when dealing directly with a prospective employer are appropriate. A brief thank-you note for help received shows consideration of the agency's efforts in your behalf.

Evaluation

What if you didn't get the job you wanted? There may simply have been someone better suited or better qualified. Still, it's helpful to review the experience in order to refine your interview skills. Were you prepared? Did you present yourself as someone sensitive to the employer's goals? Did you make known your personal strengths and objectives? Did you look your best? Sometimes discussing what happened with another person also gives you a different perspective. And there's no reason why you can't reapply another time.

CHANGING POSITIONS

It is generally expected that nurses should remain in any permanent position they accept for at least a year. Certainly, this is not too long—except in the most unusual circumstances—for you to adjust to the employment situation and find a place on the staff in which to use your ability and talents to their fullest. Furthermore, persons who change jobs too frequently may find that some employers are reluctant to hire them. However, should it be desirable or necessary to change positions, a number of points might be observed. Consider your employer and co-workers as well as yourself, and leave under friendly and constructive circumstances.

Depending on the reasons for leaving and how eager you are to make a change, some writers suggest that before you definitely accept a new position, the present employer should be informed about your desire to leave and why. It may be that, depending on the employer's concept of your value to the institution, a new, more desirable position might be offered. However, it is important to give reasonable notice of your intention to resign. If there is a contract, the length of the notice will probably be stipulated. Two weeks to a month is the usual period, depending principally on the position held and the anticipated difficulty in hiring a replacement. Don't tell everyone else before you tell your immediate superior, privately and courteously.

Try to finish any major projects you have started; arrange in good order the equipment and materials your successor will inherit; and prepare memos and helpful guides to assist the nurse who will assume your duties. Sometimes, you'll be asked to help that person before you leave. Check out employment policies about benefits, including accrued vacation or sick leave.

A letter of resignation should state simply and briefly, but in a professional manner, your intention of leaving, the date on which the resignation will become effective, and the reasons for making the change. A sincere comment or two about the satisfactions experienced in the position and regrets at leaving will close the letter graciously. There should be no hint of animosity or resentment, because this will serve no constructive purpose and may boomerang. (See Exhibit 14.3.)

EXHIBIT 14.3

Sample Letter of Resignation

240 North Street
San Diego, CA 00000
Date

Carol Winter, RN, MSN
Vice President of Nursing
West Central Hospital
20 California Avenue
San Diego, CA 00000

Dear Ms. Winter:

I will be relocating to Phoenix, Arizona, in May and have accepted a position there at General Hospital as head nurse of the pediatric unit. Therefore, I wish to resign effective April 19, 1996.

Being at West Central Hospital has been a very satisfying personal and professional experience. The atmosphere is one in which a nurse can grow, and I appreciate the support given by the staff of 4B and the head nurse, Melanie Jones. She has especially helped me to develop my managerial skills and encouraged me to take advantage of the hospital's tuition reimbursement. I expect to finish my degree in Phoenix. I am proud to have been a part of a group of practitioners and administrators who are committed to caring, competent patient care.

If there is anything I can do to help in the transition, I will be happy to do so.

Sincerely,

(Signature)
Alan Collins, RN

cc: Melanie Jones
    Head Nurse 4B

Don't burn your bridges. You may want to come back to that place at another time. At the least, you may need a reference, and if you appear vindictive or childish, the employer is unlikely to give you an enthusiastic reference, even if you did your job satisfactorily. In these days of litigation, nothing may be written specifically, but employers are adept at reading between the lines of a bland reference. The administrative network (via a personal phone call) may paint you as an undesirable employee, and you'll never know.

Terminal interviews are considered good administrative practice, and are sometimes used for a final performance evaluation and/or a means to determine the reasons for resignation. There is some question of how open employees are about discussing their resignation (unless the reason is illness, necessary relocation, and so on), perhaps because of fear of reprisal in references or even a simple desire to avoid unpleasantness. This is a decision you must make in each situation.

What if you're fired? The most common reasons for being fired are poor job performance, chronic tardiness, excessive absenteeism, substance abuse, or inappropriate behavior. Usually you are given a warning about any of these problems, and if you haven't done anything about correcting your problem (assuming that the charge is justified), you had better take a good look at yourself. Those kinds of uncorrected problems may make your future prospects look dim.

Whether or not you're caught by surprise when you're told, try to maintain your composure. If you can't pull your thoughts together, request another interview to ask questions and find out about the termination procedure. If you *are* at fault, make a clean, fast break. If you are *not* at fault, try to clarify the situation to avoid negative references. You may choose to contest the action and file a grievance, particularly if you are part of a union. This process is described in Chapter 9. However, weigh whether it's worth it. You may need to clear your name, but it might be unpleasant or impossible to stay in that setting and work productively.

In a period of downsizing in health care institutions, it is becoming more frequent to be laid off. Fewer patients and reduced budgets are major factors, especially as institutions are bought by for-profit chains or are consolidated or merged with others. Some close altogether.[13] And, in some cases, nurses are replaced by unlicensed assistive personnel, with more administrative concern for the bottom line than quality of care.

If you're called into your manager's office and told that your position is being eliminated, don't take it personally, and even more important, don't get angry and lash out at the manager; the decision is often made at a higher level and quite impersonally. Again it's a matter of not burning bridges. Clear out your locker or office, turn in your key and name-tag, if that's appropriate, and take your personal belongings and files, if any, but no hospital property. Don't try to get even by deleting important computer documents or otherwise undermining projects. Don't discuss severance pay or other details at this point.[14]

After you've had time to think, make notes about the original meeting. If possible, review your employment benefit manual and union contract. Then make an appointment with someone in the human resources department to go over your benefits. These might include retirement benefits, remaining vacation and sick leave pay, and health insurance. Federal legislation (COBRA) concerning health benefits gives you the right to remain insured for up to 18 months after you've been laid off, but you need the correct forms and information. If you are eligible for outplacement, these personnel can help with techniques of job hunting and contacts. Negotiate for severance pay, asking for twice as much as you expect to get (usually one week per year of service). It this is not forthcoming, try for additional vacation or sick-leave payout, outplacement services, or job counseling. At the same time, check on who will provide reference information and what will be said.[15]

Immediately, start planning your job hunt, but also apply for unemployment benefits; that process takes a while. Many of the same suggestions presented earlier about initiating a job search apply here. It's good if you have a "nestegg," so that you are not immediately pressed financially and don't feel desperate enough to take the first offer. Don't let the lay-off period become a time to simply "sleep-in" or avoid social gatherings, professional meetings and colleagues. All these can be useful in your job search. Use your support system of family and friends to help you psychologically and practically.[16] Keep a positive attitude about yourself. Opportunities will come!

When leaving a job is not your choice, it sometimes helps to talk with a supportive person, to ventilate and analyze what happened. Choose someone you can trust but who can help you see things as objectively as possible. Then it's time to get back to career planning. Perhaps you should look at the possibility of further education or training in a different kind of nursing. If not, be sensible about conserving your economic resources until you find another job. Try to select the next job, keeping in mind what made you unhappy in the last one and, of course, correcting those problems that got you fired, if that occurred. You need not volunteer to your prospective employer that you were fired, but if asked, don't lie. Just say that you were asked to leave and why. Don't criticize your previous employer and try to be as positive as possible about your last job. Your honesty and determination to do well could be a plus.

It's doubtful that you will stay in the same institution throughout your career. This is a very mobile society, and there are many job opportunities for nurses throughout the country (and world). Without closing the doors to unexpected opportunities, beginning early to think in terms of a career will make nursing more satisfying and interesting in the long run.

KEY POINTS

1. Assessing yourself in terms of abilities, interests, characteristics, and values is a good idea before starting a job hunt.
2. A professional résumé and appropriate letters of application are factors in being selected for a job.
3. Some of the best sources of information about the job market are advertisements, personal contacts, job fairs, and recruiters.
4. In interviewing for a job, it is important to be prepared physically and psychologically and to know, or get, as much information as possible about the position and environment.
5. Consideration of its effect on future employment is an important factor in how a job should be terminated.

REFERENCES

1. Finn MA. Discovering who you are and what you want from your career. *Healthcare Trend Trans* 3:42–44, March, 1992.
2. Hurley ML. Where will you work tomorrow? *RN* 57:31–35, August, 1994.
3. Taking the NCLEX: Information every candidate should know. *Imprint* 41:9–12, January, 1995.
4. White A. Getting the most from group study sessions. *Imprint* 41:61, 63, February–March, 1994.
5. O'Keefe N. How to open the right doors. In *Career Guide for 1994*. New York: American Journal of Nursing Company, pp 11–12.
6. Vogel D. Writing a résumé. *Imprint* 40:35–36, January, 1993.
7. Farber G. Job hunting in the world of nursing. *Imprint* 42:21–22, January, 1995.
8. Murray R. All the right moves: Winning at the job search game. *Healthcare Trend Trans* 3:30–38, November–December, 1991.
9. Muellenbach J. Mapping out your job search. *Healthcare Trend Trans* 3:14–18, November–December, 1991.
10. Filoromo T. Finding the right job. *Imprint* 37:27–35, December 1990–January 1991.
11. Vogel D, Jackson P. The interview: Reflections from the recruiter's side of the desk. *Healthcare Trend Trans* 3:24–26, March, 1992.
12. Hannan J. Site seeing: Touring prospective employers. *Healthcare Trend Trans* 3:31, 34–36, March, 1992.
13. Begany T. Layoffs: Targeting RN's. *RN* 57:37–38, July, 1994.
14. Turner S. Laid off? Now what? *Nurs 95* 25:94–98, May, 1995.
15. Ibid.
16. Russ A. Downsizing: A survival kit for employees. *Nurs Mgmt* 25:66–67, August, 1994.

15

Career Management

OBJECTIVES

After you have studied this chapter you will be able to:

1. Describe the stages of socialization through which you may go in moving from student to graduate status.
2. Define biculturalism.
3. List five symptoms of burnout.
4. Identify four things you can do to combat burnout.
5. Explain what strategies you can use to adjust successfully to the work world.
6. Discuss two workplace rights that are guaranteed to employees by the law.
7. Describe the major activities available to maintain your practice competence.
8. List funding sources for continuing your formal education.
9. Identify ways in which you can enhance your professional and personal lives as a nurse.
10. Develop your own career map even if there are major areas of uncertainty.

RESOCIALIZATION

Eventually, graduation *does* come, and for most nurses, the next step, with hardly a break, is that first nursing job. What can you expect?

The student has spent two to four years being socialized into nursing in the education setting; now resocialization into the work world is necessary. Socialization into a new role is not usually a conscious process, although both the individual being socialized and those doing the socializing consciously make certain efforts.

In reality, the educational experience for any field of work will differ from the expectations when you are being compensated for your services. For the most part, students are not integral to the systems of care, look to faculty for their cues and rewards, and are allowed to falter somewhat in their practice. Further, the socialization–resocialization phenomena (student to full-fledged professional) is often presented as a one-time occurrence. In fact, given today's rapidly changing health care system with the movement from hospitals into community practice, downsizing of hospital nursing staffs, and new markets for health services, nurses will be confronted with resocialization many times during their career life.

All of these circumstances caution that the only way to accomplish a comfortable transition time after time after time is to know yourself and the dynamics of a situation. There is nothing so unexpected or mystical about role transition and socialization. All of us have been through the process at least once (but really many times) as we took on the role of a participating member of society.

Role is an abstract idea that can be assumed only through the presence of certain cues allowing you to infer its presence. A role is a constellation of rights and responsibilities that characterize a social position. Since the individual role occupant is embedded in a social structure, the role behaviors are derived from the expectations of both the individual and the social systems with which that individual interfaces. Socialization is the process by which an individual acquires the behaviors necessary for acceptance by these interfacing groups or systems. This is accomplished through a reciprocal process of role shaping and role taking, with the eventual incorporation of the behaviors within one's self as follows:[1]

- *Step 1.* Interaction with primary groups who mirror the expected behaviors (exposure).
- *Step 2.* Development of an interpersonal attachment with significant others from that group (identification).
- *Step 3.* Clarity on expectations; covert messages are made overt (empathy).
- *Step 4.* Negotiations to resolve differences between the ideal and the real, and determine how much freedom there is to modify the role to personal preference (role shaping).
- *Step 5.* Continuing support to allow the new behaviors to become established.

Successful role transition is greatly enhanced where there is a good feeling (chemistry) between you and your group of peers (staff nurses). This alerts you to the need to meet the people you will be working with on a day-to-day basis when applying for a position. The best of organizations go further, providing a preceptorship or "buddy" arrangement with someone who is senior in the staff nurse role.[2] Make sure you ask questions until you fully understand what is expected of you, and be cautious in bending the rules until you have established yourself. However, make inquiries that help predict how much personal role shaping will be possible. Some cues of an organization that allows little flexibility in role development are:

1. Highly precise and detailed job descriptions.
2. Management by memo in situations where personal communication would have sufficed.
3. Guarded interdisciplinary boundaries that hamper smooth operation.
4. A hierarchy that is an obstacle as opposed to facilitating your work.
5. Policies, procedures, and documentation systems that are cumbersome and even inconsistent with current practice.
6. Absence of staff nurse autonomy in caring for patients.
7. Verbalized discontent from staff, but no evidence of any attempt to change things.
8. High turnover rate.

Successful role transition includes identifying with the right group, interpreting their expectations accurately, negotiating to the extent that is possible while maintaining your unique identity, and merging with the group on terms that are mutually acceptable. This is the best of worlds. In less perfect situations, you have parties that refuse to tolerate any variance; individuals who are unable to "read" the expectations accurately or refuse to become fully involved.[3]

DEALING WITH REALITY SHOCK

For all but a few graduates, the first job is as an employee in some bureaucratic setting, the antithesis of professionalism. For instance, a bureaucracy has specialized roles and tasks; professionals have specialized competence with an intellectual component. The bureaucracy is organized into a hierarchical authority structure; professionals expect extensive autonomy in exercising their special competence. The bureaucracy's orientation is toward rational, efficient implementation of specific goals and tends toward impersonality; professionals have influence and responsibility in the use of their specialized competence and make decisions governed by internalized standards.[4] On these differences alone, and there are others, professionals in a bureaucracy find themselves in conflict.

Kramer identified the problems of new graduates in resolving their role in a bureaucratic–professional conflict and called it *reality shock*, "the specific shocklike reactions of new workers when they find themselves in a work situation for which they have spent several years preparing and for which they thought they were going to be prepared, and then suddenly find that they are not."[5] Reality shock is different from, but related to, both culture shock and future shock.

Thus, when the new nurse, who has been *in* the work setting but not *of* it, embarks on the first professional work experience, there is not an easy adaptation of school-learned attitudes and behaviors, but the necessity for an entirely new socialization. Kramer has categorized and described these as follows:

1. *Skills and routine mastery.* The expectations are those of the employment setting. A major value is competent, efficient delivery of procedures and techniques to clients, not necessarily including psychological support. New graduates immediately concentrate on skill and routine mastery.

2. *Social integration.* This involves getting along with the group and being taught by them how to work and behave: the "backstage" reality behaviors. New graduates who stay at stage 1 may not be seen as competent peers. Those who try to incorporate some of the professional concepts of the educational setting and adhere to those values may alienate the group.

3. *Moral outrage.* Given the differences between what was taught and what is identified and labeled, new graduates feel angry and betrayed by both their teachers and their employers. They weren't told how it would be, and they aren't allowed to practice as they were taught.

4. *Conflict resolution.* The graduates may and do change their behavior but maintain their values; change both values and behaviors to match the work setting; change neither values nor behavior; or work out a relationship that allows them to keep their values but begin to integrate them into the new setting.[6]

In the last stage, the individuals who make the first choice may be the group with potential for making changes, but they simply slide into the bureaucratic mold or, more likely, they withdraw from nursing practice altogether. Those who choose bureaucracy take on an "it's a job" attitude, or they may eventually reject the values of both. Others become organization men and women, who move rapidly into the administrative ranks and totally absorb the bureaucratic values. Those who will change neither values nor behavior, what might be called "going it alone," either look for a place to practice where professional values are accepted or try the "academic lateral arabesque" (also used by the first group), going on to advanced education with the hope of finding new horizons or escaping. The most desirable choice, says Kramer, is the last, which she calls *biculturalism*.

It has been documented that new graduates do indeed go through variations of the socialization process described. That there has been little change in the adjustment process for decades can be seen by reviewing journals in the interim and by the nomadic patterns of nursing that must reflect deep-seated job dissatisfaction. Turnover and absenteeism are signs of boredom, lack of involvement, and apathy.

Why is this still happening? Some say that the gap in communication between educators and nursing service administrators is part of the problem; no matter how fine the students' education is, not enough schools have prepared students for evolving needs such as specialization. Educators answer that in no other professional field is the new practitioner expected to be a finished product; all have periods of training and support. In fact, the attitude of the administration is too often echoed by the staff, who may be only critical, not helpful, and do not provide the kinds of role models new graduates need. Not all behave in this way, of course, and seasoned nurses talk about how their first job was horrible or great, often depending on the kind of support they got.

The shortage of the 1980s and subsequent workplace enrichment programs greatly enhanced the retention of nurses. Those enrichments most commonly took the form of strategies to professionalize the workplace, and presumably decrease the bureaucratic–professional conflict:

1. Clinical ladders to recognize competence in direct care positions.
2. Peer review.
3. Shared governance and participatory management.
4. Increased practice autonomy.
5. Decentralization of operations.
6. Integrated documentation systems.

The realities of the workplace, albeit generally a bureaucracy, could certainly be softened if faculty were to bring more of these insights to their students, or if students had more chances for "rehearsal." The following deserve consideration:

1. A synthesis semester at the end of the educational experience that incorporates, as far as legally possible, all the ingredients of full-time employment.

' programs that alternate semesters with work placements
·ipated field.

..um that progresses toward more independence and per-
_.ı accountability with students and faculty moving to a collegial
relationship, as opposed to superiors and subordinates.

4. Service-education partnerships with faculty teaching students on their own panels of patients.
5. Summer externships, and new graduate internships or residencies.
6. Patient areas exclusively dedicated to the clinical learning needs of students.
7. Assignment of each student to a staff nurse.
8. Preceptor or "buddy" systems involving agency staff.

STRESS AND STRAIN: THE PERSISTING OCCUPATIONAL HAZARD

Stress and strain are synonymous with nursing, stress being the factors external to you and strain being those internal feelings of frustration and tension. Sometimes stress creates strain. Some individuals have the capacity to tolerate stressful conditions, putting them in perspective. In other instances strain is internally triggered and the search for external blame is fruitless. There are endless experts who can tell you how to deal with these frustrations and tensions. From Selye,[7] the father of the concept of stress, to Peplau,[8] the pioneer of psychiatric nursing, to Kobasa, who introduced the descriptor of "hardness" to explain why some people rise above it all,[9] interpretations vary. There is little predictability about who will respond negatively to stressful situations, but group cohesiveness or interpersonal support seem to have a positive effect. Your best protection against stress and strain is to be alert to those situations which usually hold jeopardy:

1. A lack of clarity of your responsibilities and reporting relationships.
2. A poor fit between your ability, attitudes or values and the expectations of your employer or co-workers.
3. Contradictory expectations of what your job responsibilities are.
4. Being caught in a situation where you are underloaded or overloaded.
5. Feelings of being under- or overqualified for a position.

The stress and strain that come with most of the service occupations can lead to codependency or burnout. In codependency, a person controls through the assurance that he or she is needed, and works to keep things that way. "Unable to determine who owns a problem, they become angry and intolerant. The natural impulse to feel for their patients and occasionally bring home their frustrations is played out with exaggeration, and eventually rejected. Where once they felt too much, they now feel too little in defense of their ego. The result is poor judgment, insensitivity and burnout."[10] The codependent personality is particularly at high risk for burnout and the severe loss of self-esteem as one's clinical competence is questioned.[11]

There's no one prescription for coming to terms with an unmanageable personal or professional life. The problems are relative to the personality of the afflicted, and solutions must be individualized. "The ultimate goal is to establish control and identity that is driven by internal strength" rather than captive to the volatility of the environment. Given that your best investment is in self-care, consider:[12]

1. Learning to use distance therapeutically. Allow people to fail and learn from their own mistakes. Find a comfortable and private place to retreat when you are stressed. If you can't physically distance yourself, try meditation techniques.
2. Decide who owns a problem. If you don't own it, you have no obligation to fix it, especially if it requires self-sacrifice.
3. Examine the quality of the peer support you give and get, and correct the situation if needed. Sometimes support systems become habits as opposed to helps.
4. Invest in upgrading yourself. Expose yourself to new experiences; learn new skills. Plan your self-care as seriously as you plan your patient care.
5. Consciously schedule routine tasks, and those requiring physical exertion as a break from complex and stressful activities.
6. Learn to trust your instincts. Every problem does not have a rational and logical solution. Sometimes think in terms of what could be the worst consequence.
7. Identify one person who would be willing to serve as your objective sounding board. This may be one way to find out how you come across to people.
8. Make contact with your feelings about situations. Feelings are neither good nor bad; they just are.
9. Create options for yourself. Identify those circumstances that you need to personally control, those that are just as well controlled for you, and those that you choose to wait out.

Today's Stressors

The stress and strain of nursing has been traditionally associated with the intensity and intimacy of our work and the feelings of helplessness which accompany the all-too-frequent position as employees in a bureaucracy. These observations continue today and are able to be qualified by some very useful description. Chapters 3 and 6 established the context for nursing as we approach the turn of the century. The health care system is laboring under severe economic pressure. Though there seems to be some doubt about this statement, unquestionably, cost-efficiency has become the mandate. Some observers are much more cynical and see the agenda as cost-reduction or cost-control, the distinction being the sacrifice or shading of quality in favor of saving dollars. Since nursing represents 55 percent of the nonphysician manpower in an industry which is labor-intensive, and given the significant (if not robust) salary increases that many nurses have experienced over recent years, nursing has been targeted for cost-cutting. Redesign, re-engineering and restructuring in many health care settings have become euphemisms for reducing the number of RNs, often those who are most highly qualified and experienced. More specifically, unlicensed assistive personnel substitute for nurses, fewer RNs and sometimes fewer workers in total are available to patients, the use of temporary and part-time workers is common, strong and principled nursing service administrators are removed or leave, and nursing often loses ground as their representation at the highest levels of management is lost.[13] There is no argument that the way we organize our work must change in these fast-moving times,[14] but most of this change has come about without "buy in" from any of those on the "front line," the bedside nurse. This leaves an angry and fretful workplace, and an uncomfortable introduction for the new graduate. Nursing positions are very hard or impossible to come by in some geographic areas, and then offer much less than you expected. This is not so in all instances; but given choices, the new graduate should ask to meet eventual co-workers, test their attitude, inquire about recent changes and the process through which they came about.

A declining number of RNs in hospitals has been associated with increased mortality, and medication errors.[15,16] Nurses report a need to adjust their practice standard, conflict between RNs and administrators, less time with their patients, less time to document properly, and minimum opportunity to consult with colleagues. How much is real and how much is a response to the frequent exclusion of nurses from the process of planning for change is uncertain. However, it is correct to say that there are new and dramatic workplace pressures and that cost-efficiency must be a constant goal (best defined as value or high quality for each dollar). Accepting this goal, nursing has become a serious economic business: every patient (regardless of setting) must be actively managed, and planning for discharge or self-care is instituted immediately on entry to the health care system. In today's best programs or facilities, you will be expected to progress your patients, often with the support of protocols, guidelines or critical paths (also sometimes called clinical paths or caremaps).[17] The use of these "clinical prompters" is not an attempt to strip nursing of autonomy or diminish creativity. They are an appropriate response to the reality that there is too much information to know everything. They make standards explicit, create a multidisciplinary focus (these paths or plans must be interdisciplinary), and reduce the burden of documentation if properly used. An example of a critical path is included in Exhibit 15.1. The optimist will see all these changes as challenge and opportunity and a new seriousness about the role of nursing.

THE WORKPLACE: RIGHTS AND HAZARDS

The prevailing theme of this chapter is successful career management through personal control. Aspects of that control are to understand how you successfully establish yourself in your role, and how you deal with stress and strain while protecting a personality that may be naturally vulnerable. An additional dimension of control is to know your rights and responsibilities as an employee—and to confront the hazardous conditions that will affect your work life from start to finish as a nurse. You have protections under the law.

A comprehensive overview of workplace rights would include issues of minimum wage, unemployment and disability, workmen's compensation, family leave, continuing health benefits after termination of employment, discrimination, job safety, pensions, unfair labor practices, and collective bargaining. The growing number of workplace concerns addressed through legislation and the courts is one circumstance that has contributed to the general decline in unionization. Unions appeared on the American scene when there were few legal workplace protections.

Given the broad range of issues the focus here will be on the most common questions:

- Can I be fired without reason?
- Is it possible to refuse an assignment?
- Are there any protections for whistle-blowing?
- What protections do I have against discrimination?
- Do I have a right to withhold information about myself from an employer?
- Are there laws that guarantee fringe benefits including health insurance, pension, and family leave?
- How dangerous is the work of nursing?

EXHIBIT 15.1

Critical/Clinical Path ... Diagnosis: Stroke

Aspect of care	Day 1	Day 2	Day 3	Day 4	Day 5 Discharge Target
Consults	Neurology, CNS, dietician, social service	Physical and occupational therapy	Physical medicine and rehab, consider speech pathologist		Consider gastroenterologist
Diagnostics	CT scan, ECG, chest plate, Chem 7 and 12, prothrombin time and partial thromboplastin time (PT/PTT), consider prealbumin	Carotid Doppler, PT/PTT if on anticoagulant	PT/PTT if indicated, consider modified barium swallow	PT/PTT if indicated	PT/PTT if indicated
Treatments	Neuro VS q2–3 hours, I&O, IV therapy	Neuro VS q2–3 hours, continency program assessment	Neuro VS q2–3 hours, continency program PRN	Neuro VS q2–3 hours, continency program PRN	Neuro VS q2–3 hours, continency program PRN
Activity	Bedrest	Up in chair 2–4 times a day, begin self-grooming, feeding	Up in chair 2–4 times a day, increase self-care	Increase OOB activity assessment for self-care potential	Increase OOB activity for self-care discharge plan
Nutrition	RN completes dysphagia assessment profile, consider dysphagia protocol	Indicate: Soft diet Dysphagia diet Tubefeeding	As for day 2	As for day 3	If tube fed, consider PEG
PT/Family education	Stroke booklet and video	Nutrition/diet/dysphagia	Incontinence	Self-care needs/ADLs	Self-care discharge plan
Discharge planning	RN gives NIH stroke scale score to LMSW	LMSW completes assessment	Disposition planned	Support as needed	Discharge

Please note:

- The path could easily be adapted to an electronic paperless system.
- The path includes provider prescriptions, and assumes that systems are in place (returned lab results, special programs and protocols, etc.), and patient outcomes (inferred in progression of plan).
- The path is integrated, providing continuity across all disciplines (this is not always the case).
- Patients who do not progress according to the path are more carefully assessed.

Source: St. Luke's Episcopal Hospital, Houston, Texas.

Can I be fired without reason?

Most employment relationships are not protected by any formal contract and are for an indefinite period of time. Such an arrangement is termed *employment-at-will*, and the relationship may be terminated by either the employee or employer at any time, with cause or for no cause at all. A growing number of court decisions in such situations have recognized employee handbooks and a variety of other internal employer-generated documents as having a quasilegal status. Thus, where an at-will dismissal violates one of these policies, the employer could be held liable. Even though you may have nothing at all in writing, an expressed contract takes shape as you discuss the terms and conditions of employment. Above and beyond this presumed contractual protection, a number of states are moving forward to protect at-will employees through legislation.

No employer is justified in an arbitrary dismissal of an employee. It is important to note what circumstances will cause an episode of dismissal to be found in favor of the employee if the situation goes to grievance, arbitration, or court. The most common conditions for a successful appeal on the employee's behalf are:[18]

1. The charges for the termination are not proved.
2. The severity of the consequence is inappropriate to the charge.
3. The reason for dismissal is unrelated to job performance.
4. Proper or customary disciplinary procedures were not used.

Most dismissals come as a result of growing dissatisfaction between employee and employer, not a single episode. The situation should have produced documentation, and a series of warnings, written notices, attempts to counsel, and so on. For more detail on the proper handling of grievances, refer to ANA's *Survival Skills in the Workplace*.

Is it possible to refuse an assignment?

That is not an idle question today as we deal with clinical situations that may be contrary to our personal conscience, hazardous, or require our participation in circumstances that are potentially unsafe for patients. This last situation is particularly common with reduced staffing and the substitution of less prepared personnel in order to cut costs.

Nursing administration has the right to assign you where needed (providing you don't have a written contract that says otherwise), but they also have the responsibility of *appropriately* assigning duties.[19] Some nurses' associations have now negotiated contracts to prevent inappropriate assignment or compulsory overtime. Others have developed a form that says, in essence, that in the nurse's professional judgment, the current assignment is unsafe and places the patients at risk, but that it will be carried out under protest. The form documents the assignment, number and condition of patients, and number and type of staff. The legality of this process has not yet been tested, and there are some other concerns. If a nurse has stated that an assignment is unsafe and then takes it, she or he is vulnerable in case of a later negligence suit. And, of course, the use of the form can be abused.

When refusing an assignment, however, one of the dangers is being accused of abandoning your patients. Just what that means in any specific case is not clear, but it could result in the loss of your license. On the other hand, supervisors use the term loosely to frighten the nurse into staying on the job. You should discuss the inappropriate assignment with the supervisor, putting her or him on notice about your limitations; to identify your options (sharing or trading the assignment); and to document the situation.[20] In the end, it is your decision, and not an easy one, but almost inevitable in many institutions. It's best to think it through ahead of time. (See Chapter 9 concerning rights of conscience in refusing an assignment.)

Whether you can safely refuse an assignment in other circumstances is not clear. Employers are usually required to offer an alternate position if the refusal is on the basis of conscience. However, if you refuse that assignment, you have little recourse. One situation that has been gaining attention is fair treatment for nurses who cannot work on certain days for religious reasons. As might be expected, rulings have differed, but in 1985, the US Supreme Court ruled that there was no constitutional right involved; that in fact it was unconstitutional for a state to legislate an unqualified right not to work on the Sabbath. From a practical point of view, the nurse may be willing to accept alternatives, such as working other holidays or weekend days.

Are there any protections for whistle-blowing?

Whistle-blowing remains a very difficult moral choice for nurses. "Whistle-blowers are employees who disclose information about an agency's violation of a law, rule or regulation; mismanagement; gross waste of funds; abuse of authority; or a substantial and specific danger to the public health or safety."[21] The range of situations for whistle-blowing is obviously broad, and in many situations the protections are few. The whistle-blower is restricted from disclosing information that is classified. It is critical to have your facts straight. Since whistle-blowers must often proceed on good faith, every effort should be made to verify the correctness of information. Since 1981, 20 states have passed legislation to protect whistle-blowers. Most of these protections are for public employees, but 10 states extend this protection to the private sector. On several occasions in the 1980s and 1990s, bills had been introduced in the Congress to preempt state laws and provide mandatory protection where no state laws apply. In 1988, a California nurse was awarded a significant cash settlement for damages incurred when she was dismissed for reporting what she considered to be an unethical termination of respiratory and nutritional support of a comatose patient. This case had a strong influence on policy development for "termination of treatment." (See Chapter 8 for more details on the ethics of whistle-blowing.)

What protections do I have against discrimination?
A host of discriminatory areas could be involved in your workplace relations. Besides the protections for race and ethnicity, gender and age are of particular interest in nursing. The discrimination against male nurses continues, especially in obstetric practice. Commentary on several cases is included in the April 1994 *American Nurse*. The US District Court in Arkansas gave the opinion that "The fact that the plaintiff is a health care professional does not eliminate the fact that he is an unelected individual who is intruding on the obstetrical patient's right to privacy. The male nurse's situation is not analogous to that of the male doctor who has been selected by the patient."[22]

There has been significant progress through federal and state laws that protect against age discrimination in the workplace. Some laws have no upper limits; others specify protection until a certain age, perhaps 65, 70, or 75. The burden of proof in age discrimination is often difficult, and nurses should be vigilant, as there is a growing trend to cut back on the numbers of nurses on staff. A typical case is reported from California where the courts awarded damages to two nurses who sued on the basis of age discrimination. These nurses, 59 and 60, respectively, were 30-year employees of the same hospital. Each had been publicly recognized for the quality of her practice. When a clinical ladder was put in place, they consciously decided to remain at a lower level of the clinical nurse category. After being told that it was mandatory for them to participate in a career advancement program and qualify for a higher status, they were both dismissed on grounds of the inability to demonstrate the competencies for the new level. Both of these nurses are now successfully employed elsewhere.[23] There is fear that these will no longer be isolated cases in nursing. This becomes an especially significant issue with the "aging" of nurses described in Chapter 4.

The Americans with Disabilities Act of 1990 extends protection in employment to individuals with HIV/AIDS, and also to people who are regarded to be infected, or in close association with persons with HIV/AIDS. The ANA has assumed the leadership role for over a decade in providing policy direction to nurses and other health care professionals in dealing with HIV/AIDS. The ANA's 1994 publication *Nursing and HIV/AIDS* is a state-of-the-art resource. Nursing's continuous presence on the health care scene and commitment to comprehensive care created the need for ANA to speak out early and loudly in the course of this pandemic. Issues of testing and disclosure of HIV status are closely linked with discrimination.

ANA opposes perpetuation of the myth that mandatory testing and mandatory disclosure of the HIV status of patients and/or nurses is a method of preventing the transmission of HIV disease, and therefore does not advocate mandatory testing or mandatory disclosure of HIV status. ANA supports the availability of voluntary anonymous or confidential HIV testing that is conducted with informed consent, and pre and posttest counseling.[24]

In every situation, the nurse's first concern is the protection of the patient. Therefore, the following policy provides direction for the HIV-infected nurse:

> Nurses who know they have a transmissible blood-borne infection should voluntarily avoid exposure-prone invasive procedures that have been epidemiologically linked to HIV or other bloodborne infection transmission. The nurse has a duty to report exposure of a patient to bloodborne infection. Support and protection of the nurse with a sero-positive status has been a long-standing position of ANA. The association supports the confidentiality of all information about the HIV-infected nurse.[25]

Sexual harassment in the workplace is a prevalent form of impermissible sex discrimination in employment. Neither the high profile of this issue in recent years nor laws prohibiting sexual harassment seem to have reduced its prevalence among nurses. Two studies, although involving small samples, should cause us to stop and consider the true extent of this form of discrimination and the responses which are most effective in confronting this type of abuse. In a survey of critical care nurses, 46 percent of the respondents had been harassed, most frequently by offensive sexual remarks and unwanted physical contact. In 82 percent of the incidents, the harassers were physicians, and 80 percent of the nurses claimed they had neither been trained to deal with the situation nor did policies exist to facilitate documentation or reporting.[26]

Reports on sexual harassment confirm the same obstacles prevent satisfactory resolution of most incidents. There is often differing opinion on what exactly falls into the category of sexually harassing behavior. Some female nurses are impatient with colleagues who consider an occasional "off color joke" or a one-time "come on" as harassment.[27] The best point of comparison is the interpretation of the US Supreme Court:[28]

> Unwelcome sexual advances, requests for sexual favors, and other forms of sexually related conduct are considered sexual harassment when:
> - acceptance of the conduct is made an explicit or implicit condition of employment
> - acceptance or rejection of the conduct affects your employment status in some way

- the conduct is so severe and pervasive that it interferes with your work performance or creates an intimidating, hostile or offensive working environment.

Besides some disagreement as to whether a harassing incident existed, nurses were generally reticent to report these situations because of a disparity in status and power between the offender and the victim. Where incidents were reported, they were frequently dismissed or ignored.[29] More assertive action was effective in most cases, but not all. The suggested response is to confront the harasser and label the behavior, report the harassment and document immediately and seek support from others.[30] Most victims who confronted the offender put a stop to the situation, others found themselves isolated, and still others gained nothing but additional hardship for taking a stand. Action offers the most hope of change; silence perpetuates the victimization. Sexual harassment policies, procedures and training to handle these situations effectively are necessary for a safe work environment.

Do I have the right to withhold information about myself from an employer?

The degree of privacy guaranteed to an employee is directly related to the information in question and its relation to the employer's interest. The need for information is considered reasonable when it relates to the "... employee's competence, reliability, and honesty as a worker, or when required by the government ..."[31] There are both limitations on the right to privacy and on the intrusions into that right. Some examples will help:

- An employer can contact a former employer and check references provided by the employee about work history.
- Employers must notify an employee and provide a report of any investigative report about an employee's credit or financial position.
- An employer can search an employee for theft of company property, but the circumstances of the detection must be reasonable (if not, the employer may be liable for false imprisonment).
- Employees can be expected to take a lie detector test, except in states where employee permission is required.
- Many employers are subject to a law that requires mandatory drug testing of their employees under certain circumstances. (Your state nurses association will be able to advise you on the laws which apply in your situation.)
- An employer may only require a physical (including HIV testing) after a conditional promise of employment has been made, and the

offer of employment may not be withdrawn unless the results interfere with the ability to perform essential job functions.

Each situation is judged on the standard of reasonableness and relevance, and interpretations vary; however, more and more case law and legislation surfaces daily. Many privacy situations are comingled with protection under civil rights and the *Americans with Disabilities Act*. State laws are also at issue here.

Are there laws that guarantee fringe benefits?

Fringe benefits and pension are of growing importance to nurses. Although most employers provide fringe benefit packages, there is no federal or state requirement, with the exception of employer contributions to Social Security, workers compensation, and unemployment insurance. However, there are a number of legislative protections that the employee should be aware of. The *Family Leave Bill* of 1993 requires that employees be allowed a time limited period for a new baby, adoption, or to care for a disabled family member. You are assured the right to return to a position comparable with the one you left, and your health benefits must be continued for the period of the leave. In a similar fashion, you are given the right to personally pay for the continuation of your health insurance for up to 36 months after you leave a job. Over the years, pensions have also increased in their protections for the worker. Benefit plans, including pensions, must satisfy nondiscriminatory requirements, treating men and women equitably. Pension benefits have mandatory vesting schedules, guaranteeing 100 percent nonforfeiture of accrued benefits after five years of service, or the option to phase in 100 percent vesting over three to seven years. In short, no benefits or pensions are guaranteed with the exception of Social Security, but where these fringes are provided there are increasing protections.

Ideally there should be a written employment contract that details conditions of employment such as salary, vacation, sick leave, holidays, social security coverage, pension, and duration of the contract. More usually, these things are shared verbally, and may be found written in personnel policies.

How dangerous is the work of nursing?

Health care personnel, including nurses, are exposed to the environmental dangers of toxic chemicals, radiation sources, and infectious agents. Nurses are also at high risk for muscle strain, back injuries, cuts, bruises and needle punctures. Psychological stress is a constant, due both to the nature of the work and to the demands of the workplace (shift rotation, overtime, and so on). Violence has also become a more frequently occurring workplace situation.

Multidrug-resistant strains of TB (MDR-TB) and HIV/AIDS have increased our awareness of workplace hazards in general and *infectious agents* in particular. The obligation of the employer is to provide environmental safety, work practice controls, and personal protective equipment to minimize or prevent exposure, and postexposure programs including counseling. The CDCP has developed guidelines for the management of health care workers following occupational exposure to HIV. A program would include information, immediate evaluation, prophylactic intervention, counseling, and supportive care. The nurse who seroconverts should be guaranteed workers' compensation and continued health insurance coverage. Workmen's compensation still presents difficulty due to probable underreporting and the burden of proving occupational transmission. Some occupational groups such as firefighters and coal miners have been successful in legislation that assumes occupational transmission for certain conditions and places the burden of proof on the employer to prove that the condition is not work-related.[32] The important observations for the new employee are what policies exist for postexposure management and whether adequate precautions are in place to reduce the risk of exposure. MDR-TB prevention requires "a high index of suspicion for TB and early recognition of symptoms which may trigger the need for respiratory precautions. ... All efforts boil down to containing the infectious agent from becoming airborne."[33] When this is impossible, most facilities are using "disposable particulate respirators that fit snugly around the face."[34]

For the protection of both patients and workers against transmission from one another, universal precautions must be used when dealing with blood and body fluids. Precautions include guidelines for handling sharps and laboratory specimens, use of gloves and gowns, hand washing, protective eyewear, disposal of linen, resuscitation procedures, and care of reusable equipment.

Ergonomic hazards, though less dramatic, are job and process design problems that are common and harmful. Examples are improper work methods and inadequate work and rest patterns or repetitive tasks that result in back injuries, carpotunnel syndrome, and stress disorders. Instruction on the proper way of bending and lifting, back support devices, psychological support groups and rotation in assignment to high-stress situations are all efforts to compensate for ergonomic effects.

Toxic substances, most particularly chemotherapeutic agents, are frequently handled by nurses, and cautions should be posted and personal protective equipment provided.

Violence has been a constant threat to nursing in the workplace. Incidents have rarely been reported because of the poor public image it would create for the health care facility. Currently caught in violent times, the incidence of workplace violence is increasing. Weapons that are easy to obtain, deinstitutionalized chronically mentally ill, substance abuse, and a generally

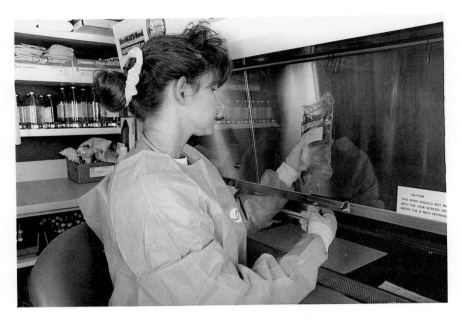

Modern diagnostics and treatment can represent workplace hazards for the nurse. (*Courtesy of Robert Wood Johnson Hospital, New Brunswick, New Jersey.*)

angry underclass all contribute to an increasing danger of violence and assault. In Los Angeles, 25 percent of trauma patients were found to be carrying lethal weapons. Assaults on inpatient units account for 13 percent of incidents in hospitals. A comprehensive review of the literature identified the following factors to be associated with assault in the health care workplace:[35]

1. Inexperienced health care workers are at increased risk of assault.
2. The largest number of injuries occur while attempting to contain patient violence.
3. Short-staffing and temporary staffing have been associated with increased assaults.
4. Assaults seem to occur during times of high activity and high emotion on patient units. Additionally, experience tells us that violence is predictable in patients who have a history of violent behavior, substance abuse, psychiatric conditions, mental retardation or bereavement.[36] The presence of policies that show sensitivity to these factors is necessary, as is the establishment of peer assistance and postassault assistance programs in environments where the incidence of violence is high.

COLLECTIVE BARGAINING:
THE PROCESS AND THE ISSUES

Collective bargaining provides individuals who are employees (not managers) the opportunity to come together as a group with one voice for the purpose of negotiating conditions of employment, salaries, benefits and other negotiable terms. For the most part, this involves appealing to a union who would then represent the employees in these matters. The details of what is negotiable may be state or work-site specific.

It was not until 1974 that nonprofit and voluntary health care employers were required to bargain collectively with their employees. This is the dominant employment sector for nurses. Despite this right, nurses were slow to turn to unions for workplace representation, seeing this option as detracting from the professionalism of the role. The attitude of nurses has changed and they are demanding decent wages and meaningful benefits. Most especially, they are concerned about their patients and become militant on behalf of safety and quality issues. Though unionizing in the health care industries has become a priority of many labor groups, the greatest number of nurses (over 170,000)[37] are represented by the state nurses associations (SNAs) who are affiliates of ANA.

The process of collective bargaining, because it is set by law, is the same regardless of the bargaining agent. A brief overview is included here which assumes that the SNA is the collective bargaining agent:

1. The nurses (or group of nurses) in an institution, discontented with a situation or conditions, and having exhausted the usual channels for correction or improvement, ask the SNA for assistance.
2. A meeting is held outside the premises of the institution and always on off-duty time. SNA staff and the nurses explore the problems, and the nurses are given advice about reasonable, negotiable issues and how to form a unit; for instance, they are told who can be included in a unit. Administrative nurses are excluded, but the question of supervisors is still being debated in some places.
3. Authorization cards, which authorize the SNA to act as the nurses' bargaining representative, must be signed by at least 30 percent of the group to be represented. Membership forms are also suggested because the SNA cannot provide service without funds. All collective bargaining activity must be carried out in nonwork areas where the employee is protected from employer interference. (There are a series of NLRB rules governing employee distribution and solicitation.)
4. If sufficient cards are signed, the SNA notifies the employer that an organizing campaign is in process, calling attention to the fact that the activity is protected. Copies of the notice are distributed to the nurses so that they know they are protected.

5. An informational meeting is held for all nurses and SNA staff.
6. If it is agreed that the SNA will represent the nurses, a bargaining unit is formed and officers are elected.
7. To seek voluntary recognition of the unit by the employer, a majority of the nurses must sign designation cards; this will probably be checked by a mutually accepted third party.
8. If the employer chooses not to recognize the unit, or if the designation is challenged by another union, a series of actions takes place, including an NLRB-conducted election. To petition for election, any union must have designation cards signed by 30 percent of the nurses in the proposed unit. The election is won or lost by the majority of nurses *voting*. They may vote for a particular union or specify none at all. The NLRB then certifies the winner or the decision to reject union representation.
9. Assuming that the SNA wins the election, the SNA representative, at the direction of the unit, attempts to settle the problems and complaints of the nurses by negotiating with administration. There are specific rules about what is negotiable. *Mandatory* subjects include salaries, fringe benefits, and conditions of employment, and both sides must bargain in good faith about these issues. *Voluntary* subjects can be almost anything else that both sides want to discuss, except for *prohibited* or illegal subjects. It should be remembered that the nurse executive, both through position and under law, is an administrator. Even though the person might be in complete support of the nurses' demands, he or she cannot join them. Quite often the director has previously tried unsuccessfully to help them achieve their goals.
10. An agreement may or may not be reached, probably with some compromise on both sides. If there is agreement, a contract is voted on and signed outlining agreed-upon conditions and the responsibility of each group. Contracts are renegotiated at set time periods, usually of several years. If no agreement can be reached, the dispute may be referred to binding or nonbinding arbitration by an outside group, or some job action such as picketing or a strike may occur. Picketing may be merely informational, to communicate the issues to the community, or it may be intended to prevent other employees or services from entering the institution. The latter, combined with a strike, is the very last resort, to be used when all other efforts fail. If such action is decided upon, sufficient notice is given to allow for disposition of patient care. Even if strikes are successful, there is often a lingering, unpleasant feeling between participants and non-participants.

　　Once a labor contract is in place, there are times when individual nurses are in dispute with the employer. A grievance procedure is generally used to resolve the problem. A grievance may be caused by "an alleged violation of a contract provision, a change in a past practice, or an employer decision that is considered arbitrary, capricious, unreasonable, unfair, or discriminatory." Simple complaints are not considered grievances. If informed discussion does not resolve the issue, a grievance procedure is followed. The steps include (1) written notice of the grievance, with a written response within a set time; (2) if the response is not satisfactory, an appeal to the director of nursing follows; (3) the employee, SNA representative, grievance chairman, and/or delegate, director of nursing, and director of personnel meet; (4) if no resolution occurs, the final step is arbitration by a neutral third party selected by both parties involved. The technique for carrying out the process involves interpersonal, adversary, and negotiating skills.

The uniqueness of nurses, the frequent choice of the SNA as their bargaining agent, and their practice patterns create some special problems in labor representation. You are referred to Chapter 30 in *Dimensions of Professional Nursing* (7th edition) for a more extensive discussion. A summary of these areas of concern is included here, but these brief statements should not minimize the seriousness or complexity of these issues:

1. Nurses, both employees and managers, have always come together in their professional associations. When those associations offer labor representation, opponents are quick to claim supervisory domination when nurse-managers hold office.
2. The RN-only bargaining unit has proved the most appropriate for the registered nurse. The hospital found it more strategic to dilute nursing issues by folding in nurses with others. The Supreme Court disagreed.[38]
3. Since nurses carry out many of their functions through other people, for example nursing assistants, there is the risk that they could be considered supervisors (managers) and lose their protected status as employees. A relevant Supreme Court decision of May 1994, involving licensed practical nurses, found them to be managers.[39]
4. Human resource techniques that build cooperation between labor and management are critical for our failing industries and health care facilities. In nursing, this observation has given rise to decentralization approaches and shared governance as discussed in Chapter 6. This necessary movement from the traditional adversarial relation in collective bargaining again challenges the employee status of nurses, and their right to unionize.

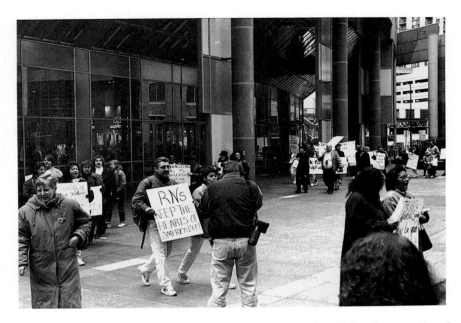

Nurses have been militant and brought their message to the public where quality of care or patient safety is in jeopardy. (*Courtesy of the American Nurses Association.*)

CAREER MAPPING

You have sought the best educational preparation to enter the field of nursing. You have hopefully done so with the intent of building a career. No field offers such variability or such opportunity to advance. Each decision you make can strategically build toward your long-term goal. Additionally, for the professional there is the obligation to remain current, which is no simple task given the rate at which the science of nursing is expanding.

The Value of Experience

You have already reviewed the process of searching and courting employment in Chapter 14. You have also been counseled to take time for a personal assessment. Identify the route in nursing you would like to take. Given today's complex clinical environment, your competence as a generalist will be short-lived.

The half-life of today's knowledge in the basic sciences is no longer than 18 months in many cases. As an applied science, can nursing hope for too much more? With your first position, you begin to develop competencies in a specialized area of practice. Given even a short period of time, you are unable to comfortably shift to new populations. For this reason it is important that you have some idea of the area of nursing which offers you the most satisfaction. Seek out a position with that population and resolve to provide the best possible care to those patients, growing through experience and keeping current with a well-planned program of continuing education. It is just as acceptable to have a vision of a lateral move into education, and formal schooling that stretches on for many years, and perhaps many degrees. It is also acceptable to fail, to reconsider and change courses many times. The only thing that is unacceptable is to have no goals at all.

While you are considering your lateral moves and vertical climbs, pay proper respect to the fact that nursing is a practice discipline. You definitely grow in your ability to care as you minister to patients and as you invest hours and years in your art. Experience is not a myth, but one essential ingredient in clinical sophistication.

CONTINUED COMPETENCE

You will maintain competency through your sensitivity and willingness to move with the times, reliable sources of continuing education, and access to information. Your employer will provide experiences to assure safety and currency and comply with state and accrediting body regulations through in-service education or staff development. But it is your personal obligation to constantly search for new and better ways to nurse. Part of that is knowing what you don't know. A first step is to identify the competencies which are basic to your area of practice, and measure yourself against this yardstick.

The term *continuing education* (CE) has been interpreted in many ways. Most agree that it includes any learning activity after the basic educational program. However, most often those programs leading to an academic degree are separated out. There is still much confusion among nurses who are sure that the renewed social and legal pressures for CE mean that they must enroll in a baccalaureate program. This is not so.

Continuing education is both provided through your employing agency, and you should also choose (or the employer may encourage you) to seek outside programs. The variety of continuing education programs is limitless. The secret is to be a discerning consumer and select those which are most immediately valuable to your practice. Continuing education need not be only clinically oriented. You must also remain conversant with current issues in the discipline, and with the thinking of nursing leaders. Employer funding and time off for continuing education is often a workplace benefit. The types of educational experiences that staff are approved to attend are often an indication of how administration views nursing, as a technical or professional field. From another perspective, it provides insights on the staff who will be your peers.

You should expect to assume at least part of the cost for your continuing education. There are those who feel that because the employers ultimately benefit from the employee's improved performance, they should provide such support as partial or full tuition payment, sabbaticals, or short-term leaves. On the other hand, hospitals and like institutions often maintain that these additional costs must be passed on unfairly to the patient, and that they have a right to expect competent practitioners. With current tight money restrictions, that philosophy is bound to prevail, although some employers do offer opportunities for CE as a fringe benefit.

With or without formal CE, nurses (and other professionals) must make a commitment to lifelong learning. Therefore, knowing how to locate needed information is essential. Fortunately, technological developments over the past 20 years have made it possible for massive bodies of data to be stored, processed, retrieved, analyzed, and transmitted electronically. To search for and obtain information in this form, a searcher needs only a computer terminal and a modem, a device to communicate over phone lines. Thus a library or nursing department, no matter how small or how limited its physical collection of journals and books or indexes, has access to most of the world's published literature. In some sites, tapes of databases are mounted on institutional mainframe computers for inhouse searching. Today, through developments in laser technology, databases on small compact discs can be searched directly. Once needed data are identified, electronic networks can be tapped to request materials not in the library from other cooperating institutions. In some cases, the full copy can be retrieved from an electronic database. There are also a variety of electronic nursing forums which allow international and national "chatter" on issues or clinical problems through e-mail. The basic requirement is an internet connection. (See Chapter 13 for specific details on electronic systems.)

For nurses, the institution's library can serve as an important vehicle for keeping up with changes in health care and in a particular specialty. In addition to literature searches, the library frequently offers valuable services for staying current. You might also begin to write yourself.

FORMAL HIGHER EDUCATION

Besides participating in CE programs, you may want to give serious consideration to formal education leading to another degree (or a first one, if you have none). Educational standards for all positions in nursing are growing steadily higher. If you really want to advance professionally to positions of greater scope and challenge, you will, in the very near future, need an advanced degree, at least a baccalaureate. The process of obtaining this and higher degrees not only will serve you well professionally but will add considerably to the enrichment of your personal life and interests. In fact, these are the reasons given most by nurses.

Although it would be difficult to denigrate the value of any good-quality educational program, give some thought to your future goals. The joy of exploring new fields and studying whatever you wish without the pressure of time or the need to fulfill requirements for a program may be especially tempting. If these interests are in any of the liberal arts or the social or physical sciences, which may be required, or can be used as electives in many programs, a dual purpose will be accomplished in that you are also started toward a degree.

Because baccalaureate programs with a nursing major have not always been available (or affordable) to nurses in a particular geographic area, a number of programs have sprung up offering a degree in nursing or another field, giving credit for the lower-division nursing courses and offering no upper-division nursing courses. Evaluate them in relation to your career goals. These programs are *not* usually acceptable for future graduate studies in nursing, and you may not be able to enroll in a graduate program without having taken upper-division nursing courses. Some nurses have found it necessary to complete a second baccalaureate program, this time with a nursing major, in order to continue into a master's program. In selecting a baccalaureate program, be sure to select one that is NLN accredited.[40]

RNs will find that they receive varying amounts of recognition or credit for their basic nursing courses, and may perhaps need to take challenge examinations. Nursing baccalaureate programs vary a great deal in this respect, but more and more nursing programs are offering some form of educational articulation, self-pacing, or other means of giving credit for previous knowledge, skill, and ability. The external degree is such a program. There are also a large number of baccalaureate programs that only admit RN students. NLN publications listing baccalaureate, master's, and doctoral programs are helpful.

Many of the same points apply to graduate education. Consider carefully what you want from a program and prepare yourself for this more competitive admission procedure. Some nurses complete graduate programs in the various sciences or education, with or without any nursing input. Again, you must consider your specific career goals. Someone with a nursing major or at least a minor may be given preference in a position requiring a graduate degree, particularly in educational positions. Many state boards of nursing require faculty in basic nursing education programs to have a graduate degree with a major in nursing. Or if you are hired now, there is no guarantee that later, when there are more nurses with graduate nursing degrees, you may not be bypassed for promotion or may be required to take a second graduate degree in nursing in order to hold the current position. These are practical considerations presented here for information. You must still make the educational decisions you wish, but with as complete a knowledge of the pros and cons as possible.

Suppose you simply don't want any degree? Or suppose you enroll in an accredited nursing program but then, in time, drop out? That's your decision. There is no reason why you can't function at an acceptable level of competence, maintaining and improving that competence through CE, thereby making a valuable contribution to the profession and society. If, however, you withdraw because of disappointment or lack of interest in that particular program, it may well be that the program is not congruent with your philosophy. Consider a second try, taking time to determine whether a program's philosophy, objectives, approaches to teaching, and attitudes are what you want. Some of this information can be obtained from the catalog, the faculty or adviser interviews, informal contact with students or *recent* graduates (programs do change). Sometimes, if some courses may be taken without need for full matriculation, a sampling of courses will prove especially informative.

Sources of Financial Aid

The problem of finances is one of the most common blocks to advanced education for able nurses. Review your financial resources realistically. If you are going to request financial aid, you will need to estimate as accurately as possible your expected income and expenses. Major educational expenses will include tuition, books, educational fees, and perhaps travel. Related personal expenses depend on where and how you live. Economizing may mean enrolling in a community college for the liberal arts and later transferring to a local or state college. Economy should not include enrolling in a poor program. Graduating from a nonaccredited nursing program may create difficulties in advancing to the next higher degree. Not all nonaccredited programs are poor, but this risk does exist.

The major sources of income for a self-supporting graduate nurse in an advanced educational program are savings or other personal resources, part-time work, scholarships, and loans. If you plan to do part-time work while attending college, make reasonably sure that a position is available at a satisfactory salary and that it seems to be professionally suitable, including offering enough flexibility to make it possible to take courses. Consider also your mental and physical health under this double load. Can you manage? One answer is cooperative education, which is part work and part school; some higher education programs function in this mode.

There are a number of scholarships, fellowships, and loans earmarked for educational purposes for which nurses are eligible. Some sources of financial assistance are well known and are used regularly; others are not used simply because people do not know about them. The financial aid officer at the institution where you plan to enroll is an excellent source of information.

The National League for Nursing, 350 Hudson Street, New York, NY 10014, sells a publication entitled *Scholarships and Loans for Nursing Education*. It contains a great deal of information that may help you decide where to apply first for financial assistance, thus saving valuable time in making applications. The Federal Student Financial Aid Information Center at (800)-433-3243 provides explanations on government loans and grants and requirements to qualify.

The professional nursing journals frequently carry news items and articles about such funds, which can be found through the annual and cumulative indexes. Most college catalogs also list sources of student financial support. Exhibit 15.2 lists some of the possible sources of funds. Some give relatively small amounts of money, but these sums do add up. Check also for special funding for ethnic and minority students.

How you apply for financial assistance may have considerable bearing on whether or not you obtain it. Correspondence, personal interviews, application forms, and references should all show the same meticulous attention that is given to an application for a new position.

EXHIBIT 15.2

Sources of Financial Aid for Education

Local	**National/international**
School alumni associations	Federal government—DHHS; Dept. of Education
District and state SNAs	Nurses Educational Funds
District and regional Leagues	American Nurses' Foundation
Other local or state nursing organizations	Sigma Theta Tau
State government	Other national nursing organizations
Chapters of national fraternities/sororities	National Student Nurses' Association Foundation
Fraternal organizations (Elks, Amvets)	Veterans Administration
Local foundations	Private foundations
Hospital associations	Military
Your place of employment	International Council of Nurses
College or university loans or scholarships	World Health Organization
Bank loans	Large corporations
Local companies	
Women's groups	

PROFESSIONAL AND COMMUNITY ACTIVITIES

Active participation in community activities is very rewarding. Some activities are directly related to nursing, such as attending alumni and nurses' association meetings and accepting appointments to committees and offices. Others include volunteer work on a regular or special basis, such as participating in student nurse recruitment programs or career days, soliciting donations for various health organizations, helping with the Red Cross blood program, assisting with inoculation sessions for children, acting as adviser to a Future Nurse Club, or volunteering time at a free clinic.

The importance of nursing input into the various community, state, and national joint provider–consumer groups that study means of improving the health care delivery system is discussed in Chapter 7. Although participation at the state or national level may not be immediately feasible for a nurse who has not yet achieved professional recognition, just showing interest and volunteering your services will often open doors at a local level. That's an important foot in the door!

Consumer activism has resulted in the formation of many groups concerned with health delivery, and nurses offering their expertise and understanding of health care service problems can make valuable contributions. Sometimes you need to convince these groups that you have a sincere interest in improved health care services and are willing to work cooperatively. In some areas, ethnic and minority groups are especially suspicious of professional health workers outside of their own group, because unfortunate experiences have shown some of them to be more concerned with defending their own interests than the consumer's well-being, as the consumer sees it. In these groups, it is even more important to listen than to talk. Participation can lead to development of free clinics, health fairs, health teaching classes, recruitment of minority students for nursing programs, tutoring sessions for students, liaison activities with health care institutions, programs for the aged, and legislative activities directed toward better health care. The opportunities, challenges, and satisfactions are unlimited.

Consumer health education is being stressed more and more today, and in what better area can nurses offer their expertise? Classes can be held under the auspices of health care institutions, public health organizations, and public and private community groups, and include teaching for wellness as well as teaching those with chronic or long-term illnesses. Nurses who like to teach and are skilled and enthusiastic can participate in programs already set up and, equally important, can work to develop other programs and involve others on the health team.

Keeping the public informed about nursing and the changes that have occurred in recent years in both education and practice is a contribution to the community. Offers to present programs about nursing are often welcome in the many community, social, business, professional, and service groups that meet frequently and are interested in community service. And yes, you *can* become a good speaker.[41]

Activities such as these involve you in the community and are stimulating and satisfying. They also require time, effort, and often patience. But besides having the satisfaction of being useful, you'll gain in personal development as a nurse and as an individual.

AS YOU ANTICIPATE THE FUTURE

Nursing is noble work, and you have chosen it wisely. You enter the profession in times of upheaval and paradox, but also at a point of its renaissance. This book has tried faithfully to portray the picture of a profession that is moving with the times. It is a profession that has often been the conscience of health care, speaking out on social issues with a fervor that has sometimes been self-destructive. Our past has been greatly influenced by the woman's movement and the growth of modern medicine and the health care industry. Through all of the change that has characterized human affairs, nursing has stayed positioned at the bedside, in the home, in the community . . . often the only human link between our patients and an intimidating experience in the health care delivery system.

Nursing will give you many benefits and allow you many choices if you are only alert to them. With the choice of nursing, you receive a distinctive role, social status, and the choice of a job or a career. For some, fuller involvement in nursing may be limited by other life circumstances such as family, school or personal interests. For others, nursing is the work of their lives. This does not eliminate the possibility of a full family, community and social life. Nurses have always balanced multiple and competing demands, and many have done so with the nagging feeling that they never do anything quite as well as they would like. Especially for women, there have been some significant changes. More attention is being given to working women and to the need for family support. Careerism is a real choice today for the nurse who wants it all.

The relatively brief accounts of civic and political opportunities have been included with a purpose. Selecting nursing as a career means more than "being a good nurse." It means bringing the sensitivities of nursing to the community in a variety of volunteer capacities and presenting yourself as a nurse.

Given the time and effort you have invested in your education, you should want to actively manage your future, yet some of you will move haphazardly through your life in nursing, neglecting to orchestrate opportunities, taking things as they come. However unwise that may be, it can offer excitement of its own. Take nursing seriously, but not so seriously that you deny yourself time to appreciate the honorable work you do.

KEY POINTS

1. There has historically been an incongruity between what you expect of the nursing workplace before graduation, and what you find when you get there.
2. Accepting that you hold different values from those in a bureaucracy and working out a relationship that accommodates both values and the reality of the workplace is a healthy way to adjust to "reality shock."
3. Nurses are considered a very costly resource and are being held to rigorous standards for actively managing the clinical care of their patients.
4. Burnout occurs when the various pressures of a job and dissatisfaction with the work situation seem to be impossible to cope with.
5. Being good to yourself, allowing for personal activities, as well as working with a support group, can relieve some aspects of stress and burnout.
6. CE for nurses may include in-service programs, self-learning, and programs offered by educational institutions and professional organizations
7. The primary purpose of CE for nurses is to ensure continued competence in practice.
8. You should take time and care in selecting the right educational program, whether for CE or for a degree, so that you don't waste your time or money.
9. Funding for formal nursing education is available from a variety of sources, but it saves time to consult first with the financial officer of the school in which you are interested.
10. Participating in nursing and community organizations is a way to enrich your life as a nurse and as a person.
11. More nurses are successfully combining family life and a nursing career, including formal education.

REFERENCES

1. Hardy ME, Conway ME. *Role Theory*. Norwalk, CT: Appleton & Lange, 1988, pp 73–110.
2. Andrusyszn MA, Maltby HR. Building on strengths through preceptorships. *Nurse Ed Tod* 13:277–281, August, 1993.

3. Reid M. Marginal man: The identity dilemma of the academic general practitioner. *Symbol Interact* 5:325, February, 1982.

4. Kramer M. *Reality Shock*. St. Louis: Mosby, 1974, p 15.

5. Ibid, pp vii–viii.

6. Ibid, pp 155–162.

7. Selye H. *Stress without Distress*. Philadelphia: J.B. Lippincott, 1974.

8. Forchuk C. *Hildegard E. Peplau: Interpersonal Nursing Theory*. Newbury Park, CA: Sage, 1993.

9. Tartasky DS. Hardiness: Conceptual and methodological issues. *Image* 25:225–229, Fall, 1993.

10. Joel LA. Maybe a pot watcher but never an ostrich. *Am J Nurs* 94:7, April, 1994.

11. Chappelle LS, Sorrentino EA. Assessing co-dependency issues within a nursing environment. *Nurs Mgmt* 24:40–42, May, 1993.

12. Joel, loc cit.

13. Shindul-Rothschild J. Restructuring, redesign, rationing, and nurses' morale: A qualitative study on the impact of competitive financing. *J Emer Nurs* 20:497–504, December, 1994.

14. Bridges W. The end of the job. *Fortune* 19:46–51, September 19, 1994.

15. Aiken LH, et al. Lower medical mortality among a set of hospitals known for good nursing care. *Medic Care* 32:8, August, 1994.

16. Leape LL, et al. Systems analysis of adverse drug events. *JAMA* 274:35–43, July 5, 1995.

17. Center for Case Management: *Case Management and Caremap Systems: Clinical Systems for Quality/Cost Outcomes*. South Natick, MA: CCM, 1992.

18. Gillies DA. *Nursing Management*, 3rd ed. Philadelphia: W.B. Saunders, 1994.

19. Fiesta J. Staffing implications: A legal update. *Nurs Mgmt* 25:34–35, June, 1994.

20. Fear of floating. *Am J Nurs* 94:56, March, 1994.

21. Flanagan L. *What You Need to Know About Today's Workplace*. Washington, DC: American Nurses Publishing, 1995, p 17.

22. Ketter J. Sex discrimination targets men in some hospitals. *Am Nurs* 26:3, 24, April, 1994.

23. Horsley J. Fighting age discrimination on the job. *RN* 57:57–60, April, 1994.

24. ANA. *Nursing and HIV/AIDS*. Washington, DC: American Nurses Publishing, 1994, p 78.

25. Ibid, p 79.

26. Kaye J, et al. Sexual harassment of critical care nurses: A costly workplace issue. *Am J Crit Care* 3:409–415, November, 1994.

27. Confronting sexual harassment. *Nursing 94* 48–50, October, 1994.

28. Outwater L. Sexual harassment issues in home care: What employers should do about it. *Caring* 13:54–60, May, 1994.
29. *Nursing 94*, loc cit.
30. Ibid.
31. Flanagan L, op cit, p 16.
32. Ketter J. Nurses, HIV exposure and the burden of proof. *Am Nurs* 26:14, 21, May, 1994.
33. Carmon M. Legal challenges of tuberculosis in the workplace. *AAOHN J* 41:96–100, February, 1993.
34. ANA. *Health and Safety in the Workplace*. Report to the 1993 ANA House of Delegates, Washington, DC.
35. Ibid.
36. Sanchez-Gallegos D, Viens DC. When the client is armed or dangerous: management of violent and difficult clients in primary care. *Nurs Pract* 20:26–32, June, 1995.
37. Personal communication, ANA, August, 1995.
38. Supreme Court upholds NLRB's rulemaking in determining RN-only bargaining units: NLRB issues guidelines. *SNA Legal Develop* July 26, 1991.
39. Joel LA. The ultimate gag rule. *Am J Nurs* 94:8, August, 1994.
40. *NLN Guide to Undergraduate RN Education*. New York: NLN, 1994.
41. Winslow EH. Overcome the fear of speaking in public. *Am J Nurs* 91:51–53, May, 1991.

Bibliography

CHAPTER 1   Care of the Sick: How Nursing Began

Benson E. On the other side of the battle: Russian nurses in the Crimean War. *Image* 24:65–68, Spring, 1992.

Berges F, Berges C. A visit to Scutari. *Am J Nurs* 86:811–813, July, 1986.

Bullough V. Nightingale, nursing and harassment. *Image* 22:4–7, Spring, 1990.

Bullough V, et al. *Florence Nightingale and Her Era: A Collection of New Scholarship*. New York: Garland Publishing, 1990.

Bullough V, Bullough B. Medieval nursing. *Nurs Hist Rev* 1:89–104, (1), 1993.

Calabria M, Macrae J. *"Suggestions for Thought" by Florence Nightingale*. Philadelphia: University of Pennsylvania Press, 1994.

Hays J. Florence Nightingale and the India sanitary reforms. *Pub Health Nurs* 6:152–154, September, 1989.

Henry B, et al. Nightingale's perspective of nursing administration. *Nurs Health Care* 11:200–206, April, 1990.

Mackenbach J. Social inequality and death as illustrated in late-medieval death dances. *Am J Pub Health* 85:1285–1292, September, 1995.

MacMillan K. Brilliant mind gave Florence her edge. *Reg Nurse* 6:29–31, April–May, 1994.

Monteiro L. Florence Nightingale and public health nursing. *Am J Pub Health* 75:181–186, February, 1985.

Nuttal P. The passionate statistician. *Int Nurs Rev* 31:24–25, January–February, 1984.

Rajabally M. Florence Nightingale's personality: psychoanalytical profile. *Int J Nurs Stud* 31:269–279, June, 1994.

Skretkowicz V. *Florence Nightingale's Notes on Nursing*. London: Scutari Press, 1992.

Slater V. The educational and philosophical influences on Florence Nightingale, an enlightened conductor. *Nurs Hist Rev* 2:137–152, 1994.

Vicinus M, Nergaard V (eds). *Ever Yours, Florence Nightingale: Selected Letters.* Cambridge, MA: Harvard University Press, 1990.

Widerquist J. Dearest friend—The correspondence of colleagues Florence Nightingale and Mary Jones. *Nurs Hist Rev* 1:25–42, 1993.

Widerquist J. The spirituality of Florence Nightingale. *Nurs Res* 41:49–55, January–February, 1992.

Woodham-Smith C. *Florence Nightingale.* New York: McGraw-Hill, 1951.

See also the sections on Nightingale in the Bullough and Bullough, Dolan, and Kalisch and Kalisch books. An outstanding collection of Nightingale's writings can be found in the Adelaide Nutting Historical Nursing collection at Teachers College, Columbia University, New York. Some of her most noted works are listed in *Dimensions of Professional Nursing*, 7th ed.

CHAPTER 2   Nursing in the United States: American Revolution to Nursing Revolution

Baas L. An analysis of the writing of Janet Geister and Mary Roberts regarding the problems of private duty nursing. *J Prof Nurs* 8:176–183, May–June, 1992.

Backer B. Lillian Wald: Connecting caring with activism. *Nurs Health Care* 14:122–129, March, 1993.

Baer E. Nursing's divided loyalties: A historical study. *Nurs Res* 38:166–171, May–June, 1989.

Buhler-Wilkerson K. Bringing care to the people: Lillian Wald's legacy to public health nursing. *Am J Pub Health* 83:1778–1786, December, 1993.

Buhler-Wilkerson K. *False Dawn: The Rise and Decline of Public Health Nursing 1900–1930.* New York: Garland Publishing, 1989.

Bullough B. Men, women, and nursing history. *J Prof Nurs* 10:127, May–June, 1994.

Bullough V, Bullough B. Achievement of eminent American nurses of the past: A prosopographical study. *Nurs Res* 41:120–124, March–April, 1992.

Bullough V, et al. *American Nursing: A Biographical Dictionary.* New York: Garland Publishing, 1988.

Bullough V, et al. *American Nursing: A Biographical Dictionary*, Vol II. New York: Garland Publishing, 1992.

Bullough V. History, nature, and nurture. *J Prof Nurs* 9:128, May–June, 1993.

Bullough B, et al. *Nursing: A Historical Bibliography.* New York: Garland Publishing, 1981.

Burton D. *Clara Barton: In the Service of Humanity.* Westport, CT: Greenwood Press, 1995.

Carnegie M. *The Path We Tread: Blacks in Nursing, 1854–1990.* New York: National League for Nursing, 1991.

Carnegie M. *The Path We Tread: Blacks in Nursing Worldwide 1850–1990.* New York: National League for Nursing, 1995.

Calhoun J. The Nightingale Pledge: A commitment that survives the passage of time. *Nurs Health Care* 14:130–136, April, 1993.

Chaney J, Falk P. A profession in caricature: Changing attitudes toward nursing in the American Medical News, 1960–1989. *Nurs Hist Rev* 1:181–202, 1993.

Dammann N. *A Social History of the Frontier Nursing Service.* Sun City, AZ: Social Change Press, 1982.

Declercq E. The trials of Hannah Porn: The campaign to abolish midwifery in Massachusetts. *Am J Pub Health* 84:1027–1028, June, 1994.

Focus: Nursing's proud history. *Imprint*, entire issue, April–May, 1990.

Doona ME. Gertrude Weld Peabody: Unsung patron of public health nursing education. *Nurs Health Care* 15:88–94, February, 1994.

Gollaher D. *Voice for the Mad: The Life of Dorothea Dix.* New York: Free Press, 1995.

Jones I. One nurse's war-life as a nurse in World War II. *Nurs Stand* 8:20–21, June 1–7, 1994.

Kaufman M (ed). *Dictionary of American Nursing Biography.* New York: Greenwood Press, 1988.

Kim M. Overview: The International Council of Nurses: The past, present, and future. *Imprint* 40:57–60, April–May, 1993.

Lewenson S. *Taking Charge: Nursing, Suffrage and Feminism in America 1873–1924.* New York: Garland Publishing, 1993.

Lipson J. Esther Lucille Brown: A memorial. *Image* 24:313–317, Winter, 1992.

Long H. D-Day remembered. *Nurs Times* 90:44–45, June 1–7, 1994.

Maker M. *To bind up the wounds.* New York: Greenwood Press, 1989.

Mayer S. Susan Greenwald: Pioneer in international public health nursing. *Nurs Health Care* 15:74–79, February, 1994.

Moments in American history. *Nurs Res* 39:126–127, March–April, 1990.

Ogren K. The risk of not understanding nursing history. *Hol Nurs Pract* 8:8–14, January, 1994.

Olson T. Laying claim to caring: Nursing and the language of training, 1915–1937. *Nurs Outlook* 41:68–72, March–April, 1993.

Pavri P. Overview: one hundred years of public health nursing: visions of a better world. *Imprint* 41:43–48, September–October, 1994.

Pilliterri A, Ackerman M. The "doctor–nurse game": A comparison of 100 years, 1888–1990. *Nurs Outlook* 4:113–116, May–June, 1993.

Progress and promise 1900–1990. *Am J Nurs*, anniversary issue, October, 1990.

Samson J. A nurse who gave her life so that others could live. *Imprint* 37:81–89, April–May, 1990.

Weinberg D, Buhler-Wilkerson K. The changing face of nursing. *Nurs Res* 41:40–42, January–February, 1992.

Wuthrow S. Our mothers' stories. *Nurs Outlook* 38:218–222, September–October, 1990.

In the text of Chapter 5 in *Dimensions of Professional Nursing*, 7th ed. (ref. 21 of this book's Chapter 2), the publisher and date of publication are cited for older studies that were widely available at that time. Many of these reports are now out of print. However, some libraries have photocopies, and microfilmed editions of most of them are also available. All of Christy's historical biographies are also listed in the bibliography of *Dimensions*. These and others are available in *Pages from Nursing History* (New York: American Journal of Nursing Company, 1984). The January–February 1995 issue of *NHC, Perspective Community* focuses on nursing history and includes articles about Staupers, Geister, Stewart, and others. Further useful references predating those cited in this edition are found in earlier editions of *The Nursing Experience*.

CHAPTER 3 The Health Care Delivery System

Aaron HJ. *Serious and Unstable Condition: Financing America's Healthcare.* Washington, DC: Brookings Institute, 1991.

Abel E, Nelson M. *Circles of Care: Work and Identity in Women's Lives.* Albany, NY: State University of New York Press, 1990.

Applebaum R, Phillips P. Assuring the quality of in-home care: The "other" challenge for long-term care. *Gerontologist* 30:444–450, April, 1990.

Baker E (ed). *Surveillance in Occupational Health and Safety.* Atlanta: Centers for Disease Control, 1989.

Baines D, et al. Primary health care and primary care: A confusion of philosophies. *Nurs Outlook* 43:7–16, January–February, 1995.

Barger SE. Establishing a nursing center: Learning from the literature and the experience of others. *J Prof Nurs* 11:203–212, July–August, 1995.

Braunstein J. National health care: Necessary but not sufficient. *Nurs Outlook* 39:54–55, March–April, 1991.

Buerhaus PI. Managed competition and critical issues facing nurses. *Nurs Health Care* 15:22–26, January, 1994.

Cossey M, Savalle–Dunn J. Sketching the future: Trends influencing nursing informatics. *JOGNN* 23:175–182, February, 1994.

Coopers and Lybrand Health Decisions Resource Group. Healthcare reform: Innovations at the state level. *Nurs Mgmt* 25:30–40, April, 1994.

Dennis KE, et al. Point of care technology: Impact on people and paperwork. *Nurs Econ* 11:229–237, July–August, 1993.

Dreifus C. Present shock. *The New York Times* 46–50, June 11, 1995.

Ehrlich P, Ehrlich A. *The Population Explosion.* New York: Simon & Schuster, 1990.

Elliott RL, et al. The effectiveness of a hospital bedside computer system. *Med Surg Nurs* 4:33–39, February, 1995.

Foust JB. Creating a future for nursing through interactive planning at the bedside. *Image* 26:129–132, Summer, 1994.

Ginzberg E. *The Medical Triangle: Physicians, Politicians and the Public.* Cambridge, MA: Harvard University Press, 1990.

Glanty K, et al. *Health Behavior and Health Education: Theory, Research and Practice.* San Francisco: Jossey-Bass, 1990.

Gold R. *Abortion and Women's Health: A Turning Point for America?* New York: Alan Guttmacher Institute, 1990.

Grau L, et al. Nursing home residents' perceptions of the quality of their care. *J Psychosoc Nurs* 33:34–41, May, 1995.

Guyette ML, Chu S. Nursing informatics: An information exchange. *Nurs Mgmt* 25:12, 14, July, 1994.

Hays BJ, et al. Informatics issues for nursing's future. *Adv Nurs Sci* 16:71–81, June, 1994.

Hendrickson G, Kovner C. Effects of computers on nursing resource use. *Comput Nurs* 8:16–22, February, 1990.

Hynes HP (ed). *Reconstructing Babylon: Essays on Women and Technology.* Bloomington, IN: Indiana University Press, 1991.

Kelly LS. Another look at the future of health care. *Nurs Outlook* 39:150–151, July–August, 1991.

Lessner MW, et al. Orienting nursing students to cost-effective clinical practice. *Nurs Health Care* 15:458–462, November, 1994.

McCracken AL. Special care units: Meeting the needs of cognitively impaired persons. *J Gerontolog Nurs* 20:41–46, April, 1994.

Mikulencak M. The "graying of America": Changing what nurses need to know. *Am Nurse* 25:1, 12, July, 1993.

Naegle MA. Drug use and HIV: Healthcare provider prospectives. *J Ass Nurse AIDS Care* 5:39–46, 51–52, May–June, 1994.

Riessman F, Carroll C. *Self-Help: Policy and Practice.* San Francisco: Jossey-Bass, 1995.

Siendwall D, Tavani C. The role of public health in providing primary care for the medically underserved. *Pub Health Rep* 106:2–4, January–February, 1991.

Stanfield P. *Introduction to the Health Professions,* 2d ed. Boston: Jones & Bartlett, 1995.

Starck PL. Health care under siege: Challenge for change. *Nurs Health Care* 12:26–31, January, 1991.

Talashek ML, et al. The substance abuse pandemic: Determinants to guide interventions. *Pub Health Nurs* 11:131–139, April, 1994.

Tappen RM, Beckerman A. A vulnerable population: Multiproblem adults in acute care. *J. Gerontolog Nurs* 19:38–42, November, 1993.

CHAPTER 4   The Discipline of Nursing

Aiken L. What nurses need to know about legal, ethical and political issues. *Revolution* 4:72–75, Summer, 1994.

Barnum B. *Nursing Theory: Analysis, Application, Evaluation*, 4th ed. Philadelphia: Lippincott, 1994.

Bernick L, Avery L. Clinical decision-making: The art and science of inquiry in caring for elders. *Perspectives* 18:2–6, Spring, 1994.

Brider P. Who killed the nursing care plan? *Am J Nurs* 91:35–39, May, 1991.

Brookfield S. On impostorship, cultural suicide, and other dangers: How nurses learn critical thinking. *J Contin Ed Nurs* 24:197–205, September–October, 1993.

Buresh B. PCAs and CTAs: Are they the beginning of the end of nursing? *Revolution* 4:8–10, Summer, 1994.

Buresh B, Gordon S. Speak up, speak out: Tell the world what you do. *Am J Nurs* 95:18–19, January, 1995.

Chang BL, Hirsch M. Nursing diagnosis research: Computer aided research in nursing. *Nurs Diag* 5:6–13, January–March, 1994.

Diers D. Learning the art and craft of nursing. *Am J Nurs* 90:65–66, January, 1990.

Foust JB. Creating a future for nursing through interactive planning at the bedside. *Image* 26:129–132, Summer, 1994.

Frisch N. Tripped up by syntax; important questions for the present and future of nursing diagnosis and nursing taxonomies. *Nurs Diag* 5:95, July–September, 1994.

George JB. *Nursing Theories*. Norwalk, CT: Appleton & Lange, 1995.

Glotz N, et al. Advancing clinical excellence: Competency-based patient care. *Nurs Mgmt* 25:42–44, January, 1994.

Gudmunsen A. Personal reflections on Martha E Rogers. *NHC: Perspectives on Community* 16:36–87, January–February, 1995.

Harrison M. Nursing care: Measuring the impact. *RN* 6:27–28, April–May, 1994.

Hull M. Your nursing image: Tending the flame. *Nurs 93* 23:116, 118, May, 1993.

Jones A. *Images of Nurses: Perspectives from History, Art and Literature*. Philadelphia: University of Pennsylvania Press, 1988.

Kalisch PA, Kalisch BJ. *The Advance of American Nursing*, 3rd ed. Philadelphia: J.P. Lippincott, 1995.

Kataoka-Yahiro M, Saylor C. A critical thinking model for nursing judgment. *J Nurs Ed* 33:351–356, October, 1994.

Kerfoot K. Changing nursing image through the media. *Imprint* 40:41–42, November–December, 1993.

Malinski V, Barrett EA. *Martha E. Rogers: Her Life and Her Work.* Philadelphia: Davis, 1994.

McQuiston C, Webb A (eds). A series titled *Notes on Nursing Theories* presents many of the major nursing theorists. Thousand Oaks, CA: Sage, 1991–1993.

Morris DL, Wykle ML. Minorities in nursing. *Ann Rev Nurs Res* 12:175–189, March, 1994.

Pillitteri A. A contrast in images: Nursing and non-nursing college students. *J Nurs Ed* 33:132–133, March, 1994.

Simpson R. Ammunition in the boardroom: The clinical nursing data set. *Nurs Mgmt* 26:16–17, June, 1995.

Tanner CA. Provocative thoughts on critical thinking. *J Nurs Ed* 33:339–342, October, 1994.

Tanner CA, et al. The phenomenology of knowing the patient. *Image* 25:273–280, April, 1993.

While AE. Competence versus performance: Which is more important? *J Adv Nurs* 20:525–531, September, 1994.

Wiens AG. Patient autonomy in care: A theoretical framework for nursing. *J Prof Nurs* 9:95–103, March–April, 1993.

CHAPTER 5   Education and Research for Practice

Bailey BI. Faculty practice in an academic nursing care center model: Autonomy, job satisfaction and productivity. *J Nurs Ed* 34:84–86, February, 1995.

Bassett C. The integration of research in the clinical setting: Obstacles and solutions. A review of the literature. *Nurse Pract* 17:4–8, January, 1992.

Bergman K, Gaitskill T. Faculty and student perceptions of effective clinical teachers: An extension study. *J Prof Nurs* 6:33–44, January–February, 1990.

Captain C. Basing practice on nursing research. *Sci Nurs* 11:111–113, December, 1994.

Deering-Flory R, Neighbors M. NLN competencies for the associate degree nurse: Are the new graduates meeting them? *Nurs Health Care* 12:474–479, November, 1991.

Donnelly GF, et al. A faculty practice program: Three perspectives. *Holistic Nurs Pract* 8:71–80, April, 1994.

Hart S. Single purpose institutions for nursing programs: To be or not to be. *J Prof Nurs* 6:55–58, January–February, 1990.

Jarvis P. Theory and practice and the preparation of teachers of nursing. *Nurs Ed Today* 12:258–265, August, 1992.

Kessenick C. Nursing research: Challenge to excellence. *Imprint* 39:84–85, September–October, 1992.

Leininger M. Transcultural nursing education: A worldwide imperative. *Nurs Health Care* 15:254–257, May, 1994.

Mitchell GJ. Discipline-specific inquiry: The Hermeneutics of theory-guided nursing research. *Nurs Outlook* 42:224–228, September–October, 1994.

Nagel L, et al. Nursing theory in perspective. *Nurs Outlook* 42:141–142, May–June, 1994.

Nugent KE, et al. Facilitators and inhibitors of practice: A faculty perspective—The role of faculty practice. *J Nurs Ed* 32:293–300, September, 1993.

Patton JG, Cook LR. Creative alliances between nursing service and education in times of economic constraint. *Nurs Connect* 7:29–37, Fall, 1994.

Rudy EB, et al. Faculty practice: Creating a new culture. *J Prof Nurs* 11:84–88, March–April, 1995.

Seidle A, Sauter D. The new non-traditional student in nursing. *J Nurs Ed* 29:13–19, January, 1990.

Stitt P. Putting practice into theory: Developing the role of the link teacher in higher education. *J Prof Nurs* 9:314, 316–317, February, 1994.

Styles M, et al. Entry: A new approach. *Nurs Outlook* 39:200–203, September–October, 1991.

Thomas SD, et al. Nursing faculty development during a time of declining resources. *J Contin Ed Nurs* 25:246–250, November–December, 1994.

Titler MG. Using NIC in nursing practice—Nursing interventions classification. *Med Surg Nurs* 3:300–302, August, 1994.

Verderber A, Urden LD. A collaborative community model for nursing research: Meeting the agenda for the 1990s. *Nurs Connect* 7:45–51, Summer, 1994.

Various journals carry a large number of articles on nursing education and research: *Journal of Nursing Education, Nurse Educator, Journal of Continuing Education, Journal of Professional Nursing, Nursing Outlook, Nursing Research,* to name a few.

CHAPTER 6   Career Opportunities

Aiken L. Charting the future of hospital nursing. *Image* 22:72–78, Summer, 1990.

American Nurses Association. *Nursing Care Report Card for Acute Care.* Washington, DC: American Nurses Publishing, 1995.

Bakker DJ, Vincensi BB. Economic impact of the CNS: Practitioner role. *Clin Nurse Spec* 9:50–53, January, 1995.

Beecroft PC. The future arrives—affirming the role of CNSs in a changing health care system. *Clin Nurse Spec* 9:1, 7, January, 1995.

Boyar DC, Marteson DJ. Intrapreneurial group practice. *Nurs Health Care* 11:28–33, January, 1990.

Burdick MB. Measuring nursing outcomes in a psychiatric setting. *Iss Ment Health Nurs* 15:137–148, March–April, 1994.

Buresh B. View from the nurses' station. *Nieman Reports* 23–25, Winter, 1993.

Bush HA, Mettler MV. NPs as entrepreneurs: Three case histories. *Am J Nurs* 94:16A-B, 16D, December, 1994.

Carroll JT, Graner ME. Hospice is managed care. *J Home Health Care Pract* 6:49–54, February, 1994.

Chaisson SF. Role of the CNS in developing a competency-based orientation program. *Clin Nurse Spec* 9:32–37, January, 1995.

Colburn K, Hiveley D. The hospice phenomenon in its second decade under Medicare. *Caring* 12:4, 7–12, November, 1993.

Glenn MJ, Smith JH. From clinical ladders to a professional recognition program. *Nurs Mgmt* 26:41–42, March, 1995.

Hawkins JW, et al. School nursing in America, 1902–1994: A return to public health nursing. *Pub Health Nurs* 11:416–425, December, 1994.

Irvine DM, Evans MG. Job satisfaction and turnover among nurses: Integrating research findings across studies. *Nurs Res* 44:246–251, July–August, 1995.

Joel LA. Entrepreneurship: A global movement. *Am J Nurs* 94:7, December, 1994.

Keane A, et al. Critical care nurse practitioners: Evolution of the advanced practice nurse role. *Am J Crit Care* 3:232–237, May, 1994.

Manion J. Nurse intrapreneurs: Heroes of health care's future: *Nurs Outlook* 39:18–21, January–February, 1991.

Murphy B. *Nursing Centers: The Time is Now.* New York: NLN, 1995.

National Student Nurses' Association. Speical issue: Nursing specialties. *Imprint* 42, April–May, 1995.

Parvi JM. Overview: One hundred years of public health nursing: Visions of a better world. *Imprint* 41:43, 45, 47–48, September–October, 1994.

Pierce S, et al. Nurses employed in non-nursing fields. *J Nurs Admin* 21:29–34, June, 1991.

Prescott PA, et al. Changing how nurses spend their time. *Image* 23:23–27, Spring, 1991.

Ray GL, Hardin S. Advanced practice nursing: Playing a vital role. *Nurs Mgmt* 26:45–47, February, 1995.

Reynolds JA. My side; Personal accounts. The best part of psychiatric nursing. *J Psychosoc Nurs Ment Health Serv* 33:41, February, 1995.

Robertson JF, Cummings CC. What makes long term care nursing attractive? *Am J Nurs* 91:41–46, November, 1991.

Rogers B. Occupational health nursing practice, education and research. *AAOHN J* 38:536–543, November, 1990.

Ross M. Adult nurse practitioner/clinical nurse specialist: Roles in health care reform. *Clin Nurse Spec* 8:291, 305, November, 1994.

Steel JE. Advanced nursing practice. *Adv Nurs Prac* 5:71–76, February, 1994.

Williams CA, Valdivieso GC. Advanced practice models: A comparison of clinical nurse specialist and nurse practitioner activities. *Clin Nurse Spec* 8:311–318, November, 1994.

Zentner J, et al. Nurse practitioner provided primary care: Managing health care costs in the workplace. *AAOHN J* 43:52–53, January, 1995.

CHAPTER 7 Leadership for an Era of Change

Alm T. Power in nursing. *J Adv Nurs* 16:503, May, 1991.

Angelini DJ. Mentoring in the career development of hospital staff nurses: Models and strategies. *J Prof Nurs* 11:89–97, March–April, 1995.

Bernhard L, Walsh M. *Leadership*, 3rd ed. St. Louis, MO: Mosby, 1995.

Collins S, Henderson M. Autonomy: Part of the nursing role? *Nurs Forum* 26:23–29, February, 1991.

Davidhizar R. Having confidence in work relationships. *Imprint* 42:23–24, January, 1995.

Hagenow NR, McCrea MA. A mentoring relationship: Two viewpoints. *Nurs Mgmt* 25:42–43, December, 1994.

Johnson R, Martin-Semeah R. Mentoring: A commitment to growth. *Nurs Allied Health J Minorities* 2:29–31, Spring–Summer, 1994.

Larson E. Nursing research and societal needs: Political, corporate and international perspectives. *J Prof Nurs* 9:73–78, March–April, 1993.

Loraine K. Leadership from the child within. *Nurs Mgmt* 26:57–58, February, 1995.

Manion J. Understanding the 7 stages of change. *Am J Nurs* 95:41–43, April, 1995.

McKnight J, Van-Dover L. Community as client: A challenge for nursing education. *Pub Health Nurs* 11:12–16, February, 1994.

Madison J. The value of mentoring in nursing leadership: A descriptive study. *Nurs Forum* 29:16–23, October–December, 1994.

Meyer C. Nurses on the political front. *Am J Nurs* 92:56–64, October, 1992.

Miner KJ, Baker JA. Health educators as environmental policy advocates. *J Health Ed* 24:141–148, May–June, 1993.

Porter-O'Grady T. Reverse discrimination in nursing leadership: Hitting the concrete ceiling. *Nurs Adm Quart* 19:56–62, Winter, 1995.

Reverby SM. Even her nursing friends see her as only a feminist and other tales of the nursing–feminism connection. *Nurs Health Care* 14:296–301, June, 1993.

Stivers C. Why can't a woman be less like a man: Women's leadership dilemma. *J Nurs Admin* 21:47–51, May, 1991.

Trudeau S. The law adds force to your voice—nurses speak up on behalf of their patients. *RN* 57:65–66, 68, January, 1994.

Weekes DP. Mentor-protégé relationships: A critical element in affirmative action. *Nurs Outlook* 37:156–157, July–August, 1989.

CHAPTER 8 Ethical Issues in Nursing and Health Care

Annas G. Ethics committees: From ethical comfort to ethical cover. *Hastings Center Rep* 21:18–21, May–June, 1991.

Bandman E, Bandman B. *Nursing Ethics Through the Life Span*, 3rd ed. Norwalk, CT: Appleton & Lange, 1995.

Baruch E, et al (eds). *Embryos, Ethics and Women's Rights: Exploring the New Reproductive Technologies*. New York: Haworth Press, 1988.

Bosek M, Baker T. Commentary: Rationing trauma care to the elderly. *Med–Surg Nurs* 4:217–219, June, 1995.

Bosek M. Doing good: An ethical quandary. *Med Surg Nurs* 4:154–156, April, 1995.

Brecht M. Nursing's role in assuring access to care. *Nurs Outlook* 38:6–7, January–February, 1990.

Calkins M. Ethical issues in the elderly ESRD patient. *ANNA J* 20:569–571, October, 1993.

Capron A. Abandoning a waning life. *Hastings Center Rep* 25:24–26, July–August, 1995.

Capron A. The burden of decision. *Hastings Center Rep* 20:36–41, May–June, 1990.

Cassel C, Meier D. Morals and moralism in the debate over euthanasia and assisted suicide. *New Engl J Med* 323:750–752, September 13, 1990.

Cassidy V, Koroll C. Ethical aspects of transformational leadership. *Holistic Nurs Pract* 9:41–47, October, 1994.

Chervenack F, McCullough L. Justified limits on refusing intervention. *Hastings Center Rep* 21:12–18, March–April, 1991.

Curtis J, et al. Use of the medical futility rationale in do-not-resuscitate orders. *JAMA* 273:124–128, January 11, 1995.

Curtin L. Collegial ethics of a caring profession. *Nurs Mgmt* 25:28–32, August, 1994.

Curtin L. Human problems: Human beings. *Nurs Mgmt* 25:38, May, 1994.

Curtin L. There's no place like home. *Nurs Mgmt* 26:26–29, January, 1995.

Devettere R. *Practical Decision Making in Health Care Ethics: Cases and Concepts*. Washington, DC: Georgetown University Press, 1995.

Dunn D. Bioethics and nursing. *Nurs Connect* 7:43–51, Fall, 1994.

Dying Well? A colloquy on euthanasia and assisted suicide. *Hastings Center Rep*, entire issue, March–April, 1992.

Ferrell B, Dean G. Ethical issues in pain management at home. *J Palliat Care* 10:67–72, Autumn, 1994.

Flack H, Pellegrino E (eds). *African–American Perspectives on Biomedical Ethics*. Washington, DC: Georgetown University Press, 1992.

Fry S. Ethical issues in research: Scientific misconduct and fraud. *Nurs Outlook* 38:296, November–December, 1990.

Fry S. Whistle-blowing by nurses: A matter of ethics. *Nurs Outlook* 37:56, January–February, 1989.

Gorlin R (ed). *Codes of Professional Responsibility*, 3rd ed. Washington, DC: Bureau of National Affairs, 1994.

Haack M, Hughes T. *Addiction in the Nursing Profession.* New York: Springer, 1990.

Hillan E. Demented elderly people: Ethical issues. *J Adv Nurs* 18:1889–1894, December, 1993.

Hoyer P, et al. Clinical cheating and moral development. *Nurs Outlook* 39:170–173, July–August, 1991.

Husted G, Husted J. *Ethical Decision Making in Nursing*, 2nd ed. St. Louis: Mosby, 1995.

Johanson W. Promoting collaboration in ethical decision making. *Crit Care Nurse* 14:96–99, October, 1994.

Jonsen A, et al. *Clinical Ethics*, 3rd ed. New York: McGraw-Hill, 1992.

Kapp M. Medical decision-making for older adults in institutional settings: Is beneficence dead in an age of risk management? *Issues Law Med* 11:29–46, Summer, 1995.

Keffer M, Keffer H. The do-not-resuscitate order: Moral responsibilities of the perioperative nurse. *AORN J* 59:641–650, March, 1994.

Lund M. Stopping treatment: Who decides? *Ger Nurs* 12:147–148, 151, May–June, 1991.

Lynch A. Ethical issues in bone marrow transplantation: A nursing perspective. *J Palliat Care* 10:23–26, Autumn, 1994.

Marsec V. Ethical dilemmas in the delivery of intensive care to critically ill oncology patients. *Semin Oncol Nurs* 10:156–164, August, 1994.

McCormick T. Ethical issues in caring for patients with renal failure. *ANNA J* 20:549–555, October, 1993.

Milner S. An ethical nursing practice model. *J Nurs Admin* 23:22–25, March, 1993.

Monagle J, Thomasma D. *Health Care Ethics: Critical Issues.* Frederick, MD: Aspen, 1994.

Olsen D. The ethical considerations of managed care in mental health treatment. *J Psychosoc Nurs Ment Health Serv* 25:8, 34–35, March, 1994.

Osgood N. Assisted suicide and older people—a deadly combination: Ethical problems in permitting assisted suicide. *Iss Law Med* 10:415–436, Spring, 1995.

Pence T, Cantrall J (eds). *Ethics in Nursing: An Anthology.* New York: National League for Nursing, 1990.

Purtilo R. *Ethical Dimensions in the Health Professions*, 2nd ed. Philadelphia: W.B. Saunders, 1993.

Rothman D. *Strangers at the Bedside: A History of How Law and Bioethics Transformed Medical Decision-making.* New York: Basic Books, 1991.

Sabin J, Daniels N. Determining "medical necessity" in mental health practice. *Hastings Center Rep* 24:5–13, November–December, 1994.

Silva M. *Annotated Bibliography for Ethical Guidelines in the Conduct, Dissemination, and Implementation of Nursing Research.* Washington, DC: American Nursing Publishing, 1995.

Silva M. *Ethical Guidelines in the Conduct, Dissemination, and Implementation of Nursing Research.* Washington, DC: American Nursing Publishing, 1995.

Schroeter K. The ethics of organ donation. *Today's OR Nurse* 17:8–12, January–February, 1995.

Starzomski R. Ethical issues in palliative care: The case of dialysis and organ transplantation. *J Palliat Care* 10:27–34, Autumn, 1994.

Trinkoff AM, et al. The prevalence of substance abuse among registered nurses. *Nurs Res* 40:172–174, May–June, 1991.

Watne K. Distinguishing between life-saving and life-sustaining treatments: When the physician and spouse disagree. *Dim Crit Care Nurs* 14:42–47 January–February, 1995.

Walters L (ed). *Bibliography of Bioethics, Vol 20.* Washington, DC: Kennedy Institute of Ethics, 1994.

Winters G, et al. Ethical issues in oncology nursing practice: An overview of topics and strategies. *Oncol Nurs Forum* 20:21–34 November–December, 1993.

Many nursing journals have monthly or periodic columns about ethics, and the Hastings Center publishes a variety of materials, as well as the *Hastings Center Report*. See also references and bibliography of Chapter 9.

CHAPTER 9 Patients' Rights; Students' Rights

Advance care planning: Priorities for ethical and empirical research. *Hastings Center Rep*, special supplement, November–December, 1994.

Annas G. Crazy-making: Embryos and gestational mothers. *Hastings Center Rep* 21:35–38, January–February, 1991.

Annas G. Editorial: Heretic prophecy and genetic privacy—can we prevent the dream from becoming a nightmare? *Am J Pub Health* 85:1196–1197, September, 1995.

Annas G. Foreclosing the use of force: A.C. reversed. *Hastings Center Rep* 20:27–29, July–August, 1990.

Annas G. One flew over the Supreme Court. *Hastings Center Rep* 20:28–30, May–June, 1990.

Avila D. Medical treatment rights of older persons and persons with disabilities: 1993–94 developments. *Iss Law Med* 10:385–400, Spring, 1995.

Backlar P. The longing for order: Oregon's medical advance directive for mental health treatment. *Commun Ment Health J* 31:103–107, April, 1995.

Capron A. Privacy: Dead and gone. *Hastings Center Rep* 22:43–45, January–February, 1992.

Cates W, et al. Topics for our times: Justice Blackmun and legal abortion—a besieged legacy to women's reproductive health. *Am J Pub Health* 185:1204–1206, September, 1995.

Chabalewski F, Norris G. The gift of life: Talking to families about organ and tissue donation. *Am J Nurs* 94:29–33, June, 1994.

Charo R. Life after *Casey*: The view from Rehnquist's "Potamkin Village". *Law Med Eth* 21:59–66, Spring, 1993.

Cruzan: Clear and convincing? Commentaries. *Hastings Center Rep* 20:5–11, September–October, 1990.

Curtin L. Abortion: A tangle of rights. *Nurs Mgmt* 24:26–31, June, 1993.

Curtin L. DNR in the OR: Ethical concerns and hospital policies. *Nurs Mgmt* 25:29–31, February, 1994.

Curtin L. Patient privacy in a public institution. *Nurs Mgmt* 24:26–27, June, 1993.

Daly B. Withholding nutrition and hydration revisited. *Nurs Mgmt* 25:30–39, May, 1995.

Danis M, et al. A prospective study of advance directives for life-sustaining care. *New Engl J Med* 324:882–895, March 28, 1991.

Fiesta J. Whistleblowers: Heroes or stool pigeons? Part I. *Nurs Mgmt* 21:16–17, June, 1990.

Fiesta J. Whistleblowers: Retaliation or protection? Part II. *Nurs Mgmt* 21:38, July, 1990.

Four easy ways to lose a job in nursing. *Am J Nurs* 90:27–28, June, 1990.

Fleischman A. Parental responsibility and the infant bioethics committee. *Hastings Center Rep* 20:21–22, March–April, 1990.

Frawley K. Confidentiality in the computer age. *RN* 57:59–60, July, 1994.

Helms L, Weiler K. Suing programs of nursing education. *Nurs Outlook* 39:158–161, July–August, 1991.

Jones L. A right to die? *Intens Crit Care Nurs* 10:278–288, December, 1994.

Leibson C. The role of the courts in terminating life-sustaining treatment. *Iss Law Med* 10:437–452, Spring, 1995.

McPherson E. Ethical implications of the human genome diversity project. *Connections* 8:36–43, Spring, 1995.

Meisel A. Legal myths about terminating life support. *Arch Int Med* 151:1497–1501, August, 1991.

Milholland K. Privacy and confidentiality of patient information: Challenges for nursing. *J Nurs Adm* 24:19–24, February, 1994.

Murphy E. Celebrating the Bill of Rights in the year of *Rust v. Sullivan. Nurs Outlook* 39:238–239, September–October, 1991.

Murphy T, Lappé (eds). *Justice and the Human Genome Project.* Berkeley and Los Angeles: University of California Press, 1994.

Nolan K. Let's take Baby Doe to Alaska. *Hastings Cent Rep* 20:3, January–February, 1991.

Pavalon E. *Human Rights and Health Care Law.* New York: American Journal of Nursing Company, 1990.

Peppin J. Physician neutrality and patient autonomy in advance directive decisions. *Issues Law Med* 11:13–28, Summer, 1995.

Pearlman R, et al. Insights pertaining to patient assessments of states worse than death. *J Clin Eth* 4:33–41, Summer, 1993.

Reigle J. Should the patient decide when to die? *RN* 58:57–60, May, 1995.

Rhodes AM. Norplant and the "coerced contraception" controversy. *MCN* 16:277, 1991.

Rhodes AM. Refusing nutrition and hydration: The Cruzan case. *MCN* 16:141, May–June, 1991.

Rhodes AM. Treatment decisions. *MCN* 16:225, July–August, 1991.

Ruholl L. Who's in charge here? *Am J Nurs* 92:21–22, June, 1992.

Rushton C. Placebo pain medication: Ethical and legal issues. *Ped Nurs* 21:166–168, March–April, 1995.

Scanlon C. Safeguarding a patient's right to self-determination. *Am Nurse* 25:20–21, November–December, 1993.

Schwarz J. Living wills and health care proxies. *Nurs Health Care* 13:92–96, February, 1992.

Seidl A. HIV testing: Patients' rights versus nurses' rights. In Bullough B, et al: *Nursing Issues for the Nineties and Beyond.* New York: Springer, 1994, pp 139–158.

Taylor R, Lantos J. The policies of medical futility. *Iss Law Med* 11:3–12, Summer, 1995.

Truog R. Triage in the ICU. *Hastings Center Rep* 22:13–25, May–June, 1992.

Vaughn M. Section 1983: Civil liability of prison officials for denying and delaying medication and drugs to prison inmates. *Iss Law Med* 11:47–63, Summer, 1995.

Weiss J, Hansell J. Substance abuse during pregnancy: Legal and health policy issues. *Nurs Health Care* 13:472–479, November, 1992.

Weiss F. The right to refuse: Informed consent and the psychosocial nurse. *J Psychosoc Nurs* 28(8):25–30, 1990.

Wintersheimer D. The role of the courts in terminating nutrition and hydration for incompetent patients. *Iss Law Med* 10:453–468, Spring, 1995.

Articles related to "rights" are often found in ethics columns in various journals because ethical issues so often become law. Other sources are the nonnursing journals that are included above and in the references of Chapter 9. See also the references and bibliography of Chapter 8.

CHAPTER 10 Politics and Public Policy

Cohen S. Health care policy and abortion: A comparison. *Nurs Outlook* 38:20–25, January–February, 1990.

Cohen DM, Wick EF. Healthcare in transition: Labor law impact on nurse-supervisor roles. *JONA* 25:35–38, June, 1995.

Congress and Health: An Introduction to the Legislative Process and its Key Participants. Washington, DC: National Health Council, revised periodically, sometimes with each Congress.

deVries C, Vanderbilt MW. Grassroots lobbying: Influencing the legislative process. *Am Nurse* 25:21, April, 1993.

Dickerson SS, Campbell-Heider N. Interpreting political agendas from a critical social theory perspective. *Nurs Outlook* 42:265–271, November–December, 1994.

Hall-Long BA. Nursing's past, present and future political experience. *Nurs Health Care Persp Comm* 16:24–28, January–February, 1995.

Leavitt JK, Mason DJ. Finding your political voice. *AJN Career Guide* 56, 58, October, 1994.

Mandell M. What you don't say can hurt you. *Am J Nurs* 93:15–16, August, 1993.

Peery BL, Rimler JH. Chemical dependency among nurses: Are policies adequate? *Nurs Mgmt* 26:52–57, May, 1995.

Wakefield, M. Influencing the legislative process. *Nurs Econ* 8:188–190, May–June, 1990.

Wold J. Worker's compensation and the occupational health nurse. *AAOHN J* 8:385–387, August, 1990.

Many publications of major nursing and health care organizations relate to legislation and politics. The ANA's *Legislative and Regulatory Initiatives* is revised yearly, and summarizes the public policy areas seen as most important by the profession. Useful government publications include the *Congressional Record* (verbatim transcript of the proceedings of the Senate and House) which can be obtained from the Congressional Record Office, H-112, Capitol, Washington, DC 20515; *Digest of Public General Bills*, from the Superintendent of Documents, Government Printing Office, Washington, DC 20401; *Committee Prints and Hearing Records*, available about two months after the close of hearings (free but requires a self-addressed label sent to the publications clerk of the committee from which the document is issued).

CHAPTER 11 Health Care Credentialing and Nursing Licensure

American College of Nurse Midwives. *An Introduction to the Continuing Competency Assessment Program.* Washington, DC: ACNM, 1994.

Archibald PJ, Bainbridge DD. Capacity and competence: Nurse credentialing and privileging. *Nurs Mgmt* 25:49–51, 54–56, April, 1994.

Brennan SJ. Recognizing and assisting the impaired nurse; Recommendations for nurse managers. *Nurs Forum* 26:12–16, February, 1991.

Carpenter MA. The impaired nurse. *Med Surg Nurs* 3:139–141, April, 1994.

Certification helps RNs achieve their goals. *Am Nurse* 23:28–29, February, 1991.

Corcoran E. Two licenses for advanced practice nurses? ENA thinks not—president's message. *J Emerg Nurs* 19:78–79, April, 1993.

Crimlisk J. Nurses need certification as well as licensure. *Nurse Pract* 19:68–69, October, 1994.

Curtin LL. Advanced licensure: A personal plum or public shield? *Nurs Mgmt* 23:7–8, August, 1992.

del Bueno DJ. Competence, criteria and credentialing. *J Nurs Admin* 23: 7–8, May, 1993.

Glotz N, et al. Advancing clinical excellence: Competency-based patient care. *Nurs Mgmt* 25:42–44, January, 1992.

How to get a license. *Am J Nurs* 95:20–27, January, 1995.

Henry P. Your due process rights in a disciplinary action. *Nurse Pract Forum* 2:210–211, December, 1991.

Hurley ML. The push for speciality certification. *RN* 36–44, June, 1944.

Inselberg L. An ethical analysis of the detection, discipline, and treatment of the alcoholically impaired nurse in practice. *Addict Nurs Netw* 3:20–23, Spring, 1991.

Kelly LS. Oh no, not again: An old ghost rises—institutional licensure. *Nurs Outlook* 38:121, May–June, 1990.

Minarik PA. Second license for advanced nursing practice? *Clin Nurse Spec* 6:221–222, Winter, 1992.

Parker J. Development of the American Board of Nursing Specialties. *Nurs Mgmt* 25:33–35, January, 1994.

Polk D, et al. The chemically dependent student nurse: Guidelines for policy development. *Nurs Outlook* 41:166–170, July–August, 1993.

Sharp N. Second license for the advanced practice nurse? *Nurs Mgmt* 23:28–29, September, 1992.

News items on changes in licensure and appropriate articles appear in almost all nursing journals. ANA, NLN, and the National Council of State Boards of Nursing all have materials about licensure in their publication lists. *Issues*, a NCSBN publication, is particularly useful.

CHAPTER 12   Legal Aspects of Nursing Practice

Anderson B. Serving justice: How to give a deposition. *Am J Nurs* 91:32–35, March, 1991.

Annas G. Not saints, but healers: The legal duties of health care professionals in the AIDS epidemic. *Am J Pub Health* 78:844–849, July, 1988.

Beckman J. *Nursing Malpractice: Implications for Clinical Practice and Nursing Education.* Seattle: University of Washington Press, 1995.

Betta P. Documenting to stay out of the courtroom. *Imprint* 38:39–40, April–May, 1991.

Blackwell M. Documentation serves as invaluable defense tool. *Am Nurse* 25:40–41, July–August, 1993.

Blouin A, Brent N. The nurse entrepreneur: Legal aspects of owning a business. *JONA* 25:13–14, June, 1995.

Bovbjerg R. Promoting quality and preventing malpractice. *J Health Polit Policy Law* 19:207–216, Spring, 1994.

Carroll P, Maher V. Legal issues in the care of patients with sickle cell disease. *AD Clin Care* 5:6, 19, September–October, 1990.

Carson W. AIDS and the nurse—A legal update. *Am Nurse* 25:18, March, 1993.

Cohn S. *Malpractice and Liability in Clinical Obstetrical Nursing.* Rockville, MD: Aspen, 1990.

Curran W, et al. *Health Care Law: Forensic Science and Public Policy.* Boston: Little, Brown, 1991.

Davis G. Your role in death investigations. *Am J Nurs* 94:39–41, September, 1994.

Davis N. Can computers stop errors? *Am J Nurs* 94:14, December, 1994.

Fiesta J. Agency nurses: Whose liability? *Nurs Mgmt* 2:16–17, March, 1990.

Fiesta J. Duty to communicate—"doctor notified." *Nurs Mgmt* 25:24–25, January, 1994.

Fiesta J. Legal Update, 1994, Part I. *Nurse Mgmt* 26:30, January, 1995.

Fiesta J. Legal Update, 1994, Part II. *Nurse Mgmt* 26:10–11, March, 1995.

Fiesta J. Legal Update, 1994, Part III. *Nurse Mgmt* 26:21, April, 1995.

Fiesta J. Legal Update, 1994, Part IV. *Nurse Mgmt* 26:18, May, 1995.

Fiesta J. Managed care: Whose liability? *Nurse Mgmt* 26:31–32, February, 1995.

Fiesta J. Malpractice and the federal employee. *Nurs Mgmt* 25:22–23, May, 1994.

Fiesta J. Nursing torts: From plaintiff to defendant. *Nurs Mgmt* 25:17–18, February, 1994.

Fiesta J. Premature discharge. *Nurs Mgmt* 25:17–20, April, 1994.

Fiesta J. The nursing shortage: Whose liability problem? Part I. *Nurs Mgmt* 21:24–25, January, 1990.

Fiesta J. The nursing shortage: Whose liability problem? Part II. *Nurs Mgmt* 21:22–23, February, 1990.

Frawley K. Confidentiality in the computer age. *RN* 57:59–60, July, 1994.

Horsley J. Does a criminal past rule out a nursing future? *RN* 57:74–76, October, 1994.

Kadzielski M. Exploring the legal aspects of quality improvement. *Am Nurse* 25:7, January, 1993.

Klein C. Malicious prosecution. *Nurse Practitioner* 10:42, June, 1985.

Klimon E. Nursing professional liability insurance: An analysis. *Nurs Econ* 3:132–159, May–June, 1985.

Koehler C. Lawsuit demands coping skills. *Am Nurse* 24:33, June, 1992.

Koehler C. The nurse as defendant. *Am Nurse* 24:17, April, 1992.

Kolodner D. Preventing malpractice. *Med Surg Nurs* 2:405–407, 424, October, 1993.

Law and aging. *Law Med Health Care*, entire issue, Fall, 1990.

Lederman R. Professional liability and obstetrical health care delivery. *Nurs Outlook* 39:14–17, January–February, 1991.

Maher V. AIDS—the legal issues. *AD Clin Care* 6:28–30, March–April, 1991.

Mahoney D. Under oath: Testifying against a physician. *Am J Nurs* 90:23–26, February, 1990.

Mandell M. What you don't say can hurt you. *Am J Nurs* 93:15–16, August, 1993.

Mantel D. The legal perils of patient discharge. *RN* 58:49–51, March, 1995.

McMullen P, Philipsen N. Fetal well-being III: Strategies to diminish liability and improve patient care in all trimesters. *Nurs Connect* 8:50–53, Spring, 1995.

Murphy E. Legal ramifications of RN staffing policies. *AORN J* 59:1064–1070, May, 1994.

Pozgar G. *Legal Aspects of Health Care Administration*, 5th ed. Rockville, MD: Aspen, 1993.

Pozgar G, et al. *Long-Term Care and the Law*. Rockville, MD: Aspen, 1992.

Quigley F. Responsibilities of the consultant and expert witness. *Focus Crit Care* 18:238–239, July, 1991.

Recent developments in health law. *J Law Med Eth* 21:117–128, Spring, 1993.

Rhodes AM. Locating case law. *MCN* 10:107, March–April, 1994.

Rhodes AM. Major legal initiatives in MCH (1975–1990). *MCN* 16:45, January–February, 1991.

Rutherford M. Small patients, big risks. *RN* 57:51–52, 56–57, September, 1994.

Scott R. *Legal Aspects of Documenting Patient Care*. Rockville, MD: Aspen, 1994.

Smith J. Occupational medical records: An intricate confidentiality issue. *AAOHN J* 42:18–21, January, 1994.

Tammelleo A. How the law protects emergency patients. *RN* 55:67–68, October, 1992.

Turley J. A framework for the transition from nursing records to a nursing information system. *Nurs Outlook* 40:177–191, July–August, 1992.

Tyler J. The internet: Legal rights and responsibilities. *Med Surg Nurs* 4:229–233, June, 1995.

The *Regan Report on Nursing Law* cited frequently in the Chapter 12 references, presents actual cases related to a number of legal problems nurses may have. Many nursing journals have monthly or occasional law columns, as well as timely articles. Checking nonnursing journals such as those cited above is also useful, since some of their articles relate specifically to nursing, and others provide a context for legal trends.

CHAPTER 13 Nursing Organizations and Publications

Fitzgerald L. Career enhancement via chapter involvement: Region 3—Sigma Theta Tau International. *Reflections* 20:14, Winter, 1994.

Fondiller S. Writing for publication. *Am J Nurs* 94:62, 64–65, August, 1994.

Fowler MDM. Professional associations, ethics, and society. *Oncol Nurs Forum* 20:13–19, November–December, 1993.

Gaines JE. Join the crowd—reasons to join a professional nursing organization. *Minority Nurse* 29–31, Summer–Fall, 1994.

Hancock C. Managing national nurses' association: The UK example. *Int Nurs Rev* 40:135–139, September–October, 1993.

Hill MJ. Urgent: New syndrome identified—writophobia. *Dermatol Nurs* 6:304, October, 1994.

Joel L. Janus in the catbird seat: In defense of the editorial. *Am J Nurs* 95:7, October, 1995.

Kirchhoff KT. Ensuring accurate references. *Nurse Author Ed* 5:1–3, Winter, 1995.

Pierson PA. No comment—all of us have an obligation to learn for ourselves what is going on in our own professional organizations. *Nurse Pract Forum* 5:59, June, 1994.

Schira MG. Conducting the literature review. *J Neurosci Nurs* 24:54–58, February, 1992.

Sharp N. American College of Nurse Practitioners: Experiment in democracy. *Nurs Mgmt* 26:22–23, January, 1995.

Swanson EA, et al. Publishing opportunities for nurses: A comparison of 92 US journals. *Image* 23:33–38, Spring, 1991.

Topp R, Utter D. Developing a reciprocal program between student nurse organizations and hospitals. *Imprint* 40:63–65, February–March, 1993.

Watson M. Marketing a new image for nursing's association—Registered Nurses' Association of Ontario. *Regist Nurse* 6:27–29, August–September, 1994.

Wink DM. Student papers: Should they publish or perish? *Nurse Educ* 19:11–12, November–December, 1994.

CHAPTER 14 Job Selection

Andrica D. Competing in the new job market: Part 2—the interview. *Nurs Econ* 13:56–57, January–February, 1995.

Andrica D. Re-engineered out of your job: What next? *Nurs Econ* 13:181, May–June, 1995.

Bleich M, Sullivan J. How to make informed employment decisions. *AD Clin Care* 4:18–21, September–October, 1989.

Davidhizar F. Feeling like a nurse. *Imprint* 41:53–54, April–May, 1994.

Davidhizar R. Is this job for you? *Imprint* 40:11–15, January, 1993.

Ketter J. Surviving layoffs. *Am Nurs* 26:25, July–August, 1994.

Marcus J. *The Complete Job Interview Handbook*. New York: Harper Perennial, 1994.

Mullin M. Where in the world are the new grad jobs? *Imprint* 41:6, 8, January, 1994.

Netherton H. Tips on successful interviewing. *Imprint* 39:27, 29, January, 1992.

Rhores J, Young M. Surviving your first job. *Healthcare Trends Transit* 3:24–27, May, 1992.

Rodriguez K. Avoid interview turn-off to ensure success. *Am Nurse* 24:19, September, 1992.

Roeder B, Oglesby S. How to prepare for employment in the '90s. *Caring* 13:52–56, April, 1994.

Sands J. Avoiding the pitfalls of job hunting. *Healthcare Trends Transit* 3:52–57, November–December, 1991.

Sills F. Five strategies to survive your first interview. *Imprint* 40:31–32, January, 1993.

Stille P. Life insurance: An important part of the benefit pie. *Healthcare Trends Transit* 3:54, March, 1992.

Study explores nurses' attitudes about career issues. *Am Nurse* 25:12, October, 1993.

Vogel D. Writing a résumé. *Imprint* 40:35–36, January, 1993.

Washington R. A practical guide to interviewing. *Imprint* 37:38–39, December 1990–January 1991.

Wheeler I. Success in your first interview. *Imprint* 41:20, 37, January, 1994.

The November–December 1991 issue of *Healthcare Trends and Transition* is almost entirely devoted to job search. There are a number of nonnursing articles and books related to job search skills in the public library. Business journals, and especially career women's magazines, have also been emphasizing these topics. Any bookstore has a section devoted to career development; some of the books are best-sellers and may be found in paperback.

CHAPTER 15 Career Management

Avery LH. Future unclear as nurses face workplace redesign and job redeployment. *AORN J* 60:99–100, 102, 104–105, July, 1994.

Bailey B. How to float safely and effectively. *Nurs 90* 20:113–116, February, 1990.

Barrett V, Phillips JA. Reproductive health in the American workplace. *AAOHN J* 43:40–51, January, 1995.

Benoliel JQ, et al. Measurement of stress in clinical nursing. *Cancer Nurs* 13:221–228, August, 1990.

Bolivar E. Hemophilia and AIDS: Dealing with nurse burnout. *Caring* 10:50–54, July, 1991.

Buchan J. Lessons from America? US magnet hospitals and their implications for UK nursing. *J Adv Nurs* 19:373–384, February, 1994.

Coston B. Fighting through an appeals process. *RN* 57–59, February, 1995.

Curtin LL. Restructuring: What works and what does not. *Nurs Mgmt* 25:7–8, October, 1994.

DiBenedetto DV. Occupational hazards of the health care industry: Protecting health care workers. *AAOHN J* 43:131–137, March, 1995.

Duquette A, et al. Factors related to nursing burnout: A review of empirical knowledge. *Iss Ment Health Nurs* 15:337–358, July, 1994.

Dienemann J, Gessner T. Restructuring nursing care delivery systems. *Nurs Econ* 10:253–258, April, 1992.

Fuszard B, et al. Rural magnet hospitals of excellence, parts 1 & 2. *J Nurs Adm* 24:21–26, January, 1994; 24:35–41, February, 1994.

Godfrey C. Downsizing: Coping with personal pain. *Nurs Mgmt* 25:90–93, October, 1994.

Grant PS. Manage nurse stress and increase potential at the bedside. *Nurs Adm Quart* 18:16–22, Fall, 1993.

Horsley J. If you're let go without getting a detailed reason. *RN* 24, January, 1995.

Ignatavicius D, Hausman K. *Clinical Pathways for Collaborative Practice.* Philadelphia: Saunders, 1995.

Joel L. Collective bargaining: A positive force in the workplace. *Revolution* 3:26–29, Winter, 1993.

Kane D. Invest in yourself. Coping with multiple roles: Mother/wife/nurse. *Nurs Forum* 28:17–21, October–November, 1993.

Kerr P. A portfolio—a good way to market your nursing skills. *Info Nurs* 25:6–7, August, 1994.

Ketter J. Surviving layoffs. *Am Nurse* 26:25, July–August, 1994.

Lathrop JP. *Restructuring Healthcare; The Patient Focused Care Paradigm.* San Francisco: Jossey-Bass, 1993.

Lindborg C, Davidhizar R. Is there a difference in nurse burnout on the day or night shift? *Health Care Superv* 11: 47–52, March, 1993.

National League for Nursing. *Scholarships and Loans for Nursing Education, 1994–1995.* New York: NLN, 1994.

Rhorer JH, Young MJ. Surviving your first job. *Healthcare Trends Transit* 3:24–27, May, 1992.

Top 10 myths about hospital restructuring and healthcare reform: Reprinted from a special issue of *California Nurse* on RNs and healthcare restructuring produced by the California Nurses Association. *Revolution* 4:24–25, Fall, 1994.

Worthington K. Workplace hazards: The effect on nurses as women. *Am Nurse* 26:15, February, 1994.

Zuffoletto J. Supreme Court rules on a landmark sexual harassment case. *AORN J* 59:529–530, February, 1994.

APPENDIXES

1. Major Studies of the Nursing Profession
2. Major Health Care Services Personnel
3. Educational Options in Nursing
4. State Boards of Nursing (1995)
5. Major Nursing and Related Organizations
6. Specialty Certifications
7. Basics of Parliamentary Procedure
8. Distinguished Nurses of the Past: Fifty Nurses Who Made a Difference

Appendix 1 Major Studies of the Nursing Profession*

Study	Year	Sponsor; Project director	Key points; Recommendations; Impact
The Educational Status of Nursing	1912	American Society of Superintendents of Training Schools for Nurses; M. Adelaide Nutting, RN	Revealed many appalling working and living conditions of students, limited and poor teaching. No real action taken, but set precedent for later studies. Highlighted need for nursing schools to be independent of hospitals.
Nursing and Nursing Education in the United States	1923	Rockefeller Foundation; Josephine Goldmark (nonnurse researcher)	Found poor educational practices and often poor quality of teachers and students. Education for public health nurses should include postgraduate courses in public health nursing. High educational standards should be maintained. The average hospital school does not adequately prepare high-grade nurses; university schools should be developed and strengthened. Resulted in founding of Yale School of Nursing.
Nurses, Patients, and Pocketbooks (first study)	1928	Committee on Grading of Nursing Schools, with members from major nursing and health care organizations; partly funded by nurses; Dr. May Ayres Burgess (statistician)	Showed oversupply of nurses; serious unemployment and maldistribution; low salaries and poor working conditions; some serious incompetence, but both the public and physicians generally satisfied with nurses' services (primarily private duty). Should secure public support for nursing education; replace student nurses with graduates in hospitals.
An Activity Analysis of Nursing (second study)	1934	Committee on Grading of Nursing Schools; Ethel Johns and Blanche Pfefferkorn (lay persons)	First large-scale attempt to find out what nurses were actually doing on the job. Included an explanation of what constitutes good nursing care and a description of basic conditions calling for the services of a nurse.
Nursing Schools Today and Tomorrow (third study)	1934	Committee on Grading of Nursing Schools; Ethel Johns	Proposed characteristics of what a "professional" nurse should know and be able to do. Set forth conditions essential for growth and functioning of a professional school, including types of control, funding, and qualifications of faculty.

* Considerable detail on these studies is found in Kelly and Joel, *Dimensions of Professional Nursing*, 7th ed. New York: McGraw-Hill, 1995, Chapter 5.

Study	Year	Sponsor; Project director	Key points; Recommendations; Impact
Study of Incomes, Salaries and Employment Conditions Affecting Nurses (exclusive of those engaged in public health nursing)	1938	American Nurses Association (ANA)	Data from 11,000 questionnaires returned by private-duty, institutional, and office nurses. Had considerable bearing on the development of the ANA economic security program.
Administrative Cost Analysis for Nursing Service and Nursing Education	1940	National League of Nursing Education (NLNE); American Hospital Association (AHA); ANA	Provided data on the cost of a school of nursing to the hospital and the economic value of services rendered by students. No real action taken.
The General Staff Nurse	1941	ANA, NLNE, AHA, Catholic Hospital Association (CHA) (joint committee)	Indicated that staff nurses had little status, as reflected by their hours of duty (often split shifts), salaries, and personnel policies. Gave impetus to the movement to upgrade staff nurses' status.
Nursing for the Future	1948	Carnegie Foundation; Russell Sage Foundation; National Nursing Council (representatives of various health organizations); Esther Lucile Brown, PhD (social anthropologist)	Pointed out continued inadequacies of schools of nursing; emphasized need for official examination of all, with publication of names of accredited schools and pressure to eliminate those not accredited. Found nursing education "not professional." Nursing education should be part of the mainstream of education. Nurses could be divided into "professional" and "practical" categories. Mixed reviews. Similar recommendations given in other reports 20 years later.

Appendix 1 (continued)

Study	Year	Sponsor; Project director	Key points; Recommendations; Impact
Nursing Schools at the Mid-Century	1950	National Committee for the Improvement of Nursing Services (committee of members of all six national nursing organizations); Russell Sage Foundation; Margaret Bridgman, RN EdD (former Academic Dean)	Reported on practices of over 1000 schools of nursing (organization, cost, curriculum content, clinical resources, student health). Gave schools the opportunity to evaluate their performance; stimulated improvement in baccalaureate schools.
Twenty Thousand Nurses Tell Their Story	1958	ANA and American Nurses Foundation (ANF); Dr. Everett C. Hughes (professor of sociology)	Part of a five-year sequence of 34 studies of nursing functions. Funded in part by individual nurses. Intended to produce better patient care; revealed what nurses actually did, their attitudes about the job, and job satisfaction. Formed basis for development of ANA nursing functions, standards, and qualifications.
Community College Education for Nursing	1959	Institute of Research and Service in Nursing Education Teachers College, Columbia University; Mildred Montag, RN EdD (nursing professor)	Report of five-year Cooperative Research Project in Junior and Community College Education for Nursing, based on Montag's doctoral study. Included evaluation of seven two-year nursing programs leading to an associate degree (AD) in nursing. A second part presented data from 811 graduates. Influenced establishment of more AD programs.
Toward Quality in Nursing: Needs and Goals	1963	Consultant Group on Nursing—panel of nurses, others in the health field and the public; Apollinia Adams, RN (special assistant to Division of Nursing Chief)	Report to US Surgeon General to advise him on nursing needs and to identify the role of the federal government in ensuring adequate nursing service for the nation. Noted qualitative and quantitative shortages of nursing personnel, problems in recruiting and retaining nurses, need for more nursing research, and improvement of nursing education and administration. Recommended study of nursing education and federal funding for nursing.

Study	Year	Sponsor; Project director	Key points; Recommendations; Impact
An Abstract for Action (Report of the National Commission on Nursing and Nursing Education)	1970	ANA, ANF, National League for Nursing (NLN), Avalon (Mellon) and Kellogg Foundations; Jerome Lysaught EdD (nonnurse educator)	Analyzed current practices and patterns of nursing and assessed future needs. Included observations and analysis of findings from other studies. Feedback from various groups reiterated many of Brown's findings and recommendations from 1948. Recommended joint practice committees of physicians and nurses, state master planning committees for nursing education, federal funding for nursing research and education, different approaches to nursing curriculum, degree programs in diploma schools. Got mixed reviews. Followed by new federal funding (for a short time), short term joint practice committees. Later follow-up showed little lasting impact.
Extending the Scope of Nursing Practice: A Report of the Secretary's Committee to Study Extended Roles	1971	US Deparment of Health Education and Welfare (DHEW); Faye Abdellah, RN, EdD (Assistant Surgeon General)	Appointed by Secretary Elliott Richardson. Reviewed current responsibilities of nurses; noted nurses' role on the health team. Recommended: curricular innovations demonstrating physician-nurse team concept in health care delivery; financial support for educating nurses in extended role; economic studies to assess impact of extended nursing practice on health care system. Resulted in federal funding and growth of nurse practitioner programs.
The Study of Credentialing in Nursing: A New Approach	1979	ANA; Inez Hinsvark, RN, EdD (nursing professor)	Consisted of a comprehensive review of credentialing, especially health care and nursing. (Contains excellent information.) Followed by appointment of a Task Force to implement recommendations. Reaffirmed earlier recommendation to establish free-standing credentialing center for nursing. Not accepted by nursing organizations.

Appendix 1 (continued)

Study	Year	Sponsor; Project director	Key points; Recommendations; Impact
Magnet Hospitals: Attraction and Retention of Nurses	1983	American Academy of Nursing (AAN), AAN Task Force on Nursing Practice; Margaret McClure, RN, EdD, chair (nurse executive)	Identified US hospitals able to attract and retain RNs. Studied 41 (questionnaires, interviews). Findings included the importance of well-prepared nurse managers and chief nurse executives; good nurse executives (seen as strong, supportive, visible); clearly enunciated high standards; participatory management; good personnel policies and competitive salaries; career development opportunities.
Nursing and Nursing Education; Public Policies and Private Actions	1983	DHHS contracted to the Institute of Medicine (IOM) Study Committee; included some nurses; Dr. Katharine Bauer (nonnurse)	Mandated by PL 96-76, the Nurse Training Act Amendments of 1979, to determine whether further substantial outlays of federal monies for nursing education were needed to ensure an adequate supply of nurses. Recommended in part that various combinations of public and private support be applied to financial aid for nursing students in basic programs, graduate programs and students in NP programs, to upgrade skills of RNs, LPNs, and aides in LTC facilities; improvement of supply and job tenure by addressing employment conditions; continued support for collection and analysis of nursing data; establishment of a federal organizational entity for nursing research. Seen as influential in establishment of National Center for Nursing Research (NCNR).

Study	Year	Sponsor; Project director	Key points; Recommendations; Impact
National Commission on Nursing Study	1983	American Hospital Association (AHA); Hospital Research and Educational Trust; American Hospital Supply Corporation. Independent Commission; members from various fields, including nursing; Marjorie Beyers, RN, PhD	Primarily initiated in response to the nursing shortage. Final report much weaker than initial report, probably due to need for compromise to further implementation. Stated need for all types of nursing programs, with baccalaureate education as an "achievable goal"; promoted educational mobility. Omitted statement urging utilization of nurses according to educational background. Other recommendations: high priority for nursing research; strong affiliations between academic institutions and practice settings; involvement of nursing in hospital policymaking; recognition of nursing as a clinical practice; salaries and benefits commensurate with nurses' education, experience, and performance.
Secretary's Commission on Nursing	1988	DHHS; Lillian Gibbons, RN, PhD	Established in response to widespread nursing shortage, to advise the DHHS Secretary, Dr. Otis Bowen. Documented pervasive and serious nursing shortage and reinforced themes of previous nursing shortage studies concerning need for improvement of status and working conditions of nurses. Demand for nurses seen as increasing. To increase supply, saw need for increased financial support for education, improved program accessibility, promoting nursing as a career.
Nursings' Vital Signs: Shaping the Profession for the 1990s	1989	Tri-Council, made up of ANA, NLN, American Association of Colleges of Nursing (AACN), American Organization of Nurse Executives (AONE); Vivien De Back, RN, PhD	NCNIP was launched (1984–1991) with Kellogg Foundation funding to implement selected recommendations of the IOM and the National Commission on Nursing Reports. Described innovative approaches and strategies developed by the work groups on education, management and practice, research, and development. Distributed a number of brochures and documents offering recommendations for the future of nursing.
Report of the National Commission on Nursing Implementation Project (NCNIP)	1991		

Appendix 1   (continued)

Study	Year	Sponsor; Project director	Key points; Recommendations; Impact
			Also noted that NPs and CNMs not used to fullest, in part due to lack of reimbursement. Held number of conferences on differentiated practice (nursing assignments according to competence, experience, and educational background); nursing information systems; and nurses' contribution to health care. Developed proposal for Advertising Council to clarify image of nursing. Successful National Nursing Image Campaign seen as partially responsible for increasing nursing school enrollments. Project concluded in 1991; seen as fostering coalitions between nursing and other groups.
Secretary's Commission on the National Nursing Shortage (CONNS)	1990	DHHS; 15 member committee representing nursing, other providers, third party payers, data policy field representatives, the public and ex-officio government representatives; Caroline Burnett, RN ScD.	Appointed for one year by DHHS Secretary, Dr. Louis Sullivan, to advise federal officials on projects to implement the recommendations of the 1988 report. Analyzed ongoing public and private sector initiatives related to 3 focal areas; developed 4 projects and 10 recommendations. First project focused on recruitment, educational pathways, retention and career development in long-term care facilities. Two projects in second focal area (restructuring nursing service, use of nursing personnel, information systems and related technology). One, a study of nurse-midwives in primary care settings; the other on case management. Recommendations were made related to the third focal area, data collection and analysis requirements as well as first 2 areas. Follow-through on recommendations not evident, perhaps because nursing shortage eased.

Study	Year	Sponsor; Project director	Key points; Recommendations; Impact
Health Professions Education for the Future: Schools in Service to the Nation	1993	Pew Health Professions Commission (funded by Pew Charitable Trusts); E.H. O'Neill	Follow-up on 1991 report that declared education and training of health professions not adequate to meet health needs of American people. This report reinforced that belief, with sections on various health professions, including nursing. Listed competencies needed for 2005. Pointed out difficulties in making these changes, particularly reluctance of academics. Cited value of nurse-midwives and nurse practitioners, importance of nurses in care of aging, in health promotion and disease prevention, in providing cost-effective care, and in management of care. Proposed 6 strategies for nursing education. Also made strong policy recommendations for federal and state governments, the health professions, and higher education.

Appendix 2 Major Health Care Services Personnel

Occupation/ profession	Estimated active supply[a]	Basic education[b]			
		One year or less	Associate degree, or 2- or 3- year program	Baccalaureate	Professional/ graduate[c]
Primary Care					
Chiropractor (DC)	53,000			×	4 years
Clinical psychologist	57,000			×	4 years +
Dentist (DD)	149,000			3 years min.	3–4 years +
Doctor of medicine (MD)	653,062			3 years min.	5 years +
Doctor of optometry (OD)	30,770			3 years min.	4 years
Doctor of osteopathy (DO)	34,050			3 years min.	4 years +
Doctor of podiatric medicine (DPM) (Podiatrist)	12,500			3 years min.	4 years
Nurse-midwife (CNM)[f]	6,000		(×)	(×)	×
Nurse practitioner (NP)[f]	49,000		(×)	(×)	×
Nursing (all areas except primary care)					
Registered nurse (RN)	Approximately 2.2 million		(×)	(×)	(1–3 years)

Salaries[d] ($ per yr/1994)	State regulation:[e] licensure; certification; registration	Major issues and trends
	× [g]	Not accepted as legitimate by some health care providers, especially MDs. After battle, recognized in all states as primary care providers, with reimbursement, including Medicare and Medicaid.
	× [g]	Competing with psychiatrists and others in mental health for patients. Seeking prescriptive authority.
88,000	× [g]	Oversupply. Some dental schools closing or admitting fewer. Emphasis on specialization, notably preventive dentistry.
171,380	× [g]	Oversupply predicted by 2000, especially specialists. Others encroaching on their practice. Less control. More becoming employees. More are marketing services.
82.500	× [g]	Education expanding to prepare better for diagnosis and treatment; MDs object. Growth in pediatric, rehabilitative, and geriatric optometry.
	× [g]	Still growing; oversupply not reported, perhaps because most in primary care as opposed to specialties.
	× [g]	Struggling with MDs to expand practice. Residency programs (advanced training) expanding, although not required. Want more liberal hospital privileges. Concern about wages, autonomy, federal funding.
43,636	× [g]	More middle-class women want their services; more MDs trying to limit their practice. Major insurance crisis with soaring rates resulted in first nurse self-insurance. Only half employed in practices that include deliveries. Lay midwives are seeking legal recognition.
43,636	× [g]	More states allowing for expanded practice, prescriptive authority, reimbursement and clinical privileges. Still difficult to have independent practice. MD opposition continues. New employment market in hospitals.
39,332	× [g]	Greater movement to higher education. New opportunities outside of hospitals. Oversupply in some geographic areas.

Appendix 2   **(continued)**

Occupation/ profession	Estimated active supply[a]	Basic education[b]			
		One year or less	Associate degree, or 2- or 3-year program	Baccalaureate	Professional/ graduate[c]
Licensed practical nurse (LPN)	644,000	×			
Clinical nurse specialist (CNS)[f]	58,000			×	1–2 years
Nurse anesthetist (CRNA)[f]	25,000			×	1–2 years
Nursing assistant (NA), home health aid (not including mental health)	850,000+	×			
Others providing direct services or therapy					
Art, music, dance therapists	NA			(×)	(×)
Dental assistant	201,000	(×)	(×)		
Dental hygienist	100,000		×		
Dietitians	67,000			×	1 year
Dietetic technician Assistant	16,000	(×)	(×)		
Emergency medical technician (EMT)	100,000	(×)	(×)		
Pharmacist	161,900			5 years	1–2 years (PharmD)

Salaries[d] ($ per yr/1994)	State regulation:[e] licensure; certification; registration	Major issues and trends
22,880	× [g]	Fewer being employed in hospitals. Nursing homes major employer. Longer educational program being suggested. More continuing to RN.
41,226	× [g]	In public policies to allow for expanded practice, reimbursement, prescriptive authority, and clinical privileges have been included with NPs under the title of advanced practice registered nurse. Some beginning to assume primary care role with the chronically ill. Mostly salaried in health care facilities, and sometimes seen as unnecessary when finances become tight.
80,900	×	Proven history of safety and effectiveness, but constant struggle to remain free of anesthesiologist oversight.
	×	Many in nursing homes. Low salaries continue. Some increase in hospital employment to reduce numbers of higher paid workers. Being encouraged to continue education to LPN, then RN level. Requirements for training and certification to work in nursing homes and as homehealth aides in some states.
		Growing market with the aged and disabled. Therapeutic role is not fully understood. Often seen as a frill in hard economic times.
18,304	×	
38,480	× [g]	More seeking independent practice, not controlled by dentist, and role expansion; dentists objecting. Some giving anesthesia.
35,900		Some see need for licensure; achieved in few states. Concern about image, third-party reimbursement.
20,350		More delegation from dietitian in management and routine diet instruction; assistants suggested for broader role in nursing home.
27,600	× [g]	Some struggle with nursing because of their use as nurse substitutes, especially in emergency rooms.
45,430	× [g]	Looking for ways to expand role. Some as clinical pharmacists, some in primary care (like the NP). PharmD wanted as entry-level degree. External degree programs for pharmacists who want PharmD. Lobbying for prescriptive authority.

Appendix 2 (continued)

Occupation/ profession	Estimated active supply[a]	Basic education[b]			
		One year or less	Associate degree, or 2- or 3-year program	Baccalaureate	Professional/ graduate[c]
Pharmacy assistant	53,885	(×)	(×)		
Physician's assistant (PA)	23,000		(×)	(×)	
Psychiatric mental health technician	71,508	(×)	(×)		
Respiratory therapist	73,529	(×)	(×)	×	
Surgical technologist (OR technician)	43,689	(×)	(×)		
Therapeutic recreational specialist	30,201		(×)	(×)	
Diagnostic Services					
Clinical laboratory technicians			×		
Technologists	267,675				×
EEG technician	6,349	(×)	(×)		
EKG technician	16,470	(×)	(×)		
Nuclear medicine technologist	12,197		×		
Radiologic technologist (x-ray technician)	162,044	(×)	(×)	(×)	
Administration, Business, Record-keeping					
Health services managers and administrators	274,000			(×)	(×)
Medical records administrator (RRA)	18,000			(×)	(×)
Technician (HRT)	69,000	×			

Salaries[d] ($ per yr/1994)	State regulation:[e] licensure; certification; registration	Major issues and trends
49,500	× [g]	Programs expected to grow. Being used in hospitals instead of residents. Must work under direction of MD. Many states permit prescribing. Some competition with NPs. Some going on to nursing or public health. Now equal number of women and men.
	×	Much used in state, local government hospitals. RN concern about overuse, competence. Low salary.
31,200	×	Disagreement as to whether nurses should reassume some of these responsibilities. Increased demand in hospitals.
22,880		Disagreement as to whether OR nursing should include this role; report to nurse or MD. Low salary.
33,600		Growing market with the elderly and disabled.
33,800	×	More complex technology and computers being used. Some leaving because of fear of AIDS.
26,520	×	Low salaries at technician and assistant level.
25,792		Low salaries.
25,792		Low salaries, and anticipated decline in job market due to new technology.
31,350		More complex technology.
33,000	× [g]	Becoming more complex with subspecialization in field. Major shortage, due to increase in nonintrusive testing.
		Oversupply in hospitals as they reduce administrative and middle management positions. Need for strategic planners, financially astute people cited.
	×	Great need predicted, especially because of importance of records for reimbursement; more
24,800		computer use.

Appendix 2 (continued)

Occupation/ profession	Estimated active supply[a]	Basic education[b]			
		One year or less	Associate degree, or 2- or 3-year program	Baccalaureate	Professional/ graduate[c]
Medical secretary-unit clerk	NA	(×)	(×)		
Unit (ward) manager	NA	(×)	(×)	(×)	

Rehabilitation, Counseling, and Social Support

Denturist (dental technician)	70,000		(×) or apprenticeship		
Occupational therapist (OT)	37,600			(×)	(×)
Assistant	8,000	(×)	(×)		
Optician	63,070	(×)	(×) or apprenticeship		
Physical therapist (PT)	90,242			(×)	(×)
Technician	61,003	×			
Rehabilitation counselor	NA			×	
Speech pathologist/ audiologist	86,700			×	×
Medical social worker	60,000			(×)	(×)
Vocational rehabilitation therapist	NA			×	

Public/Community Health; Environment

Community/school health educator	NA			×	

Salaries[d] ($ per yr/1994)	State regulation:[e] licensure; certification; registration	Major issues and trends
		Computer affecting how a job is done.
		May be entering position for management career ladder.
	×	Looking for independent practice, free of dentists.
37,250	×	More needed in home care. Major shortage now.
27,500		
43,680	× ×	Great demand; many have private practices; more needed in home care where they often assume the role of primary provider. Major shortage, yet admissions to educational programs are very competitive. Cardiac rehab and sports medicine are growth areas.
		Some competition with other rehabilitation groups.
44,000	×[g]	Growing fields; more with graduate education.
27,250	×[g]	Looking for ways to expand role. Overlap with others. Competing with nurses in case management. Move towards doctorates. More needed.
		Some competition with social workers; governmental positions may decrease with budget cuts.
		Expanding role as prevention/health promotion is funded; some competition with nurses.

Appendix 2   (continued)

Occupation/ profession	Estimated active supply[a]	Basic education[b]			
		One year or less	Associate degree, or 2- or 3- year program	Baccalaureate	Professional/ graduate[c]
Environmentalist (sanitarian)	NA			(×)	(×)
Industrial hygienists and safety technicians	NA		(×)	(×)	

[a] Figures cited are from the eighth *Report to Congress on Health Personnel in the United States.* Washington, DC: DHHS, PHS, HRSA, 1992. These numbers represent individuals. Other figures have been obtained from occupational/professional associations and from the US Department of Labor's Bureau of Labor Statistics, Office of Employment Projections. Numbers from the latter source represent jobs, but in general are an adequate proxy for estimating the number of individuals in an occupation. Where there was a choice, the individual count from HRSA or the occupational association has been used.

[b] (×) indicates optional routes to occupational preparation. An absence of brackets notes the prevailing or required education for entry into practice.

[c] Usually assumes liberal arts or other baccalaureate that does not include clinical work; thus, number of years of preprofessional study or a cross, indicating the completion of an undergraduate degree, will also appear.

Salaries[d] **($ per yr/1994)**	**State regulation:**[e] **licensure; certification; registration**	**Major issues and trends**
29,000		More complex problems to deal with because of new discoveries of environmental dangers.
		May be under pressure in work situations because of adversarial relations between labor and management.

[d] Salaries cited come from the *Occupational Outlook Handbook* (May 1994) of the US Department of Labor, and from the occupational/professional associations representing these groups. The variation in salaries based on geography, specialization and employer (public/private sector/self-employed) was significant, but there was an attempt to average across areas. In many instances there was no salary information, or reporting was so varied as to be useless. Where official information gave hourly earnings, they were converted to an annual salary to allow comparison between groups. The assumption in that case was a 40 hour week and a 52 week year.

[e] Either voluntary or mandatory credentialing in at least one state. States can vary dramatically.

[f] Have a basic license as an RN, but may be required to hold a second governmental credential as a CNM, NP, CRNA, or CNS. In each instance, basic nursing education may be from AD to baccalaureate or higher, and specialty preparation for the CNM and NP may be nondegree or graduate.

[g] Mandatory continuing education in at least one state; again inconsistent state to state.

Appendix 3 Educational Options in Nursing

Types	Approximate number of programs (1995)	Program sites	Program length	Admission require-ments[a]	Cost per year tuition and fees (1996)
Practical/ vocational nursing education	1090	Vocational/ technical school; junior college; hospital; high school/in-dependent agency/ college (rarely)	9–12 months	High school or equivalent unless program is in high school.	$1585 public; $4731 private
Associate degree (AD) education	868	Junior/ community, technical college;	2 aca-demic years (12–18	College require-ments. High school or	$500–1800 public; $7000 private

Curriculum	Credential[b]	Educational mobility	Competencies at graduation[c]
Basic theory on illness and health. Introductory biological and social sciences. About two-thirds of time in clinical settings.	Certificate; diploma; associate degree[d], LPN/LVN license after NCLEX-PN.	Career ladder usually with testing into RN programs. External AD or BSN degrees available.	1. Practices in a variety of settings including hospitals, nursing homes and home care, functioning under the guidance and supervision of an RN, physician, or dentist, to provide basic therapeutic, rehabilitative and preventive care to patients with well-defined health problems. 2. Directs the activities of personnel assistive to nursing in long-term care facilities and nursing homes. 3. Assesses basic physical, emotional, spiritual, and sociocultural needs of the health care client and provides appropriate nursing care. 4. Collects data within established protocols and guidelines from various sources. 5. Utilizes knowledge of normal values to identify deviations in health status. 6. Documents data collection. 7. Communicates findings to appropriate health care personnel, recording accurately. 8. Contributes to the development of nursing care plans utilizing established nursing diagnoses for clients with common, well-defined health problems. 9. Prioritizes nursing care needs of clients. 10. Assists in the review and revision of nursing care plans to meet the changing needs of clients. 11. Establishes and maintains therapeutic relationships with clients, families, and significant others.

Adapted from K. Beaver et al, *Entry-level Competencies of Graduates of Educational Programs in Practical Nursing*, 2nd ed. New York: National League for Nursing, 1989 (currently under revision).

Basic natural and social sciences, ˙umanities;	Associate degree. Licensure after passing	Most of non-nursing courses transfer to baccalaureate. May	1. Functions as a generalist in a structured setting where policies, procedures, and protocols for health care are established.

Appendix 3 **(continued)**

Types	Approximate number of programs (1995)	Program sites	Program length	Admission require-ments[a]	Cost per year tuition and fees (1996)
Associate degree (*continued*)		senior college; hospital (rarely)	months) to 2 calendar years	equivalent. Specific courses may be required to enter nursing program.	
Diploma education	124	Hospital	Usually 24–30 months;	High school or equiva-lent. Good	$2826 public; $5500 private

Curriculum	Credential[b]	Educational mobility	Competencies at graduation[c]
nursing courses; supervised experiences in hospital and other agencies. About half program is general education.	NCLEX-RN. Some certification later if exams passed.[g]	need to test for advanced standing in nursing. Some programs have direct articulation. External BSN degree available	2. Develops, implements, and evaluates a nursing plan, using established nursing diagnoses and data related to the client's cultural, spiritual, psychosocial, and physical needs, to promote, maintain, and restore health; revises plan as needed. 3. Provides direct care for clients with common well-defined diagnoses, using the nursing process; establishes priorities for care. 4. Administers and monitors the medical regimen for clients undergoing therapeutic and/or diagnostic procedures. 5. Communicates effectively, verbally and in writing, concerning client's response to treatment, and uses communication techniques that assist client and significant others to cope with and resolve problems. 6. Modifies and implements teaching plan as needed, collaborating with other health care workers. 7. Recognizes need for referral, confers with other appropriate personnel, and makes referral. 8. Delegates aspects of care appropriately to LPNs and ancillary personnel, and is accountable for care delegated. 9. Provides for continuity of care in management of chronic health care needs. 10. Recognizes the importance of nursing research.

Adapted from *Educational Outcomes of Associate Degree Nursing Programs: Roles and Competencies.* New York: National League for Nursing, 1990 (currently under revision); and *Defining and Differentiating ADN and BSN Competencies* (MAIN, 1985).

Natural and social sciences,	Diploma. Licensure after passing	College courses may transfer. May need to test	1. Provides nursing care for individuals, families, and groups by utilizing the nursing process.

Appendix 3   **(continued)**

Types	Approximate number of programs (1995)	Program sites	Program length	Admission require-ments[a]	Cost per year tuition and fees (1996)
Diploma education (*continued*)			could be three years	academic achieve-ment. Pre-requisite courses.	
Baccalaureate education	509	College; university; hospital[e]	4 aca-demic years	Admission requirement for institution and program. Good academic standing.	$2,845 public; $11,000 private

Curriculum	Credential[b]	Educational mobility	Competencies at graduation[c]
sometimes from a college. Nursing courses, early clinical experience focused on hospital nursing.	NCLEX-RN.[d] Some certification later if pass exam.[g]	for advanced standing in nursing, BSN external degree available.	2. Provides for the promotion, maintenance, and restoration of health, and support and comfort to the suffering and dying. 3. Utilizes management skills including collaboration, coordination, and communication with individuals, families, groups, and other members of the health care team. 4. Assumes a leadership role within the health care system. 5. Teaches individuals, families, and groups based on identified health needs. 6. Functions as an advocate for the consumer and the health care system to improve the quality and delivery of care. 7. Practices nursing based on a theoretical body of knowledge, ethical principles, and legal standards. 8. Evaluates nursing practice for improvement of nursing care. 9. Accepts responsibility and accountability for professional practice. 10. Utilizes opportunities for continuing personal and professional development. 11. Participates in health-related community services. 12. Utilizes critical thinking in professional practice.

Adapted from *Role and Competencies of Graduates of Diploma Programs in Nursing*, 2d ed. New York: National League for Nursing, 1989 (currently under revision).

			AD competencies plus:
About one-half liberal arts and sciences. Nursing theory and practice last 2 years. Clinical	Bachelor of Science. Other baccalaureate. Licensure after passing NCLEX-RN.	Can advance directly to graduate work if other qualifications met.	1. Practices as a generalist in all settings. Provides comprehensive services of assessing, promoting, and maintaining physical and mental health of individuals, families, groups, and aggregates (populations with shared characteristics of environment).

Appendix 3   **(continued)**

Types	Approximate number of programs (1995)	Program sites	Program length	Admission require-ments[a]	Cost per year tuition and fees (1996)
Baccalaureate education (*continued*)					
Graduate education (entry into practice)	2 doctorate programs	University	2–3 academic years	Baccalaureate in any field. May require prerequisite courses. Mature; high academic standing or other achievements.	(Relates to all) Graduate education tuition varies greatly according to type of program and region. Annual tuition may be anywhere from $3500 to $25,000 more or less.

Curriculum	Credential[b]	Educational mobility	Competencies at graduation[c]
experience in many settings including public health.	Certification later if pass exam.[g]		2. Plans, implements evaluates, and directs care for clients, including those with complex health care needs, assuming a leadership role. 3. Interprets medical plan of care into nursing activities. 4. Evaluates nursing research for applicability to nursing actions and incorporates appropriate findings after consulting with nurse researcher. 5. Collaborates with colleagues and citizens in identifying and effecting needed changes in health care. 6. Synthesizes theoretical and empirical knowledge from nursing, scientific, and humanistic disciplines with practice. 7. Enhances the quality of nursing and health practices within practice settings through the use of leadership skills and a knowledge of the political system. 8. Evaluates research for the applicability of its findings to nursing practice.

Adapted from *Characteristics of Baccalaureate Education in Nursing.* New York: National League for Nursing, 1987 (currently under revision) and *Defining and Differentiating ADN and BSN Competencies* (MAIN 1985).

| Nursing theory and practice. Nursing sciences if not prerequisite. Clinical experience in diverse settings. | Doctor of Nursing (ND). Licensure after passing NCLEX-RN. Certification later if pass exam. | Continue to specialization master's and doctorates. | Similar to baccalaureate, but some of the time may be devoted to specialization. ND particularly geared to scientific inquiry. |

Appendix 3 **(continued)**

Types	Approximate number of programs (1995)	Program sites	Program length	Admission requirements[a]	Cost per year tuition and fees (1996)
Graduate education (*continued*)					Part-time $330 per credit mean. Can be much higher.
Master's (advanced)	278	University	1–3 academic years	Nursing baccalaureate usually necessary;[f] good academic standing; standardized tests; and samples of writing are commonly required.	
Doctorate	60	University	1–2 academic years beyond master's plus dissertation	Same as master's, but have good academic standing in graduate study and research capabilities. Other special requirements such as standardized tests (GRE Millers analogy), and samples of writing or master's-level research acumen are common.	

Curriculum	Credential[b]	Educational mobility	Competencies at graduation[c]
Nursing theory and practice in clinical specialization, administration, or education. Research and theory development courses. Research, advanced theory, and practice in selected field. Science and interdisciplinary courses (cognates) to support area of specialization.	Master of science. Other Master's. Certification if pass test.[g] DNS, PhD, Ed.D. other doctorates.	After masters acceptance to doctoral study if qualified. Post-doctoral study available.	Builds on baccalaureate plus: 1. Practices in a specialized health care setting as clinical specialist/ nurse practitioner or clinician with specialized clinical knowledge and skills caring for individuals, family, groups, or aggregates. Nurse administrators or nurse educators may have and use some or all of these clinical skills in performing their functions. 2. Acts as consultant to colleagues in nursing, other health disciplines, agencies, and organizations. 3. As clinician, provides additional insight in coordinating medical and nursing care plans. 4. Collaborates as equal with other disciplines. 5. Initiates nursing research and collaborates in research with nursing and other colleagues. 6. Improves nursing and health care through expert practice and through the advancement of theory in practice. 7. Assumes leadership role in development of nursing as profession and as influential part of health care delivery and policy making. 8. Collaborates with colleagues and citizens in identifying and effecting needed changes in health care.

[a] Most programs require references and some indication of motivation to succeed in a field. This becomes very important in acceptance for advanced education. Many require a standardized test.
[b] All nursing programs have the option of seeking accreditation by the National League for Nursing.
[c] All speak to ethical and legal practice and accountability.
[d] North Dakota requires AD for LPN and BSN for RN. Other states may follow.
[e] A few states have permitted some hospital based schools to give degrees.
[f] Some programs accept nurses with nonnursing baccalaureates, requiring completion of prerequisite courses.
[g] Certification for practice competency is possible without the baccalaureate in some specialty areas, but the BSN is fast becoming the standard. Certification as a specialist requires the master's degree. Both levels award the credential after successful testing and documented specialty practice and educational experiences.

Appendix 4   State Boards of Nursing (1995)

Alabama

Alabama Board of Nursing
PO Box 303900
Montgomery, Alabama 36130–8900

Street address:
RSA Plaza, Suite 250
770 Washington Avenue
Montgomery, Alabama 36130–8900

Alaska

Alaska Board of Nursing
PO Box 110806
Juneau, Alaska 99811–086

Street address:
Department of Commerce and
   Economic Development
Div. of Occupational Licensing
3601 C Street, Suite 722
Anchorage, Alaska 99503

American Samoa

American Samoa Health Service
Regulatory Board
LBJ Tropical Medical Center
Pago Pago, American Samoa 96799
Telex No. 782-573-LBJ TMC

Arizona

Arizona State Board of Nursing
1651 E. Morten Ave., Suite 150
Phoenix, Arizona 85020

Arkansas

Arkansas State Board of Nursing
University Tower Building, Suite 800
1123 South University
Little Rock, Arkansas 72204

California–RN

California Board of Registered
   Nursing
PO Box 944210
Sacramento, California 94244–2100

Street address:
400 R. Street, Suite 4030
Sacramento, California 95814–6200

Colorado

Colorado Board of Nursing
1560 Broadway, Suite 670
Denver, Colorado 80202

Connecticut

Connecticut Board of Examiners
   for Nursing
150 Washington Street
Hartford, Connecticut 06106

For exam information:
Examinations and Licensure Div.
   of Medical Quality Assurance
Connecticut Dept. of Health
   Services
150 Washington Street
Hartford, Connecticut 06106

Delaware

Delaware Board of Nursing
Margaret O'Neill Building
PO Box 1401
Dover, Delaware 19903

District of Columbia

District of Columbia Board
   of Nursing
614 H Street, NW
Washington
District of Columbia 20001

Florida

Florida Board of Nursing
111 Coastline Drive East
Suite 516
Jacksonville, Florida 32202

For exam information:
Florida Dept. of Professional
   Regulation
1940 N. Monroe Street
Tallahassee, Florida 32399–0750

Georgia–RN

Georgia Board of Nursing
166 Pryor Street, SW
Atlanta, Georgia 30303

Guam

Guam Board of Nurse Examiners
PO Box 2816
Agana, Guam 96910

Hawaii

Hawaii Board of Nursing
PO Box 3469
Honolulu, Hawaii 96801

Idaho

Idaho Board of Nursing
PO Box 83720
Boise, Idaho 83720–0061

Illinois

Illinois Dept. of Professional
   Regulation
320 West Washington Street
3rd Floor
Springfield, Illinois 62786

Illinois Dept. of Professional
   Regulation
100 West Randolph, Suite 9-300
Chicago, Illinois 60601

Indiana

Indiana State Board of Nursing
   Health Professions Bureau
402 West Washington Street
Room #041
Indianapolis, Indiana 46204

Iowa

Iowa Board of Nursing
State Capitol Complex
1223 East Court Avenue
Des Moines, Iowa, 50319

Kansas

Kansas State Board of Nursing
Landon State Office Building
900 SW Jackson, Suite 551-S
Topeka, Kansas 66612–1230

Kentucky

Kentucky Board of Nursing
312 Wittington Parkway, Suite 300
Louisville, Kentucky 40222–5172

Louisiana

Louisiana State Board of Nursing
912 Pere Marquette Building
150 Baronne Street
New Orleans, Louisiana 70112

Maine

Maine State Board of Nursing
State House Station #158
Augusta, Maine 04333–0158

Maryland

Maryland Board of Nursing
4140 Patterson Avenue
Baltimore, Maryland 21215–2299

Massachusetts

Massachusetts Board of
   Registration in Nursing
Leverett Saltonstall Building
100 Cambridge Street, Room 1519
Boston, Massachusetts 02202

Michigan

Bureau of Occupational &
   Professional Regulation
Michigan Department of Commerce
Ottawa Towers North
611 West Ottawa
Lansing, Michigan 48933

For exam information:
Office of Testing Services
Michigan Dept. of Commerce
PO Box 30018
Lansing, Michigan 48909

Minnesota

Minnesota Board of Nursing
2700 University Avenue
   West 108
St. Paul, Minnesota 55114

Mississippi

Mississippi Board of Nursing
239 N. Lamar Street, Suite 401
Jackson, Mississippi 39201

Missouri

Missouri State Board of Nursing
PO Box 656
Jefferson City, Missouri 65102

Street address:
3605 Missouri Blvd.
Jefferson City, Missouri 65109

Montana

Montana State Board of Nursing
111 North Jackson
PO Box 200513
Helena, Montana 59620–0513

Nebraska

Bureau of Examining Boards
Nebraska Department of
Health.
PO Box 95007
Lincoln, Nebraska 68509

Street address:
301 Centennial Mall South
Lincoln, Nebraska 68508

Nevada

Nevada State Board of Nursing
PO Box 46886
Las Vegas, Nevada 89114

Street address:
4335 S. Industrial Road, Suite 430
Las Vegas, Nevada 89103

New Hampshire

New Hampshire Board of Nursing
Health & Welfare Building
6 Hazen Drive
Concord, New Hampshire
03301–6527

New Jersey

New Jersey Board of Nursing
PO Box 45010
Newark, New Jersey 07101

Street address:
124 Halsey Street, 6th Floor
Newark, New Jersey 07102

New Mexico

New Mexico Board of Nursing
4206 Louisiana Blvd N.E.
Suite A
Albuquerque, New Mexico 87109

New York

New York State Board of Nursing
State Education Department
Cultural Ed. Center, Room 3023
Albany, New York 12230

North Carolina

North Carolina Board of Nursing
PO Box 2129
Raleigh, North Carolina 27602

Street address:
3724 National Drive
Raleigh, North Carolina 27612

North Dakota

North Dakota Board of Nursing
919 South 7th Street, Suite 504
Bismarck, North Dakota 58504–5881

Northern Mariana Islands

Commonwealth Board of
   Nurse Examiners
Public Health Center
PO Box 1458
Saipan, MP 96950

Telex 783–744
Ask for Public Health Center
Answerback code PNES PN 744

Ohio

Ohio Board of Nursing
77 South High Street, 17th Floor
Columbus, Ohio 43266–0316

Oklahoma

Oklahoma Board of Nursing
2915 North Classen Blvd, Suite 524
Oklahoma City, Oklahoma 73106

Oregon

Oregon State Board of Nursing.
Suite 465
800 NE Oregon Street, Box 25
Portland, Oregon 97232

Pennsylvania

Pennsylvania State Board of Nursing
PO Box 2649
Harrisburg, Pennsylvania 17105–2649

Street address:
124 Pine Street
Harrisburg, Pennsylvania 17101

Puerto Rico

Commonwealth of Puerto Rico
Board of Nurse Examiners
Call Box 10200
Santurce, Puerto Rico 00903

Rhode Island

Rhode Island Board of Nurse
   Registration & Nursing Education
Cannon Health Building
Three Capitol Hill, Room 101
Providence, Rhode Island 02908–5097

South Carolina

South Carolina State Board of
   Nursing
220 Executive Center Drive
Suite 220
Columbia, South Carolina 29210

South Dakota

South Dakota Board of Nursing
3307 South Lincoln Avenue
Sioux Falls, South Dakota 57105–5224

Tennessee

Tennessee State Board of Nursing
283 Plus Park Blvd
Nashville, Tennessee 37217–1010

Texas–RN

Texas Board of Nurse Examiners
PO Box 140466
Austin, Texas 78714

Street address:
9101 Burnet Road
Austin, Texas 78758

Utah

Utah State Board of Nursing
Division of Occupational & Prof.
   Licensing
PO Box 45805
Salt Lake City, Utah 84145-0805

Street address:
Heber M. Wells Building, 4th Floor
160 East 300 South
Salt Lake City, Utah 84111

Vermont

Vermont State Board of Nursing
109 State Street
Montpelier, Vermont 05609-1106

For mailing UPS or Fed Ex:
81 River Street
Montpelier, Vermont 05602-1106

Virgin Islands

Virgin Islands Board of Nurse
   Licensure
PO Box 4247, Veterans Drive Station
St. Thomas, US Virgin Islands 00803

Street address:
Plot #3 Kongens Gade
St. Thomas, US Virgin Islands 00803

Virginia

Virginia Board of Nursing
6606 West Broad Street, 4th Floor
Richmond, Virginia 232309-1717

Washington

Washington State Nursing Care
Quality Assurance Commission
Department of Health
PO Box 47864
Olympia, Washington 98504–7864

West Virginia–RN

West Virginia Board of Examiners
for Registered Professional Nurses
101 Dee Drive
Charleston, West Virginia
25311–1620

Wisconsin

Wisconsin Dept. of Regulation &
Licensing
1400 East Washington Avenue
PO Box 8935
Madison, Wisconsin 53708–8935

Wyoming

Wyoming State Board of Nursing
Barrett Building, 2nd Floor.
2301 Central Avenue
Cheyenne, Wyoming 82002

Appendix 5 Major Nursing and Related Organizations

Organization and year established[a]	Membership eligibility[b]	Primary purpose	Membership size (approximate)
General Nursing Organizations			
American Nurses Association (ANA) 600 Maryland Ave. S.W., Washington, DC 20005 [1897]	Only state and territorial nurses' associations (SNA) are members. RN licensure for individual membership in SNA.	Work for improvement of health standards and availablity of care for all; foster high standards of nursing; stimulate and promote professional development of nurses and advance their economic and general welfare.	53 SNAs with a total of 200,000 members.
International Council of Nurses (ICN) 3, Place Jean-Marteau 1201, Geneva, Switzerland [1900]	National nurses' associations (NNAs).	Share knowledge so nursing practice throughout the world is improved; provide a medium through which NNAs may share common interests to promote health of people and care of the sick.	114 NNAs
National League for Nursing (NLN) 350 Hudson St., New York, NY 10014 [1893]	Anyone interested in fostering development and improvement of nursing service and education, and nursing service and education agencies.	Foster development and improvement of nursing services and nursing education through coordinated action of nursing and others, so that nursing needs of the people are met. Accredit nursing education and service agencies.[g]	41 state-affiliated leagues for nursing 1,950 agency members 11,672 individuals
National Student Nurses' Association (NSNA) 555 W. 57th St., New York, NY 10019 [1953]	Students in state approved programs leading to RN licensure or RNs enrolled in baccalaureate nursing programs.	Contribute to nursing education to provide for highest quality health care; CE; aid in development of student.	37,339

	Activities[c]					
Certifi-cation[d]	Standards set and published	Legislative activities[e]	Research activities[f]	Members of NFSNO[i]	NOLF	Publications[h] (journals, newsletters)
×[g]	×	×	×		×	*American Nurse; American Journal of Nursing; Capital Update; Center for Ethics and Human Rights Communique; Legal Developments; E&GN Update*
	×		×			*International Nursing Review*
[g]	×	×	×		×	*Nursing and Health Care: Perspectives on Community*
		×	×	×	×	*Imprint; Dean's Notes*

Appendix 5 (continued)

Speciality Nursing Organizations

Organization and year established[a]	Membership eligibility[b]	Primary purpose	Membership size (approximate)
Academy of Medical–Surgical Nurses (AMSN) East Holly Ave., Box 56 Pitman, NJ 08071 [1992]	RNs interested in the specialty.	Advance the practice of medical–surgical nursing through continuing education, establishing standards, providing peer support and a forum for the management of issues.	2,800
American Association of Critical-Care Nurses (AACN) 101 Columbia, Aliso Viejo, CA 92656 [1969]	RNs, LPNs, students and all those interested in care of the acutely and critically ill and their families.	Improve practice; provide CE for critical-care nurses; promote environments that facilitate comprehensive nursing practice for people with critical illness or injury.	78,000 in 270 chapters
American Association of Diabetes Educators (AADE) 444 N. Michigan Ave., Suite 1240 Chicago, IL 60611-3901	RNs interested in the specialty.	Support development of the specialty and maintenance of quality care.	10,032
American Association of Neuroscience Nurses (AANN) 218 N. Jefferson, Suite 204, Chicago, IL 60606 (related to World Federation of Neurosurgical Nursing) [1968]	RNs active or interested in neurological, neurosurgical nursing.	Foster and promote interest, education, research, and high standards in neurosurgical nursing and promote growth of nursing.	3,000
American Association of Nurse Anesthetists (AANA) 222 South Prospect Ave., Park Ridge, IL 60068 [1931]	Certified Registered Nurse Anesthetists (CRNA) and student NAs.	Advance science and art of anesthesia; promote cooperation with other disciplines; CE; develop standards.	26,500

			Activities[c]			
Certifi-cation[d]	Standards set and published	Legislative activities[e]	Research activities[f]	Members of NFSNO[i]	NOLF	Publications[h] (journals, newsletters)
			×	×	×	Med–Surg Nursing; AMSN News
×	×	×	×	×	×	Critical Care Nurse; Am J Critical Care; AACN Critical Issues; AACN Nursing Scan in Critical Care
×	×			×		NA
×	×	×	×	×	×	J of Neuroscience Nursing; Synapse
×[g]	×	×	×	×	×	AANA Journal; AANA Newsletter

Appendix 5   (continued)

Organization and year established[a]	Membership eligibility[b]	Primary purpose	Membership size (approximate)
American Association of Occupational Health Nurses (AAOHN) 50 Lenox Point Atlanta, GA 30324 [1942]	RNs employed in occupational health.	Maintain professional excellence in OHN through education and research programs; promote OHN; stimulate interest and provide forum for issues in field.	12,500
American Association of Spinal Cord Injury Nurses (AASCIN) 75–20 Astoria Blvd. Jackson Heights, NY 11370-1178 [1983]	RNs engaged in care of patients with spinal cord injury.	Promote excellence in meeting needs of those with spinal cord injury; disseminate information; promote education and research.	1,500
American College of Nurse Midwives (ACNM) 818 Connecticut Ave. Washington, DC 20006 [1955: 1929 AANM 1955 merger]	ACNM certified nurse-midwives or RN students in accredited nurse-midwifery programs.	Set standards for education and practice and evaluate these. Facilitate efforts of CNMs who provide quality service to individuals and child-bearing families. Promote research.	4,800
American Holistic Nurses Association (AHNA) 4101 Lake Boone Trail, Suite 201 Raleigh, NC 27607 [1980]	Nurses and others interested in holistically oriented health care.	Promote education of nurses in concepts and practice of the health of the whole person; serve as an advocate of wellness.	NA
American Nephrology Nurses Association (ANNA) East Holly Ave., Box 56, Pitman, NJ 08071 [1969]	RNs interested in care of patients with renal disease; Associate: dieticians, social workers, LPN/LVNs, technicians.	Develop and update standards of practice in this field; to promote individual growth, promote research and development in field; CE.	9,000 in 66 chapters

| | Activities[c] | | | | | Publications[h] |
Certifi-cation[d]	Standards set and published	Legislative activities[e]	Research activities[f]	Members of NFSNO[i]	NOLF	(journals, newsletters)
×	×	×	×	×	×	*AAOHN Journal*; *AAOHN News*
	×	×	×	×	×	*SCI Nursing*
×[g]	×	×	×	×	×	*Journal of Nurse Midwifery*; *Quickening*
			×	×	×	*Journal of Holistic Nursing*; *Beginnings*
×	×	×	×	×	×	*ANNA Journal*; *ANNA Update*

Appendix 5 (continued)

Organization and year established[a]	Membership eligibility[b]	Primary purpose	Membership size (approximate)
American Psychiatric Nurses Association (APNA) 1200-19th St., NW, Suite 300 Washington, DC 20036	RNs in the field.	Advance the practice of psychiatric nursing through continuing education, setting standards, peer support and providing a forum for management of issues.	2,800
American Public Health Association (APHA) Public Health Nursing Section, 1015 15th St. N.W., Washington, DC 20005 [APHA 1872; PHN section 1923]	RNs practicing or interested in PH nursing.	Improve nursing service and education in broad perspective of public health.	2,200
American Radiological Nurses Association (ARNA) 2021 Spring Road, Suite 600 Oark Brook, IL 60521 [1981]	RNs.	Define the functions, qualifications and educational criteria for radiology nurses; recommend standards; evaluate practice; disseminate research.	1,393
American Society for Parenteral and Enteral Nutrition (ASPEN) 8630 Fenton St., Suite 412 Silver Springs, MD 20910-3805 [1975]	Multidisciplinary: MDs, RNs, dieticians, pharmacists; Associate: students and individuals who do not belong to core disciplines.	Promote quality patient care, education and research in field of nutrition and metabolic support.	7,200
American Society of Ophthalmic Registered Nurses (ASORN) P.O. Box 193030, San Francisco, CA 94119 [1976]	RNs engaged in ophthalmic nursing.	Unite RNs in field to promote excellence in ophthalmic nursing; CE.	1,800

	Activities[c]					
Certifi-cation[d]	Standards set and published	Legislative activities[e]	Research activities[f]	Members of NFSNO[i]	NOLF	Publications[h] (journals, newsletters)
		×	×	×	×	*Journal of Psychosocial Nursing*
	×	×	×	×	×	*American Journal of Public Health; Nation's Health*
	×		×	×		*ARNA Images*
×	×		×		×	*Journal of Parenteral and Enteral Nutrition; Nutrition in Clinical Practice*
×	×			×	×	*Insight*

Appendix 5   (continued)

Organization and year established[a]	Membership eligibility[b]	Primary purpose	Membership size (approximate)
American Society of Plastic and Reconstructive Surgical Nurses (ASPRSN) East Holly Ave., Box 56, Pitman, NJ 08071 [1975]	LPNs, RNs engaged in field of plastic and reconstructive surgery.	Promote highest professional standards for better and safer care; CE.	1,500
American Society of Post Anesthesia Nurses (ASPAN) 11512 Allecingie Pkwy, Richmond, VA 23235 [1980]	RNs with primary practice in post anesthesia care.	CE. Upgrade standards of care; promote professional growth; facilitate cooperation with others in field; encourage specialization and research.	11,087 in 41 state and regional associations
American Urological Association, Allied (AUAA) 11512 Allecingie Pkwy, Richmond, VA 23235 [1972]	Persons in health care profession engaged in care of urologic patient.	Serve as vehicle for distribution of all available information in field; point way to advanced nursing technique and equipment; help nurses to become specialists.	2,400 in 44 chapters
Association for Professionals in Infection Control (APIC) 1016 Sixteenth St., NW Washington, DC 20036-5703 [1972]	All individuals involved in infection control activities.	Improve patient care, support development of effective and rational infection control programs, promote quality research in field.	10,443
Association for Women's Health, Obstetric and Neonatal Nurses (AWHONN) 700-14th St., Suite 600 Washington, DC 20005-2019 [1969]	RNs interested in the field.	Promote excellence in nursing practice with women and newborn.	28,000

		Activities[c]				
Certifi- cation[d]	Standards set and published	Legislative activities[e]	Research activities[f]	Members of NFSNO[i]	NOLF	Publications[h] (journals, newsletters)
×	×			×	×	*Journal of Plastic and Reconstructive Surgical Nursing*
×	×			×	×	*Breathline*; *Journal of Post Anesthesia Nursing*
×	×	×	×	×	×	*Urologic Nursing*, *Urogram*
×	×	×		×	×	*American Journal of Infection Control*; newsletter
×	×	×	×	×	×	*Journal of Obstetric, Gynecological and Neonatal Nursing*

Appendix 5 (continued)

Organization and year established[a]	Membership eligibility[b]	Primary purpose	Membership size (approximate)
Association of Child and Adolescent Psychiatric Nurses (ACAPN) 1211 Locust St. Philadelphia, PA 19107	RNs and students interested in the field.	Recognize the uniqueness of and promote communication among child psychiatric nurses, and improve the mental health of infants, children, adolescents and their families through advocacy, practice, education and research.	NA
Association of Nurses in AIDS Care (ANAC) 704 Stony Hill Road, Suite 106 Yardley, PA 19067 [1987]	RNs; Associates: LPNs and students.	Develop this area of specialty practice and promote quality care for patients.	2,600 in 33 chapters
Association of Operating Room Nurses (AORN) 2170 S. Parker Rd., Suite 300 Denver, CO 80231 [1954]	Nurses employed in perioperative practice, education, research.	Enhance professionalism of perioperative nurses; improve their performance; provide a forum for interaction and idea exchange.	47,000 in 380 chapters worldwide
Association of Pediatric Oncology Nurses (APON) 11512 Allecingie Pkwy, Richmond, VA 23235 [1976]	RNs interested in or engaged in pediatrics, oncology, pediatric oncology.	Promote optimal care of children with cancer and their families.	1,990
Association of Rehabilitation Nurses (ARN) 5100 Old Orchard Rd., Skokie, IL 60077 [1974]	RNs in rehabilitation nursing.	Advance quality of rehabilitation nursing; CE.	10,000 in 88 chapters worldwide

		Activities[c]				Publications[h] (journals, newsletters)
Certifi-cation[d]	Standards set and published	Legislative activities[e]	Research activities[f]	Members of NFSNO[i]	NOLF	
		×	×		×	*Journal of Child and Adolescent Psychiatric and Mental Health Nursing; ACAPN Newsletter*
		×	×		×	*Journal of the Association of Nurses in AIDS Care*
×	×	×	×	×	×	*AORN Journal*
	×		×	×		*Journal of Pediatric Oncology Nursing*
×	×	×		×	×	*Rehabilitation Nursing; ARN News; Rehabilitation Nursing Research*

Appendix 5 (continued)

Organization and year established[a]	Membership eligibility[b]	Primary purpose	Membership size (approximate)
Consolidated Association of Nurses in Substance Abuse (CANSA) 303 W. Katella Ave., Suite 202 Orange, CA 92667 [1979]	RNs, LP/LVNs, LPTs; Student membership, Associate membership, Corporate membership.	Establish and promote standards for the practice of nursing in the field of chemical dependency.	NA
Dermatology Nurses' Association (DNA) East Holly Ave., Box 56, Pitman, NJ 08071 [1982]	RNs, LPNs and technicians in dermatology nursing.	Develop and foster highest standards of dermatologic nursing care; enhance professional growth through education and research; promote interdisciplinary collaboration; enhance communication.	2,000
Developmental Disabilities Nurses' Association (DDNA) 1720 Willow Creek Circle, Suite 515 Eugene, Oregon 97402	RNs practicing in or having interest in the field.	Support practice with the developmentally disabled as a specialty.	880
Emergency Nurses' Association (ENA) 216 Higgins Rd., Park Ridge, IL 60068 [1970]	RNs in emergency care with special skills or knowledge in emergency nursing. Associate: any other health professional	Provide optimum care to patients in emergency departments.	23,350
International Society of Psychiatric Consultation-Liaison Nurses (ISPCLN) 437 Twin Bay Drive Pensacola, FL 32534 [1994]	RNs practicing or interested in the area.	Promote psychiatric consultation liaison as a subspecialty of psychiatric and mental health nursing.	NA

	Activities[c]					Publications[h]
Certifi-cation[d]	Standards set and published	Legislative activities[e]	Research activities[f]	Members of NFSNO[i]	NOLF	(journals, newsletters)
×	×			×	×	*Behavioral Health Management*; *Dove Newsletter*
				×	×	*Focus*; *Dermatology Nursing*
						NA
×	×	×	×	×	×	*Journal of Emergency Nursing*
						NA

Appendix 5 (continued)

Organization and year established[a]	Membership eligibility[b]	Primary purpose	Membership size (approximate)
Intravenous Nurses Society (INS) Two Brighton St., Belmont, MA 02178 [1973]	RNs in specialty practice of IV therapy.	Enhance the practice of an IV nurse through research, education, and standards.	9,123
National Association of Neonatal Nurses (NANN) 1304 Southpoint Blvd., Suite 280 Petaluma, CA 94954-6859 [1984]	RNs; Associates: other health care workers.	Advance the practice of neonatal nursing and safeguard the quality of care to the consumer.	13,000
National Association of Nurse Practitioners in Reproductive Health (NANPRH) 2401 Pennsylvania Ave., NW Washington, DC 20037 [1980]	NPs in obstetrics, gynecology, family planning, reproductive health, endocrinology and infertility practice.	Assure quality reproductive health services that guarantee reproductive freedom and to protect and promote service delivery by NPs.	2,000
National Association of Orthopaedic Nurses (NAON) East Holly Ave., Box 56, Pitman, NJ 08071 [1980]	RNs/LPNs involved in orthopedic nursing.	Enhance personal and professional growth of members through continuing education.	7,000 in 130 chapters
National Association of Pediatric Nurse Associates and Practitioners (NAP-NAP) 1101 Kings Hwy Rd., Suite 206, Cherry Hill, NJ 08034 [1973]	RNs who are primary care specialists in pediatrics.	Support legislation to improve the quality of health care to children and adolescents.	4,465 in 40 chapters

	Activities[c]					
Certification[d]	Standards set and published	Legislative activities[e]	Research activities[f]	Members of NFSNO[i]	NOLF	Publications[h] (journals, newsletters)
×	×	×	×	×	×	*Journal of Intravenous Nursing*; *INS Newsline*
	×	×	×		×	*Neonatal Network*; *Journal of Neonatal Nursing*
[g]	×	×		×		*Newsletter*
×	×	×	×	×	×	*Orthopaedic Nursing*
×	×	×	×	×	×	*Journal of Pediatric Health Care*; newsletter

Appendix 5   (continued)

Organization and year established[a]	Membership eligibility[b]	Primary purpose	Membership size (approximate)
National Association of School Nurses (NASN) Box 1300, 16e Route One, Scarborough, ME 04070-7300 [1969]	School nurses employed by boards of education, institutions of higher learning and state departments of education.	Strengthen education of children by providing leadership in promotion and delivery of adequate health services by qualified school nurses.	8,500
National Flight Nurse Association (NFNA) 6900 Grove Road Thoroughfare, NJ 08086-9447 [1981]	RN flight nurses.	Support the development of flight nursing as a specialty.	1,525
National Gerontological Nursing Association (NGNA) 1250 Parkway Drive, Suite 510 Hanover, MO 21076 [1984]	RNs, students, nursing assistants; Associate: nonnurses.	Provide a forum in which gerontological nursing issues are identified and explored; public education.	1,700
National Nurses' Society on Addictions (NNSA) 4101 Lake Boone Trail, Suite 201 Raleigh, NC 27607 [1975]	RNs, senior nursing students interested in chemical dependency problems.	Extend knowledge, disseminate information; promote quality care for the addicted patients and their families; become involved in social issues and public policy concerning addiction.	1,142
Oncology Nursing Society (ONS) 1016 Greentree Rd., Pittsburgh, PA 15220 [1975]	RNs engaged in or interested in oncology.	Develop new knowledge in cancer detection and improvement of care; encourage nurses to specialize in cancer nursing.	25,500 in 179 chapters

	Activities[c]					Publications[h] (journals, newsletters)
Certification[d]	Standards set and published	Legislative activities[e]	Research activities[f]	Members of NFSNO[i]	NOLF	
×	×	×		×		*School Nurse*; newsletter
				×		*Aeromedical Journal; Across the Board*
			×		×	*Geriatric Nursing; New Horizons*
×	×	×		×	×	*NNSA* newsletter
×	×	×	×	×	×	*Oncology Nursing Forum; ONS News*

Appendix 5 (continued)

Organization and year established[a]	Membership eligibility[b]	Primary purpose	Membership size (approximate)
Respiratory Nursing Society (RNS) 5700 Old Orchard Road, Skokie, IL 60077 [1990]	RNs interested in the specialty.	Promote coordinated, comprehensive high-level nursing care for respiratory patients through fostering nurses' development.	NA
Society for Vascular Nursing (SVN) 309 Winter Street Norwood, MA 02062-1333 [1982]	Licensed nurses; Associate: nonnurse health professionals; Corporate members.	Promote excellence in the compassionate and comprehensive management of persons with vascular disease.	900
Society of Gastroenterology Nurses and Associates (SGNA) 1070 Sibley Tower Rochester, NY 14604 [1974]	RNs, LP/LVNs, medical technologists, x-ray technicians, PAs.	Advance the science and practice of the specialty through education, research, advocacy and collaboration.	6,500
Society of Otorhinolaryngology and Head-Neck Nurses (SOHN) 116 Canal Street, Suite A, New Smyrna Beach, FL 32168-7004 [1976]	RNs working in the field.	Support the development of the specialty in the public interest.	1,092
Society of Pediatric Nurses (SPN) 7250 Parkway Drive, Suite 510 Hanover, MD 21076 [1990]	Staff nurses, school and outpatient nurses, CNSs, NPs, administrators, educators and researchers.	Improve nursing care of children and their families and develop pediatric nursing as a subspecialty.	2,000
Society of Urologic Nurses and Associates (SUNA) East Holly Ave., Box 56 Pitman, NJ 08071	RNs working in the field.	Support the development of the specialty in the public interest.	2,202

	Activities[c]					Publications[h]
Certifi-cation[d]	Standards set and published	Legislative activities[e]	Research activities[f]	Members of NFSNO[i]	NOLF	(journals, newsletters)
	×		×		×	*Perspectives in Respiratory Nursing; RNS Bulletin*
	×		×		×	*Journal of Vascular Nursing; SVN . . . prn*
×	×			×	×	Newsletter
×	×			×	×	*ORL-Head and Neck Nursing; Update*
			×		×	*SPN Newsletter*
×	×			×		NA

Appendix 5   (continued)

Organization and year established[a]	Membership eligibility[b]	Primary purpose	Membership size (approximate)
Wound, Ostomy and Continence Nurses Society (WOCN) 2755 Bristol St., Suite 110 Costa Mesa, CA 92626	RNs working in the field.	Support the development of the specialty in the public interest.	3,693

Organizations Related to Leadership and Scholarship

Organization and year established[a]	Membership eligibility[b]	Primary purpose	Membership size (approximate)
Alpha Tau Delta, National Fraternity for Professional Nurses 5207 Mesada St., Alta Loma, CA 91701 [1921]	Students in accredited baccalaureate or higher degree programs; based on scholarship, personality, and character. Also alumnae chapters.	Further professional and education standards, develop leadership, encourage excellence.	6,000
American Academy of Nursing (AAN) 600 Maryland Ave. SW, Washington, DC 20005 [1973]	Elected by current members, based on contributions to nursing; members are called fellows (FAAN).	Advance role of nursing in health care delivery; identify and explore issues in health care, the professions and society; and propose resolutions; disseminate scholarly concepts; formulate strategies to improve health care.	1100 active; 113 emeritus
Sigma Theta Tau International Honor Society of Nursing 550 W. North St., Indianapolis, IN 46202 [1922]	High academic achievement and leadership qualities as student in baccalaureate and higher degree programs. Also community leaders.	Recognize superior achievement, leadership qualities, foster high professional standards, encourage creative work; support scholarliness in nursing.	105,000

| Activities[c] | | | | | | Publications[h] |
Certifi-cation[d]	Standards set and published	Legislative activities[e]	Research activities[f]	Members of NFSNO[i]	NOLF	(journals, newsletters)
×	×			×	×	NA
					×	*Captions of Alpha Tau Delta*
		×	×		×	Newsletter
			×		×	*Image: The Journal of Nursing Scholarship; Reflections*

Appendix 5   (continued)

Organization and year established[a]	Membership eligibility[b]	Primary purpose	Membership size (approximate)
Chi Eta Phi Society 3029 13th St. N.W., Washington, DC 20029 [1932]	Interested RNs and students in US and Africa; focus is on black nurses.	Recruit into nursing, identify corps of nursing leaders who will be agents of social change.	70 chapters in US, US Virgin Islands, Africa

Organizations with Ethnic, Racial, Religious Interests

American Assembly for Men in Nursing (AAMN) 437 Twin Bay Dr. Pensacola, FL 32534 [1974]	Men nurses.	Provide support to men nurses; encourage men into nursing.	NA
Association of Black Nursing Faculty in Higher Education (ABNF) 1708 North Roxboro Rd., Durham, NC 20009	Nursing faculty of African–American background and those interested in their issues.	NA	NA
National Association of Hispanic Nurses (NAHN) 1501 Sixteenth St., NW, Washington, DC 20036 [1976]	Hispanic nurses, any RN interested.	Improve care of Hispanic patients; educate about health care needs; recruitment and retention of Hispanic students; assure equal opportunities for Hispanic nurses.	NA
National Black Nurses' Association (NBNA) 1012 Tenth St. NW, Washington, DC 20001 [1971]	RNs, LPNs, students.	Improve care for black consumers; influence legislation about blacks; recruit blacks into nursing; unify black nurses.	NA
Nurses Christian Fellowship (NCF) P.O. Box 7895, 6400 Schroeder Rd., Madison, WI 53707 [1948]	Christian nurses and students.	Help students and nurses grow spiritually; focus on ministering to whole person.	NA

		Activities[c]				Publications[h]
Certifi-cation[d]	Standards set and published	Legislative activities[e]	Research activities[f]	Members of NFSNO[i] NOLF		(journals, newsletters)
					×	Newsletter
					×	*Interaction*
					×	NA
		×	×		×	*El Faro*
		×			×	NA
						Journal of Christian Nursing

Appendix 5   (continued)

Organization and year established[a]	Membership eligibility[b]	Primary purpose	Membership size (approximate)
Philippine Nurses Association of America (PNAA) 7728 Hillandale Ave. San Diego, CA 92120 [1979]	RNs and others interested in the issues of Filipino nurses.	Uphold the image and foster the welfare of Filipino nurses as a professional group.	NA

Job-Related Special Interest Groups

American Academy of Ambulatory Care Nursing Administration (AAACN) East Holly Ave., Box 56, Pitman, NJ 08071 [1978]	Any RN interested in ambulatory nursing care.	Promote high standards of ambulatory care nursing administration and practice through education, exchange of information, and scientific investigation.	1,400
American Association of Colleges of Nursing (AACN) One Dupont Circle, Suite 530, Washington, DC 20036 [1969]	Institutions with baccalaureate or higher degree nursing programs represented by dean or comparable chief administrator.	Promote academic leadership in nursing; disseminate information about higher education in nursing; advance the quality of baccalaureate and higher nursing education; promote research.	460 schools of nursing
American Association of Nurse Attorneys (AANA) 720 Light St., Baltimore, MD 21230 [1982]	Nurse attorneys, nurses in law school.	Facilitate information sharing; develop the profession; educate nurses about law; influence health policy.	600
American Association of Office Nurses (AAON) 109 Kinderkamack Rd., Montvale, NJ 07645 [1988]	RNs in office practice and others interested in their issues.	Development of the specialized field of the office nurse.	4,000

		Activities[c]				
Certifi-cation[d]	Standards set and published	Legislative activities[e]	Research activities[f]	Members of NFSNO[i]	NOLF	Publications[h] (journals, newsletters)
					×	
	×		×	×		Viewpoint
		×	×			Journal of Professional Nursing; AACN Newsletter
		×	×	×	×	Inside TAANA
						The Office Nurse

Appendix 5   (continued)

Organization and year established[a]	Membership eligibility[b]	Primary purpose	Membership size (approximate)
American Organization of Nurse Executives (AONE) 840 North Lake Shore Dr., 10E, Chicago, IL 60611 [1967]	Nurse executives; nurse managers; graduate faculty in nursing administration.	Provide leadership for advancement of nursing practice and patient care in organized health care systems, through achievement in excellence in nurse executive practice; shape policy in health care.	NA
Home Health Nurses Association (HHNA) 437 Twin Bay Drive Pensacola, FL 32534-1350 [1993]	RNs in any aspect of home health care.	Develop the specialty of home care nursing in pursuit of quality services for the public.	3,000
Hospice Nurses Association (HNA) 5512 Northumberland St. Pittsburgh, PA 15217-1131 [1986]	RNs in hospice practice; Associate and student membership.	Foster excellence in hospice nursing.	NA
International Association of Forensic Nurses (IAFN) 6900 Grove Rd. Thoroughfare, NJ 08086	RNs in forensic work; Associate, student and retired statuses.	Access information about the science of forensic nursing.	NA
National Association for Health Care Recruitment (NAHCR) P.O. Box 5769 Akron, OH 44372 [1975]	Those working in hospitals or health care agencies actively involved in health care recruiting.	Promote and exchange principles of professional health care recruitment.	1,500

		Activities^c				Publications^h
Certifi-cation^d	Standards set and published	Legislative activities^e	Research activities^f	Members of NFSNO^i	NOLF	(journals, newsletters)
		×	×			Nurse Executive
			×			Home Healthcare Nurse; HHNA News
×	×		×		×	Fanfare
						Journal of Forensic Nursing
			×	×		Recruitment Directions

Appendix 5   (continued)

Organization and year established[a]	Membership eligibility[b]	Primary purpose	Membership size (approximate)
National Association of Directors of Nursing Administration in Long Term Care (NADONA/LTC) 10999 Reed Hartman Hwy., Suite 229 Cincinnati, OH 45242	Nurses in long-term care administration or management.	Support development of the practice area.	2,800
National Council of State Boards of Nursing 676 N. St. Clair, Suite 550 Chicago, IL 60611 [1978]	Boards of nursing in states and territories.	Develop licensing exams; assist boards in administering them; develop model licensure laws and regulations; disseminate information.	61 boards of nursing
National Nurses in Business (NNB) 1000 Burnett Ave., Suite 450 Concord, CA 94520	RN-entrepreneurs.	Support for nurse-owned businesses.	1,000
National Nursing Staff Development Organization (NNSDO) 437 Twin Bay Dr. Pensacola, FL 32534-1350 [1989]	Nurses in staff development practice.	Foster the art and science of staff development through research, standard setting and issues management.	NA
Nurses Organization of Veteran's Affairs (NOVA) 1726 M Street., NW, Suite 1100 Washington, DC 20036	RNs working in the VA system.	NA	NA

		Activities[c]				
Certifi-cation[d]	Standards set and published	Legislative activities[e]	Research activities[f]	Members of NFSNO[i]	NOLF	Publications[h] (journals, newsletters)
×	×				×	NA
		×	×			*Issues*
						NA
×	×		×		×	*Trendlines*
					×	NA

Appendix 5   (continued)

Organization and year established[a]	Membership eligibility[b]	Primary purpose	Membership size (approximate)
Other Special Interest Groups			
American Association for the History of Nursing (AAHN) P.O. Box 90803 Washington, DC 20090 [1982]	Anyone interested in purpose of the association.	Educate public about history and heritage of nursing; support historical research; promote development of centers for preservation of historical materials; disseminate information on nursing history.	NA
North American Nursing Diagnosis Association (NANDA) 1211 Locust St. Philadelphia, PA 19107 [1982]	Any RN interested in nursing diagnosis.	Develop a taxonomy of nursing diagnosis.	900
Nurses Environmental Health Watch (NEHW) 181 Marshall St. Duxbury, MA 03443 [1979]	Nurses interested in environmental health concerns.	Provide education about actual and potential health hazards.	NA
Regional Nursing Organizations			
Midwest Alliance in Nursing (MAIN) 2511 E 46th St., Suite E-3 Indianapolis, IN 46205 (Midwest Nursing Research Society is independent affiliate) [1979]	Nursing education programs and health care institutions/ agencies providing nursing care in 13-state Midwest region.	Facilitate regional investigation, planning, communication; collaborate to obtain shared goals and resolve issues in order to achieve maximum utilization of resources for cost-effective care.	NA

		Activities[c]				
Certifi-cation[d]	Standards set and published	Legislative activities[e]	Research activities[f]	Members of NFSNO[i] NOLF		Publications[h] (journals, newsletters)
			×			Bulletin
			×		×	Nursing Diagnosis
		×				Health Watch
		×	×			Mainlines

Appendix 5   (continued)

Organization and year established[a]	Membership eligibility[b]	Primary purpose	Membership size (approximate)
Northeast Organization for Nursing (NEON) Hewitt Hall University of N.H. Durham, NH 03824 [1983]	Nursing education programs and health care agencies with identifiable nursing department in 6-state New England region and Mid-Atlantic region.	Bring about cooperative planning and collaboration between nursing education and service to improve health care of the region.	NA
Southern Council on Collegiate Education for Nursing, affiliated with Southern Regional Education Board (SREB) 1340 Spring St. NW, Atlanta, GA 30309 [SREB 1948; Council 1962]	AD, Baccalaureate and higher degree programs in nursing in SREB 14-state region.	Generate and implement projects related to improvement of nursing education; provide forum for college-based programs to receive information and conduct regional planning.	200 institutions
Western Institute of Nursing (WIN) P.O. Box Drawer P, Boulder, CO 80301 [1986]	Individual RN nursing education programs and nursing service agencies in 13 Western states, including Alaska and Hawaii.	Influence the quality of health care in the West through monitoring issues and trends and designing, implementing, evaluating regional, action-oriented, nursing strategies in education, practice, research.	NA

Health-Related Organizations

National Association for Practical Nurse Education and Service (NAPNES) 1400 Spring St., Suite 310, Silver Spring, MD 20910 [1941]	LPNs/LVNs, RNs, nurse educators, physicians, administrators and consumers interested in practical nursing; agency members.	Improve and extend PN education to meet public needs.	NA

| | | Activities[c] | | | | Publications[h] |
Certifi-cation[d]	Standards set and published	Legislative activities[e]	Research activities[f]	Members of NFSNO[i]	NOLF	(journals, newsletters)
		×	×			Newsletter
	×	×	×			Newsletter
	×	×	×			Newsletter; *Western Journal of Nursing Research*
	×	×	×			*Journal of Practical Nursing*

Appendix 5   (continued)

Organization and year established[a]	Membership eligibility[b]	Primary purpose	Membership size (approximate)
National Federation of Licensed Practical Nurses (NFLPN) 1418 Aversboro Rd., Garner, NC 27529 [1949]	State organizations made up of LPNs/LVNs and individual LPNs.	Secure recognition and effective utilization of LPNs; promote LPN welfare; improve standards of practice and education.	NA

[a] The organization may have been established under another name.

[b] Many organizations have associate membership for students and interested LPN/LVNs or others, and corporate membership. Some of these special categories have been noted, for more detailed information on others, make direct contact.

[c] All organizations have meetings or conventions, provide continuing education and carry out public relations activities of some sort to educate or influence the public about themselves. Many offer other benefits such as insurance, credit cards, travel discounts, and so on.

[d] Certification is often done by a separately incorporated organization.

[e] Legislative activities usually include staying on top of legislative and governmental issues and actions, informing members on these, and providing information to legislators. Not all organizations actively lobby (often inappropriate to their mission or tax status). Others have lobbyists on staff or subcontract for these services.

		Activities[c]				Publications[h]
Certifi-cation[d]	Standards set and published	Legislative activities[e]	Research activities[f]	Members of NFSNO[i]	NOLF	(journals, newsletters)
	×	×	×			*Licensed Practical Nurse*

[f] Research activities may include data collection and/or dissemination, research projects, funding for research, and educating on research.

[g] Accreditation also done (this may be through a separate corporation).

[h] Write to the organization for more detail on the frequency of periodicals, and a complete list of other publications.

[i] Only specialty practice organizations qualify for membership in NFSNO; although others may join as an affiliate. Even those who qualify may choose affiliate status.

Note: An extensive list of nursing organizations is available electronically on the AJN-NETWORK.

Appendix 6   Specialty Certifications[a]

Specialty	Credential	Eligibility[b]
Addictions Nursing	CARN	Practicing as RN for 3 years, 4000 hours in addiction practice in last 5 years
Case Manager (multidisciplinary)	CCM	24 months in case management
Childbirth Education (multidisciplinary)	ACCE	3 years childbirth education teaching in last 5 years, 30 hours CE in last 3 years
Continence Nursing	CCCN	Baccalaureate degree, specialty education program accredited by WOCN, or 2 years full-time practice in specialty
Critical Care Nursing • Adult • Neonatal • Pediatric	CCRN	1750 hours in specialty in last 2 years, with half of hours during most recent year
Diabetes Educator (multidisciplinary)	CDE	2 years or 2000 hours of direct diabetes patient education
Dialysis Nursing • Hemodialysis • Peritoneal	 CHN CPDN	One year of specialty experience and current employment in the field
Emergency Nursing	CEN	2 years experience in specialty and Emergency Nurses Assn. membership
Enterostomal Therapy Nursing	CETN	Accredited enterostomal therapy course that requires BSN
Flight Nursing	CFRN	2 years experience in specialty

Certifying organization	Recertification	Numbers Certified (1995)	Fee[c]
Addiction Nursing Cert. Board, 4101 Lake Boone Trail, Raleigh, NC 27607	Every 4 years by CE or retest	1,200	$165–250
Certification of Insurance Rehabilitation Specialist Commission, 1835 Rohlwing Road, Rolling Meadows, IL 60008	Every 5 years by CE	15,800 (85% RNs)	$275
ASPO/Lamaze, 1200 19th St., NW, Washington, DC 20036	N/A	3,600	$225–350
Wound Ostomy & Continence Nsg. Certification Board, 2755 Bristol St., Suite 110, Costa Mesa, CA 92626	Every 5 years by retest	4	$200–250
American Assoc. of Critical Care Nurses Cert. Corp., 101 Columbia, Aliso Viejo, CA 92656	Every 3 years by CE or retest	51,307 385 1,388	$150–225
National Certification Board for Diabetes Educators, 444 N. Michigan Ave., Suite 1240, Chicago, IL 60611	Every 5 years by retest	6,600	$160–210
Board of Nephrology Examiners, PO Box 44085, Madison, WI 53744	Every 4 years by retest or CE	1,745	$140
Board of Certification for Emergency Nursing, 216 Higgins Road, Park Ridge, IL 60068	Self-assessment including CE or retest	23,000	$100–220
Wound, Ostomy & Continence Nsg. Certification Bd., 2755 Bristol St., Suite 110, Costa Mesa, CA 92626	Every 5 years by retest	1,816	$200–250
Board of Certification for Emergency Nursing, 216 Higgins Road, Park Ridge, IL 60068	Self-assessment including CE or retest	758	$140–260

Appendix 6   **(continued)**

Specialty	Credential	Eligibility[b]
Gastroenterology Nursing	CGA	4000 hours in last 5 years in GI specialty
Hospice Nursing	CRNH	2 years hospice experience
Infection Control (multidisciplinary)	CIC	Practice in area for 2 years, baccalaureate in health care field or waiver
Intravenous Nursing	CRNI	1600 hours IV experience in last 2 years
Lactation Consultant	IBCLC	CE related to breastfeeding in last 3 years and 2500 to 4000 practice hours
Nephrology Nursing	CNN	2 years nephrology experience in last 3 years
Neuroscience Nursing	CNRN	2 years in specialty and active clinical practice
Nurse Anesthetist	CRNA	Graduate of accredited educational program (post-baccalaureate)
Nurse Midwifery	CNM	Graduate of accredited educational program, and testing within 12 months of completion
Nursing Service Administration-LTC	C	12 months experience in LTC administration in last 10 years
Nursing Director-LTC	CNDLTC	12 months in a variety of managerial capacities in LTC

Certifying organization	Recertification	Numbers Certified (1995)	Fee[c]
Certifying Board of Gastroenterology Nurses and Associates, 720 Light St., Baltimore, MD 21230	Every 5 years by CE or retest	2,350	$200–270
National Board for Certification of Hospice Nurses, 1211 Ave. of the Americas, New York, NY 10036	Every 4 years	980	$200–275
Certification Board of Infection Control, PO Box 14661, Lenexa, KS 66285	Every 5 years by retest	2,800	$230
IV Nurses Certification Corp., Two Brighton St., Belmont, MA 02178	Every 3 years by retest or CE	3,000	$225–380
International Board of Lactation Consultant Examiners, Box 2348, Falls Church, VA 22042	Every 5 years by retest or CE; 10 years must retest	6,000	$370
Nephrology Nursing Certification Board, East Holly Ave., Box 56, Pitman, NJ 08071	Every 3 years by CE or retest	N/A	$175–225
American Board of Neuroscience Nsg., 475 Riverside Dr., New York, NY 10115	Every 5 years by retest	823	$175–195
Council on Certification of Nurse Anesthetists, 222 S. Prospect Ave., Park Ridge, IL 60068	Every 2 years by CE and active practice	26,000	$425
ACNM Certification Council, 8401 Corporate Dr., Suite 630, Landover, MD 20785	Every 5 years by CE or retest	4,194	$385
NADONA/LTC Certification Registrar, 10999 Reed Hartman Hwy., Suite 630, Cincinnati, OH 45242	Every 5 years by CE	3,000	$100–180
American Society for LTC Nursing, 660 Lonely Cottage Dr., Upper Black Eddy, PA 18972	Every 5 years by CE	100	$120–210

Appendix 6   (continued)

Specialty	Credential	Eligibility[b]
Nutrition Support Nursing	CNSN	2 years experience in specialty
Obstetrical/ Gynecological Nursing • Ambulatory Women's Health • Hi-Risk OB • Inpatient ON • Lo-Risk Neonatal • Maternal Newborn • Neonatal Intensive Care • Reproductive/ Endocrine/ Infertility • Neonatal Nurse Practitioner • Women's Health Care Nurse Practitioner	RNC	Specific clinical practice and in some instances educational requirements
Occupational Health Nursing	COHN	Specific courses related to occupational health nursing in past 5 years, experience and BSN
Oncology Nursing • Generalist • Advanced	OCN	30 months of practice in last 5 years, 2000 hours in oncology in last 5 years, BSN for generalist by 1999, masters for advanced
Ophthalmic Nursing	CRNO	4000 hours experience in specialty
Orthopaedic Nursing	ONC	2 years experience as RN, 1000 hours in specialty in last 3 years
Ostomy Care Nursing	COCN	Baccalaureate degree, specialty education program accredited by WOCN, or 2 years full-time practice in specialty

Certifying organization	Recertification	Numbers Certified (1995)	Fee[c]
National Board for Nutrition Support Certification, 8630 Fenton St., Suite 412, Silver Spring, MD 20910	N/A	N/A	N/A
National Certification Board OB/GYN and Neonatal Nursing Specialties, 645 N. Michigan Av., Chicago, IL 60611	Every 3 years by CE or retest	36,367 combined 612 247 21,680 2,840 401 7,528 494 1,929 6,760	$250
American Board for Occupational Health Nurses, 9944 South Roberts Rd., Palos Hills, IL 60465	Every 5 years by CE and experience	7,580	$250
Oncology Nursing Certification Corporation, 501 Holiday Dr., Pittsburgh, PA 15220	Every 4 years by retest	16,000	$210–285
National Certifying Board for Ophthalmic Registered Nurses, 655 Beach St., Box 193030, San Francisco, CA 94119	Every 5 years by retest	470	$175–250
Orthopaedic Nurses Certification Board, East Holly Ave., Box 56, Pitman, NJ 08071	Every 5 years by CE or retest	2,646	$180–225
Wound, Ostomy and Continence Certification Board, 2755 Bristol St., Suite 110, Costa Mesa, CA 92626	Every 5 years by retest	4	$200–250

Appendix 6 (continued)

Specialty	Credential	Eligibility[b]
Otorhinolaryngology and Head-Neck Nursing	CORLN	6000 hours in specialty in last 3 years
Pain Management (multidisciplinary)	CNOR	Diplomate, fellow, or clinical associate status, requiring doctorate, masters, or bachelor's degree and experience
Pediatric Nursing • General • Nurse Practitioner	 CPN CPNP	 Recent experience, BSN by 1997 Masters or post-masters PNP program
Pediatric Oncology Nursing	CPON	2 years experience in last 5 years
Perioperative Nursing • RN First Assistant • Perioperative Nursing	 CRNF CNOR	 CNOR, 2000 hours in role Immediate past 2 years in OR nursing
Plastic and Reconstructive Surgical Nursing	CPSN	2 years experience in specialty within last 5 years
Post-Anesthesia Nursing	CPAN	1800 hours experience in last 3 years
Rehabilitation Nursing	CRRN	2 years practice in specialty in last 5 years
School Nursing	CSN	Baccalaureate degree, 3 years experience in school nursing

Certifying organization	Recertification	Numbers Certified (1995)	Fee[c]
National Certifying Board for Otorhinolaryngology and Head-Neck Nurses, 1211 Avenue of the Americas, New York, NY 10036	Every 5 years by CE and practice or retest	N/A	N/A
American Academy of Pain Management, 3600 Sisk Rd., Suite 2D, Modesto, CA 95356	Every 4 years by CE	N/A	$250
National Certification Board of Pediatric Nurse Practitioners and Nurses, 416 Hungerford Dr., Rockville, MD 20850	Every 5 years by CE or retest	3,163 5,161	$195
Certification Corporation of Pediatric Oncology Nurses, 11512 Allecingie Pkwy., Richmond, VA 23235	Every 5 years by CE or retest	470	N/A
National Certification Board of Perioperative Nursing, 2170 S. Parker Rd., Suite 295, Denver, CO 80231	Every 5 years by retest Every 5 years by CE or retest	548 27,216	$375–500 $150–225
Plastic Surgical Nursing Certification Board, East Holly Ave., Box 56, Pitman, NJ 08071	Every 3 years by retest or CE	243	$175–275
American Board of Post-Anesthesia Nursing Certification, 475 Riverside Dr., New York, NY 10115	Every 3 years by retest or CE	1,000	$235–300
Rehabilitation Nursing Certification Board, 5700 Old Orchard Rd., Skokie, IL 60077	Every 5 years by retest or CE	11,000	$185–265
National Board for Certification of School Nurses, Box 1300, Scarborough, ME 04070	N/A	1,025	$150–200

Appendix 6   (continued)

Specialty	Credential	Eligibility[b]
Urology Nursing	CURN	One year of experience in specialty
Wound Nursing	CWCN	Baccalaureate degree, specialty education accredited by WOCN, or 2 years full-time practice in specialty

Certifying organization	Recertification	Numbers Certified (1995)	Fee[c]
American Board of Urologic Allied Health Professionals, East Holly Ave., Box 56, Pitman, NJ 08071	Every 3 years by retest or CE	291	$195–250
Wound, Ostomy & Continence Certification Board, 2755 Bristol St., Suite 110, Costa Mesa, CA 92626	Every 5 years by retest	26	$200–250

[a] Certifications offered by the American Nurses Credentialing Center (ANCC) are not included in this appendix, but presented in Exhibit 13.2 of Chapter 13. ANCC offers 26 certifications, and currently certifies over 100,000 nurses. Information on eligibility requirements can be obtained from ANCC, 600 Maryland Avenue, SW, Suite 100 West, Washington, DC 20024-2571.
[b] The RN is assumed for eligibility, except if noted as multidisciplinary.
[c] The fee cited here is for initial certification; renewal fees are generally less; reduced rates are commonly offered to members of specialty associations.

Appendix 7   Basics of Parliamentary Procedure

By-laws. An organization's by-laws are the basis on which it functions. They include:

- Name
- Purposes
- Functions
- Requirements for membership
- Dues
- The officers
- Governing body
- Committees
- Other organizational units and their responsibilities
- How elected or appointed
- How amendments are made
- The parliamentary authority used to conduct business (often *Robert's Rules of Order Newly Revised*)

Usual *order of business* at a meeting (may have additional parts at a convention):

1. Call to order
2. Minutes of previous meetings
3. Reports of officers, boards, standing committees
   Executive reports
   Executive announcements
   Reports of:
       President
       Vice President
       Secretary
       Treasurer
       Board of Directors
       Standing committees
4. Reports of special committees
5. Announcements
6. Unfinished business
7. New business
8. Adjournment

Motions are proposals or suggestions that initiate action or enable the assembly to express itself. To make a motion:

1. Stand or raise your hand or go to a microphone when indicated.
2. Wait for the chair's signal to go ahead.
3. Address the presiding officer as "Madame (or Mister) Chairman," "Chairperson," "President," or "Speaker."
4. Identify yourself by name and whatever else is customary in that organization, such as office, affiliation, city, or state.

5. State the motion clearly and as briefly as possible. Write out a motion if time permits, for accuracy and the record. Frequently a written motion is given to the secretary for the minutes.
6. Ask to speak to the motion after making it. Don't speak first and then make the motion. Wait for the second before presenting your statement.
7. The chair will call for a second. (Not required if it is a committee motion.)
8. For seconding, rise, identify yourself and say "I second the motion."
9. If no one seconds, the motion is automatically lost and not recorded.
10. If the motion is seconded, the chair says, "It has been moved and seconded that . . . Is there any discussion?"
11. If there is a discussion, it may take the form of comments and/or a motion suggesting an amendment. The maker of the motion speaks first.
12. An amendment, if any, is voted on first, then the original motion with the amendment, if it was accepted.
13. Discussion may be stopped by saying, "I move to close debate" or "I call for the question." This is not debatable and if carried, the motion on the floor is voted on immediately.
14. There may be motions to table a motion (set it aside temporarily— sometimes permanently), to postpone action, or to refer it to a committee. All avoid further action at that time.
15. If an action is taken (motion passed or rejected) that, for whatever reason, people regret, someone on the *prevailing* side may ask to bring it before the assembly again. Anyone can second. This takes precedence and is acted on at once, following the usual procedure. The result may be the same or different, usually different.

Resolutions are indications of the organization's position on key issues.

1. Resolutions are submitted to a resolutions committee by any member, committee or other organizational entity.
2. The format usually begins with: Whereas (giving one or more reasons) and ends with Therefore be it resolved: (stating one or more resolutions related to the "whereas").
3. Resolutions are reviewed by the committee, and sometimes edited or combined with a similar resolution, with permission of the originators.
4. Resolutions usually go the board, but do not necessarily have to be approved by them, depending on policy.
5. A rejected resolution can usually be presented from the floor.
6. At conventions, there may be an open resolutions committee hearing in which resolutions are discussed and debated without formal parliamentary procedure. They may then be changed before formal presentation at the business meeting, saving time and confusion.
7. Resolutions are voted on like motions.
8. Courtesy resolutions at the end of the meeting are usually formalities, showing appreciation to various people or groups.

Appendix 8 Distinguished Nurses of the Past: Fifty Nurses Who Made a Difference*

Name, dates, place of birth	Education and selected honors	Key events; Contributions
Alline, Anna (later Brown, 1923) 1864–1935 East Machias, ME	Normal school in Iowa; Brooklyn Homeopathic Hosp. Trng Sch for Nsg, 1893; Post-grad study Gen. Mem. Hosp. NYC 1896; Enrolled in Teachers College (TC) Columbia U, NYC 1900.	Pioneer in nsg. ed.; studied under Richards and served as her asst. One of first two students to enroll in new, hospital economics courses at TC. Stayed as director and teacher; helped to ensure continuity of program. First inspector of nsg schools for NY state board. Treasurer Am Society of Superintendents of Training Schools for nursing (ASSTSN) later NLNE and NLN. Life member NLNE. Numerous articles in *American Journal of Nsg (AJN)*
Arnstein, Margaret 1904–1972 New York City	AB, Smith College, 1925; Presbyterian Hosp Sch Nsg, 1928; AM, TC, 1929; MS, Johns Hopkins U, 1934; Honorary degrees: Smith College, 1950; Wayne State U, 1964; U of Mich, 1972. Number of honors: first woman to receive Rockefeller Public Service Award (Lasker Award); USPHS Distinguished Service Award; APHA Sedgwick Mem Medal.	Leader and educator in public health nursing, US and abroad. Encouraged by Wald, close friend of family. As nurse-researcher and head of nsg div. of USPHS, increased its ability to provide statistical information. (25 year career with USPHS.) Helped launch plan to increase nsg students for WW II. Worked with WHO to prepare guide for surveying nsg services in various countries. Influential in improving health care and developing nsg services in Balkans after WW II. Sr advisor for intl health (AID and Rockefeller Foundation) 1945. Dean, Yale Sch of Nsg. Author: many articles; coauthor *Communicable Disease Control* 1962.

---

* For further information about these and other nursing leaders, see Chapters 1 and 2, as well as References and Bibliography for these chapters.

Name, dates, place of birth	Education and selected honors	Key events; Contributions
Austin, Anne 1891–1986 Philadelphia, PA	Homeopathic Hospital Trng Sch for Nsg, Buffalo, NY 1927; BS in nsg and teachers certificate, TC, 1932. AM, sociology, U Chicago, 1934.	Best known for work on history of nursing and enthusiasm for preservation of historical documents. Had been public health nurse; served with ANC in France (WW I); taught in diploma and bacc nsg schools from coast to coast. Author, many articles and books on nursing history.
Barton, Clarissa (Clara) 1821–1912 N. Oxford, MA	Liberal Institute, Clinton, NY 1850–51, No nsg ed. More than 25 honors, including Iron Cross (Germany); Medal of Intl RC; Sultan's decoration (Turkey).	Founder of Am Red Cross (ARC). Major contrib to nsg in disaster nsg. Early Civil War nurse, present at many battles, known as "Angel of the Battlefield." With support of Pres Lincoln in 1865, set up office to locate MIA's. Later, went to Europe for health, studied work of Intl Red Cross (IRC). Served as volunteer nurse in Franco-Prussian War. In 1881, was successful in persuading US govt of need for an ARC. As president, participated in numerous disaster relief activities in US and abroad. Author: reports, books, articles about RC. Kept more than 40 diaries.

Appendix 8   (continued)

Name, dates, place of birth	Education and selected honors	Key events; Contributions
Bickerdyke, Mary Ann 1817–1901 Knox Co, OH	Possibly studied under Dr. Hussey, who ran Physio-Botanic Med College, Cinn. Honors: Mother Bickerdyke Day, Kansas, 1897; statue in Galesburg, IL, "Victory freighter," WW II named after her.	Volunteer nurse in Civil War. Known as "Mother" or "General" Bickerdyke and "cyclone in calico," as she nursed Union soldiers. Enraged Army doctors because she was advocate of soldiers; saw that they were cared for as well as possible. Became friend of Grant and Sherman, who supported her against them; eg. campaigned for women nurses in army, physicians objected, Grant approved; found supplies for wounded not reaching them, remedied situation with Grant's support. Rode ambulance wagon with Sherman's march through Georgia, and cared for freed Union prisoners from Andersonville. Throughout war, searched battlefields for wounded. Successfully raised funds throughout North for US Sanitary Commission, between battles.
Breckenridge, Mary 1881?–1965 Memphis, TN	St. Luke's Hospital Sch Nsg, 1910; Postgrad course in pub health nsg, TC, 1921; certified nurse-midwife, and postgrad trng in London, 1923–24. Honorary LLD, U of Kentucky. Honors: French medal; NLN Nutting Award; other awards from natl and community groups. ANA Hall of Fame. Women's Hall of Fame (Seneca Falls, NY).	Best known as founder of Frontier Nsg Service of Kentucky, offering maternal-child care to people in isolated mountains. Director, 40 yrs. Also founded school of midwifery there. Earlier: retired from nsg in 1918 to bear children. After their death, worked for US Children's Bureau. Eventually went to France, organizing relief for pregnant women and children. Organized child hygiene and visiting nurse association (VNA) there.

Name, dates, place of birth	Education and selected honors	Key events; Contributions
Browne, Mother de Sales (Frances Browne) 1826–1910 Westmoreland, PA	Home education. No formal nsg ed.	Entered Convent of Mercy, Pgh, PA; was moved to DC to take charge of new infirmary for sick poor. Ordered to Vicksburg to establish school; organized parishioners to visit and care for sick and poor. In Civil War, cared for Confederate soldiers under harsh conditions in various hospitals, escaping as Yankees captured towns, and nursing in next place. Eventually Mother Superior for 30 yrs.
Craig, Leroy 1887–1976 Dixmont, ME	McLean Hospital Trng Sch for Nurses, Waverly, MA 1912. Honors: Pa Nurses Assn citation for contrib to psych nurs and promoting legislation affecting status of men (1956).	In vanguard of political and educational activities promoting professional recognition and opportunities for men nurses. Instrumental in federal legislation allowing male nurses to be commissioned as officers in armed services at parity with women. (Wife was Army nurse recruiter.) Appointed as founding director and supt of nurses in Men's Nursing Dept, Pa Hosp for Mental and Nervous Diseases, concurrently serving as 1st director, Pa Hosp Sch of Nsg for Men (1914), remaining active in both until retirement (1956). Established innovations in nursing curriculum; wrote several articles noting contributions of men nurses.

Appendix 8   (continued)

Name, dates, place of birth	Education and selected honors	Key events; Contributions
Curtis, Namahyoke Gertrude (Sockum) 1861–1935	Snell Seminary, San Francisco, 1888. No formal nsg ed. Honors: Given high official commendation for leadership of "immune nurses."	Noted for being commissioned by War Dept. to serve as contract nurse in Spanish American War, recruiting also 30 additional "immune nurses," black women who had had yellow fever. (Later received lifetime gov't pension for this). Descended from family of German, Afro-American and Native American stock. Married secretly at 18 to man who later graduated from Northwestern University Medical School, Chicago. There, became instrumental in efforts to found Provident Hospital; became active in local, state, and national politics and held number of politically appointed government positions in Chicago and Washington DC, where husband was CEO of Freedman's Hospital. Served under Clara Barton in Galveston Flood in Texas as ARC volunteer. Remained in public service during WW I. Buried in Arlington Cemetery.
Cumming, Kate c. 1833–1909 Edinburgh, Scotland	Ed not known. No nsg ed.	Refined southern lady who volunteered for service as nurse with Confederate Army. When these nurses received official status, became matron of military hospital. Published journal about nsg and hospitals after war that gave good information on the care given, activities, and analysis of problems.

Name, dates, place of birth	Education and selected honors	Key events; Contributions
Davis, Mary E.P. c. 1840–1924 New Brunswick, Canada	Mass Gen Hosp Trng School for Nurses, Boston 1878. Honors: ANA Hall of Fame.	Largely responsible, with Palmer, for planning the organization and financing of *AJN*. As business manager, made it self-supporting. One of the founders of ASSTSN. Previously supt. of hospital and training school, Hosp. Univ. of Penn; Progressive attitude about ed. Helped found Mass Nurses Assn; wrote many journal articles.
Delano, Jane 1862–1919 Montour Falls, NY	Bellevue Trng Sch for Nurses, NYC, 1886. Honors: Disting Service Medal (US and ARC). Sculpture in ARC hdq, DC. ANA Hall of Fame.	Appointed Supt Army Nurse Corps (ANC) 1910. As director of Dept. Nsg, ARC (held simultaneously with ANC position), perfected plan, with ANA, to have 9000 qualified nurses ready when US declared war on Germany. (Supplied 20,000 nurses). Said to have rendered greatest service of any US woman to help win WW I. Previously held major positions at U of PA and Bellevue Hospitals. Author: book on home care of sick. Died in France making final inspection of hospitals. Buried with military honors at Arlington Natl cemetery.

Appendix 8   (continued)

Name, dates, place of birth	Education and selected honors	Key events; Contributions
Dix, Dorothea 1802–1887 Hambden, ME	School in Boston, then studied privately and in libraries, public lectures. Honors: US stamp in her honor; named park in Hambden; ANA Hall of Fame.	Spearheaded national reforms in treatment of mentally ill and disabled. Opened school for small children at age 14 and continued to teach. Outraged at treatment of women in a "house of correction" most of whom were mentally ill; began campaign for improvement with varying success. Was recognized, and when volunteered, was appointed Supt of US Army Nurses for Civil War; set up infirmaries and recruited and screened nurses. Was undermined by requirement that nurses responsible only to doctors. Never regained momentum after war ended.
Dock, Lavinia 1858–1956 Harrisburg, PA	Bellevue Trng Sch for Nurses, NY, 1886. Honors: ANA Hall of Fame.	Active in early development of nursing organizations in US, and of ICN. Edited "Foreign Dept" of *AJN* for 23 years. Militant woman suffragist and ardent crusader for rights of poor and workers; pacifist. Supported concept of "one world." Held key positions at Bellevue, Johns Hopkins, IL Trng Sch for Nurses; worked with Wald at Henry Street Settlement; also nurse in several social organizations. Held office in ASSTSN and ICN. Author of books on materia medica, nsg history, Red Cross history, "Hygiene and Morality" (about venereal disease, then very daring), and numerous articles.

Name, dates, place of birth	Education and selected honors	Key events; Contributions
Drown, Lucy 1848–1934 Providence, RI	Salem Normal School, MA; Boston City Hosp Sch of Nsg, 1884.	Considered by some as pioneer in trng sch org, development of private duty, state and nat'l org, and state licensing laws. Supt of nurses 30 years Boston City Hosp. Mentored many future leaders. Charter member ASSTSN and first treasurer.
Franklin, Martha 1870–1968 New Haven, CT	Women's Hosp Trng Sch for Nurses, Philadelphia, 1898. Honors: ANA Hall of Fame.	Only Afro-American graduate of her class. Over next 10 years, recognized and fought discrimination in nursing as well as society. One of earliest to pass state registration exams. Primarily did private duty, but campaigned nationally for racial equality in nsg. Founded and first president of Nat'l Assn Colored Grad Nurses (NACGN).
Freeman, Ruth 1906–1982 Methuen, MA	Mt. Sinai Sch Nsg NYC, 1927; BS Columbia U, NY, 1934; MA, NYU, 1939; EdD, NYU, 1951. Many honors incl: ANA McIver Award; NLN Nutting Award; APHA Bronson Award; and named award by nsg section; IRC Nightingale Medal; honorary member, Sigma Theta Tau.	Leader in public health nsg; helped professionalize field through teaching, writings, work in prof orgs. Worked at Henry St. Visiting Nurse Service; then taught NYU, U. Minn, Johns Hopkins. Stressed interdisciplinary practice and communication. Pres, NLN, Nat'l Health Council; VP; NOPHN; key positions, APHA. Several books; many articles.

Appendix 8   **(continued)**

Name, dates, place of birth	Education and selected honors	Key events; Contributions
Gardner, Mary 1871–1961 Newton, MA	Newton Hosp Sch Nsg RI, 1905; Honorary MA, Brown U, 1918. Honors: NOPN Medal for distinguished service; ANA Hall of Fame.	One of earliest directors and organizers of a visiting nurse association (VNA). One of founders of NOPHN, first secretary and second president. Key positions in Providence District Nurses Assn (RI), ARC Town and Country Nsg Service: As special advisor to ARC, surveyed public health nsg in Eastern Europe (1920). Considered int'l authority on pub health nurs. Prolific writer including *Public Health Nursing* first text on subject; translated into many languages; book on phn admin; novel, *Katherine Kent*, and numerous articles.
Goodrich, Annie 1866–1954 New Brunswick, NJ	New York Hosp Trng Sch for Nsg, NYC, 1892. Honorary Degrees: DSC, Mount Holyoke, 1921; MA, Yale, 1923; LLD Russell Sage College, 1936. Many honors incl: NLN Nutting Award; US Disting Service Award; several from France and Belgium; ANA Hall of Fame.	Distinguished educator and inspiring leader, who aroused public to need for higher educational standards for nurses. First dean, Yale University School for Nursing. Key positions in various hospitals/schools in New York City, asst professor, TC, NY, Dir of Nsg, Henry Street Settlement, Dean, Army School of Nursing. Held major offices in ANA, ASSTSN, and other US nursing organizations and ICN. Author, *Social and Ethical Significance of Nursing,* 1932.

Name, dates, place of birth	Education and selected honors	Key events; Contributions
Gretter (Mrs.), Lystra 1858–1951 Bayfield, Ontario, Canada	Buffalo Gen Hosp Trng Sch for Nurses, Buffalo, NY, 1888.	Leader in many forward trends: first 8-hour day for student nurses; one of first to employ graduate nurses to supervise and teach students (instead of doctors). "Moving Spirit" of group that wrote Nightingale Pledge. Principal, Trng School, Harper Hospital, Detroit, Director, Detroit VNA. Major offices in state and national nsg org; Charter member, NOPHN.
Hall, Lydia 1906–1969 NYC, NY	Gettysburg College; NY Hosp Sch Nsg 1927; BS in PHN, TC, 1937; MA, TC, 1942; doctoral study TC. Honors: TC alumni Dist Achievement Award; hospital named after her (NY); ANA Hall of Fame.	Known for professional care model, considered by some as a type of nsg theory. At Montefiore Hosp, NY, developed unit (Loeb Center) in which nurses selected pts for their potential for rehab, gave prof care, assessing pt needs on one-to-one basis. Had been at VNS of NY, Fordham Hosp Sch Nsg, and NY Heart Assn. Actively involved in ANA, NLN, NOPHN and volunteer committees in NY. Sought-after speaker, prolific author particularly about Loeb Center concept.
Kimber, Diana (Sister Mary Diana) ?–1928 Oxfordshire, England	Bellevue Hosp Trng School, 1885? Previous: broad education in England and Germany.	Recognized as author of first scientific book written by a nurse for nurses (anatomy and physiology); repeated editions between 1893 and 1948. Asst supt under Robb in Ill., then Old Charity Hospital in NYC. Returned to England; joined Anglican Sisterhood, whose chief work was public health nsg. Also contributed to welfare of sick nurses.

Appendix 8   **(continued)**

Name, dates, place of birth	Education and selected honors	Key events; Contributions
Kuehn, Ruth Perkins 1900–1986 Sharon, WI	Children's Memorial Hosp, Chicago, 1925; BS 1931, MA 1934; PhD 1942, Ohio State U. Honors include: Sigma Theta Tau; received first mentor award 1985, from one of her protégés who was then president; also named endowed research award at Pitt.	Founder and first dean, University of Pgh. Sch of Nsg, (1939), after demanding it be an autonomous school of nursing. Initiated nation's first CE workshop. First US dean to hold PhD. Developed masters and doctoral programs; pioneer in nursing research especially on method improvement and utilization of personnel. Pitt became first PA nursing school to admit Afro-American students and first to allow students to marry and complete program, (was herself married to MD); mentor to future leaders. Previous positions as faculty at Ohio State. President of Sigma Theta Tau; VP; ANA; involved with ICN (had recruited international students since she became dean). Held other offices and committee assignments in nursing and nonnursing organizations; international consultant. Author, pediatric textbook 1933, and coauthor, *Patterns of Patient Care*, first on team nursing research; also articles.
Maas, Clara 1876–1901 E. Orange, NJ	Newark German (Memorial) Hosp, Newark, NJ 1895. Honors: commemorative stamp, (Cuba and US) and medal (Franklin Mint); ANA Hall of Fame; NJ hospital named after her.	Young army nurse martyr who volunteered to participate in investigation of yellow fever transmission, in Cuba. Bitten by infected mosquito and died. Had offered services in Cuba and Philippines during Spanish-American War. Buried with military honors.

Name, dates, place of birth	Education and selected honors	Key events; Contributions
Mahoney, Mary 1845–1923 Boston, MA	N Eng Hosp for Women and Children, 1879 Boston. Honors: Mary Mahoney Award: named by NACGN, now given by ANA; ANA Hall of Fame.	First "Negro" nurse in US. Inspired black nurses to strive for better working conditions and facilities in "Negro" nursing schools and work toward combatting racial discrimination. Primarily worked as private duty nurse in Boston. Life member of Nat'l Assn Colored Grad Nurses (NACGN).
Markolf, Ada (Stewart) 1870–1945 Braintree, MA	Waltham Trng Sch for Nurses, Waltham, MA, 1893. Later, passed course on massage.	Best remembered as first industrial nurse hired by employer in US (VT Marble Co), followed by sister. Matron of hosp opened by Company (1896), for 2 years; then 20 years practicing massage and private duty. Retired at 47 to marry.
Maxwell, Anna 1851–1929 Bristol, NY	Boston City Hosp Trng Sch for Nurses, 1880. Many honors including: ANA Hall of Fame; Medal of Honor from France for organizing the nsg service of Presbyterian Hosp Unit in WW I. Buried with military honors in Arlington Cemetery.	Made nursing a more desirable occupation for women with high social standing, interpreting nsg to those outside the profession. Instituted standardization of nursing techniques and procedures. Active in ASSTSN, ANA, AJN; ICN. Key positions: Boston Trng School, St. Luke's and Presbyterian, NYC. In charge of Steinberg Hospital, GA, during Spanish-Am War. Coauthor of book on practical nursing.

Appendix 8   (continued)

Name, dates, place of birth	Education and selected honors	Key events; Contributions
McGarvah Mary Eleanor 1886–1979 Windsor, Ontario, Canada	Farrand Trng Sch for Nurses, Harper Hosp, Detroit, 1911; Bachelor of Law, University of Detroit, 1929. Honors: Named Humanitarian Award established by Am Assn Nurse Attorneys.	First nurse attorney; expert in public health law and regulation. After graduation from nsg school, did private duty, then joined Detroit Health Dept. Helped to establish prenatal clinics and registration of midwives. As supervisor in new special investigation division, found Health Dept needed legal/legislative clout, so became attorney. Was promoted to dir div and served Health Dept for 41 years, also maintaining private practice. Many accomplishments in public health. Coauthored 2nd and 3rd edition of *Jurisprudence for Nurses* (1935, 1945), believed to be first book on nursing and the law.
McIsaac, Isabel 1858–1914 Waterloo, IA	IL Trng Sch for Nurses (ITS), 1888. Honors: Named loan fund.	Excellent teacher and administrator, playing major roles in early days of nursing. First to institute clinical demonstration; designed CE for graduate nurses, including arguing for CE, at nsg conventions. Wrote several important textbooks on nursing technique, bacteriology, hygiene for nurses and public schools. As supt, ITS, increased ed prog to 3 years. Charter member and VP of alumnae assn of ITS, first in US. As president, established what might be the first code of ethics. Later, held major offices in nat'l nsg org and became traveling field secretary visiting schools and hospitals throughout US. Among first nurses to lobby for ANC, replacing Delano in 1912. Suffragette. Key spokesperson for nursing.

Name, dates, place of birth	Education and selected honors	Key events; Contributions
McIver, Pearl 1893–1976 Lowery, Minn	Minn State Teacher's College, 1912; BS, U of Minn Sch Nurs, 1919; MA, in phn admin, 1932; Hon degree, Western Reserve, 1957. Honors: APHA Lasker Award; ANA, PHN Award, later named for her; ICN: F. Nightingale Medal; Honorary member, Sigma Theta Tau; U Minn outstanding achievement award.	As chief, expanded public health nursing in USPHS into modern and extensive agency. First PHN on staff in 1933. First chief, 1944–1957. Initiated census of PHN's. Administered nsg ed program, 1941–43, and traveled extensively to other countries after WW II as part of US technical assistance program. Key roles in PH and nsg org. As pres, ANA, initiated census of all prof nurses. Pres *AJN* Co, later ex dir. Wrote many articles for *AJN* and *Public Health Nursing.*
McManus, N. Louise 1906–1993 N. Smithfield, MA	Diploma, Institutional Mgt Prog, Pratt Instit (NY); Diploma, Mass Gen Hosp; Bacc, Masters, TC, NY; PhD ed res Columbia U, 1947. Many honors, incl: NLN Nutting Award; first recipient of TC alumni award, named after her; CU Bicentennial Medal; Medals, Greek RC; Women's Hall of Fame (Seneca Falls, NY).	Major contrib to nsg ed, incl: first org unit for research in nsg ed (TC, 1953); leader in dev of AD nsg progs; resp for dev of nat'l state board lic exam pool. One of first nurses to receive PhD. Assist dir NLNE study leading to curriculum guide. At TC for 36 years, 14 as dir, nurs ed div, following Stewart. Consulted internationally in Turkey, Kenya, others, with AID and ICN. Past chair, Florence Nightingale Intl Foundation. Many benchmark publications (books, articles) primarily on nsg ed and research.

Appendix 8   (continued)

Name, dates, place of birth	Education and selected honors	Key events; Contributions
Nutting, Mary Adelaide 1858–1948 Waterloo, Alta, Canada	Johns Hopkins Hosp Sch of Nsg, Baltimore, 1891 Many honors incl: Medals, historical collection at TC, 4 funds, ed unit at Johns Hopkins, all named after her. ANA Hall of Fame.	First nurse to hold professorship in a university. First head of what was later the Dept of Nursing Education at TC. (Persuaded Dean Russell to introduce courses for nurses). Attracted nurses from around world. Great influence on education of nurses, particularly colleges and universities. Key offices in ASSTSN, ANA, ICN, and other nursing org. Helped establish *AJN*, mem of committee that published Goldmark Report. Coauthor, *History of Nursing*, and book on economics of nursing schools.
Osborne, Estelle (Massey) Riddle 1901–1981 Palestine, TX	2 yr course at Prairie View State College, TX; City Hospital Number 2, St Louis, MO, 1923; BS, 1930, and MA, 1931 TC, NYC. Honors: Mary Mahoney Award (NACGN) 1946; Nurse of the Year NYU; 1st black nurse as honorary fellow AAN; ANA Hall of Fame; NEF named scholarship for black nurses seeking master's degree in nsg.	Leader in nurs ed and development of nsg org. Faced prejudice throughout her education. Resigned early jobs because of discrimination. Studied part-time at TC, while teaching at Lincoln Hosp and Harlem Hospitals. After MA, became 1st dir of nsg ed at Freedman's Hospital (DC); established closer relations with Howard U. Other educational positions incl NYU, then asst dir, later assoc gen director, at NLN. Retired in 1967, but continued to speak extensively on role of black nurses. Many firsts for a black nurse: NOPHN Committee, ANA Board of Directors, Rep to ICN, Director Philips Hosp, St. Louis. Active as pres, NACGN and various Afro-American organizations.

Name, dates, place of birth	Education and selected honors	Key events; Contributions
Palmer, Sophia 1853–1920 Milton, MA	Mass Gen Hosp Trng Sch for Nurses, Boston *c.* 1900. Also studied journalism. Honors: Several nursing libraries named after her. ANA Hall of Fame.	Helped establish *AJN*; first editor from first issue to death. Leader in movement to secure state licensure for nurses. Helped organize ASSTSN and ANA. Previously, organized St. Luke's Trng School, Bedford, MA. Reorganized Garfield Memorial, DC and established school; supt Rochester City Hosp; first pres, NY State Bd of Nurse Examiners. Member local and national RC committees.
Reiter, Frances 1904–1977 Smithton, PA	Johns Hopkins Hosp Trng Sch for Nurses, 1931; BA, nsg ed TC 1941; MA, TC, 1942. Many honors include: ANA honorary membership; IRC Nightingale Medal; NLN disting service award; Honorary fellow, AAN.	Chiefly known for concept and term "nurse clinician." Strong believer in bacc ed, Chair of ANA committee that wrote "position paper." Main contrib in nsg ed and research; held key admin and teaching positions in Montefiore, (Pgh) Johns Hopkins, Boston U, Mass Gen, TC, First Dean, Grad Sch Nsg, NY Med College. Proj dir, US PHS study on quality of nsg care; on ex comm, *Nsg Research*; major roles in nsg orgs.
Richards, Linda 1841–1930 Near Potsdam, NY	St Johnsburg Academy, VT N Eng Hosp for Women and Children, Boston, 1873. Numerous honors include: Likeness engraved on corporate seal of ANA. In 1948, 63 cities and 48 states observed Linda Richards day in honor of her graduation 75 years previously. NLN named award; ANA Hall of Fame. Women's Hall of Fame (Seneca Falls, NY).	Taught school in Vermont. Entered nurse trng, inspired by Nightingale's writings. Known as America's "first trained nurse." Primarily organizer and supt of many trng schools and nursing services, usually only staying 2 years. Also pioneer in establishing trng schools for nurses in mental hospitals. Active in founding national nsg organizations: first president ASSTSN; organized first trng school for nurses in Japan, under missionary auspices. Part of committee approaching TC re courses for nurses. Wrote reminiscences on being first trained nurse, 1911.

Appendix 8   (continued)

Name, dates, place of birth	Education and selected honors	Key events; Contributions
Robb, Isabel Hampton 1860–1910 Welland, Ont., Canada	Teaching certif: Collegiate Institute of St. Catherine's Ontario, Canada. Bellevue Trng School for Nurses, NY, 1883; course at St. Paul's House, Rome 1883–85. Honors: Several scholarships and funds named after her; ANA Hall of Fame.	Brilliant leader who did much to improve and develop curriculum in early nursing schools, including lengthening program, inaugurating a regular class schedule, providing for holidays, eliminating stipend. Supt, ILL Trng Sch for Nurses, Chicago; organizer and supt Johns Hopkins. One of founders and first pres Nurses Associated Alumni (NAA); pres ASSTSN; helped found *AJN*; ICN committee member. One of earliest nursing authors: books on practice and ethics. Continued to participate in nursing (but not practice) after marriage.
Roberts, Mary 1877–1959 Sheboygan, MI	Jewish Hosp Sch of Nsg, Cincinnati, OH, 1899; BS, TC, NYC, 1921. Honors: Bronze Medal, France; Nutting award for leadership; IRC Nightingale medal; named awards; ANA Hall of Fame.	Brilliant writer and editor of *AJN* for 28 years. Considered great teacher and investigator who had insight into nursing movements. Traveled throughout Europe visiting nsg centers under sponsorship of Rockefeller Foundation. Established trng sch for nurses, Savannah Hosp GA. Supt of several other hosps. Dir, Army Sch of Nsg and Bureau of Nsg, Lake Denison, ARC, WW I. Many committees of national nsg orgs, ICN, and Nsg Council on Nat'l Defense, WW I. Author of books on nsg history and ANC.

Name, dates, place of birth	Education and selected honors	Key events; Contributions
Rogers, Martha 1914–1994 Dallas, TX	U of Knoxville, 1931–33; Knoxville Gen'l Hosp Sch of Nurs, 1936; BSN in public health nsg, George Peabody College, Nashville, 1937; MA, public health supervision, TC, 1945; MPH, Johns Hopkins, 1952; ScD, Johns Hopkins, 1953; Numerous honorary degrees. Honors: many awards: Fellow, AAN; ANA Hall of Fame.	Primarily known as originator of the nursing theory, "Science of Unitary Human Beings" or "Rogerian Science." Professor and head of NYU Div Nsg Ed from 1954–1975. After retirement, continued to teach (professor emeritus). Consultant to US govt. Prolific author/speaker and nsg gadfly re "anti-educational archaisms." In nursing education, president of number of natl ed orgs plus Sigma Theta Tau. Active in nsg org committees. Prior to 1954, had been involved in public health nursing and supervision.
Sanger, Margaret 1879–1966 Corning, NY	Claverack College, NY. White Plains Hosp, NY, 1902; postgrad, Manhattan Eye and Ear, 1902; Self-study on pop problems; Hon LLD, Smith College, 1949; Hon LLD, U Ariz, 1966. Many honors incl: Am Women's Assn Medal of Achievement; Gold Medal, Emperor of Japan, 1962; Pl Parenthood, Albert and Mary Lasker Award, and medal named after her; ANA Hall of Fame.	Nurse leader of Am birth control movement; founder, Planned Parenthood. Was teacher; after postgrad course, married, had 3 children. Constant flare-ups of TB. Doing home nsg, became concerned by women on Lower East Side (NY), who died of childbirth or illegal abortions and could get no information about birth control. During years of battle for reform, was arrested for disseminating such information, much of which she had gotten in Europe. Started birth control clinics and research; got support of wealthy. Fought many court battles, wrote many books. Finally got AMA support. Retired to Arizona: new leaders of movement deemed her brand of feminism counterproductive.

Appendix 8   (continued)

Name, dates, place of birth	Education and selected honors	Key events; Contributions
Shaw, Mrs. Clara Weeks 1857–1940 Sanbarton, NH	NY Hosp Trng Sch for Nurses, 1880. Previously graduated, RI State Normal School	Credited with being first nurse to write a nursing textbook in US (1885). Became standard text for many schools. Supt, Paterson Gen Hospital, Paterson, NJ. No further nursing work after marriage in 1888.
Staupers, Mabel 1890–1989 Barbados, W. Indies	Freedman's Hosp Sch of Nsg, DC, 1917. Many honors, incl: Spingarn Medal, NAACP, NLN Linda Richards Award; ANA Mahoney Award; Medgar Evans Human Rights Award; Urban League Award; ANA Hall of Fame.	Strong integrationist and feminist. Through political and public pressure, and help of Eleanor Roosevelt, forced Army and Navy to accept black nurses without quotas (WW II). Helped black MD's organize 1st private facility in Harlem, allowing black doctors to treat pts. Served as administrator and dir of nsg. Conducted survey of health needs of Harlem; Led to NYTB and Health Assn; became first ex sec (12 yrs). Became first ex sec NACGN, 1934–1946. Pres, NACGN later. Wrote significant book on integration of "Negroes" into American nursing.
Stewart, Isabel Maitland 1878–1963 Fletcher, Ontario, Canada/Manitoba	Normal School, Winnipeg Genl Hosp Trng Sch 1902; BS (1911), MA (1913), TC. Number of hon doctorates in US and Canada. Many honors from US, Canada, Finland. One of 23 "women of achievement," NY League of Nat Fed Bus and Prof Women, 1936. ANA Hall of Fame.	Helped shape development of 20th century nsg ed and practice. Instrumental in developing first program for preparing nurse faculty at TC; aided in educational research, promoting use of objective tests. Revived interest in study of nsg sch's by outside group, resulting in valuable 1926 report (Appendix 1). Prof of Nurs Ed and Dir of Dept at TC for 22 years. Involved in natl and intl nsg ed orgs. Member Women's Board of Henry St, VNA. Coauthor, with Dock, of nsg history text, 1920. Author, *Education of Nurses*, 1943; editor, *AJN* Dept of Nsg Ed.

Name, dates, place of birth	Education and selected honors	Key events; Contributions
Stimson, Julia 1881–1948 Worcester, MA	NY Hosp Sch of Nsg, NYC, 1908; BA, Vassar College; MA, Washington U, St. Louis, 1917. Honors: Many honors from US, Britain, Belgium, France. Also: ANA Hall of Fame; IRC Nightingale Medal.	First woman given rank of major in US (Colonel, 1945). Came to natl notice through spectacular achievement of organizing and administering work of nurses at Gen Hosp in Rouen, France, WW I. Recruited nurses for ANC and ARC; longest tenure in history of ANC. Chief nurse ARC, France 1918 and dir nurs service, Am Expeditionary Forces 1918, Supt ANC 1919–37, also dean, Army Sch of Nsg. Had been supt of nurses several hosp. Pres ANA; many ARC, army and nsg committees. Author, *Handbook of Drugs and Solutions*, many articles.
Taylor, Susie King 1848–1912	Secret tutoring to read and write.	Born a slave; escaped to area under Union control; married Union soldier at 14. Known as nurse during Civil War, having made rounds with Clara Barton at about age 15. Services never compensated after war. Started schools after war, then domestic employment. In Boston, helped organize, and involved with, Woman's Relief Corps (for Union veterans), but never nursed officially again. Wrote insightful reminiscences of camp life in Civil War, which she published herself.

Appendix 8   (continued)

Name, dates, place of birth	Education and selected honors	Key events; Contributions
Thoms, Adah c. 1870–1943 Richmond, VA	Normal School, Richmond; Woman's Infirmary and Sch of Therapeutic Massage, NYC, 1900; then Lincoln Hosp and Home Trng Sch., NYC, 1905; courses in various NYC institutions. Honors: First to receive NACGN's Mahoney Award; ANA Hall of Fame.	Known chiefly for seeking equal opportunity for black nurses, particularly getting 18 accepted in army with full rank and pay. (Surgeon General had refused, but her persistence and shortage of nurses in flu epidemic of 1918, forced him to accede.) Asst Dir, Lincoln Hosp, 18 yrs. Helped organize NACGN. Among first to add pub health nsg course to curriculum at Lincoln. Participated in intl affairs—one of first 3 black delegates to ICN. Apptd by Asst Surg Gen to key advisory council, 1921. Actively involved in many nsg and other org. Wrote first history of black nurses.
Truth, Sojourner (Isabella Von Wagener) c. 1797–1883? Hurley, NY	No formal education. Honors: Michigan Women's Hall of Fame; Nat'l Women's Hall of Fame, Seneca Falls, NY. Mars Robot (US) named Sojourner to honor her (1995).	Amazing, brave, and resourceful Afro-American, best known for her abolitionist activities and stirring speeches although she was a lifelong illiterate. Born a slave, she escaped and was given refuge by a family whose name she took. In 1843, took name of Sojourner (will travel) Truth (will tell) and began preaching, raising money for her causes. At 77, traveled to DC, met with president, eventually appointed to work with Freedman's Hospital. For 2 years, cared for black soldiers, brought order to filthy, chaotic conditions. Continued campaigning for freed slaves' rights and women's rights.

Name, dates, place of birth	Education and selected honors	Key events; Contributions
Tubman, Harriet (Araminta) c. 1820–1913 Bricktown, MD	No formal education. Honors: Commemorative stamp; Monument in Auburn	Escaped abused slave known as the "conductor of the underground railroad" for the secret trips she made to lead more than 300 slaves to freedom. During Civil War served as nurse in Sea Islands and other camps, as needed, caring for sick and wounded regardless of color; was also spy and scout for Union Army (for which she later received a pension). Helped develop Freedmans' Colony in SC and worked in that hosp using it as a base; also served in hospitals in NC and FL. In Auburn, NY, later used her home as shelter for needy black people. Given military funeral.
Wald, Lillian 1867–1940 Cincinnati, OH	NY Hosp Trng Sch, 1891; studied at Women's Medical College, NYC. Honorary Degrees: LLD, Mount Holyoke, 1912; Smith, 1930. Numerous honors and medals incl: recognition by Mayor LaGuardia in 1936 as "citizen rendering greatest service to NYC." Memorial tributes by Pres Roosevelt, NY governor, 2 NYC mayors and leaders of health and social service agencies; ANA Hall of Fame; Women's Hall of Fame (Seneca Falls, NY); Hall of Fame for Great Americans, NYU.	Founded Henry St VNA in NYC, first nonsecretarian publ health service in US. Promoted publ health and social welfare concepts entire life. Started school nsg, NYC. Fought for better housing in slums; initiated idea for US Children's Bureau. Taught at TC. One of organizers and 1st pres, NOPHN. Served on numerous local, natl, intl committees. Author, 2 books about Henry St.

Appendix 8　**(continued)**

Name, dates, place of birth	Education and selected honors	Key events; Contributions
Yellowtail, Susie 1903–1981 Crow Agency, MT	Bacone College, OK; E. Northville Hosp Trng Sch, Springfield, MA, with internships, Boston Hosp, 1926. Honors: President's Award for Outstanding Nsg and Health Care. Mrs. Indian America.	One of first Native American RNs. Strong, effective advocate for better ed and health on reservations. Worked for USPHS, various reservations, then 30 yrs for own people (Crow Agency); nsg and midwife services. With husband, medicine man, reintroduced aspects of traditional healing ceremony. Apptd by Pres Kennedy to PH, Ed, and Welfare Board, 1961; served through several presidencies, fought for improvement of health services for her people; traveled nationally.

Index

ISBN 0-07-105483-9